Cerebellar Disorders

A Practical Approach to Diagnosis and Management

Cerebellar Disorders

A Practical Approach to Diagnosis and Management

Mario Ubaldo Manto
Fonds National de la Recherche Scientifique Neurologie
Université Libre de Bruxelles, Hopital Erasme
Laboratoire de Neurologie Expérimentale
Brussels, Belgium

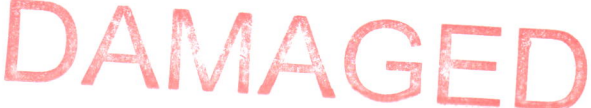

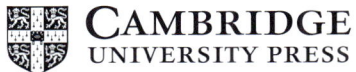 CAMBRIDGE
UNIVERSITY PRESS

CAMBRIDGE UNIVERSITY PRESS
Cambridge, New York, Melbourne, Madrid, Cape Town,
Singapore, São Paulo, Delhi, Dubai, Tokyo

Cambridge University Press
The Edinburg Building, Cambridge CB2 8RU, UK

Published in the United States of America by
Cambridge University Press, New York

www.cambridge.org
Information on this title:
www.cambridge.org/9780521878135

© M. U. Manto 2010

First published 2010

Printed in the United Kingdom
at the University Press, Cambridge

*A cataloge record for this publication is available from the
British Library*

ISBN 978-0-521-87813-5 Hardback

To Ana Maria, Valentin, and Aurélie

Contents

Foreword   ix
Preface   xi
Acknowledgments   xii

Introduction   1

1 Embryology and anatomy   2

2 Physiology of the cerebellum   23

3 Symptoms of cerebellar disorders   36

4 Clinical scales   53

5 Diagnosis of cerebellar disorders as a function of age   69

6 Overview of the general management of cerebellar disorders   75

7 Malformations   78

8 Cerebellar stroke   88

9 Immune diseases   102

10 Endocrine disorders   113

11 Infectious diseases   118

12 Corticobasal degeneration   133

13 Tumors and paraneoplastic disorders   135

14 Trauma of the posterior fossa   149

15 Toxic agents   157

16 Autism spectrum disorders and ataxia   171

17 Progressive myoclonic epilepsies   174

18 Multiple system atrophy   179

19 Essential tremor   184

20 Autosomal recessive cerebellar ataxias   189

21 Mitochondrial disorders   229

22 X-linked ataxias   237

23 Dominant ataxias   242

Index   284

The Color Plates will be found between pages 52 and 53.

Foreword

When I was on staff at the Peter Bent Brigham Hospital in Boston, we had a weekly Neurology Grand Rounds together with the Children's Hospital and the Beth Israel Hospital. Dr. Charles Barlow was Chief at Children's Hospital and Professor of the Harvard Neurology Department at Children's and the Brigham. At the Grand Rounds, a wide variety of neurological cases were presented, but we were not permitted to present a patient with degenerative ataxia. Dr. Barlow certainly admitted that the patients were interesting, but he got too frustrated with the presentations, since we never made a clear diagnosis. Times have certainly changed. The differential diagnosis of identified conditions is now huge, and advances in genetics and molecular biology have begun to give detailed insights into the pathophysiology. Neurodegeneration is still not without mystery, but medicine is hot on the trail to understand a variety of pathways by which it occurs.

The cerebellum has the most neurons of any part of the brain, and it interacts with all parts of the brain. Its beautiful cellular architecture seen throughout the structure suggests a common mode of information processing, which is still not fully determined. When malfunctioning, there are gross motor problems, and more recently, it has become clear that there are more subtle problems with other brain functions, including cognition and emotion. Advances are being made here also.

This book on cerebellar disorders by Dr. Mario U. Manto begins with our current understanding of the anatomy and physiology of the cerebellum, and then dives into the diagnosis and treatment of the many different disorders. As virtually all pathological processes can affect the cerebellum, the book actually covers much of neurology. Dr. Manto has been devoted to the study of the cerebellum in his career. His contributions are numerous in many areas, and his enthusiasm led him to found and edit the journal, *The Cerebellum*, which has rapidly become quite distinguished with an impact factor approaching 4. He is almost uniquely qualified to write an authoritative text covering the whole subject.

When dealing with the different disorders, the book approaches the patient in multiple ways. What is the differential diagnosis by age or by pathologic entity? What is the differential diagnosis for recessive, dominant, or X-linked disorders? What laboratory tests should be done to clarify the situation? What scales can be used to quantify the disorder? And then, what can be done for treatment? There is no reason to take a dim view of treatment when the possibilities are taken as a whole for all the ataxias.

The text is written in a clear way without excessive material. The facts, the important ones, are easy to find, and can serve to educate and advise when dealing with a specific patient. The book can be helpful not only for students and neuroscientists, but for neurologists at all levels of expertise. It is a welcome addition to the neurology library.

Mark Hallett, MD
Human Motor Control Section
National Institute of Neurological
Disorders and Stroke
National Institutes of Health
Bethesda, Maryland

Preface

Our knowledge of cerebellar functions and cerebellar disorders has increased tremendously during the past century. With the advent of new technologies, important pathophysiological mechanisms have been deciphered or are being elucidated. The twenty-first century will be the century of treatment for the large spectrum of cerebellar disorders. This book aims to provide updated information both at the clinical and fundamental levels. It is written to provide an integrated view of cerebellar functions, facilitate diagnostic strategies, and become a companion for students and neuroscientists dealing with the cerebellum or cerebellar ataxias.

Acknowledgments

I am particularly grateful to Nick Dunton for his enthusiasm, professionalism, and encouragements, which have made the preparation of this book a rewarding experience. It has been a real pleasure working with the editorial staff of Cambridge University Press, especially Nisha Doshi. She has been invaluable in helping finalize this book. Many thanks to Rebecca Kerins for her precious help. I am indebted to Ken Karpinski for handling the proofs. I thank my teachers and mentors Jean Jacquy, Emile Godaux, and Jerzy Hildebrand for their willingness to share their knowledge. They have introduced me to the field of cerebellar disorders. I am also grateful to my colleagues for sharing information and materials. My research is supported by the Fonds National de la Recherche Scientifique, to whom I extend my gratitude.

Introduction

The terminology of cerebellar ataxias encompasses a wide range of disorders. The advances in neuroimaging, the progress in translational neurosciences, the recent discoveries in molecular biology, and the availability of genetic testing have revolutionized the field of cerebellar disorders. In particular, the identification of the causative mutations of many hereditary ataxias has influenced daily practice worldwide. Since the clinical diagnosis of subtypes of ataxias is often complicated by the salient overlap of the phenotypes between genetic subtypes, and given the numerous disorders affecting the cerebellum, many students, biologists, clinicians, and researchers often experience difficulties in the discipline of cerebellar diseases. Making the right diagnosis remains a major goal when facing a growing number of disorders which look apparently similar. This book aims to provide a framework for the diagnosis and management of cerebellar ataxias, with explanations on the pathophysiological basis to bridge the gap between basic medical sciences and clinical problems. In particular, I have reviewed the literature of these last 15 years and tried to gather the most relevant information in the field, often published in papers scattered throughout the scientific literature. The most critical tests to be performed are underlined.

The book is divided into 23 chapters, starting with the embryology and anatomy of the cerebellum. These chapters remain essential for the appraisal of cerebellar ataxias. The chapter on physiology reviews the theories and mechanisms underlying cerebellar function. The most commonly used clinical scales for evaluating ataxic disorders are discussed in Chapter 4. Diagnosis and general management of cerebellar ataxias are discussed in Chapters 5 and 6, respectively. The following chapters discuss the sporadic forms and inherited diseases encountered in daily practice. Each chapter describes the disorder and its pathogenesis, emphasizing the research aspects which have direct clinical implications. Autosomal recessive cerebellar ataxias, autosomal dominant cerebellar ataxias (spinocerebellar ataxias [SCAs]), and X-linked ataxias are reviewed. The sections on inherited ataxias have been expanded to include the most recently discovered genetic ataxias. The last decades have brought a growing number of demonstrations that the cerebellum participates in non-motor activities. The contributions of cerebellar circuitry in the so-called cognitive operations, including executive functions, learning, and language, and in emotional symptoms are also discussed.

I have attempted to take into account the numerous comments received following the publication of *The Cerebellum and Its Disorders* in 2002. In particular, I have included tables to facilitate the differential diagnosis of cerebellar ataxias. Disorders occurring in children had been overlooked. They are now presented, so that most of the cerebellar disorders relevant in a general neurologist's practice will be explained. I have also attempted not to duplicate material in order to keep the text as concise as possible. In particular, I had to be selective for the animal models of cerebellar ataxias, selecting those with a potential clinical application.

Embryology and anatomy

Embryology

Origin of the cerebellum

The cerebellum originates from the metencephalon and the caudal mesencephalon (dorsal rhombomere 1) and reaches its final configuration several months after birth (Koop et al., 1986; Lechtenberg, 1993). The superior vermis begins to be formed at about 7 to 8 weeks of gestation, and the fusion of the inferior vermis continues up to about 18 weeks. The superior rhombic lip and the adjacent parts proliferate to generate the rudiment of the cerebellum. The central cavity of the rhombencephalon becomes the fourth ventricle. In the following weeks, the cerebellum will expand rostrally, caudally, dorsally, and laterally. Cerebellar hemispheres can be identified at the fifth month as two lateral masses.

Transverse fissures appear progressively on the surface (Figure 1.1). The posterolateral fissure is the first to appear, enabling the identification of the flocculi and the nodulus. The flocculus and the superior cerebellar peduncle are identified at day 45 (O'Rahilly et al., 1988). The posterolateral fissure is clearly discernible at week 9. At the end of the third month, the primary fissure emerges, demarcating the anterior lobe. Two grooves can be distinguished: the secondary fissure and the prepyramidal fissure.

Generation of cerebellar neurons

The ventricular neuroepithelium is responsible for the generation of nuclear cells and Purkinje cells. Interneurons of the cerebellar cortex originate from the metencephalon and the mesencephalon, while granule cells emerge solely from the external granular layer (EGL) originating from the metencephalon. The migration of primitive cells over the surface of the cerebellum begins at about 11 to 12 weeks of gestation. Three stages can be identified: (1) generation of nuclear neuroblasts from the ventricular epithe-

lium, deep nuclei appearing at weeks 11 to 12, and an intense growth of dentate nuclei between week 20 and week 25 (Mihajlovic & Zecevic, 1986); (2) radial outward migration of Purkinje neuroblasts and tangential migration of the EGL, with the Purkinje cell layer becoming apparent between weeks 17 and 28 and synapses between Purkinje cells and parallel fibers being formed at week 24; and (3) inward migration of the external granular layer starting at week 30 and persisting after birth. EGL cells will migrate through the Purkinje cell layer to form the internal granular layer.

During the development of the cerebellum, the number of Purkinje cells determines the size of the population of granule neurons. Purkinje cells control the mitotic activity of granule cell neuroblasts within the EGL. Indeed, the Purkinje cell layer located underneath the EGL continuously secretes a mitotic signal sonic hedgehog (SHH), which drives the extensive proliferation of granular cells such that granule cells become the most abundant neurons in the cerebellum (Wechsler-Reya & Scott, 1999) (Figure 1.2). SHH also acts on Bergmann glia differentiation. The SHH overall expression profile in early post-natal stages is directly responsible for the final size of the cerebellum, being required for full lobe extent (Vaillant & Monard, 2009). The external granular layer will disappear progressively during the first year of life (Lechtenberg, 1993).

Projections to the cerebellum display a parasagittal and striped organization, perpendicular to the fissures, forming compartments in the cerebellar circuitry (Gravel & Hawkes, 1988; Voogd & Ruigrok, 2004). Cells in limited regions of the inferior olive send climbing fibers in a band-like manner to a specific compartment of Purkinje neurons, and mossy fibers project to the granule cell layer in specific regions of the bands (Hawkes et al., 1993; Zagrebelsky et al., 1997). Parasagittal bands of Purkinje neurons are preprogrammed intrinsically during development (see also section The inferior olivary complex).

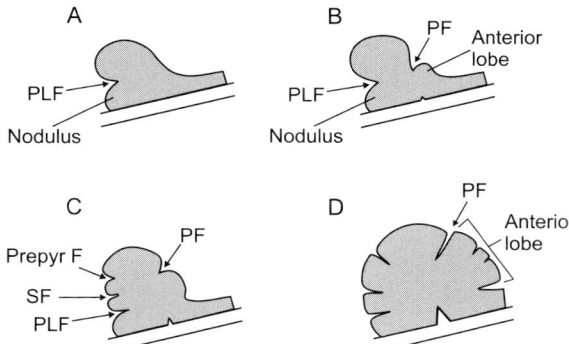

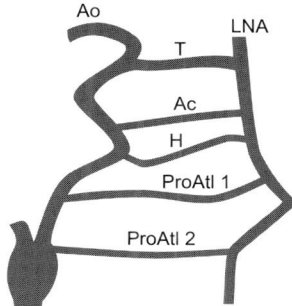

Figure 1.3 Representation of the embryonic carotid-vertebrobasilar anastomoses on the right side. Abbreviations: Ao: aorta; LNA: longitudinal neural artery; T: trigeminal artery; Ac: acoustic (otic) artery; H: hypoglossal artery; ProAtl 1: type 1 proatlantal artery; ProAtl 2: type 2 proatlantal artery. Adapted from: Pasco et al., 2004.

Figure 1.1 Genesis of fissures. The first fissure appearing is the posterolateral fissure (PLF). The second is the primary fissure (PF), which delineates the superior part of the anterior lobe. The prepyramidal fissure (Prepyr F) and the secondary fissure (SF) appear subsequently, followed by a development of the anterior lobe.

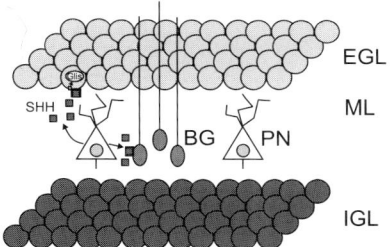

Figure 1.2 Development of the cerebellar cortex. SHH (Sonic hedgehog, represented with red squares) is secreted by Purkinje neurons (PN). SHH triggers the mitosis of cerebellar granular neuronal precursors in the external granular layer (EGL). SHH also promotes differentiation of Bergmann glia (BG). SHH acts through a patched protein and a transmembrane protein called SMO, triggering the activation of transcription factors. EGL cells will migrate to form the internal granular layer (IGL). Adapted from Vaillant and Monard, 2009.

Vertebrobasilar system embryogenesis

The vertebrobasilar system arises from collaterals of the dorsal aorta (which will give rise to the internal carotid artery) (Padget, 1954). Three embryonic arteries contribute to the intracranial portions of the vertebrobasilar system: the trigeminal artery, the acoustic artery, and the hypoglossal artery (Figure 1.3). At the cervical level, the first six segmental arteries will form the vertebral arteries. The first segmental artery is called the proatlantal artery. At 30 days, a longitudinal neural artery appears on each side, supplied by the trigeminal artery, the acoustic artery, the hypoglossal artery, and the proatlantal artery. At 31 days, the two longitudinal neural arteries merge to become the

basilar artery. This latter communicates with the posterior communicating arteries originating from the internal carotid arteries. Simultaneously, the ventral trunks of the trigeminal, acoustic, and hypoglossal arteries disappear. The posterior-inferior cerebellar artery is a remnant of the embryological hypoglossal artery. At day 33, the proatlantal artery is linked to the basilar artery by its cranial branch. The ventral trunks of the first six segmental arteries will disappear. Disruption of the embryogenesis of the vertebrobasilar system leads to persistent carotid-vertebrobasilar anastomoses (Pasco et al., 2004):

- The persistent trigeminal artery is found – usually incidentally – in about 0.2% of angiograms in adults. The artery arises from the posterior side of the intracavernous internal carotid artery and joins the basilar artery in its distal part. The ipsilateral vertebral artery and the proximal basilar artery are often hypoplastic. Patients may complain of diplopia due to abducens nerve (nerve VI) irritation in the cavernous sinus or may complain of facial neuralgias. Aneurysms may develop.

- The persistent hypoglossal artery is found in about 0.05% of angiograms. It arises from the posterior side of the cervical internal carotid in front of the C1–C2 space. The ipsilateral vertebral and posterior communicating arteries are hypoplastic.

- The persistent acoustic artery is very rare. It originates from the internal carotid artery in the intrapetrous carotid canal and reaches the caudal portion of the basilar artery.

Genes, signaling, and development of the cerebellum

Several genes involved in the regulation of brain and cerebellar development have been identified, in

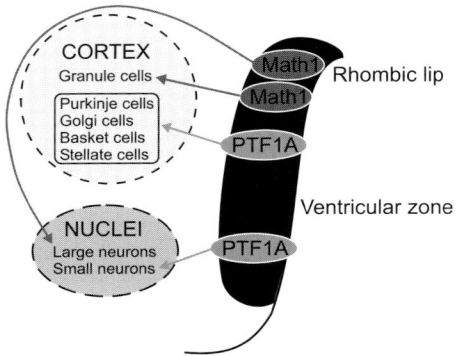

Figure 1.4 Cerebellar neurons are generated from two anatomically distinct progenitor zones within the primordia. Math1 expressing neuroepithelium (rhombic lip) generates glutamatergic neurons (red arrows). PTF1A-expressing neuroepithelium (ventricular zone) generates GABAergic neurons (blue arrows). Cells leaving the rhombic lip migrate over the anlage and form an external layer of cells which continue to proliferate. Granule neuron progenitors form the external granular layer (EGL). Inward radial migration of EGL generates the internal granular layer (IGL). Cerebellar Purkinje neurons are post-mitotic as they leave the ventricular zone. Adapted from: Hoshino, 2006. (See color section).

particular, microcephalin, ASPM, and FOXP2 (Evans et al., 2006). Microcephalin plays a critical function in brain size regulation during the proliferation phase of neurogenesis. FOXP2, a transcription factor, affects the development of several regions of the brain. Experiments with mice show that FOXP2 regulates cerebellar development and neural migration (Shu et al., 2005).

The Math1 gene encodes a transcription factor specifically expressed in the precursors of the EGL and is required for granule cell lineage (Ben-Arie et al., 1997). All known glutamatergic neurons of the cerebellum derive from the Math1-positive rhombic lip, including unipolar brush cells and the glutamatergic subset of neurons in cerebellar nuclei (Figure 1.4). PTF1A (pancreas transcription factor 1A) is implicated in the genesis of cerebellar GABAergic neurons (Hoshino et al., 2005). Mutations of the PTF1A gene on chromosome 10p13-p12.1 is associated with pancreatic and cerebellar agenesis (Sellick et al., 2004; see also Chapter 7). In absence of PTF1A, failure to generate GABAergic neurons will lead to a massive pre-natal death of all glutamatergic neurons because the GABAergic synaptic partners are absent (Millen & Gleeson, 2008). The so-called zinc finger family of transcrip-

tion factors (ZIC) includes ZIC1, whose activity is required to maintain the EGL cells in a progenitor state.

Notch proteins are transmembrane proteins which participate in the process of cell-fate assignation during development (Artavanis-Tsakonas et al., 1999). The activation of Notch signaling is dependent on the interaction with Delta, Serrate, and Lag-2 ligands expressed on neighboring cells. Notch undergoes proteolytic cleavages. The resulting Notch1 intracellular domain translocates to the nucleus and activates transcription of target genes involved in cellular differentiation and development (Bailey & Posakony, 1995). Delta-Notch–like epidermal growth factor–related receptor, a Notch ligand on neurons, is abundantly expressed in Purkinje neurons and moderately expressed in granule cells. It contributes to the maturation of Bergmann glia via Purkinje neurons–glia interactions (Eiraku et al., 2002; Saito & Takeshima, 2006). Notch1 signaling regulates the responsiveness of progenitor cells to bone morphogenetic proteins secreted from the roof plate of the fourth ventricle. In the absence of Notch1, cerebellar progenitors are depleted during the early production of hindbrain neurons, resulting in a severe decrease in the deep cerebellar nuclei that are normally born subsequently (Machold et al., 2007).

SHH acts on gene expression through the activity of the GLI transcription factor family (Vaillant & Monard, 2009). Its transmembrane receptor Patched 1 allows the translocation of a protein called SMO to the cilia (see also Joubert syndrome in Chapter 7). SHH needs to be cholesterol-modified in order to be active. Inhibition of this step causes abnormal development (Lanoue et al., 1997). The Smith-Lemli-Opitz syndrome is an example of association of cerebellar hypoplasia (see also Chapter 7) and impaired cholesterol metabolism (Porter, 2008).

The reelin signaling pathway guides neuroblast migration in the developing cerebral cortex and cerebellum (D'Arcangelo et al., 1995). In the cerebellum, the granule cells secrete reelin, which guides migration of Purkinje neurons. Very low density lipoprotein receptor and apolipoprotein E receptor type 2 are transmembrane receptors for reelin (see also dysequilibrium syndrome in Chapter 20). With reelin binding, an intracellular signaling cascade is triggered, allowing neuroblasts to complete migration and adopt their ultimate positions in laminar structures in the CNS.

Neurotrophins

Neurotrophins, such as nerve growth factor, neurotrophin 3, and brain-derived neurotrophic factor (BDNF), play important functions in the development and maturation of the nervous system. Their effects are mediated by binding to specific high-affinity tyrosine kinase receptors (Trks). Nerve growth factor is a ligand for TrkA type receptors, BDNF targets TrkB receptors, and neurotrophin 3 is a ligand for TrkC receptors. BDNF is highly expressed in the cerebellum. Granule cells express BDNF, and both granule and Purkinje cells express TrkB receptors (Wetmore et al., 1990; Segal et al., 1995). BDNF is found in the adult cerebellum, especially in Purkinje neurons. BDNF promotes survival and axonal elongation of granule cells and promotes survival and differentiation of Purkinje neurons (Larkförs et al., 1996). BDNF not only regulates cerebellar post-natal development and dendritic maturation, but also participates in synaptic plasticity (Richardson & Leitch, 2005). Development of GABAergic synapses is also under the control of BDNF (Rico et al., 2002). Neural activity tunes the release of neurotrophins. Therefore, neurotrophins participate in activity-dependent synaptogenesis of inhibitory synapses (Drake-Baumann, 2006).

Imaging and fetal development

Ultrasound and fetal MRI have become two major techniques to assess cerebellar development in the fetus (Triulzi et al., 2006). The ultrasound technique has several advantages: easy access, low cost, portability, and real-time assessment. The technique provides accurate brain and ventricular morphometric measurements, with fairly good intra- and inter-reader reliability. Nevertheless, for the qualitative assessment of brain parenchyma and anatomy, it is operator-dependent. It also suffers from a lack of resolution. MRI is superior to ultrasound in this regard. It is very accurate for identifying morphologically the development of the cerebellum. Its limitations include the resolution, although improvements are occurring. Fetal MRI allows an accurate estimation of cerebellar development from about week 19 (Figure 1.5). Vermis height and length and cerebellar transverse diameter can be identified easily. Quantitatively, the cerebellum will roughly double its diameters between week 19 and week 37. After 21 weeks, posterior fossa structures are well defined on MRI. At this time, the tentorium has reached its final orientation, and the typical shape of the brainstem is recognizable. Primary fissure is well discernible in sagittal sections at week 21 or 22, and vermis folia start to be visible after week 24. Fetal MRI can be used also to assess indirectly the processes of myelination and synaptogenesis. Myelination starts during midgestation from the spinal cord to progress cranially. Sensory pathways are the first to myelinate. The archicerebellum and the paleocerebellum are myelinated in a newborn, while cerebellar hemispheres are not. T2-weighted techniques are particularly suited to monitor the progression of myelination due to the high contrast between the unmyelinated and the myelinated white matter. A slight hypointense signal can be recognized by week 21 in the deep white matter of the cerebellum, corresponding to cerebellar nuclei.

Anatomy

Nomenclature

In humans, Jansen proposed to divide the cerebellum in three parts: the anterior lobe, the posterior lobe, and the paraflocculus/flocculus (Figure 1.6). Dow has suggested to divide the cerebellum in three areas on the basis of the mossy fiber projections: the vestibulocerebellum corresponds to the flocculonodular lobe, the paleocerebellum corresponds to the vermal anterior and posterior lobes with mainly spinal projections, and the neocerebellum refers to the mediolateral part with essentially corticopontocerebellar projections (Dow, 1942). The nomenclature of Larsell is widely used in animals. The cerebellum is divided in 10 lobules (I to X according to the nomenclature of Larsell), illustrated in Figures 1.6 and 1.7. Fissures separating the lobules are shown in Figure 1.8. Although individual lobules are easily identified in the human cerebellum, the overall shape of the cerebellum may vary between subjects (Diedrichsen et al., 2009). For instance, lobule IX may appear downwards near the opening of the foramen magnum in some subjects, whereas in others it will appear upwards to lobule VIII. The proportion of the cerebellar gray matter assigned to each lobule is illustrated in Figure 1.9. Lobule VII, consisting of crus I, crus II, and crus VIIb, accounts for nearly 50% of the gray matter volume (Diedrichsen et al., 2009). The left hemisphere is larger than the right hemisphere in the majority of subjects. Anterior lobules III and IV are larger on the right side. The reverse is observed for lobule VI. This asymmetry might be related to handedness (Snyder et al, 1995).

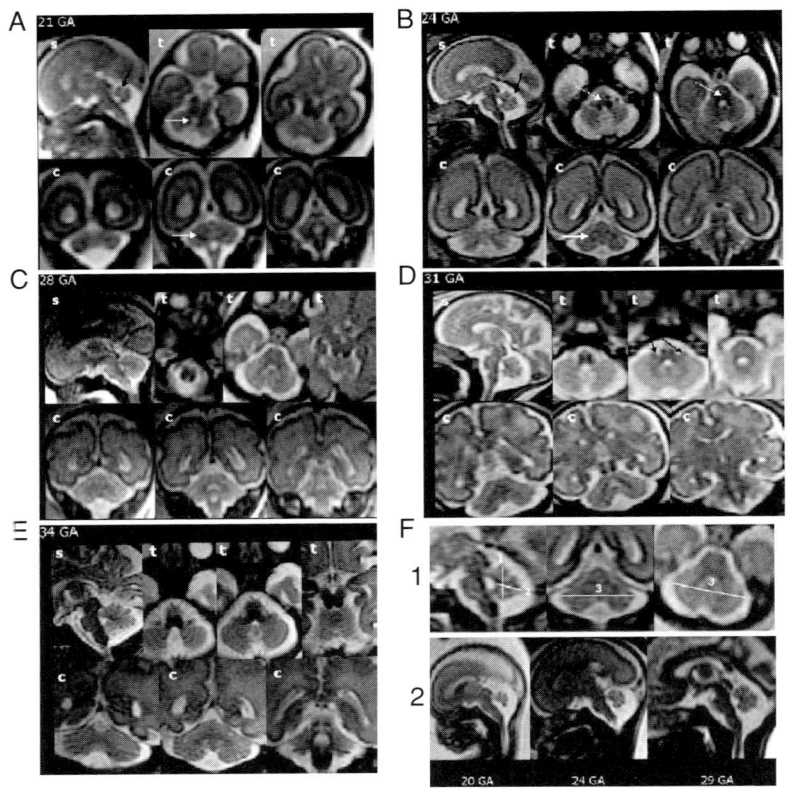

Figure 1.5 Steps of cerebellar development in the fetus on brain MRI. (A) Cerebellar development at 21 weeks gestational age (GA). MRI in the sagittal (s), transverse (t), and coronal (c) planes. Primary fissure (black arrow) is already detectable on the sagittal image. A slight hypointense signal, most likely due to dentate nuclei, can be recognized on the deep cerebellar white matter (white arrows). (B) Cerebellar development, 24 weeks GA. Primary fissure (black arrow) and cerebellar nuclei (white arrows) are detectable. T2 hypointensity in dorsal medulla and pons is also detectable (white dotted arrow). (C) Cerebellar development, 28 weeks GA. A rapid increase of vermian size (s) in comparison with A and B is well detectable. (D) Cerebellar development, 31 weeks GA. Hypointense cerebellar flocculi are visible (black arrows). (E) Cerebellar development, 34 weeks GA. Cerebellar folia are easily detectable also in coronal and transverse section. (F) Measurements on brain MRI. Upper panels: Measurements of vermis height, vermis anteroposterior diameter, Transverse cerebellar diameter. Bottom panels: isolated mild inferior vermian hypoplasia detected at 20 weeks GA, and follow-up studies at 24 and 29 weeks GA demonstrate a progressively normal development of cerebellar vermis. From: Triulzi, 2006. With permission.

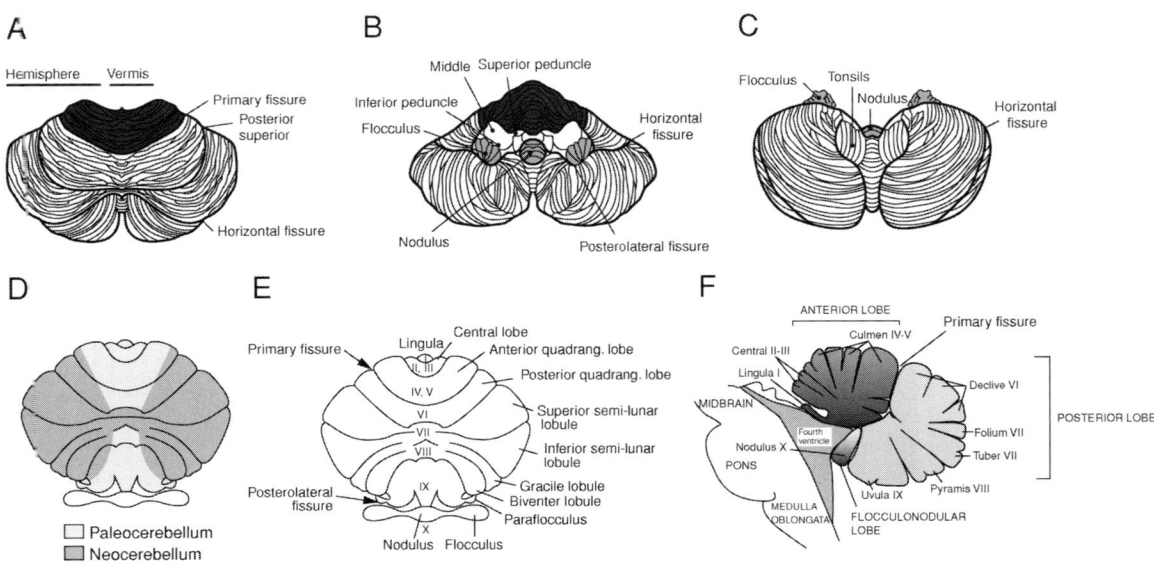

Figure 1.6 Illustration of the human cerebellum. (A) Superior view. The anterior lobe is demarcated from the posterior lobe by the primary fissure. (B) Anterior-inferior view showing the cerebellar peduncles. The flocculonodular lobe, delineated by the posterolateral fissure, is visible. (C) Inferior view showing the posterior part of the posterior lobe and the flocculonodular lobe. (D) Phylogenetic division of the cerebellum in paleocerebellum (medially), neocerebellum (laterally), and archicerebellum (flocculonodular lobe) represented on an unfolded cerebellum. (E) Division in 10 lobules. (F) Components of the vermis. From: Colin et al., 2002. With permission. (See color section).

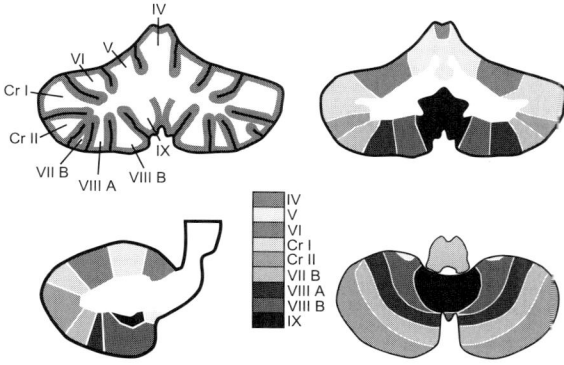

Figure 1.7 Parcellation of the cerebellum in individual lobules. Upper panels, coronal sections; lower left, parasagittal section; lower right, inferior view of the cerebellum. (See color section).

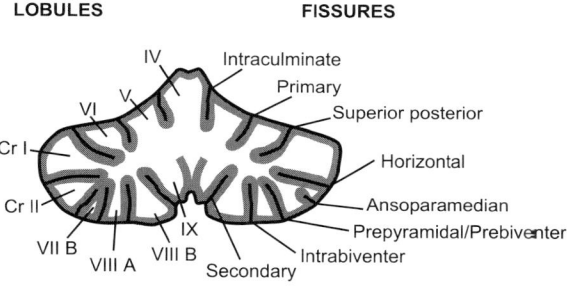

Figure 1.8 Lobules of the cerebellum in a coronal section and the corresponding fissures.

The cerebellum is highly stereotyped in its cellular circuitry, but the organization of input–output pathways differs according to the cerebellar region, leading to a functional compartmentalization.

Afferent fibers

Three pairs of cerebellar peduncles allow the afferent fibers to reach their targets: the inferior cerebellar peduncle (also called restiform body), the middle cerebellar peduncle (brachium pontis), and the superior cerebellar peduncle (brachium conjunctivum). Tracts passing through the cerebellar peduncles are listed in Table 1.1. The number of afferent fibers is very high as compared with cerebellar efferent fibers (ratio of about 40:1). The cerebellum receives three types of fibers: climbing fibers emerging exclusively from the contralateral inferior olive and ascending in the inferior cerebellar peduncle, mossy fibers arising from a large number of sources, and the diffusely distributed cholinergic/monoaminergic afferents (often called "the third afferent system"). While climbing fibers are thin and relatively slow-conducting fibers, mossy fibers are large and fast conducting fibers (Colin et al., 2002; see also Chapter 2).

The afferent synaptic projections are organized in parasagittal stripes: (1) mossy fiber inputs from the

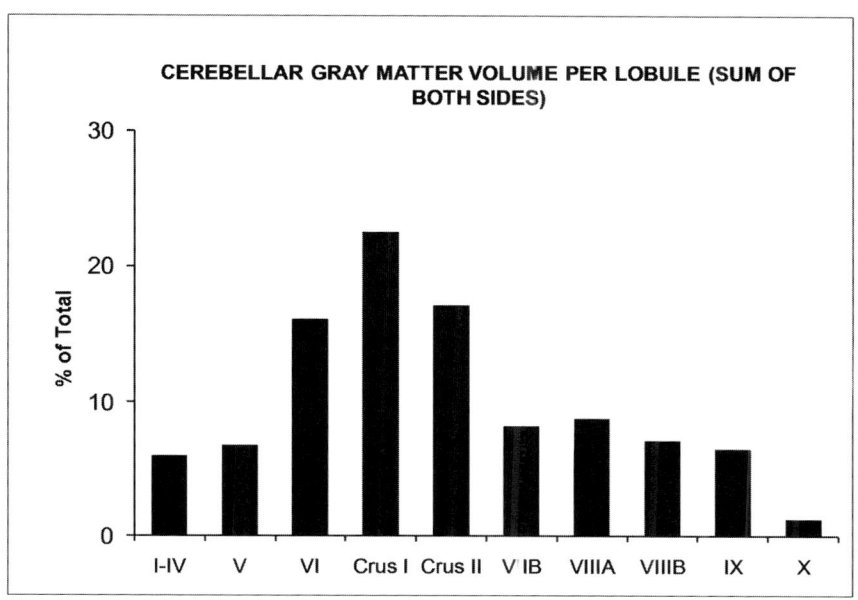

Figure 1.9 Volume of lobules in percentage of the total estimated cerebellar gray matter volume in healthy adults (total = 100%). Volumes of left and right side are considered together. Adapted from: Diedrichsen et al., 2009. (See color section).

Table 1.1 Tracts passing in the cerebellar peduncles

Peduncle	Afferents	Efferents
Inferior cerebellar peduncle (restiform body)	Olivocerebellar tract Vestibulocerebellar tract Cuneocerebellar tract[a] Reticulocerebellar tract Dorsal spinocerebellar tract[a] Trigeminocerebellar tract	Cerebelloolivary tract Cerebellovestibular tract Cerebellospinal tract Cerebelloreticular tract
Middle cerebellar peduncle (brachium pontis)	Pontocerebellar tract	
Superior cerebellar tract (brachium conjunctivum)	Ventral spinocerebellar tract[b] Tectocerebellar tract	Dentatorubral tract Cerebellotegmental tract Cerebellovestibular tract Cerebelloolivary tract

[a]Uncrossed. [b]Crossed.

spinocerebellar and cuneocerebellar tracts, (2) striped muscarinergic receptors in the Purkinje and molecular layers complemented with mossy fiber rosettes stained with acetylcholinesterase, and (3) zonal and prealbumin/calcitonin gene-related peptide reactive climbing fiber inputs (Hamamura et al., 2004). Stripes of these inputs alternate and monoclonal antibodies against a membrane fraction clearly show a parasagittal stripe organization of Purkinje neurons, with alternating zebrin-positive and -negative bands. These zebrin compartments could represent a fundamental unit of organization in the cerebellum (see also section The inferior olivary complex).

Cerebellar circuitry

The cerebellum is highly stereotyped in its cellular circuitry (Figure 1.10). The highly folded cerebellar cortex projects to (relatively) small nuclei, the sole output of the cerebellum.

The cerebellar cortex

Purkinje neurons

The cerebellar cortex is divided in three layers. Purkinje cells make a monolayer (ganglionic), which separates the molecular layer (outer) from the inner granular layer. The estimation of the number of Purkinje neurons for a human cerebellum is about 15 million. These neurons have a typical pear-shaped soma, with a single axon leaving the lower pole. The agranular endoplasmic reticulum is extremely developed. Its membrane contains inositol 1,4,5-triphosphate and ryanodine receptors. In the granular layer, numerous collaterals are oriented perpendicularly to the axis of the folium. Purkinje neurons are GABAergic (Ito & Yoshida, 1964). They inhibit deep nuclei and vestibular nuclei. Also, branches of the supra-ganglionic and infra-ganglionic plexus inhibit the basket/stellate cells and the Golgi/Lugaro cells, respectively.

The primary dendrite emerging from the outer pole makes an arbor, with the terminal part of the dendrite being covered by numerous spines making excitatory synapses with parallel fibers. Purkinje neurons have one of the most extensive dendritic domains, composed of a dense network of spines along distal shafts. Climbing fibers target Purkinje neurons in an exclusive one-to-one relationship. The connection between one ascending climbing fiber and a Purkinje neuron represents a very powerful synapse (see Chapter 2).

Granule cells

Granule cells have an oval shape, with typical naked nuclei due to the thinness of the cytoplasm. There are about 3 to 7 million granule cells/mm^3 in humans, which equals between 10^{10} and 10^{11} cells/cerebellum. Terminals of mossy fibers end up in the granular layer, giving rise to clubby enlargements, called "rosettes" (Figure 1.11), which are parts of a complex globular enlargement (glomerulus). Rosettes give rise to special "en marron" excitatory synaptic contacts with terminal branches of the granule cell dendrites. One rosette makes about 90 to 100 synapses with dendrites, with each granule cell presenting four to five dendrites. Axons of Golgi neurons make inhibitory synapses on the branches of the granule dendrites. Granule cells are the origin of an ascending thin axon which penetrates in the molecular layer to bifurcate in two parallel

A

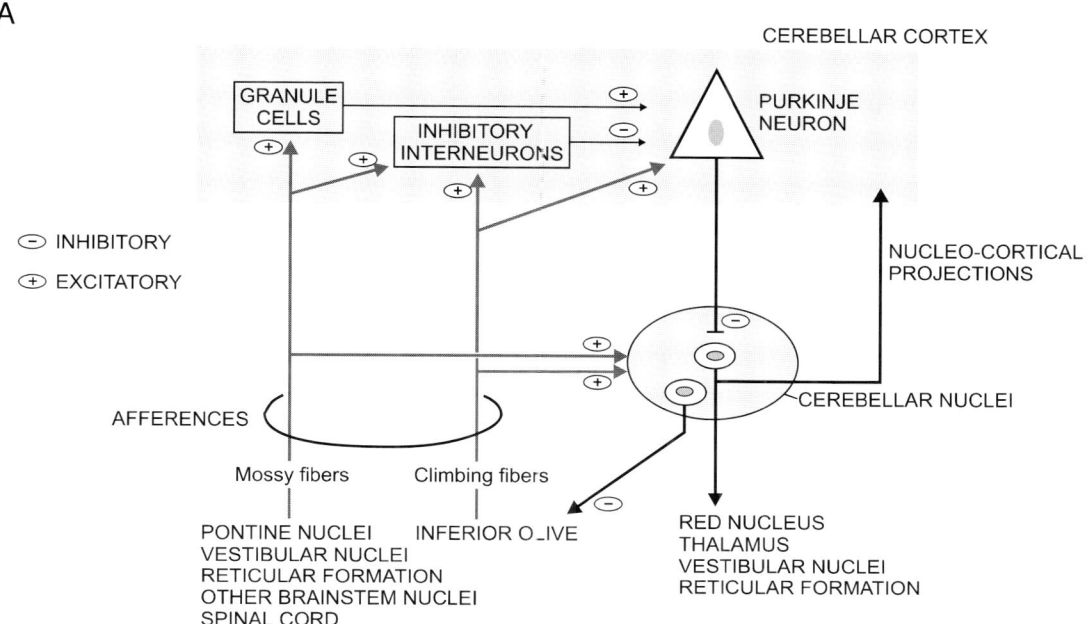

B

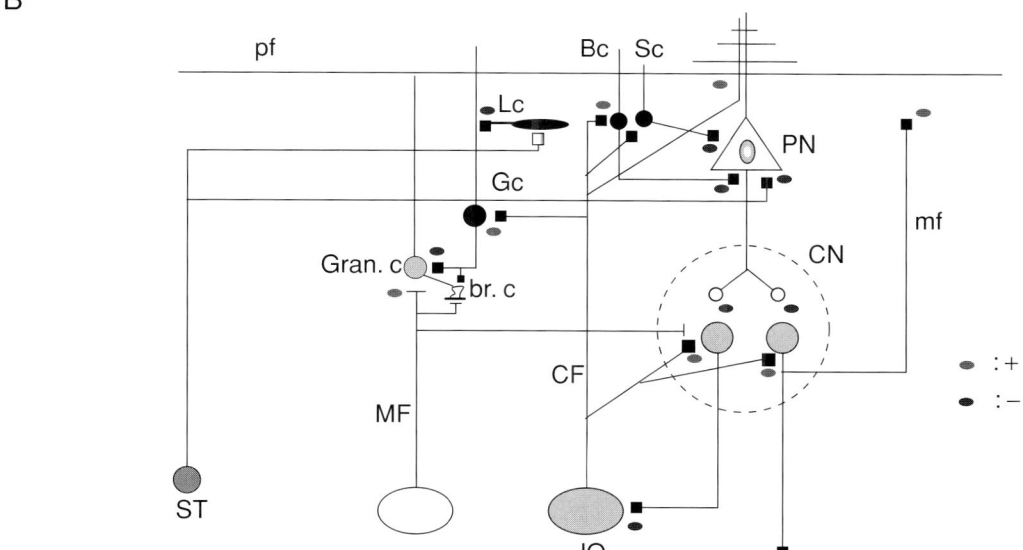

Figure 1.10 Wiring and connections of the cerebellar circuitry. (A) Mossy fibers (blue) and climbing fibers (red) project to cerebellar cortex (gray area) and cerebellar nuclei. The Purkinje neuron interacts with granule cells and inhibitory interneurons of the cerebellar cortex. Purkinje cells represent the output of the cerebellar cortex. Purkinje neurons inhibit cerebellar nuclei, which are the origin of the output emerging from the cerebellum. (B) Neurons of cerebellar circuitry. Abbreviations: MF: mossy fiber; CF: climbing fiber; IO: inferior olive; Gran. c: granule cell; br. c: brush cell; Gc: Golgi cell; Lc: Lugaro cell; Bc: basket cell; Sc: stellate cell; PN: Purkinje neuron; CN: cerebellar nuclei. +: excitatory; – : inhibitory. (See color section.)

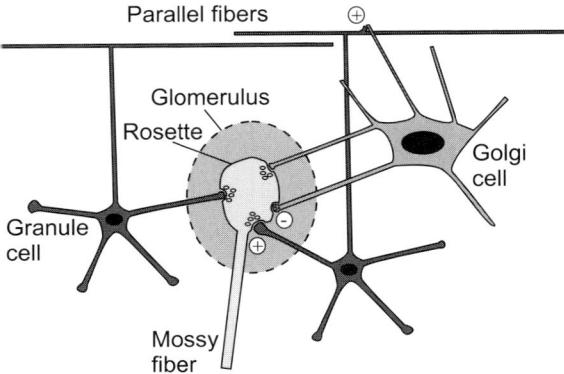

Figure 1.11 The glomerulus. The enlarged extremity of a mossy fiber (represented in yellow), called "rosette," is connected with dendrites of the granule cells (shown in blue) and a Golgi cell (illustrated in green). It also receives an axonal projection from the latter. Therefore, Golgi cells regulate mossy fiber inputs. Golgi cells are themselves excited by parallel fibers emerging from the granule cells. (See color section.)

branches running parallel to the axis of the folium in opposite directions. Parallel fibers have a diameter of about 0.25 μm, with a length estimated at 2 to 7 mm. Varicose swellings form excitatory synapses with dendritic spines of Purkinje neurons, which are dynamic small protuberances bearing the postsynaptic components of the synapses. Their shape and number are sensitive to numerous physiological conditions, such as learning (Federmeier et al., 2002). Parallel fibers liberate nitric oxide (NO), which activates guanylate-cyclase.

Unipolar brush cells

Unipolar brush cells are found in the granular layer. Their size is between a granule cell and a Golgi cell (Mugnaini & Floris, 1994). They are densely stained with anti-serum against calretinin, a calcium-binding protein. A main feature of unipolar brush cells is their thick dendrite terminating in a brush-like tip, hence their name. They are found mainly in the vestibulo-cerebellum and the lingula. Their density is moderate-to-low in other folia of the vermis and in the intermediate cortex. They are found rarely in lateral regions of the cerebellum. Mossy fiber terminals form a special synapse with the dendrites of unipolar brush cells. There is a long synaptic cleft, with many sites of vesicle clustering. The neurotransmitter is trapped in the cleft, a single spike in the mossy fiber producing a 500-msec spike burst. The axons branch in the granular layer and end with a rosette.

Inhibitory interneurons

Inhibitory interneurons are located in the molecular and granular layers. Basket cells are located just above the Purkinje layer. Their dendrites have long spines. The axon runs perpendicular to the long axis of the folium above Purkinje neurons and gives off descending collaterals surrounding the Purkinje cell soma in a basket-like shape. The end of the basket connects with the Purkinje cell in a structure called "pinceau." This is an inhibitory synapse, one basket cell inhibiting up to nine Purkinje neurons. Stellate cells occupy the outer two-thirds of the molecular layer. They have a short axon. Their dendrites make inhibitory synapses with the Purkinje cell dendrites outside the basket. Golgi cells and stellate cells share parallel fiber inputs with the Purkinje neurons. Golgi cells are inhibited by collaterals of Purkinje neurons and inhibit the synaptic transmission between mossy fiber rosettes and granule cell dendrites, regulating mossy fiber inputs. Lugaro cells are characterized by a small fusiform soma and a dendrite expanding horizontally under Purkinje cells. Both their soma and dendrites receive a massive innervation from collaterals of the axon of Purkinje neurons. Lugaro cells have an ascending axon, making numerous inhibitory synapses with the soma and dendrites of basket and stellate cells.

Bergmann glial cells

Bergmann glial cells are specialized astrocytes closely associated with Purkinje cells. Astrocytes are extensively coupled by gap junctions (Giaume & McCarthy, 1996). These latter participate in electrical coupling and intercellular signaling. They are formed by two hemichannels, each of which comprises six protein subunits called connexins. Connexin43 (Cx43), the major constituent of astrocytic gap junctions, is highly expressed in astrocytes throughout the brain. Another group of proteins, called pannexins and contributing to gap junctions, are expressed in particular in Purkinje cells.

Cerebellar nuclei

The cerebellar nuclei are the main target of Purkinje neurons. In humans, the medial nucleus corresponds to the fastigial nucleus, the globosus/emboliformis to the anterior/posterior interpositus nucleus, and the lateral nucleus to the dentate nucleus. This latter contains the majority of neurons. It looks like a folded band, with a hilus located medially. It can be identified on high-resolution MRI (Figure 1.12). The dentate nucleus is composed of a rostromedial zone (magnocellular) and a posterolateral zone (parvocellular). While neurons in the dentate nucleus are mainly composed of large multipolar cells, the interpositus nucleus and the fastigial nucleus are composed of both large and small multipolar neurons.

Nucleofugal fibers are excitatory and use glutamate as a neurotransmitter, except for the GABAergic nucleo-olivary projections, which exert a strong inhibition on the contralateral inferior olive, regulate Purkinje cell firing, and might be involved in the gating of sensory input to the olive. Nuclear neurons receive a dense projection from Purkinje neurons. The excitatory input on nuclear cells emerges from collaterals of climbing and mossy fiber afferents. It is currently accepted that the input from mossy fibers is the major excitatory input to nuclei. Nucleofugal fibers emit collaterals ending in the granular layer (nucleocortical fibers). These projections have a somatotopic organization (Provini et al., 1998). They are often considered as providers of negative feedback loops.

The fastigial nucleus projects bilaterally to the vestibular and reticular nuclei, controlling reticulospinal and vestibulospinal tracts (Figure 1.13). Crossed (uncinate fasciculus or hook bundle, which arches around the brachium conjunctivum) and uncrossed fibers emerge from the fastigial nucleus.

The interpositus nucleus, divided in anterior and posterior parts, projects to the contralateral thalamus and adjacent areas of the ventral anterior (NVA), area X, and ventral posterolateralis nucleus (VPLN). Fibers send collaterals to the red nucleus. The interpositus nucleus also sends collaterals to the nuclear reticularis tegmenti pontis (NRTP), the pontine nuclei, and the superior colliculus.

The dentate nucleus projects mainly to the thalamus (NVL, VPLN, area X, intralaminar nuclei) and the red nucleus.

The inferior olivary complex

The inferior olivary complex includes the principal olive, medial and dorsal accessory olive, and medial lamina. The inferior olive comprises about 1.5 million cells. As mentioned earlier, the white matter of the cerebellum can be divided in longitudinal strips: eight major bands (A, X, B, C1, C2, C3, D1, D2) project to well-defined regions of cerebellar nuclei and receive climbing fibers from specific areas of the inferior olive

(Voogd & Glickstein, 1998). Zones A, X, and B are found in the vermis. Zones C1–C3 project to the anterior interposed nucleus, the C2 zone projects to the posterior interposed nucleus, and the D1–D2 zones project to the caudoventral and rostrodorsal portions of the dentate. The flocculus is also divided into eight longitudinal strips, which are related to four small parts of the inferior olive. Anatomically and functionally, the olivocerebellar system can be considered as composed of a sagittal band of cortex receiving climbing fibers from a small part of the inferior olive and sending an output to a well-defined zone of nuclei. In other words, a small area in the inferior olive is linked to a definite area of the cerebellar output. Such an input–output topographical link is absent for the mossy fibers. Purkinje neurons exhibit biochemical and immunological heterogeneities which fit with this sagittal distribution. Cells in the inferior olive are organized in groups which tend to discharge simultaneously and project to the same sagittal band. The inferior olive is particularly enriched in neuronal gap junctions, which serve to underlie synchronous activity in the olivocerebellar system (Llinas et al., 1974; Sotelo et al., 1974; Marshall et al., 2007). Gap junctions are formed mostly by connexin36 proteins.

The inferior olive receives projections from the spinal cord (crossed ventral and dorsal spinoolivary tracts), the brainstem (especially red nuclei), cerebellar nuclei (interpositus and dentate nuclei exert an inhibitory effect), pretectal nuclei (relaying optokinetic information), layer V of motor cortex area 4 and premotor cortex area 6, and visual and vestibular areas. Zona incerta of the thalamus also projects to the inferior olive and might be a relay not only for the projections from the motor cortex, but also from prefrontal, cingulated, parietal, and temporal areas (Schmahmann & Pandya, 1997).

Spinocerebellar tracts

Spinocerebellar tracts end mainly in the anterior lobe, the paramedian lobule, and the pyramis of the posterior lobe. The dorsal spinocerebellar tract (DSCT; Flechsig tract) takes its origin in the Clarke column in the thoracic and lumbar segments. DSCT conveys information from the hind limbs. DSCT is uncrossed and enters the cerebellum via the inferior cerebellar peduncle. DSCT neurons are either proprioceptive or exteroceptive. DSCT transmission is characterized by a high level of accuracy in time and space.

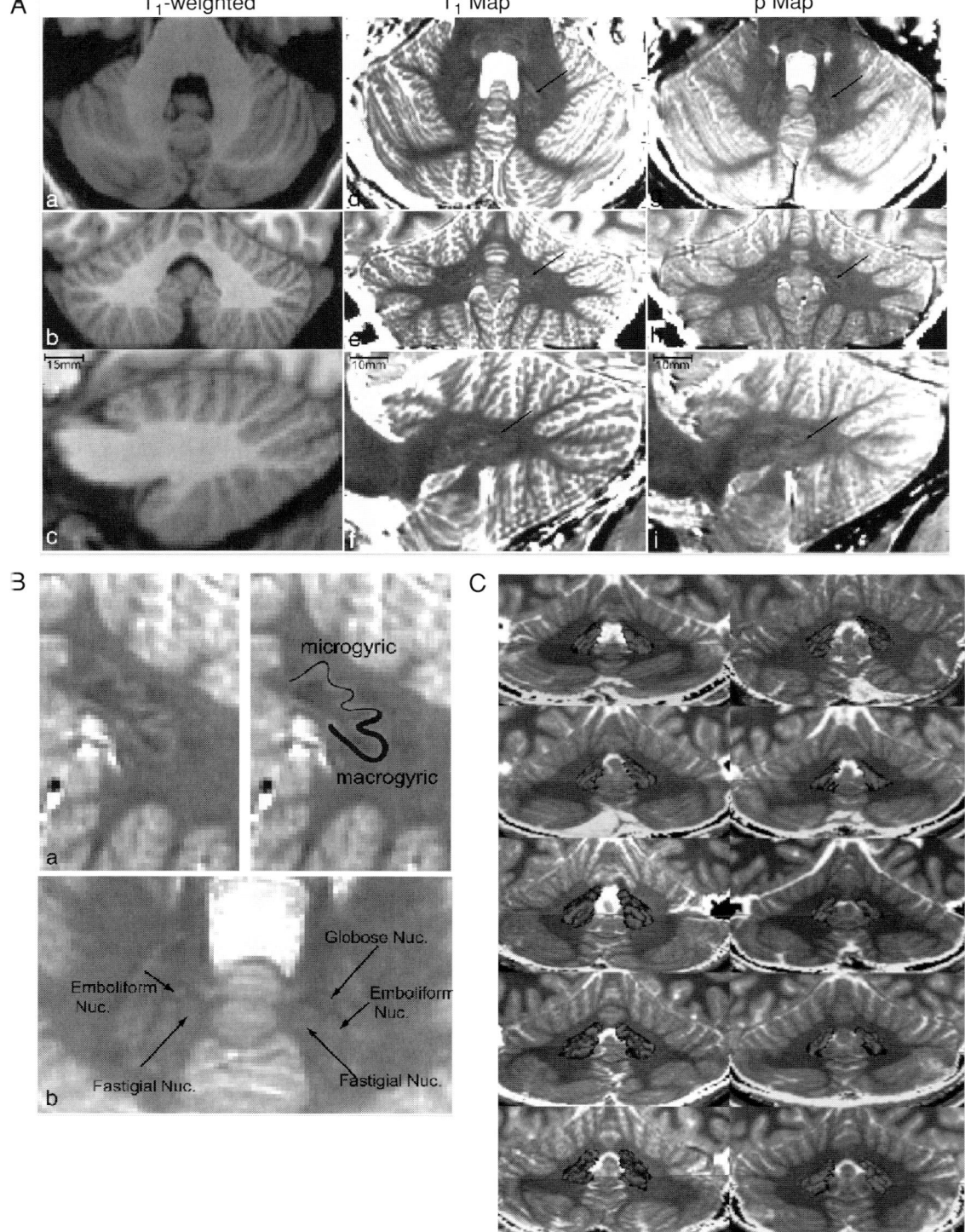

Figure 1.12 Imaging of cerebellar nuclei in adults using high-resolution MRI. (A) (a–c) Axial, coronal, and sagittal slices of the human cerebellum and corresponding slices through the high-resolution (0.7 × 0.7 × 0.7 mm 3 voxels) ρ (d–f) and T1 (g–i) maps calculated from multi-averaged data requiring 40 min of scan time. The dentate, as well as globose and emboliform nuclei of the interposed nucleus, can be clearly delineated on both the T1 and ρ maps, allowing their anatomy to be fully appreciated. Arrows indicate the dentate nucleus on each image. (B) Anatomy of the deep cerebellar nuclei. Upper row, the dentate nucleus is composed of two parts: a dorsomedial and rostral region with narrow dentations (microgyric dentate) and a ventrolateral and caudal portion with wide and subdivided gyrations (macrogyric dentate). Lower picture: identification of the fastigial, globose, and emboliform nuclei. (C) Volume renderings of the dentate nuclei of each of 10 adults, superimposed on their corresponding T1 maps. The images are taken from the superior-anterior viewpoint. From: Deoni and Catani, 2007. With permission. (See color section.)

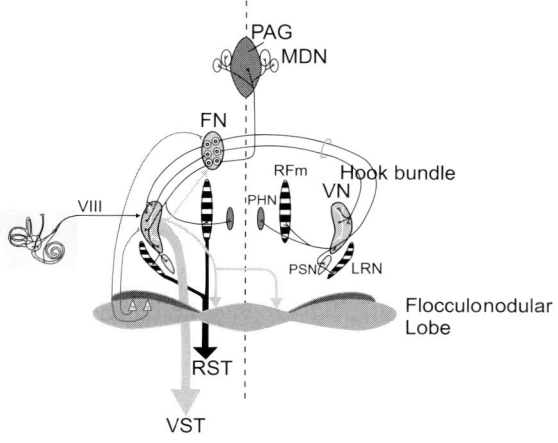

Figure 1.13 Connections of the fastigial nucleus (FN). FN projects bilaterally to vestibular nuclei (VN) and projects to the periaqueductal gray (PAG) and the mesodiencephalic nuclei (MDN: interstitial and Darkschewitsch nuclei). FN also projects to bulbar reticular formation: medial bulbar reticular formation (RFm) and lateral reticular nuclei (LRN), at the origin of the reticulospinal tract (RST). Reticular nuclei project back to cerebellar nuclei (cerebello-reticulocerebellar loops, not illustrated) and receive afferents from the spinal cord. FN is also connected with the parasolitarius nuclei (PSN) and the perihypoglossal nuclei (PHN). VN projects to the spinal cord via the vestibulospinal tract (VST) and projects back to the FN and the flocculonodular lobe. Interrupted line: midline. (See color section).

Proprioceptive cells are stimulated by Ia, Ib, and II fibers. Exteroceptive cells are activated by cutaneous pressure receptors.

The ventral spinocerebellar tract (VSCT; Gowers tract) emerges from the third to sixth lumbar segments. VSCT crosses the midline, ascends ventrally to DSCT in the spinal cord, and crosses a second time in the superior cerebellar peduncle. VSCT also conveys information from the hind limbs. VSCT neurons receive a dense polysynaptic input from the ipsilateral flexor reflex afferents, predominantly exciting fibers evoking flexor reflexes, including cutaneous fibers, groups II and III muscle afferents, and joint afferents (Oscarsson, 1973). They are also influenced by group I muscle receptors.

The cuneocerebellar tract conveys information from the forelimb. It includes proprioceptive cells found in the external cuneatus nucleus and exteroceptive cells. The rostral spinocerebellar tract is the equivalent of the VSCT for the forelimb. Cell bodies are located in the rostral Clarke column. Axons enter the cerebellum via the superior and the inferior cerebellar peduncles.

Vestibular afferents

Primary afferents from vestibular nerves/vestibular nuclei project to the ipsilateral vestibulocerebellum. Fibers from the vestibular nuclei project diffusely to the vermis, the flocculus and paraflocculus, the paramedian lobule, and the fastigial and interpositus nucleus.

Acoustic, visual, and trigeminal afferents

Sounds and stimulation of the visual cortex induce responses in lobules VI to VIII, the audiovisual representation of the cerebellum. Trigeminal afferents project to the posterior lobe.

Reticular nuclei

The lateral reticular nucleus (LRN), located lateral to the inferior olive, emits projections ascending via the superior cerebellar peduncle. Mossy fibers are bilaterally distributed, with an ipsilateral dominance. Spinal tracts project upon the LRN. These nuclei also receive collaterals from propriospinal neurons, which stimulate the motoneurons. This is seen as a source of information for the cerebellum about motor commands. Both the pyramidal tract and the rubrospinal tract stimulate the LRN, which also receives afferent fibers from the superior colliculus and the lateral vestibular nucleus.

The LRN receives a powerful excitatory input from the cerebellar nuclei, to which it sends excitatory projections (Dietrichs, 1983). Ringing has been shown in this reciprocal excitatory connection (Ito, 1984). The projections to cerebellar nuclei would provide a controlled excitatory background activity averaged over multiple spinal and supra-spinal inputs, modulated by the inhibition from Purkinje cells.

The nuclear reticularis tegmenti pontis (NRTP), located dorsally to the medial lemniscus, receives its main input from Brodmann areas 1 to 6. NRTP projects to the contralateral anterior lobe and the paramedian lobule and medial parts of lobules VI/VII, sending collaterals to the dentate and interpositus nuclei. These nuclei send massive projections back to the NRTP. The NRTP relays visual information to the flocculus.

The paramedian reticular nucleus, located near the raphe, receives numerous afferents from the spinal cord. Projections reach the anterior lobe, the vermal posterior lobe, and the flocculus.

One of the perihypoglossal nuclei, called the nucleus prepositus hypoglossi, projects to the oculomotor nuclei, has connections with vestibular and cerebellar nuclei, and receives visual plus somesthetic inputs. The nucleus prepositus hypoglossi plays a key role in the control of gaze.

Pontine nuclei

Projecting neurons to the cerebellum give off mossy fibers. Areas 4 and 6 are a major input of the corticopontocerebellar connections. Primary sensory areas 3, 1, and 2; parietal areas 5 and 7; and supratemporal areas also contribute. Brodmann areas project to slabs oriented rostrocaudally in the pons. Each slab projects mainly contralaterally to the cerebellar hemisphere in a defined area. Because a small area of the cortex may project to several points in a slab and in the cerebellar surface, the terminology of "fractured somatotopy" is commonly used. This patchy projection of the mossy fiber system contrasts with the sagittal strip projection of the climbing fiber system. About 10% of the pontocerebellar projection is ipsilateral.

The thalamocortical projections

The thalamic nuclei NVL/VPLN/NVA are key targets of cerebellar projections. Inputs from contralateral dentate and interpositus nuclei terminate densely in these nuclei. Inputs from fastigial nuclei are restricted and bilateral. A fine somatotopic organization has been suggested for the cerebello-thalamocortical projection, with separate output channels from the cerebellar nuclei being linked to distinct regions of the motor cortex (Middleton & Strick, 1997). Thalamic nuclei project to motor cortex, premotor cortex, supplementary motor area, and prefrontal, posterior parietal, and temporal regions. Intralaminar nuclei project towards association areas and limbic cortices (Schmahmann & Pandya, 1997). Projections to the motor and premotor cortex originate from the dorsal portions of the dentate nucleus, whereas projections to the prefrontal and posterior parietal areas of the cortex originate from the ventral portions of the dentate nucleus (Dum & Strick, 2003) (Figure 1.14). Purkinje cells of the ansiform lobule receive inputs from the prefrontal area 46 and project to the same area (Kelly & Strick, 2003).

Table 1.2 Origin and targets of aminergic pathways in the cerebellum

Amine	Source	Targets
5-HT	Medullary and pontine reticular formation	Cerebellar cortex: dense plexus in granular and Purkinje cell layers
	Raphe nuclei	Cerebellar nuclei: dense plexus
NE	Dorsal and ventral parts of the locus coeruleus	Cerebellar cortex: around glomeruli and around dendrites of Purkinje cells Cerebellar nuclei
ACh	Pedunculopontine tegmental nucleus Lateral paragigantocellular nucleus Raphe nuclei	Cerebellar cortex Cerebellar nuclei
DA	Ventral mesencephalic tegmental area	Cerebellar cortex
Histamine	Tuberomammillary nucleus	Cerebellar cortex

Abbreviations: ACh: acetylcholine; DA: dopamine; 5-HT: serotonin; NE: noradrenaline.

OUTPUT CHANNELS OF THE DENTATE NUCLEUS

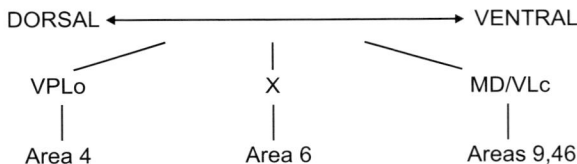

Figure 1.14 Output channels of the dentate nucleus. Distinct areas of the dentate nucleus project predominantly upon different regions of the contralateral cerebral cortex, via thalamic nuclei (MD/VLc: medial dorsal/ventralis lateral pars caudalis nuclei; area X, VPLo: nucleus ventralis posterior lateralis pars oralis). Dorsal portions of the dentate nucleus project mainly upon area 4. With permission from: Manto, 2009. (See color section.)

Aminergic and cholinergic inputs to the cerebellum

Both the cerebellum and the inferior olive receive a diffuse aminergic innervation. Table 1.2 lists the main sites of origin of these inputs, as well as their targets in the cerebellar circuitry. Aminergic fibers are neuromodulators in cerebellar circuits. Neuromodulation is defined by chemical communication between neurons that is not fast, not point-to-point, or not simply

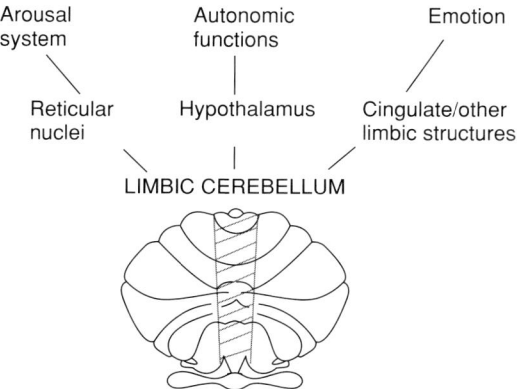

Arousal system → Reticular nuclei
Autonomic functions → Hypothalamus
Emotion → Cingulate/other limbic structures

LIMBIC CEREBELLUM

Figure 1.15 Connections of the so-called "limbic cerebellum." Medial zones of the cerebellum are connected with reticular nuclei, hypothalamus, and limbic areas. Reciprocal connections with the limbic structures include the amygdala, the hippocampus, and the septum. These pathways would be the substratum of a limbic cerebellum, according to which the vermis and fastigial nuclei participate in the regulation of the arousal system, autonomic functions, and emotions.

Table 1.3 Neurotransmitters and neuromodulators of the cerebellum

Glutamate
Aspartate
GABA
Glycine
Taurine

Neuromodulators
    Serotonin
    Noradrenaline
    Acetylcholine
    Dopamine

Histamine
Nitric oxide

Peptides
    Opioids (enkephalin)
    Corticotropin releasing factor
    Secretin/PACAP/VIP
    Cholecystokinin
    Calcitonin gene-related peptide
    Tachykinins
    Somatostatin
    Motilin

Endocannabinoids
Purinergic signaling (ATP, adenosine)
Zinc (?)

Abbreviations: ATP: adenosine triphosphate; PACAP: pituitary adenylate cyclase–activating polypeptide; VIP: vasoactive intestinal peptide.

excitation or inhibition (Schweighofer et al., 2004). See also section Neurotransmitters.

Autonomic centers

Stimulation of the vagal nerve evokes responses in the cerebellar cortex, and the cerebellum receives projections from the sensory nuclei of nerve IX. Cerebellar circuitry projects to the hypothalamus, with a reciprocal connectivity. Projections arise from multiple hypothalamic nuclei and terminate in all layers of the cerebellar cortex, as well as in cerebellar nuclei. There is a preferential distribution in the flocculus and vermis (Haines et al., 1990).

Connections with the limbic system

The cerebellum is connected with multiple elements of the Papez limbic circuit subserving emotion (see also the section Cognitive abnormalities and emotional disorders in Chapter 3) (Figure 1.15). Cerebellar stimulation of the fastigial nucleus evokes responses in the hippocampus and the amygdala (Heath & Harper, 1974).

Neurotransmitters

Table 1.3 lists the neurotransmitters and neuromodulators of cerebellar circuitry. Glutamate is a transmitter for both the mossy fiber and the climbing fiber system. The post-synaptic element of the synapse mossy fiber-granule cell presents N-methyl-D-aspartate (NMDA) and amino-3-hydroxyl-5-methyl-4-isoxazole-proprionate (AMPA) receptors. Some mossy fibers contain choline acetyl transferase and use acetylcholine as a transmitter. Moreover, several peptides having a modulatory role have been identified in the mossy fibers, such as enkephalin or corticotrophin-releasing factor. Corticotrophin-releasing factor, cholecystokinin, and calcitonin gene-related peptide may be gathered in mossy fibers. Climbing fibers are strongly enriched in glutamate and can retrogradely transport aspartate to the inferior olive (Wiklund et al., 1984). It was thought initially that climbing fibers might use homocysteic acid as a neurotransmitter for some of them, but immunoreactivity studies indicate that homocysteic acid is mostly confined to glia. Transporters removing transmitters from the synaptic cleft for climbing fibers are excitatory amino acid transporter type 4 (EAAT4), concentrated in Purkinje cell spines, and EAAT3, which has a wider distribution (Rothstein et al., 1994).

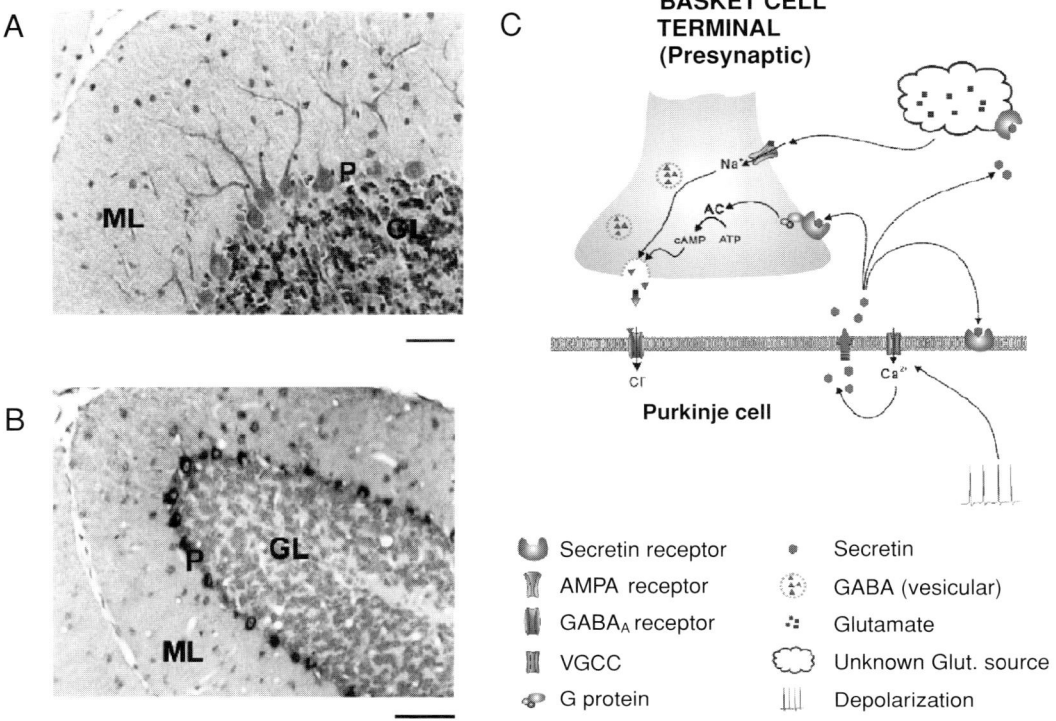

Figure 1.16 A–B. Expression of secretin and secretin receptor in the rat cerebellar cortex. (A) In the cerebellar cortex, only Purkinje neurons are immunopositive to secretin antibody, indicating that these cells are the source of endogenous secretin. Positive signal is indicated by brown reaction product. Scale bar: 40 µm. (B) In situ hybridization technique reveals that both Purkinje neurons and interneurons within the molecular layer express secretin receptor mRNA and therefore synthesize the receptor. Positive signal is indicated by deep blue reaction product. Scale bar: 100 µm. ML, molecular layer; P, Purkinje cell layer; GL, granule cell layer. (C) Proposed model of the actions of secretin in the cerebellum. Increased firing of Purkinje neurons opens voltage-gated calcium channels and triggers the release of secretin from the somatodendritic region. Secretin then facilitates GABA release from interneuron terminals directly via activation of presynaptic secretin receptor, and indirectly via the release of glutamate from an unknown source and involving presynaptic AMPA receptors. Secretin could also bind to secretin receptors located on Purkinje cells. The exact function of this interaction remains to be identified, but may be related to neurotrophic action of secretin, especially in immature brain, and modulation of long-term synaptic plasticity. From: Yung et al., 2006. With permission.

Glutamate is also the transmitter of parallel fibers. Purkinje cell spines contain high densities of AMPA receptors (Baude et al., 1994). Post-synaptic densities are also enriched in delta2-receptors, involved in synaptic plasticity and cerebellar development (Kurihara et al., 1997). A mutation of this receptor has been identified in Lurcher mice. GLAST, the predominant glial glutamate transporter in the cerebellum, is abundant around parallel fiber–Purkinje cell synapses, suggesting that glial glutamate transport contributes significantly to the termination of transmitter action.

Purkinje cells are enriched in glutamic acid decarboxylase, a GABA-synthesizing enzyme. The first evidence of an inhibitory action of Purkinje cells came from the work of Ito and Yoshida (1964). Taurine is

also enriched in Purkinje cells and is considered to play a role in osmoregulation. Taurine could regulate the volume of Purkinje neurons during an osmotic stress via an interaction with glia.

Purkinje cells also contain the pituitary adenylate cyclase–activating polypeptide (PACAP), involved in apoptosis and cerebellar development. PACAP increases proliferation of granule cells and stimulates their migration (Vaudry et al., 1999). Secretin, a 27–amino acid peptide belonging to the secretin/PACAP/VIP superfamily, is present and neuroactive in several regions of the brain, including the cerebellum (Yung et al., 2006). Within the cerebellar cortex, both secretin and secretin receptor are expressed in Purkinje neurons (Figure 1.16). Secretin

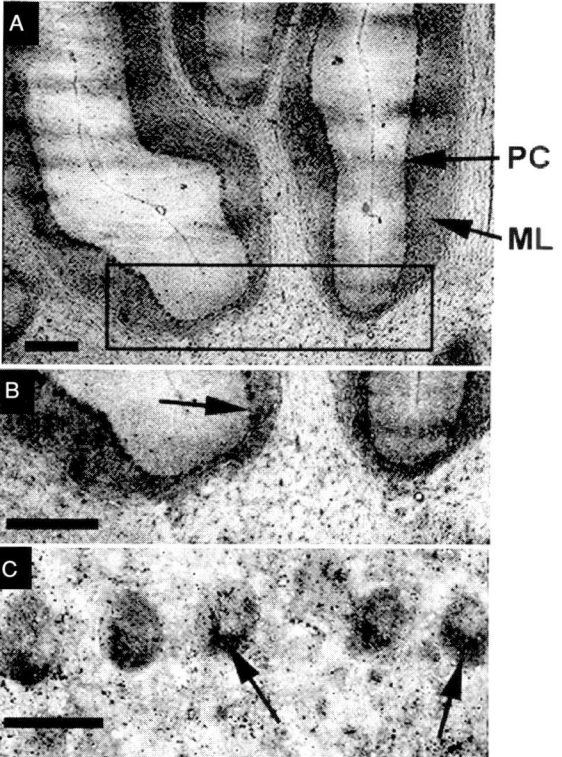

Table 1.4 Effects of aminergic neuromodulators on cerebellar neurons and synapses

	5-HT	NE	ACh	DA	Histamine
Purkinje cells[a]	−	−			+
GABA-Purkinje cells	+,++	+,++	++		
Lugaro cells	+				
Basket cells/stellate cells		+			
Granule cells→ Purkinje cells	-, −	−	+	−	
Granule cells	- (variable)				+
Mossy fiber→ granule cell	-				
Parallel fiber→ Purkinje cells	-				
Nuclei	-	-			
Inferior olive	+	-			

Abbreviations: Ach: acetylcholine; DA: dopamine; 5-HT: serotonin; NE: noradrenaline; +: short-term facilitation; ++: long-term facilitation; -: short-term depression; −: long-term depression.
[a]The net effect of serotonin on Purkinje cells is a decrease in responsiveness to its inputs. Adapted from: Schweighofer et al., 2004.

Figure 1.17 Staining for cannabinoid type 1 (CB1) immunoreactivity in the cerebellum. (A) The molecular layer (ML) and Purkinje cell layer (PC) are intensely CB1-immunoreactive. The inset shows the area from which subsequent images are taken. (B) The arrow indicates Purkinje cells detailed in (C). (C) Purkinje cells show a polarized distribution of CB1, with greater CB1-immunoreactivity adjacent to the granule layer (arrows). Scale bars: (A, B) 200 μm; (C) 20 μm. CB1–cerebellum. From: Ashton et a ., 2004. With permission.

is also expressed in basket cells. Co-expression of secretin and secretin receptor mRNA has been detected in cerebellar nuclei. Secretin modulates GABAergic synaptic transmission, acting as a retrograde messenger. Tachykinins constitute another group of endogenous neuropeptides, including substance P, neurokinin A, and neurokinin B. These three neuropeptides bind with G-protein–linked receptors. They act synergistically with glutamate transmission (Severini et al., 2003). In particular, tachykinins interact with AMPA receptors on granule cells (Pieri et al., 2005). They may participate in excitotoxicity by inducing an overactivation of AMPA receptors.

Recent studies have demonstrated that another group of retrograde messengers, the endocannabinoids, is released by Purkinje cells. Type 1 cannabi-noid receptors (CB1Rs) are expressed presynaptically at all studied synaptic inputs to the Purkinje neurons (Diana et al., 2002). A high proportion of CB1 receptors are located at inhibitory interneurons throughout the molecular layer (Ashton et al., 2004) (Figure 1.17). Labeling studies are consistent with their presence in basket cell and stellate cell inhibitory interneurons. Endocannabinoids may participate in the regulation of Purkinje cell inputs in order to promote synaptic plasticity (Safo et al., 2006).

GABA is the predominant transmitter of cerebellar interneurons (basket cells, stellate cells, Golgi cells, Lugaro cells). Glycine is also thought to be involved in the inhibitory processes controlled by cerebellar interneurons. About 70% of Golgi neurons co-express GABA and glycine. Both molecules could be transported by the same vesicular carrier. The unipolar brush cells are an exception in the population of cerebellar interneurons. They are glutamatergic.

Table 1.4 summarizes the main effects of the aminergic neuromodulators on cerebellar neurons and synapses. Regarding serotonin input, fibers are distributed in all parts of the cerebellum, except lobule X. Serotoninergic fibers inhibit glutamate release from mossy fibers, tune cellular responses to GABA,

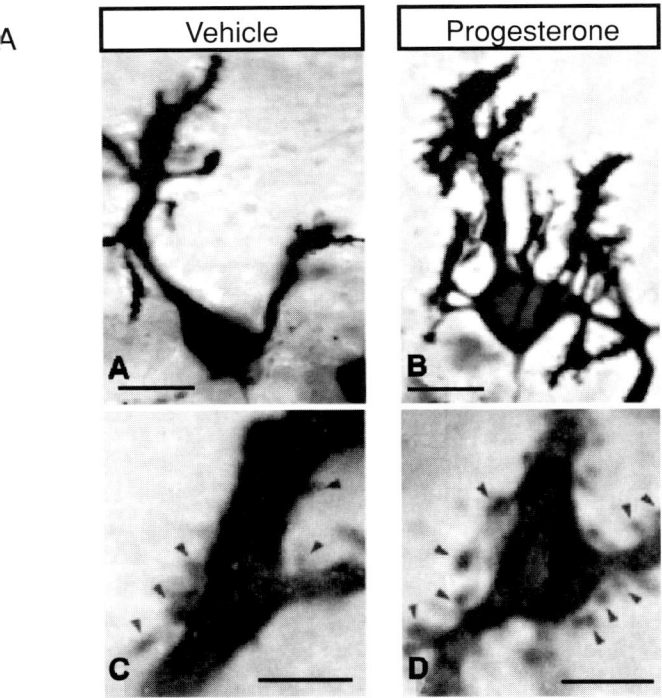

A

Figure 1.18 Top panels: dendritic growth and spinogenesis in response to progesterone in the developing Purkinje cell. Cerebellar cultures from newborn rats grown for 5 days in vitro and immunostained for calbindin. (A, B) Purkinje cell dendrites in the progesterone-treated group appear to be well developed compared with the control group. Scale bars: 20 mm. (C, D) Progesterone treatment induced the greater density of dendritic spines of the Purkinje cell. Arrowheads indicate spine structures. Scale bars: 5 μm. Bottom: Potential mechanisms for organizing actions of progesterone produced in the developing Purkinje cell. Progesterone acts on the Purkinje cell through intracellular receptor–mediated mechanisms that promote dendritic growth, spinogenesis, and synaptogenesis in this neuron by genomic mechanisms. Progesterone may induce the expression of neurotrophic factors which directly promote Purkinje dendritic growth, spinogenesis, and synaptogenesis during neonatal life. Reproduced in part from: Tsutsui, 2006. With permission.

B

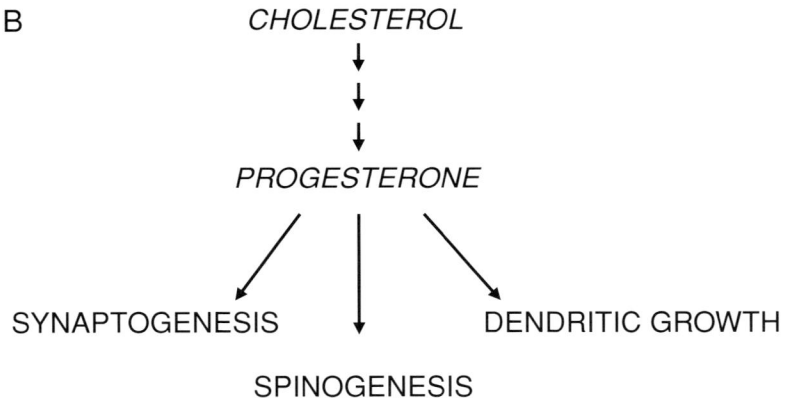

and regulate the activity of glial GABA transporters (Voutsinos et al., 1998). Local application of serotonin modulates the firing rate of Purkinje cells both in vivo and in vitro. Lugaro cells are also responsive to serotonin. The noradrenergic input modulates the responses of cerebellar neurons to GABA and glutamate. A genuine dopaminergic innervation is also found in the cerebellum. Dopamine and dopamine transporters are found in the three layers of the cerebellar cortex, with the highest densities in the molecular layer (Panagopoulos et al., 1991; Ikai et al., 1992). Cerebellum expresses all dopamine receptors (D_{1-5}) belonging to the two D1-like and D2-like superfamilies (Giompres & Delis, 2005).

The hypothalamus projects to the cerebellum using histamine as a transmitter. Histaminergic fibers are found in all cortical layers of the cerebellum. H1 receptors are preferentially expressed on Purkinje cell dendrites.

Activation of NMDA receptors in the cerebellum stimulates the production of nitric oxide (NO). Granule cells are a main source of NO. Granule cells, parallel fibers, and basket cells are equipped with the neuronal isoform of NO synthase. Release of NO from parallel fibers is involved in long-term depression (see Chapter 2). Production of cyclic guanosine monophosphate (cGMP) results indirectly from NO production. cGMP immunoreactivity is found mainly in Bergmann glia and astrocytes.

Adenosine triphosphate (ATP) is released from both neurons and glial cells as a transmitter or as a co-transmitter. In the cerebellar cortex, ATP acts on presynaptic inhibitory interneurons. ATP can be degraded in adenosine, which itself can activate adenosine receptors (Deitmer et al., 2006). Overall, ATP is considered as an endogenously released transmitter, enhancing the spontaneous activity of Purkinje neurons via P2 receptors. Adenosine A1 receptor activation decreases the excitatory output of granule cells and increases their excitability (Courjaret et al., 2009).

The possibility that zinc is involved in cerebellar synaptic transmission has been raised. This is supported by the expression of zinc transporters in Purkinje neurons, granule cells, inhibitory interneurons of the cerebellar cortex, and Bergmann glia of the Purkinje cell layer (Wall, 2005). Multiple zinc transporters are present in Bergmann glia, suggesting that these cells might represent a zinc pool in the cerebellar cortex (Wang et al., 2005). Zinc could modulate synaptic transmission in cerebellar glomeruli (Wang et al., 2002). However, a genuine role of zinc in cerebellar synaptic transmission remains to be established.

Neurosteroids

Recent data show that the brain is capable of synthesizing steroids de novo (Tsutsui, 2006) (Figure 1.18). Purkinje neurons are a main site of neurosteroid formation. They are equipped with several steroidogenic enzymes. Purkinje cells synthesize progesterone and allopregnanolone de novo from cholesterol during neonatal life. Progesterone promotes spinogenesis and synaptogenesis via nuclear receptors. Allopregnanolone is involved in Purkinje and granule

cell survival. Estrogen formation also occurs in the neonate.

References

Artavanis-Tsakonas S, Rand MD, Lake RJ. Notch signaling: cell fate control and signal integration in development. *Science* 1999;**284**(5415):770–6.

Ashton JC, Appleton I, Darlington CL, Smith PF. Immunohistochemical localization of cannabinoid CB1 receptor in inhibitory interneurons in the cerebellum. *Cerebellum* 2004;**3**(4):222–6.

Bailey AM, Posakony JW. Suppressor of hairless directly activates transcription of enhancer of split complex genes in response to Notch receptor activity. *Genes Dev* 1995;**9**(21):2609–22.

Baude A, Molnar E, Latawiec D, McIlhinney RA, Somogyi P. Synaptic and nonsynaptic localization of the GluR1 subunit of the AMPA-type excitatory amino acid receptor in the rat cerebellum. *J Neurosci* 1994;**14**:2830–43.

Ben-Arie N, Bellen HJ, Armstrong DL, et al. Math1 is essential for genesis of cerebellar granule neurons. *Nature* 1997;**390**(6656):169–72.

Colin F, Ris L, Godaux E. Neuroanatomy of the cerebellum. In *The Cerebellum and Its Disorders*, ed. M. Manto and M. Pandolfo. Cambridge, UK: Cambridge University Press, 2002, pp. 6–29.

Courjaret R, Tröger M, Deitmer JW. Suppression of GABA input by A1 adenosine receptor activation in rat cerebellar granule cells. *Neuroscience* 2009;**164**(4):946–58.

D'Arcangelo G, Miao GG, Chen SC, et al. A protein related to extracellular matrix proteins deleted in the mouse mutant reeler. *Nature* 1995;**374**(6524):719–23.

Deitmer JW, Brockhaus J, Casel D. Modulation of synaptic activity in Purkinje neurons by ATP. *Cerebellum* 2006;**5**(1):49–54.

Deoni SC, Catani M. Visualization of the deep cerebellar nuclei using quantitative T1 and rho magnetic resonance imaging at 3 Tesla. *Neuroimage* 2007;**37**(4):1260–6.

Diana MA, Levenes C, Mackie K, Marty A. Short-term retrograde inhibition of GABAergic synaptic currents in rat Purkinje cells is mediated by endogenous cannabinoids. *J Neurosci* 2002;**22**:200–8.

Diedrichsen J, Balsters JH, Flavell J, Cussans E, Ramnani N. A probabilistic MR atlas of the human cerebellum. *Neuroimage* 2009;**46**:39–46.

Dietrichs E. Cerebellar nuclear afferents from the lateral reticular nucleus in the cat. *Brain Res* 1983;**288**:320–4.

Dow RS. The evolution and anatomy of the cerebellum. *Biol Rev* 1942;**17**:179–220.

Drake-Baumann R. Activity-dependent modulation of inhibition in Purkinje cells by TrkB ligands. *Cerebellum* 2006;**5**(3):220–6.

Dum RP, Strick PL. An unfolded map to the cerebellar dentate nucleus and its projections to the cerebral cortex. *J Neurophysiol* 2003;**89**:634–9.

Eiraku M, Hirata Y, Takeshima H, Hirano T, Kengaku M. Delta/notch-like epidermal growth factor (EGF)-related receptor, a novel EGF-like repeat-containing protein targeted to dendrites of developing and adult central nervous system neurons. *J Biol Chem* 2002;**277**(28):25400–7.

Evans PD, Mekel-Bobrov N, Vallender EJ, Hudson RR, Lahn BT. Evidence that the adaptive allele of the brain size gene microcephalin introgressed into Homo sapiens from an archaic Homo lineage. *Proc Natl Acad Sci USA* 2006;**103**(48):18178–83.

Federmeier KD, Kleim JA, Greenough WT. Learning-induced multiple synapse formation in rat cerebellar cortex. *Neurosci Lett* 2002;**332**(3):180–4.

Giaume C, McCarthy KD. Control of gap-junctional communication in astrocytic net-works. *Trends Neurosci* 1996;**19**:319–25.

Giompres P, Delis F. Dopamine transporters in the cerebellum of mutant mice. *Cerebellum* 2005;**4**(2):105–11.

Gravel C, Hawkes R. Parasagittal organization of the rat cerebellar cortex: direct correlation between antigenic Purkinje cell bands revealed by mabQ113 and the organization of the olivocerebellar projection. *J Comp Neurol* 1988;**273**:399–420.

Habas C. Functional imaging of the deep cerebellar nuclei: a review. *Cerebellum* DOI 10.1007/s12311-009-0119-3. In press.

Haines DE, May PJ, Dietrichs E. Neuronal connections between the cerebellar nuclei and hypothalamus in Macaca fascicularis: cerebello-visceral circuits. *J Comp Neurol* 1990;**299**;106–122.

Hamamura M, Watanabe S, Fukumaki Y. Selective changes in the shapes of parasagittal bands of Aldoc (Zebrin) mRNA in the rat vermis of the cerebellum after repeated methamphetamine injections. *Cerebellum* 2004;**3**(4):236–47.

Hawkes R, Blyth S, Chockkan V, et al. Structural and molecular compartmentation in the cerebellum. *Can J Neurol Sci* 1993;Suppl **3**:S29–35.

Heath RG, Harper JW. Ascending projections of the cerebellar fastigial nucleus to the hippocampus, amygdala, and other temporal lobe sites: evoked potential and histological studies in monkeys and cats. *Exp Neurol* 1974;**45**:2682–7.

Hoshino M. Molecular machinery governing GABAergic neuron specification in the cerebellum. *Cerebellum* 2006;**5**(3):193–8.

Hoshino M, Nakamura S, Mori K, et al. Ptf1a, a bHLH transcriptional gene, defines GABAergic neuronal fates in cerebellum. *Neuron* 2005;**47**(2):201–13.

Ikai Y, Takada M, Shinonaga Y, Mizuno N. Dopaminergic and non-dopaminergic neurons in the ventral tegmental area of the rat project, respectively, to the cerebellar cortex and deep cerebellar nuclei. *Neuroscience* 1992;**51**(3):719–28.

Ito M. *The Cerebellum and Neural Control.* New York: Raven Press, 1984.

Ito M, Yoshida M. The cerebellar-evoked monosynaptic inhibition in Deiters' neurones. *Experientia* 1964;**20**;515–6.

Kelly RM, Strick PL. Cerebellar loops with motor cortex and prefrontal cortex of a nonhuman primate. *J Neurosci* 2003;**23**:8432–44.

Koop M, Rilling G, Herrmann A, Kretschmann HJ. Volumetric development of the fetal telencephalon, cerebral cortex, diencephalon, and rhombencephalon including the cerebellum in man. *Bibl Anat* 1986;**28**:53–78.

Kurihara H, Hashimoto K, Kano M, et al. Impaired parallel fiber-Purkinje cell synapse stabilization during cerebellar development of mutant mice lacking the glutamate receptor delta2 subunit. *J Neurosci* 1997;**17**:9613–23.

Lanoue L, Dehart DB, Hinsdale ME, et al. Limb, genital, CNS, and facial malformations result from gene/environment-induced cholesterol deficiency: further evidence for a link to sonic hedgehog. *Am J Med Genet* 1997;**73**(1):24–31.

Lärkfors L, Lindsay RM, Alderson RF. Characterization of the responses of Purkinje cells to neurotrophin treatment. *J Neurochem* 1996;**66**(4):1362–73.

Lechtenberg R. Embryogenesis of the cerebellum. In *Handbook of Cerebellar Diseases*, ed. R. Lechtenberg. New York: Marcel Dekker, 1993, pp. 13–16.

Llinas R, Baker R, Sotelo C. Electrotonic coupling between neurons in cat inferior olive. *J Neurophysiol* 1974;**37**;560–71.

Machold RP, Kittell DJ, Fishell GJ. Antagonism between Notch and bone morphogenetic protein receptor signaling regulates neurogenesis in the cerebellar rhombic lip. *Neural Dev* 2007;**2**:5.

Manto M. Mechanisms of human cerebellar dysmetria: experimental evidence and current conceptual bases. *J Neuroeng Rehabil* 2009;**6**:10.

Marshall SP, Van Der Giessen RS, de Zeeuw CI, Lang EJ. Altered olivocerebellar activity patterns in the connexin36 knockout mouse. *Cerebellum* 2007;1–13.

Middleton FA, Strick PL. Cerebellar output channels. In *The Cerebellum and Cognition*, ed. J.D. Schmahmann. San Diego, CA: Academic Press, 1997, pp. 61–82.

Mihajlovic P, Zecevic N. Development of the human dentate nucleus. *Hum Neurobiol* 1986;**5**:189–97.

Millen KJ, Gleeson JG. Cerebellar development and disease. *Curr Opin Neurobiol* 2008;**18**:12–9.

Mugnaini E, Floris A. The unipolar brush cell: a neglected neuron of the mammalian cerebellar cortex. *J Comp Neurol* 1994;**339**:174–180.

O'Rahilly R, Mullet F, Hutchins GM, Moore GW. Computer ranking of the sequence of appearance of 40 features of the brain and related structures in staged human embryos during the seventh week of development. *Am J Anat* 1988;**182**:295–317.

Oscarsson O. Functional organization of spinocerebellar paths. In *Handbook of Sensory Physiology, Vol. 2, Somatosensory System*, ed. A. Iggo A. Berlin: Springer Verlag, 1973, pp. 339–80.

Padget DH. Designation of the embryonic intersegmental arteries in reference to the vertebral artery and subclavian stem. *Anat Rec* 1954;**119**(3):349–56.

Panagopoulos NT, Papadopoulos GC, Matsokis NA. Dopaminergic innervation and binding in the rat cerebellum. *Neurosci Lett* 1991;**130**(2):208–12.

Pasco A, Papon X, Bracard S, et al. Persistent carotid-vertebrobasilar anastomoses: how and why differentiating them? *J Neuroradiol* 2004;**31**(5):391–6.

Pieri M, Severini C, Amadoro G, et al. AMPA receptors are modulated by tachykinins in rat cerebellum neurons. *J Neurophysiol* 2005;**94**(4):2484–90.

Porter FD. Smith-Lemli-Opitz syndrome: pathogenesis, diagnosis and management. *Eur J Hum Genet* 2008;**16**(5):535–41.

Provini L, Marcotti W, Morara S, Rosina A. Somatotopic nucleocortical projections to the multiple somatosensory cerebellar maps. *Neuroscience* 1998;**83**(4):1085–104.

Rothstein JD, Martin L, Levey AI, et al. Localization of neuronal and glial glutamate transporters. *Neuron* 1994;**13**:713–25.

Richardson CA, Leitch B. Phenotype of cerebellar glutamatergic neurons is altered in stargazer mutant mice lacking brain-derived neurotrophic factor mRNA expression. *J Comp Neurol* 2005;**481**(2):145–59.

Rico B, Xu B, Reichardt LF. TrkB receptor signaling is required for establishment of GABAergic synapses in the cerebellum. *Nat Neurosci* 2002;**5**(3):225–33.

Safo PK, Cravatt BF, Regehr WG. Retrograde endocannabinoid signaling in the cerebellar cortex. *Cerebellum* 2006;**5**:134–45.

Saito SY, Takeshima H. DNER as key molecule for cerebellar maturation. *Cerebellum* 2006;**5**(3):227–31.

Schmahmann JD, Pandya DN. The cerebrocerebellar system. *Int Rev Neurobiol*. 1997;**41**:31–60

Schweighofer N, Doya K, Kuroda S. Cerebellar aminergic neuromodulation: towards a functional understanding. *Brain Res Brain Res Rev* 2004;**44**(2–3):103–16.

Segal RA, Pomeroy SL, Stiles CD. Axonal growth and fasciculation linked to differential expression of BDNF and NT3 receptors in developing cerebellar granule cells. *J Neurosci* 1995;**15**(7 pt 1):4970–81.

Sellick GS, Barker KT, Stolte-Dijkstra I, et al. Mutations in PTF1A cause pancreatic and cerebellar agenesis. *Nat Genet* 2004;**36**(12):1301–5.

Severini C, Ciotti MT, Mercanti D, Barbato C, Calissano P. A tachykinin-like factor increases glutamate toxicity in rat cerebellar granule cells. *Neuropharmacology*. 2003;**44**(1):117–24.

Shu W, Cho JY, Jiang Y, et al. Altered ultrasonic vocalization in mice with a disruption of the FOXP2 gene. *Proc Natl Acad Sci USA* 2005;**02**:9643–8.

Snyder PJ, Bilder RM, Wu H, Bogerts B, Lieberman JA. Cerebellar volume asymmetries are related to handedness: a quantitative MRI study. *Neuropsychologia* 1995;**33**:407–19.

Sotelo C, Llinas R, Baker R. Structural study of inferior olivary nucleus of the cat: morphological correlates of electrotonic coupling. *J Neurophysiol* 1974;**37**(3):541–59.

Triulzi F, Parazzini C, Righini A. Magnetic resonance imaging of fetal cerebellar development. *Cerebellum* 2006;**5**(3):199–205.

Tsutsui K. Biosynthesis and organizing action of neurosteroids in the developing Purkinje cell. *Cerebellum* 2006;**5**:89–96.

Vaillant C, Monard D. SHH pathway and cerebellar development. *Cerebellum* 2009;**8**:291–301.

Vaudry D, Gonzalez BJ, Basille M, Fournier A, Vaudry H. Neurotrophic activity of pituitary adenylate cyclase-activating polypeptide on rat cerebellar cortex during development. *Proc Natl Acad Sci USA* 1999;**96**:9415–20.

Voogd J, Glickstein M. The anatomy of the cerebellum. *Trends Neurosci* 1998;**21**:370–5.

Voogd J, Ruigrok TJ. The organization of the corticonuclear and olivocerebellar climbing fiber projections to the rat cerebellar vermis: the congruence of projection zones and the zebrin patterns. *J Neurocytol* 2004;**33**:5–21.

Voutsinos B, Dutuit M, Reboul A, et al. Serotoninergic control of the activity and expression of glial GABA transporters in the rat cerebellum. *Glia* 1998;**23**:45–60.

Wall MJ. A role for zinc in cerebellar synaptic transmission? *Cerebellum* 2005;**4**(4):224–9.

Wang Z, Danscher G, Kim YK, Dahlstrom A, Mook Jo S. Inhibitory zinc-enriched terminals in the mouse cerebellum: double-immunohistochemistry for zinc transporter 3 and glutamate decarboxylase. *Neurosci Lett* 2002;**321**(1–2):37–40.

Wang ZY, Stoltenberg M, Huang L, et al. Abundant expression of zinc transporters in Bergman glia of mouse cerebellum. *Brain Res Bull* 2005;**64**(5):441–8.

Wechsler-Reya RJ, Scott MP. Control of neuronal precursor proliferation in the cerebellum by Sonic Hedgehog. *Neuron* 1999;**22**(1):103–14.

Wetmore C, Ernfors P, Persson H, Olson L. Localization of brain-derived neurotrophic factor mRNA to neurons in the brain by in situ hybridization. *Exp Neurol* 1990;**109**(2):141–52.

Wiklund L, Toggenburger G, Cuénod M. Selective retrograde labelling of the rat olivocerebellar climbing fiber system with D-[3H]aspartate. *Neuroscience* 1984;**13**:441–68.

Yung WH, Chan YS, Chow BKC, Wang JJ. The role of secretin in the cerebellum. *Cerebellum* 2006;**5**:43–8.

Zagrebelsky M, Strata P, Hawkes R, Rossi F. Reestablishment of the olivocerebellar projection map by compensatory transcommissural reinnervation following unilateral transection of the inferior cerebellar peduncle in the newborn rat. *J Comp Neurol* 1997;**379**(2):283–99.

Physiology of the cerebellum

The output of the cerebellum is directed to all components of the motor systems, except for the basal ganglia. It tunes the activities of voluntary muscles, coordinating the timing, durations, and magnitudes of muscle discharges. The cerebellum participates in the planning of activities, in the learning of new motor skills, and in the updating of motor schemes acquired earlier. Moreover, it contributes to various aspects of cognitive operations and might regulate emotional processes.

The three functional divisions

Three rostrocaudal longitudinal zones have been identified in the cerebellar cortex: a vermal zone projecting to the fastigial nucleus, an intermediate zone projecting to the interpositus nucleus, and a lateral zone projecting to the dentate nucleus (Figure 2.1; see also Chapter 1). Theories of cerebellar functions suggest that the intermediate cerebellum is more involved in monitoring of ongoing movement, while the lateral cerebellum is more active during anticipatory control.

Activities in the cerebellar nuclei

A complete body map is found within each of the cerebellar nuclei (Figure 2.2). There is somatotopic representation, with the hind limb located rostromedially. Cerebellar nuclei are under the inhibitory control of Purkinje cells. Purkinje neurons and cerebellar nuclei change their firings in advance of changes in the firing of their downstream targets such as the motor cortex, indicating a key role in prediction. In absence of movement, nuclear cells fire at high discharge rates of about 40 to 50 Hz (Bastian & Thach, 2002). There is a fine modulation of firing rates during sensorimotor tasks. Vestibular and fastigial nuclei control eye movements, stance/posture, and gait. The interpositus nucleus contributes to modulation of reflexes, including stretch and placing. The dentate nuclei are involved in the control of voluntary movements of the extremities, including reaching and grasping.

Functional imaging studies show that the fastigial nucleus is activated during repetitive movements in relation to task complexity/postural adjustment (Tracy et al., 2001). Pronation/supination tasks (diadochokinesia) activate the medial areas of the cerebellum. The globose/emboliform nucleus shows increased activity during sequential distal movements (Dimitrova et al., 2006). Valsalva maneuver, thirst satiation, and nociception also activate the fastigial and globose/emboliform nuclei. However, there are difficulties in delineating the activation of these nuclei. This is due to several factors: they are very thin, they are closely related to the gray matter of lobules VIII and IX, and imaging techniques like functional MRI (fMRI) underestimate the activation due to partial volume effects and statistical thresholding problems. These technical issues are also valid for the activation of dentate nuclei, keeping in mind that activation reflects synaptic and dendritic processing and not just spiking of neurons. The tasks associated with activation of dentate nuclei are summarized in Table 2.1. The dentate nucleus is predominantly recruited during complex motor, sensorimotor, and cognitive tasks. It is strongly activated during sequential movements of fingers and tongue, drawing, and coordination of eye and hand during tracking movements (Jueptner & Weiller, 1998; Dimitrova et al., 2006). Activation is also observed during performance of intentional eye movements, such as saccades. Hyperactivation of the dentate nucleus is also observed in patients with palatal tremor, possibly due to inferior olivary discharges (Boecker et al., 1994). Ipsilateral activation of the dentate nucleus is preferential during polymodal cue-guided and complex motor activity. The dentate is also active during active tactile discrimination and passive sensory discrimination without finger movements (Seitz et al., 1991; Liu et al., 2000). The activity is strongly modulated by cognitive factors such as the

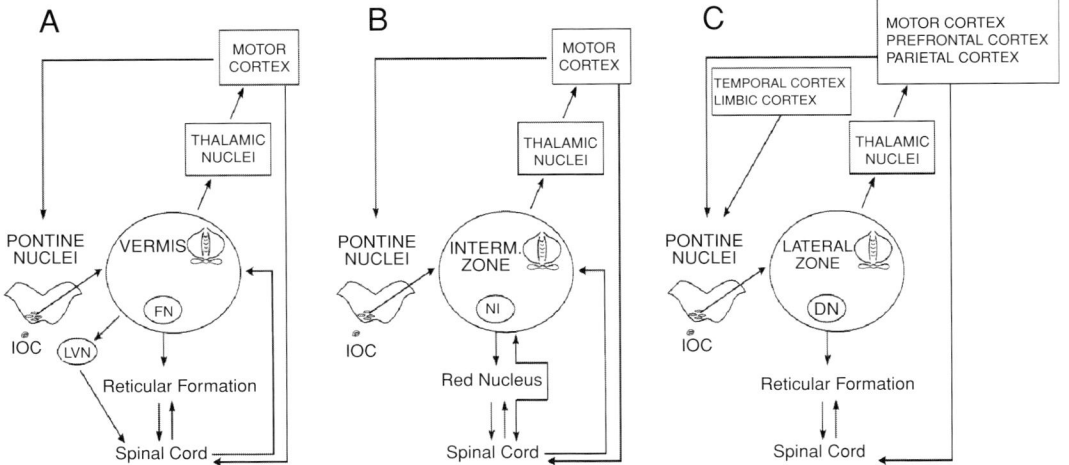

Figure 2.1 Comparison of the anatomical connections of the three functional zones of the cerebellum: the vermal zone (A), the intermediate zone (B), and the lateral zone of the cerebellum (C). The midline zone and the intermediate zone receive direct information from the spinal cord, unlike the lateral cerebellum. Abbreviations: IOC: inferior olivary complex; LVN: lateral vestibular nucleus; FN: fastigial nucleus; NI: nucleus interpositus; DN: dentate nucleus. With permission from: Manto, 2009.

MULTIPLE BODY MAPS

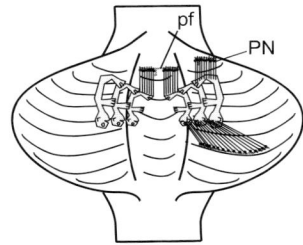

Figure 2.2 Multiple body maps are represented in each cerebellar nucleus. Abbreviations: pf: parallel fibers; PN: Purkinje neurons. With permission from: Manto, 2009.

attentional load and the involvement of working memory. Foci of activation predominate in ventrocaudal and mediocentral parts in these tasks.

Activities of Purkinje neurons

Beams of parallel fibers excite dendrites of inhibitory interneurons in the cerebellar cortex (basket, stellate, and Golgi cells). Basket and stellate axons run tangential to either side of the transverse parallel fiber beam, inhibiting the Purkinje neurons in the flanks of the beam. Purkinje neuron simple spike activity is driven by mossy fiber input to granule cells. Via parallel fibers, Purkinje neurons receive a massive convergence of inputs. Purkinje cell simple spikes are influ-

enced by direction of movement and motion speed (Coltz et al., 1999).

Incoming spikes from climbing fibers produce large excitatory post-synaptic potentials which generate repetitive responses at the level of the soma, called complex spikes (Thach, 1967). Purkinje neuron complex spike activity occurs at rates of 1 to 3 Hz. According to the Marr-Albus-Ito theory, the complex spike informs of an error or provides a teaching signal to the Purkinje neuron, helping a trial-and-error learning mechanism (Marr, 1969; Albus, 1971; Ito, 1984). This is supported by studies showing an increase in complex spike activity during the learning phase. Complex spikes occurring early during a reaching task could participate in the encoding of direction and destination of the arm (Kitazawa et al., 1998). Another hypothesis is that complex spikes provide an internal motor clock (Lang et al., 1999).

The complex spikes activate voltage-controlled calcium channels, and calcium triggers a major calcium-to-calcium release from the reticulum. However, the synapse-climbing fiber Purkinje neuron is not just excitatory. The climbing fiber also carries an inhibition signal, and when the climbing fiber is stimulated simultaneously with the parallel fibers, the responsiveness of parallel fibers decreases after the conjunctive stimulation (long-term depression [LTD]). This is considered to be a chemical memory trace which could be involved in the storage of key parameters underlying

Table 2.1 Tasks associated with activation of dentate nuclei

Motor tasks	Procedural learning	Sensory tasks	Cognitive tasks
Bimanual movements	Writing ideograms	Tactile discrimination of objects	Procedural learning
Finger/tongue/foot movements	Visuomotor learning	Tactile exploration	Working memory
Sequences of movements	Sequential movements		Navigation
Tracking tasks	Isometric tasks		Semantic tasks
Drawing			
Eye–hand coordination			
Voluntary eye movements			
Adapted from: Habas et al. (in press).			

motion control. Stimulation of parallel fibers alone can trigger a long-term potentiation of the synapse parallel fiber/Purkinje neuron.

Activities of the inferior olivary complex

Olivary cells have low discharge rates. They rarely exceed 5 to 10 spikes/sec. Indeed, olivary neurons are refractory for about 100 msec following discharge, which limits their abilities to fire at high rates (Gibson et al., 2004). Inferior olivary neurons display spontaneous oscillatory activity and respond as nonlinear oscillators to afferent signals (Marshall & Lang, 2004). The great majority of olivary cells respond to somatosensory stimulation, but not as a direct consequence during active movement. Recordings suggest that the inferior olivary complex associates arbitrary sensory stimuli with somatosensory events (see also discussion of eyeblink conditioning in section Learning) (Gibson et al., 2004). Although the cerebellum receives a massive mossy fiber input from muscle spindles, the direct projection of primary spindle afferents to the inferior olive is very small. The dorsal accessory olive is more sensitive to somatosensory stimuli than the principal olive or the medial accessory olive. Interestingly, olivary neurons often respond to more than one modality of stimulation (somatosensory, vestibular, visual, nociceptive, visceral), which provides a property of modality convergence to the inferior olivary complex (Gibson et al., 2004). Neurons of the inferior olivary complex are sensitive to amines. Serotonin increases the average firing rate of inferior olivary neurons while slowing their oscillation

frequency and increasing the coherence of oscillations (Sugihara et al., 1995).

Control of eye movements

Anatomically, the flocculonodular lobe and the paraflocculus are strongly interconnected with the vestibular nuclei (see Chapter 1). The cerebellum controls the vestibuloocular reflex (VOR) and the optokinetic reflexes. The VOR stabilizes vision during head turning by counter-rotating the eyes in the orbit. The gain (eye velocity/head velocity) can be adapted by visual-vestibular mismatch. Flocculectomy impairs gain adaptation. Visual suppression of the VOR by fixating a target moving simultaneously is reduced in cerebellar patients. The initiation of the optokinetic nystagmus, evoked when watching a target moving rapidly in one direction, is often characterized by either exaggerated or decreased excursions. Smooth pursuit depends on the integrity of the cerebellum.

Single-unit recordings show a major role of the fastigial nucleus related to eye movements, control of head position, and regulation of muscle activities during stance and gait. The rostral fastigial nucleus controls head orientation and eye–head gaze shifts (Pelisson et al., 1998). The caudal fastigial nucleus controls oculomotor aspects, such as saccades or smooth pursuit (Fuchs et al., 1994).

Control of speech

Lesions of the superior paravermal region are commonly associated with speech deficits (Lechtenberg & Gilman, 1978). Recent studies point towards two separate networks subserving speech motor control

25

(Riecker et al., 2005). A preparative loop includes the supplementary motor area, dorsolateral frontal cortex including Broca area, anterior insula, and superior cerebellum. The executive loop comprises the sensorimotor cortex, basal ganglia, thalamus, and inferior cerebellum.

Control of limb movements

Single-unit recordings in the intermediate cerebellar cortex and the interpositus nucleus have demonstrated that they control reflex movements when a holding position is suddenly perturbed (Frysinger et al., 1984).The interpositus nucleus is implicated in somesthetic reflexes that control antagonist muscles to damp joint oscillations and to correct movements via feedback initiated by the movement itself (Vilis & Hore, 1980). It contributes to the excitability of both the motor cortex and the stretch reflex by controlling the gamma motor neurons (Gilman, 1969).

The dentate nucleus regulates reaction time through initiation of movements triggered by vision or mental percepts and accuracy of single-joint and multi-joint goal-directed movements, such as reaching. Lesions of the dentate nuclei are associated typically with an overshoot of the target (hypermetria) and a decomposition of multi-joint movements (Thach et al., 1992; Bastian et al., 1996). Rapid limb movements towards a fixed target (called ballistic movements) are normally characterized by high peak velocities and bell-shaped velocity profiles, with a triphasic pattern of electromyographic activity: a first agonist burst is followed by an antagonist burst, with a subsequent second agonist burst. The lateral cerebellum plays a major role in the programming of several parameters: preparation time, peak acceleration, rate of rise of the agonist and antagonist muscle activities, and onset latency of the antagonist activity (Hore et al., 1991; Manto et al., 1994; see also Chapter 3). Overall, cerebellar circuits exert a facilitatory effect upon motor cortical areas of agonist and antagonist muscles.

The lack of coordination observed during multijoint movements is not explained by a simple summation of the elemental deficits observed during single-joint movements. Interaction torques generated in the multi-degree of freedom human arm require a very accurate central control (Topka & Massaquoi., 2002). The net torque (NET) takes into account forces aris-ing from muscle activities (MUS), external forces such as gravity (EXT), and dynamic inertial and interaction forces (DYN) according to the following equation: $NET = MUS + EXT + DYN$. One main function of the cerebellum would be to predict and compensate for dynamic interaction forces during voluntary movement. Intensities of forces are scaled to the square of movement speed, providing a possible explanation for the increase in clumsiness when patients perform quicker movements. Cerebellar circuitry might keep an internal representation of the biomechanical properties of each body segment, regularly updated by peripheral sensory information (Sainburg et al., 1999). This representation might be defective in cerebellar disorders.

Posture and gait

Due to its anatomical connections, the medial cerebellar zone can integrate spinal and vestibular inputs to influence vestibulospinal and reticulospinal tracts. The intermediate zone can integrate spinal and cortical inputs to influence walking via projections to motor cortical areas. Regarding the lateral cerebellum, it influences walking via cortical interactions and contributes to the voluntary modifications of the locomotor cycle (Bastian & Morton, 2007).

Sitting, stance, and gait are usually impaired in midline cerebellar lesions. Lesions in the medial and intermediate zones of the cerebellum, especially in the anterior lobe, disturb movements linked to an equilibrium function (Horak & Diener, 1994). Lack of coordination of trunk and legs leads to an irregular gait in cerebellar patients. Lower vermal lesions tend to be associated with pluridirectional increased body sway at low frequency and high amplitudes, and lesions in the upper vermal zone tend to increase anterior-posterior body oscillations at higher velocities and lower amplitudes (Dichgans & Fetter, 1993; Bastian & Morton, 2007; see also Chapter 3).

The cerebellum regulates step and stride length and cadence and attenuates the variability of gait during successive cycles. Walking trajectory veers erratically in cerebellar patients, with difficulties in initiation, stops, or turns. Abnormal patterns of gait include irregular timing of peak flexion at one joint with respect to the other joints and/or joint–joint decomposition, which can be seen as a reduction in the movement at one joint during movement of another joint (Bastian & Morton, 2007). The cerebellum

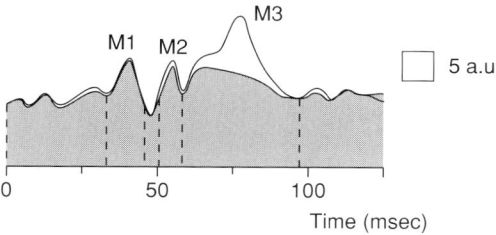

Figure 2.3 Cerebellar control of long-latency reflexes (LLR). Illustration of long-latency electromyographic (EMG) responses to stretches of the first dorsal interosseous muscle in a cerebellar patient (black line) and in a control subject (gray line). Latencies of averaged rectified EMG responses are normal, but the M3 response is increased in the cerebellar patient. Surface EMG rectified and averaged 200 times. Responses are calibrated in arbitrary units (a.u.). With permission from: Manto, 2009.

allows the adequate scaling of anticipatory postural responses during standing postural perturbations (Horak & Diener, 1994). The analysis of goal-directed leg placement shows that the interposed and the adjacent dentate nuclei are more frequently affected (Ilg et al., 2008). The intermediate zone seems to play an important role for multi-joint limb control both in goal-directed leg movements and in locomotion. Regarding the posterior cerebellar vermis, it might control the coordination of bilateral movements of the legs (Bastian et al., 1998).

The cerebellum modulates the magnitudes of long-latency reflexes (LLRs) in four limbs. LLRs are involved in the stabilization of postural activities in four limbs and contribute to stability of stance. The cerebellum controls the M2/M3 components of LLRs (Friedemann et al., 1987). In particular, the cerebellar cortex decreases the amplitude of the M3 component, which corresponds to a transcortical loop (Figure 2.3). These cerebellar-cortical loops are especially involved in adapting postural responses based on prior experience (Jacobs & Horak, 2007).

Learning

The cerebellum plays several key roles in learning. It is established that multiple memory systems operate in parallel. The cerebellar circuits are involved in many aspects of memory, in particular, in non-declarative memory. This latter includes procedural learning (skills and habits), priming and perceptual learning, basic associative learning (including simple classical conditioning of emotional and skeletal muscle responses), and non-associative learning (Gerwig

et al., 2007). Performance of activities is the method to convey procedural memory.

While the corticostriatal system deals with learning of new sequences, the cerebrocerebellar systems are primarily engaged in the motor adaptation phases of learning (Doyon et al., 2003). Cerebellar circuits coordinate event sequences. Cerebellar patients have difficulties in serial reaction time tasks (SRTTs), showing marked impairments in the acquisition of procedures (Torriero et al., 2007). The classical paradigm in SRTT is a choice reaction time with four possible responses. The subject is asked to respond as quickly as possible to a series of stimuli which consists of a repeating sequence of about 10 elements. Control subjects become faster with practice, even if they are not aware that there is a sequence. The subject may recognize that there is a sequence (shift from implicit learning to explicit learning). The identification of the sequence will be associated with an improvement in performance. Cerebellar patients have an abnormal implicit learning (Pascual-Leone et al., 1993).They do not improve in reaction times and fail to develop explicit knowledge, even when clues about the sequences are provided. The left lateral cerebellum might be more active in procedural learning through the ipsilateral hand, whereas the right lateral cerebellum would be involved equally regardless of hand (Torriero et al., 2004).

The cerebellum is essential to the adjustments required when facing environmental changes or perturbations (Morton & Bastian, 2004). The prototype of adaptation learning is the gain of the vestibuloocular reflex (VOR), which refers to the amplitude of eye movements due to head motion. The cerebellum and brainstem are key players in the adaptation of the VOR. Selection of the gain is a learning phenomenon, but no apparent new skill is required when the gain changes (Hallett & Grafman, 1997). VOR adaptation aims to minimize image movement on the retina, tuning the trajectory of the compensatory eye movement. When the eye-movement command is inaccurate, the image on the retina will move (the so-called retinal slip). Retinal slip can be seen as a sensory consequence of inaccurate motor commands in the VOR (Highstein et al., 2005). Climbing fiber input to floccular Purkinje cells carries a retinal slip signal (Maekawa & Simpson, 1973). In this way, VOR adaptation is an example of how the cerebellum uses the sensory consequences of inaccurate movement commands to learn precise motor commands (Highstein et al., 2005).

In practice, the VOR operates in conjunction with other systems, such as smooth pursuit. The sites of plasticity for VOR adaptation are multiple (Boyden et al., 2004). The brainstem (especially vestibular nuclei) and the cerebellar cortex are two main locations. Having multiple sites of plasticity offers the advantage of improving the performance of the VOR given the delayed slip signal (Highstein et al., 2005). In addition, multiple plasticity mechanisms may provide the flexibility required to store memories over different time scales (Boyden et al., 2004).

One paradigm which is used to estimate the adaptation motor learning in arm movements is the following (Deuschl et al., 1996): the subject is facing a screen showing a target moving repeatedly between two positions. The subject has to match a ballistic movement of the elbow (or hand) to the target (or to match the isometric force during a pinch task). After a first block of trials, the gain of the system is modified (the relation between the arm movement and its visual feedback is changed), and a second block of trials is recorded. The absolute movement amplitude and movement duration are analyzed. An exponential function is fitted to the amplitude values obtained after change of the gain. This function is an estimation of the speed of learning. Errors show typically exponential learning curves during adaptation. The number of trials necessary to adapt to the new condition is higher in cerebellar patients.

Another typical example of adaptation to environmental change is the prism adaptation. In this task, the subject has to adjust movements while wearing prism glasses, which displace vision. Subsequently, the prisms are removed and the subject has to re-adjust movement once again. Cerebellar patients have difficulties in both tasks. The recalibration of misaligned reference frames due to perturbed visual input is dependent upon a network of cortical (anterior cingulate, anterior intraparietal region) and cerebellar regions (Danckert et al., 2008).

One model which has been extensively studied is classical conditioning of eyeblink responses (Thompson, 2005; Delgado-García & Gruart, 2006; Gerwig et al., 2007). A corneal airpuff or periorbital shock (the unconditioned stimulus, US) is delivered to the eye (Figure 2.4). This stimulus elicits a reflexive blink (the unconditioned response, UR), which consists of closure of the eyelid in humans. When a neutral conditioned stimulus (CS) such as a tone is repeatedly paired with a corneal airpuff, subjects learn to blink the eye to the tone. This conditioned response (CR) occurs in a timed manner, so that the eyelid is lowered and the cornea protected at the time of the airpuff. The CS enters in the circuitry mainly through the pontine nuclei. The US projects to the dorsal accessory inferior olive via the trigeminal nucleus. Simultaneously, the US is projected from the trigeminal nucleus through brainstem areas to cranial nerves, including the facial nucleus. The brainstem generates the UR. Mossy fibers originating from the pontine nuclei carry CS information into the cerebellum. Climbing fibers originating from the inferior olive carry US information into the cerebellum. Plastic changes occur in the cerebellar cortex and cerebellar nuclei, resulting in increased interpositus nucleus activity after paired CS-US presentation. Plastic changes also occur in the pontine nuclei and trigeminal complex (Bracha, 2004). Repeated tone/airpuff pairings cause long-term depression (LTD) of the excitatory synapses between parallel fibers and Purkinje cells in which activity immediately precedes climbing fiber activation. This may reduce tone-evoked Purkinje cell activity. The consequence is a reduced inhibition from Purkinje cells to the cerebellar nuclei, enhancing the activity in the cerebellar nuclei which is thought to drive the learned eyeblink (Linden, 2003). Human studies have allowed better delineation of the contribution of the cerebellar components in the control of eyeblink conditioning. Cerebellar lesions are associated with impaired eyeblink conditioning (Solomon et al., 1989; Gerwig et al., 2003). Acquisition of eyeblink conditioning is impaired in various disorders in which the cerebellum plays a key role, such as essential tremor. Impairment of more complex forms of eyeblink conditioning (e.g. trace eyeblink conditioning) and delayed conditioning of other aversive responses (e.g. limb flexion response) in cerebellar subjects suggest a more general role of the cerebellum in associative learning (Gerwig et al., 2007). Overall, the cerebellum is involved in acquisition, timing, and extinction of conditioned eyeblink responses. Cortical areas of the ipsilateral superior cerebellum contribute to the acquisition and timing of CR. Moreover, the ipsilateral cerebellar cortex participates in extinction of CRs. Cortical areas important for CR acquisition overlap with areas related to the control of the unconditioned eyeblink response. Likewise, cortical lesions are followed by increased amplitudes of unconditioned eyeblinks (Gerwig et al., 2007). These findings are in good accordance with those of animal studies.

Figure 2.4 Cerebellar circuit for classical eyeblink conditioning. The conditioned stimulus CS (tone) enters the circuit through the pontine nuclei. The unconditioned stimulus (US; an airpuff or shock) is projected via the trigeminal nucleus to the inferior olive, and at the same time to the facial nucleus, forming a brainstem pathway responsible for production of the unconditioned response (UR). Mossy fibers originating from the pontine nuclei carry CS information, while climbing fibers originating from the inferior olive carry US information into the cerebellum. Excitability changes occur in cerebellar neurons that receive input from the CS mossy fibers and US climbing fibers both in the cerebellar cortex (for example long-term depression – LTD – of parallel fiber-Purkinje cell synapses) and in nuclei. The net effect of plasticity in these two areas is to increase interpositus nucleus activity, which may be capable of driving activity in brainstem neurons that control eye blinking. CR: conditioned response. Adapted from: Gerwig et al., 2007.

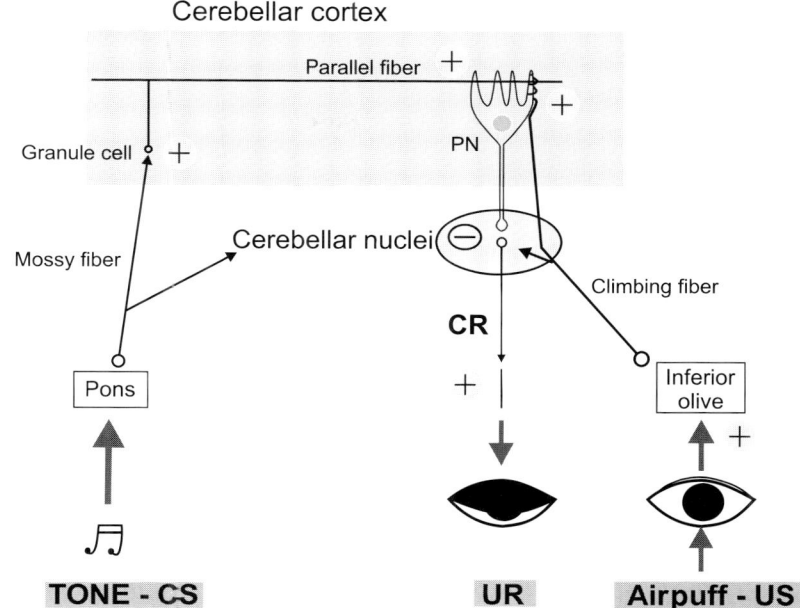

"Sensory" processing

One of the basic cerebellar functions could be the online monitoring of sensory information (Gao et al., 1996). The cerebellum could facilitate the use of sensory information for the brain or could detect sensory sequences rather than controlling timing aspects (Miall, 1997). Although cerebellar circuits are activated by numerous sensory stimuli (proprioceptive, exteroceptive, etc.), sensory deficits in cerebellar patients are extremely subtle and are outside the classical testing of sensations used in daily practice for neurological patients.

Cerebellum and timing

The cerebellum has been considered as a provider of the internal timing system required to perform sensorimotor tasks accurately (Ivry et al., 1988). Cerebellar circuits would provide the precise temporal representation to execute motion smoothly (Yarom & Cohen, 2002). Interactions between the cerebellum and the inferior olive would endow the system with the ability to generate complex temporal patterns, producing consistent intervals between movements. Nevertheless, neuroimaging studies suggest that the function of timing is under the control of distributed networks composing the cerebellum, the dorsolateral prefrontal cortex, the intraparietal sulcus region, and the caudate

nucleus. The specific role of the cerebellar circuitry might be related to the anticipatory responses and the ability to learn predictive relationships between sequences of events (see section Learning).

Computational models of cerebellar function

Optimal strategies are mandatory to perform motion with accuracy, given the highly complex non-linear biomechanical features of the human body, including the muscles and joints, and the numerous interactions with the environment. The CNS copes permanently with noise and delays. Therefore, a high degree of modifiability in the operational mechanisms underlying motor control is mandatory.

The works of Marr and Albus have strongly influenced the computational models of cerebellar function these last decades (Ito, 2006). This theory proposes that a subset of the parallel fiber synapses contacting any Purkinje cell controls its output. This would be accomplished by weakening the strength of the synapses activated during an erroneous motor command. The error signal leading to such weakening was proposed to be the climbing fiber input. The cerebellum would gain the control of movement through trial-and-error practice, linking a given motor context to a new motor response. The theory predicts a plasticity of the parallel fiber synapse if it is active at the same time as the climbing fiber (see also LTD). Another attractive model is based upon the adaptive filter hypothesis. The adaptive filter is a signal-processing device transforming sets of signals varying temporally (Fujita, 1982). One main goal of adaptive filters is to decorrelate inputs from outputs (Dean et al., 2004). From the computational standpoint, the adaptive filter advantageously deals with the unavoidable noise encountered in biological systems.

Internal models

Expectations and estimates of future motor states are critical for performing fast coordinated movements. Predictions are necessary because the cerebral cortex cannot respond solely on the basis of slowly evolving sensory and perceptual feedback. One of the main theories addresses a central issue in motor control, namely, the intrinsic time delay of sensory feedback associated with motor commands and motion. Sensorimotor delays vary according to the modality and context and may be in the range of 50 to 400 msec. The cerebellum has been proposed to contain the neural representations or "internal models" in order to emulate fundamental natural processes such as body motion (Ramnani, 2006). This theory is supported by fMRI studies, transcranial magnetic stimulation (TMS) experiments, and psychophysical studies. Clumsiness would be due to a malfunction in the predictive feedforward control and/or to a disorder in the accurate appraisal of the consequences of motor commands. According to this theory, the brain precisely controls the movement without the need for sensory feedback.

The cerebellum may function similarly to a "forward model" by using efference copies of motor orders to predict sensory effects of movements. Accurate predictions would decrease the dependence on time-delayed sensory signals. Cerebellar circuitry would be necessary to learn how to make appropriate predictions using error information about the discrepancies between the actual and predicted sensory consequences, not only for limb movements, but also for postural adjustments (Ioffe et al., 2007). The cerebellum would compute an expected sensory outcome, which would be sent to cerebral cortical areas via excitatory connections to the thalamus and to the inferior olive via inhibitory connections (Figure 2.5). The inferior olive could operate as a sort of comparator,

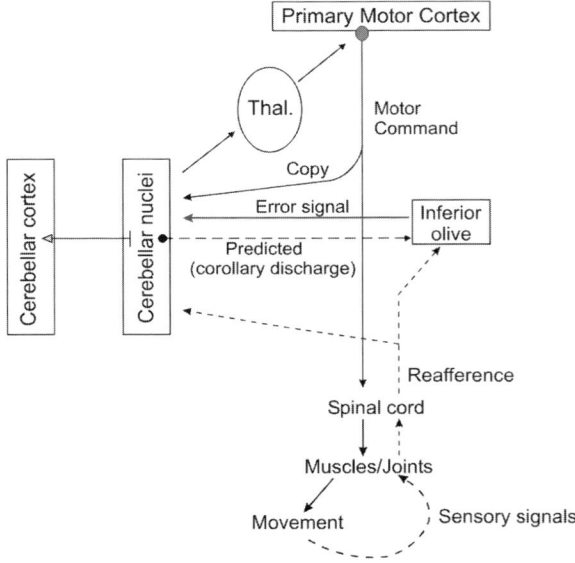

Figure 2.5 Forward models. Communication flows for information processing in forward models of motor coding. Cerebellar modules receive an efference copy of motor commands via the cortico-pontocerebellar tract, in order to make predictions. Reafference signals and corollary discharges reach the comparator (inferior olive), which generates an error signal updating the plastic cerebellar microcircuits. Expected sensory outcomes are conveyed to the primary motor cortex via excitatory connections and to the inferior olive via inhibitory pathways. With permission from: Manto, 2009.

signaling errors back to the cerebellar cortex and training it to make correct predictions. Purkinje cell firings have several of the characteristics of a forward internal model of the arm. Indeed, Purkinje cell firing heralds the kinematics of motion. Experimental data suggest that Purkinje neurons from lobules IV to VI encode position, directional parameters, and velocities of arm movements (Roitman et al., 2005). The cerebellum takes information and adapts it to a given sensorimotor context and, through repetitions, will make the appropriate adjustments to make the behavior more and more efficient.

Some of the most convincing evidence that the CNS uses internal forward models in human motor behavior comes from studies dedicated to the control of grasping forces during manipulation of objects (Nowak et al., 2007). The rate of grip force development and the balance between the grip and load forces when grasping/lifting an object are programmed in order to meet the requirements due to physical object properties, such as weight, surface friction, or shape. Cerebellar patients generate excessive grip forces in relation to loads, suggesting a distorted predictive force control.

Inverse models

According to this theory, the cerebellum would lodge an "inverse model." Here the input to the cerebellum would be the aimed trajectory, and the output would be a motor command. In order to train this type of model, error information would best be characterized in motor coordinates in three directions. In the laboratory, cerebellar patients exhibit difficulties in adapting to external force field, in agreement with the inverse dynamics hypothesis (Maschke et al., 2004). Neurophysiological data support the existence of inverse models. Shidara and colleagues have shown that Purkinje cell activity during ocular movements is consistent with signals of an inverse model (Shidara et al., 1993). Although studies of the changes in Purkinje cell firings that occur when an external force load is changed from resistive to assistive during elbow movements are suggestive of an inverse dynamics model, it should be noted that these experiments have not controlled limb kinematics or modified the magnitude of external loads (Yamamoto et al., 2007). To test the hypothesis that Purkinje cell firing is the output of an inverse dynamics model, forces must be changed while kinematics is kept constant. Purkinje neurons might code for kinematic (i.e. sensory state) but not dynamic information (i.e. muscle commands) (Pasalar et al., 2006). A majority of Purkinje cells do not exhibit any modulation in the patterns of discharges as a function of force type or load. In addition, the spatial tuning pattern seems unaffected, strengthening the idea of uncoupling between Purkinje cell firing and electromyographic activity in limbs. Two of the differences between cerebellar simple spike responses and those of motor cortical cells are the non-uniform distribution of preferred directions and the extensive overlap in the timing of the correlations. These differences suggest that Purkinje cells handle kinematic information in a different way as compared with motor cortical neurons.

Forward models and inverse models can be seen as two inter-related models. Forward models are required for the acquisition of a behavior. During learning of a given behavior, an inverse model is created, allowing skilled motion at an unconscious level (Ito, 2008). The cerebellum interacts permanently with supra-tentorial areas, especially the premotor cortex, the motor cortex, the posterior parietal cortex, and the primary sensory cortex, in order to generate the appropriate encoding of force and direction of motion (Figure 2.6).

Cerebellum and cognitive operations

The cognitive regions of the cerebellum receive projections from the non-primary frontal, parietal, and occipital association cortex and send projections back via the thalamus. A similar operational mechanism could underlie both motor processing and cognitive operations, given the similar architecture of the circuits. A closed cerebrocerebellar communication loop is present for the cerebellum with the prefrontal cortex, supporting the hypothesis that cerebellar circuitry provides a forward model for mental operations of the cerebral cortex. Ito has suggested that internal models could apply also to cognitive functions such as thought (Ito, 2006). In thought, a mental model of an image, idea, or concept is presumably formed in the temporoparietal association cortex. In a second stage, mental models are controlled as an object by the prefrontal cortex. The prefrontal cortex would manipulate mental models just as the motor cortex regulates motion of body segments (Ito, 2006). In a third stage, the cerebellar circuitry would copy a mental model to form an internal model.

Evidence that the cerebellum contributes to executive functions is growing (see also Chapter 3). Executive control refers to the ability to orchestrate various cognitive tasks to achieve a specific goal. Executive functions are closely linked to the prefrontal cortex in human subjects. Accumulating data suggest that different regions of the prefrontal cortex are related to distinct aspects of executive control. The lateral prefrontal cortex, which is strongly connected with the cerebellum, plays an important role. Response inhibition (assessed, for instance, by the Stroop test), multitasking (assessed by the digit span), set shifting (assessed by the Wisconsin Card Sorting Test), and working memory are all executive control subcomponents under the supervision of the prefrontal cortex.

Anatomical connections of the cerebellum with reticular nuclei and thalamic nuclei projecting widely throughout cerebral hemispheres open the possibility of a role of cerebellar circuitry in arousal and nociception (Schmahmann, 2002).

31

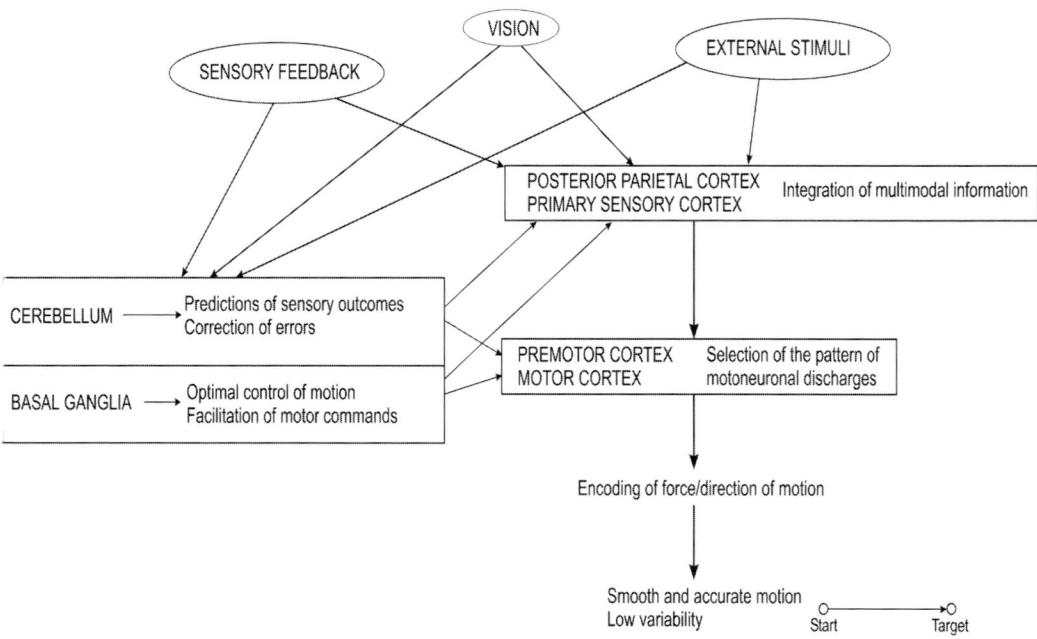

Figure 2.6 Overview of the motor control strategy for limb movements. Cerebellum builds internal models and corrects motor commands, comparable to a system identification function. Basal ganglia ensures an optimal control of motion, facilitating motor commands. The parietal cortex integrates proprioceptive and visual outcomes, as well as sensory feedback, playing a role of state estimator. Premotor cortex and motor cortex transforms predictions into sets of motoneuronal discharges, encoding for force and direction of movement. With permission from: Manto, 2009.

Cerebellum, mood, and depression

Cerebellar activation in lobules IV, V, and VI has been reported in conditions associated with happiness or sadness (Lane et al., 1997). Morphologic differences in the cerebellum of patients with depression have been suspected. In particular, unipolar depression and bipolar disorder have been associated with smaller size of the cerebellum (Soares & Mann, 1997). Moreover, decreased size of the vermis has been reported in major depression (Shah et al., 1992). A reduction of the size of vermal lobules VIII to X has been found in patients with multiple episodes of depression (DelBello et al., 1999). Further studies are required to confirm these findings and provide a definite link between cerebellar operations and control of mood.

References

Albus JS. A theory of cerebellar function. *Math Biosci* 1971;**10**:25–61.

Bastian AJ, Morton S. Mechanisms of cerebellar gait ataxia. *Cerebellum* 2007;**6**(1):79–86.

Bastian AJ, Martin TA, Keating JK, Thach WT. Cerebellar ataxia: abnormal control of interaction torques across multiple joints. *J Neurophysiol* 1996;**76**:492–509.

Bastian AJ, Mink JW, Kaufman BA, Thach WT. Posterior vermal split syndrome. *Ann Neurol* 1998;**44**:601–10.

Bastian AJ, Thach WT. Structure and function of the cerebellum. In *The Cerebellum and Its Disorders*, ed. M. Manto and M. Pandolfo. Cambridge, UK: Cambridge University Press, 2002, pp 49–66.

Boecker H, Kleinschmidt A, Weindl A, et al. Dysfunctional activation of subcortical nuclei in palatal myoclonus detected by high-resolution MRI. *NMR Biomed* 1994;**7**:327–9.

Boyden ES, Katoh A, Raymond JL. Cerebellum-dependent learning: the role of multiple plasticity mechanisms. *Annu Rev Neurosci* 2004;**27**:581–609.

Bracha V. Role of the cerebellum in eyeblink conditioning. *Prog Brain Res* 2004;**143**:331–9.

Coltz JD, Johnson MT, Ebner TJ. Cerebellar Purkinje cell simple spike discharge encodes movement velocity in primates during visuomotor arm tracking. *J Neurosci* 1999;**19**:1782–1803.

Danckert J, Ferber S, Goodale MA. Direct effects of prismatic lenses on visuomotor control: an event-related functional MRI study. *Eur J Neurosci* 2008;**28**(8):1696–704.

Dean P, Porrill J, Stone JV. Visual awareness and the cerebellum: possible role of decorrelation control. *Prog Brain Res* 2004;**144**:61–75.

DelBello MP, Strakowski SM, Zimmerman ME, Hawkins JM, Sax KW. MRI analysis of the cerebellum in bipolar disorder: a pilot study. *Neuropsychopharmacology* 1999;**21**:63–8.

Delgado-García JM, Gruart A. Building new motor responses: eyelid conditioning revisited. *Trends Neurosci* 2006;**29**:330–8.

Deuschl G, Toro C, Zeffiro T, Massaquoi S, Hallett M. Adaptation motor learning of arm movements in patients with cerebellar disease. *J Neurol Neurosurg Psychiatry* 1996;**60**(5):515–9.

Dichgans J, Fetter M. Compartmentalized cerebellar functions upon the stabilization of body posture. *Rev Neurol (Paris)* 1993;**149**:654–64.

Dimitrova A, de Greiff A, Schoch B, et al. Activations of cerebellar nuclei comparing finger, foot and tongue movements as revealed by fMRI. *Brain Res Bull* 2006;**71**:233–41.

Doyon J, Penhune V, Ungerleider LG. Distinct contribution of the cortico-striatal and cortico-cerebellar systems to motor skill learning. *Neuropsychologia* 2003;**41**(3):252–62.

Friedemann HH, Noth J, Diener HC, Bacher M. Long latency EMG responses in hand and leg muscles: cerebellar disorders. *J Neurol Neurosurg Psychiatry* 1987;**50**(1):71–7.

Frysinger RC, Bourbonnais D, Kalaska JF, Smith AM. Cerebellar cortical activity during antagonist cocontraction and reciprocal inhibition of forearm muscles. *J Neurophysiol* 1984;**51**:32–49.

Fuchs AF, Robinson F, Straube A. Participation of the caudal fastigial nucleus in smooth-pursuit eye movements: I. Neuronal activity. *J Neurophysiol* 1994;**72**:2714–28.

Fujita M. Adaptive filter model of the cerebellum. *Biol Cybern* 1982;**45**:195–206.

Gao JH, Parsons LM, Bower JM, et al. Cerebellum implicated in sensory acquisition and discrimination rather than motor control. *Science* 1996;**26**:545–7.

Gerwig M, Dimitrova A, Kolb FP, et al. Comparison of eyeblink conditioning in patients with superior and posterior inferior cerebellar lesions. *Brain* 2003;**126**:71–94.

Gerwig M, Kolb FP, Timmann D. The involvement of the human cerebellum in eyeblink conditioning. *Cerebellum* 2007;**6**:38–57.

Gibson AR, Horn KM, Pong M. Activation of climbing fibers. *Cerebellum* 2004;**3**(4):212–21.

Gilman S. The mechanism of cerebellar hypotonia. *Brain* 1969;**92**:621–38.

Habas C. Functional imaging of deep cerebellar nuclei: a review. *Cerebellum* 2009, June 10 [Epub ahead of print].

Hallett M, Grafman J. Executive function and motor skin learning. In *The Cerebellum and Cognition*, ed. J. Schmahmann. San Diego, CA: Academic Press, 1997, pp. 297–323.

Highstein SM, Porrill J, Dean P. Report on a workshop concerning the cerebellum and motor learning, held in St Louis October 2004. *Cerebellum* 2005;**4**(2):140–50.

Horak FB, Diener HC. Cerebellar control of postural scaling and central set in stance. *J Neurophysiol* 1994;**72**:479–93.

Hore J, Wild B, Diener HC. Cerebellar dysmetria at the elbow, wrist and fingers. *J Neurophysiol* 1991;**65**:563–71.

Ilg W, Giese MA, Gizewski ER, Schoch B, Timmann D. The influence of focal cerebellar lesions on the control and adaptation of gait. *Brain* 2008;**131**(Pt 11):2913–27.

Ioffe ME, Chernikova LA, Ustinova KI. Role of cerebellum in learning postural tasks. *Cerebellum* 2007;**6**:87–94.

Ito M. Cerebellar circuitry as a neuronal machine. *Prog Neurobiol* 2006;**78**:272–303.

Ito M. *The Cerebellum and Neural Control*. New York: Raven Press, 1984.

Ito M. Control of mental activities by internal models in the cerebellum. *Nat Rev Neurosci* 2008;**9**(4):304–13.

Ivry RB, Keele SW, Diener HC. Dissociation of the lateral and medial cerebellum in movement timing and movement execution. *Exp Brain Res* 1988;**73**:167–80.

Jacobs JV, Horak FB. Cortical control of postural responses. *J Neural Transm* 2007;**114**(10):1339–48.

Jueptner M, Weiller C. A review of differences between basal ganglia and cerebellar control of movements as revealed by functional imaging studies. *Brain* 1998;**121**:1437–49.

Kitazawa S, Kimura T, Yin PB. Cerebellar complex spikes encode both destinations and errors in arm movements. *Nature* 1998;**392**:494–7.

Lane RD, Reiman EM, Ahern GL, Schwartz GE, Davidson RJ. Neuroanatomical correlates of happiness, sadness, and disgust. *Am J Psychiatry* 1997;**154**:926–33.

Lang EJ, Sugihara I, Welsh JP, Llinas R. Patterns of spontaneous Purkinje cell complex spike activity in the awake rat. *J Neurosci* 1999;**19**:2728–39.

Lechtenberg R, Gilman S. Speech disorders in cerebellar disease. *Ann Neurol* 1978;**3**:285–90.

Linden DJ. Neuroscience: from molecules to memory in the cerebellum. *Science* 2003;**301**:1682–5.

Liu Y, Pu Y, Gao JH, et al. The human red nucleus and lateral cerebellum supporting roles for sensory information processing. *Hum Brain Mapp* 2000;**10**:147–59.

Maekawa K, Simpson JL. Climbing fiber responses evoked in vestibulocerebellum of rabbit from visual system. *J Neurophysiol* 1973;**36**(4):649–66.

Manto M. Mechanisms of human cerebellar dysmetria: experimental evidence and current conceptual bases. *J Neuroeng Rehabil* 2009;**6**:10.

Manto M, Godaux E, Jacquy J. Cerebellar hypermetria is larger when the inertial load is artificially increased. *Ann Neurol* 1994;**35**:45–52.

Marr DA. A theory of cerebellar cortex. *J Physiol (London)* 1969;**202**:437–70.

Marshall SP, Lang EJ. Inferior olive oscillations gate transmission of motor cortical activity to the cerebellum. *J Neurosci* 2004;**24**(50):11356–67.

Maschke M, Gomez CM, Ebner TJ, Konczak J. Hereditary cerebellar ataxia progressively impairs force adaptation during goal-directed arm movements. *J Neurophysiol* 2004;**91**:230–8.

Miall RC. Sequences of sensory predictions. *Behav Brain Sci* 1997;**20**:258–9.

Morton SM, Bastian AJ. Prism adaptation during walking generalizes to reaching and requires the cerebellum. *J Neurophysiol* 2004;**92**(4):2497–509.

Nowak DA, Topka H, Timmann D, Boecker H, Hermsdorfer J. The role of the cerebellum for predictive control of grasping. *Cerebellum* 2007;**6**:7–17.

Pasalar S, Roitman AV, Durfee WK, Ebner TJ. Force field effects on cerebellar Purkinje cell discharge with implications for internal models. *Nat Neurosci* 2006;**9**:1404–11.

Pascual-Leone A, Grafman J, Clark K, et al. Procedural learning in Parkinson's disease and cerebellar degeneration. *Ann Neurol* 1993;**34**(4):594–602.

Pelisson D, Goffart L, Guillaume A. Contribution of the rostral fastigial nucleus to the control of orienting gaze shifts in the head-unrestrained cat. *J Neurophysiol* 1998;**80**:1180–96.

Ramnani N. The primate cortico-cerebellar system: anatomy and function. *Nat Rev Neurosci* 2006;**7**:511–22.

Riecker A, Mathiak K, Wildgruber D, et al. fMRI reveals two distinct cerebral networks subserving speech motor control. *Neurology* 2005;**64**:700–6.

Roitman AV, Pasalar S, Johnson MT, Ebner TJ. Position, direction of movement, and speed tuning of cerebellar Purkinje cells during circular manual tracking in monkey. *J Neurosci* 2005;**25**:9244–57.

Sainburg RL, Ghez C, Kalakanis D. Intersegmental dynamics are controlled by sequential anticipatory, error correction and postural mechanisms. *J Neurophysiol* 1999;**81**:1045–56.

Schmahmann JD. The role of cerebellum in affect and psychosis. In *The Cerebellum and its Disorders*, ed. M. Manto and M. Pandolfo. Cambridge, UK: Cambridge University Press, 2002, pp. 136–57.

Seitz RJ, Roland PE, Bohm C, Greitz T, Stone-Elander S. Somatosensory discrimination of shape: tactile exploration and cerebral activation. *Europ J Neurosci* 1991;**3**:481–92.

Shah SA, Doraiswamy PM, Husain MM, et al. Posterior fossa abnormalities in major depression: a controlled magnetic resonance imaging study. *Acta Psychiatr Scand* 1992;**85**:474–9.

Shidara M, Kawano K, Gomi H, Kawato M. Inverse-dynamics model eye movement control by Purkinje cells in the cerebellum. *Nature* 1993;**365**:50–2.

Soares JC, Mann JJ. The anatomy of mood disorders: review of structural neuroimaging studies. *Biol Psychiatry* 1997;**41**:86–106.

Solomon PR, Stowe GT, Pendlbeury WW. Disrupted eyelid conditioning in a patient with damage to cerebellar afferents. *Behav Neurosci* 1989;**103**:898–902.

Sugihara I, Lang EJ, Llinás R. Serotonin modulation of inferior olivary oscillations and synchronicity: a multiple-electrode study in the rat cerebellum. *Eur J Neurosci* 1995;**7**(4):521–34.

Thach WT. Discharge of Purkinje and cerebellar nuclear neurons during rapidly alternating arm movements in the monkey. *J Neurophysiol* 1967;**31**:785–96.

Thach WT, Goodkin HG, Keating JG. Cerebellum and the adaptive coordination of movement. *Ann Rev Neurosci* 1992;**15**:403–42.

Thompson RF. In search of memory traces. *Annu Rev Psychol* 2005;**56**:1–23.

Topka H, Massaquoi S. Pathophysiology of clinical cerebellar signs. In *The Cerebellum and its Disorders*, ed. M. Manto and M. Pandolfo. Cambridge, UK: Cambridge University Press, 2002, pp. 121–35.

Torriero S, Oliveri M, Koch G, Caltagirone C, Petrosini L. Interference of left and right cerebellar rTMS with procedural learning. *J Cogn Neurosci* 2004;**16**(9)1605–11.

Torriero S, Oliveri M, Koch G, et al. Cortical networks of procedural learning: evidence from cerebellar damage. *Neuropsychologia* 2007;**45**(6):1208–14.

Tracy JI, Faro SS, Mohammed FB, et al. Cerebellar mediation of the complexity of bimanual compared to unimanual movements. *Neurology* 2001;**57**: 1862–9.

Vilis T, Hore J. Central neuronal mechanisms contributing to cerebellar tremor produced by limb perturbations. *J Neurophysiol* 1980;**43**:279–91.

Yamamoto K, Kawato M, Kotosaka S, Kitazawa S. Encoding of movement dynamics by Purkinje cell simple spike activity during fast arm movements under resistive and assistive force fields. *J Neurophysiol* 2007;**97**:1588–99.

Yarom Y, Cohen D. The olivocerebellar system as a generator of temporal patterns. *Ann N Y Acad Sci* 2002;**978**:122–34.

Symptoms of cerebellar disorders

Cerebellar function is usually affected through several mechanisms, which often combine (Gilman et al., 1981): reduced blood flow, edema, mechanical compression, invasion of cerebellar parenchyma, inflammatory response, immune process, cytotoxic effect, and neurodegeneration. Brainstem and meninges are commonly affected also.

Five general principles apply (Manto, 2002):

1. Lateral focal cerebellar lesions induce ipsilateral signs, although expanding lesions may produce a false localization of clinical signs.
2. Diffuse cerebellar disorders, such as degenerative ataxias, are usually responsible for relatively symmetric deficits.
3. Cerebellar deficits due to non-progressive disease tend to undergo attenuation with time.
4. Lesions involving the afferent or efferent cerebellar pathways outside the cerebellum may generate cerebellar-like deficits.
5. Cerebellar symptoms are influenced more by the location and rate of progression of the disease than by the pathological characteristics (Gilman et al., 1981; Lechtenberg, 1993). Slowly progressive lesions may be remarkably asymptomatic for a long time, while rapidly expanding lesions are associated with severe symptoms in most cases (Dow & Moruzzi, 1958; Gilman et al., 1981).

Table 3.1 lists the symptoms commonly encountered in patients exhibiting a cerebellar ataxia, with lesions affecting mainly the cerebellum itself. Cognitive and emotional deficits are discussed in the section Classification of clinical signs, under "Cognitive abnormalities" and emotional disorders. Gait difficulties, headache, nausea/vomiting, and dizziness are the most common symptoms. In patients presenting lesions restricted to the cerebellum, the main symptoms are gait difficulties, headache, dizziness, limb clumsiness, speech difficulties, blurred vision, feebleness, and fatigability.

Table 3.1 Symptoms associated with cerebellar disorders[a]

Symptom
Gait difficulties
Headache
Nausea/vomiting
Dizziness
Clumsiness in limbs
Speech difficulties
Tremor
Blurred vision, impaired visual acuity
Diplopia
Feebleness
Sensory complaints
Fatigability
Memory difficulties
Impotence
Swallowing difficulties
Illusion of movement in environment
Hearing loss
Tinnitus
Limb or facial weakness
Urinary incontinence

[a]Cognitive and emotional symptoms are discussed in section "Cognitive abnormalities" and emotional disorders.

Headaches are reported very early in many patients. They can be influenced by postural changes. Headaches may be the sole symptom in cases of tumor, abscess, or stroke. Pain may be restricted to a region around or behind the eye(s) or to the parietal or occipital region. Occipital pain may be associated with sensations of neck stiffness (Gilman et al., 1981). A cerebellar tumor must be ruled out in all children complaining of headache in the morning in association or not with nausea, vomiting, clumsiness, or gait difficulties. Vomiting may be projectile with

Table 3.2 Clinical signs as a function of the sagittal zone affected

Vermal zone	Paravermal zone	Lateral zone
Oculomotor deficits	Dysarthria	Oculomotor deficits
Dysarthria		Dysarthria
Head tilt		Head tilt
Ataxia of stance		Dysmetria
Ataxic gait		Kinetic tremor
Titubation		Action tremor
		Hypotonia
		Dysdiadochokinesia
		Decomposition of movements
		Dysrhythmokinesia
		Impaired check/rebound
		Ataxia of stance
		Ataxic gait

no warning. Severe abrupt dull headache associated with gait ataxia and vomiting in a hypertensive patient suggests an intracerebral hemorrhage.

Ataxia: definition

Ataxia is a term originally used to describe dysequilibrium in tabes and is currently applied to describe the jerky or irregular character of movement or posture, when a disorder of coordination cannot be explained by strength or sensation deficits (Holmes, 1917). Asynergia was defined by Babinski as an inability to combine each element of a movement into a complex motor action (Babinski, 1899). Dysmetria is a term coined to describe the errors in metrics of motion: hypermetria designates an overshoot and hypometria an undershoot. The inability to perform rapid successive movements is called adiadochokinesia or dysdiadochokinesia (Babinski, 1902).

Clinical signs and sagittal zone affected

Table 3.2 lists the clinical signs depending on the sagittal zone affected (Gilman et al., 1981; Dichgans, 1984). The combination of oculomotor deficits with ataxia of stance and gait suggests a midline zone disorder. There is no syndrome associated with a lesion restricted to the intermediate zone, but isolated dysarthria has been

reported (Amarenco et al., 1991). Combinations of dysmetria, kinetic tremor, hypotonia, and dysdiadochokinesia are indicative of lateral lesions.

Classification of clinical signs

Cerebellar signs can be assigned to one of the six following categories:

- oculomotor disturbances
- dysarthria/speech deficits
- deficits in limbs movements
- deficits in gait/posture
- autonomic signs
- "cognitive abnormalities"

Oculomotor disturbances

Clinical examination

The examiner checks the stability of gaze (by holding the index finger at about 30 cm in front of the patient), looks for a static ocular misalignment, and looks for a nystagmus by maintaining the index finger motionless laterally (left/right) and in an upwards and downwards position. Saccades are assessed by putting the index fingers in each of the patient's temporal visual fields. The patient is asked to keep the eyes in a primary position and then to look laterally at one of the fingers (Trouillas et al., 1997). Latency, accuracy, and velocity of saccades are estimated. To assess the vestibuloocular reflex (VOR), the patient is seated on a rotating chair, fixating on an object which moves synchronously with head movements. Movements of the eyes are observed while the chair is rotated at a constant velocity. Normally, the subject can suppress the VOR by fixating on the object. The rotation of the chair is then stopped suddenly, and a post-rotatory nystagmus is specifically looked for. The rotating drum is used to assess the optokinetic response (the drum test also evaluates the pursuit) by asking the patient to count the stripes. Finally, Frenzel goggles allow the estimation of eye movements without fixation. Table 3.3 lists the oculomotor deficits observed in cerebellar patients.

Table 3.4 indicates the correlation between the topography of the lesion and the observed deficits. In cerebellar patients, oculomotor disorders usually result from lesions of the dorsal vermis or fastigial nucleus, the flocculus/paraflocculus, and/or the uvula and nodulus (Lewis & Zee, 1993). The dorsal vermis and the fastigial nuclei are primarily involved in

37

Table 3.3 Oculomotor deficits observed in cerebellar disorders

Fixation deficits
    Unsteady fixation (instability of gaze)
    Flutter
    Macrosaccadic oscillations

Ocular misalignment
    Skew deviation

Disorders of pursuit
    Saccadic pursuit

Deficits of saccades
    Hypermetric/hypometric saccades

Nystagmus
    Gaze-evoked nystagmus
    Centripetal nystagmus
    Rebound nystagmus
    Primary-position upbeat nystagmus
    Periodic alternating nystagmus

VOR and OKR deficits

Abbreviations: OKR: optokinetic reflex; VOR: vestibuloocular reflex.

Table 3.4 Correlation between the topography of the cerebellar lesion and oculomotor deficits

Structure	Deficits
Dorsal vermis/fastigial nucleus (lobules VI, VII)	Saccadic dysmetria Flutter Macrosaccadic oscillations Saccadic pursuit
Flocculus/paraflocculus	Gaze-evoked nystagmus Rebound nystagmus Saccadic pursuit Abnormal gain of VOR Abnormal optokinetic response
Nodulus	Periodic alternating nystagmus
Ventral uvula	

Abbreviation: VOR: vestibuloocular reflex.

initiation, accuracy, and dynamics of saccades, whereas the flocculus/paraflocculus is involved mainly in stabilization of a visual image on the retina (Fetter et al., 1994).

Fixation deficits

Flutter typically refers to conjugate brief oscillations of the eyes during a fixation or during movement of the eyes (Cogan, 1954; see Figure 3.1). Oscillations are usually horizontal. Macrosaccadic oscillations refer to cycles of square wave jerks, defined as spontaneous small saccades in opposite directions during fixation. Opsoclonus ("dancing eyes") is defined as involuntary, multidirectional, and conjugate saccadic oscillations (Orzechowski, 1927). Opsoclonus and myoclonus are symptoms of the "Kinsbourne syndrome" (Kinsbourne, 1962; see Chapter 11).

Skew deviation

Skew deviation is characterized by a static ocular misalignment, with one eye being higher than the other (Lewis & Zee, 1993). It results from an imbalance between otolith inputs. This misalignment can be associated with lesions of the mesencephalic region, pontomesencephalic area, cerebellum, medulla, or peripheral vestibular apparatus, or in the vestibular cortex. Skew deviation should be considered when faced with any vertical diplopia which cannot be explained by cranial nerve palsies, myasthenia, or disease of extraocular muscles.

Ocular tilt reaction

Ocular tile reaction (OTR) is an eye–head postural reaction combining head tilt, conjugated eye cyclotorsion, skew deviation, and impaired vertical perception (tilt of the subjective visual vertical). Partial OTR may occur following lesions of the caudal parts of the cerebellum, such as cerebellar infarction in the territory of the posterior inferior cerebellar artery (Mossman & Halmagyi, 1997). The dentate nucleus is involved in vestibular processing, such as the perception of verticality (Baier et al., 2008). Lesions of the dentate nucleus can lead to tilts of the subjective visual vertical in the contraversive direction (i.e. a vestibular tone imbalance to the contralateral side), while cerebellar lesions excluding the dentate nucleus and involving the biventer lobule, the middle cerebellar peduncle, the tonsil, and the inferior semilunar lobule can induce a tone imbalance to the ipsilesional side (Baier et al., 2008).

Disorders of pursuit

Lack of smoothness during a pursuit task is very common in cerebellar patients, but is not specific for cerebellar disorders. Movements are decomposed into fast and slow movements, called "catch-up saccades." A superimposed nystagmus is usually observed.

Figure 3.1 Oculomotor disturbances in cerebellar patients recorded with electrooculography (EOG). Upwards deflections: eye movement to the right, downwards deflections: eye movement to the left. From: Manto, 2002. With permission.

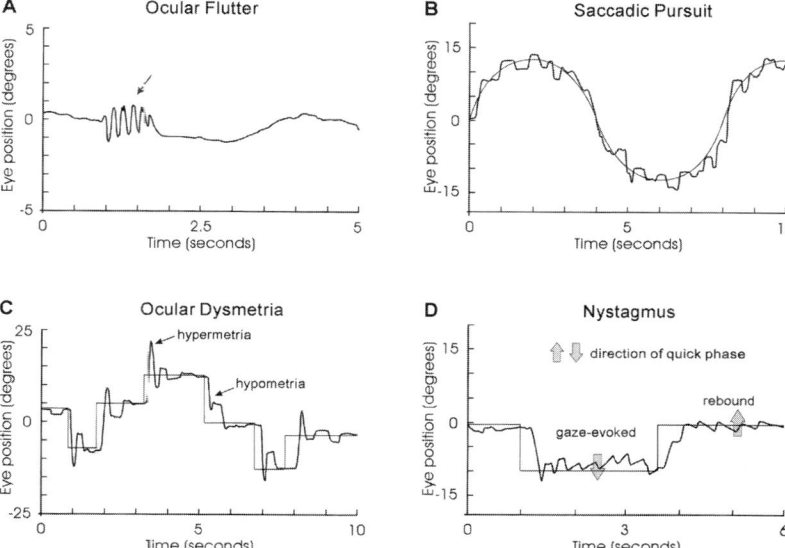

Disorders of saccades

The overshoot of a target (hypermetric saccade) is very common in cerebellar disorders (Selhorst et al., 1976). In most cases, centripetal saccades are more dysmetric than centrifugal saccades. When the dysmetria is more severe for one eye, the term of disconjugate dysmetria is used. Hypermetric saccades may be followed by corrective saccades or glissadic movements. Glissades are very common in patients presenting a diffuse cerebellar atrophy. Hypometria designates the undershoot and is less specific than hypermetria.

Nystagmus

Nystagmus is made of oscillations of the eyes, with alternating fast and slow movements. Gaze-evoked nystagmus (also called gaze-paretic), which is very common in cerebellar disorders, consists of a slow drift of the eyes followed by saccades tending to return the gaze towards an eccentric position (Gilman et al., 1981). When the fast component has a large amplitude, it is often called a "coarse" nystagmus. Rebound nystagmus is a transient nystagmus occurring during the return to a primary position after maintaining an eccentric gaze. Although relatively specific, it lacks any localizing value. Down-beat nystagmus is a primary-position nystagmus with fast ocular movements downwards. It is observed mainly in diseases of the cervicomedullary junction such as Chiari mal-

formations, in hereditary ataxic diseases (in particular, spinocerebellar ataxia type 6), and in immune disorders (Yee et al., 1984). Lateral gaze and convergence usually exacerbate down-beat nystagmus. Down-beat nystagmus occurs when physiological inhibitory cerebellar input, in particular of the flocculus, to the vestibular nuclei is inhibited. When the nystagmus is provoked by extension/rotation of the head, a cerebellar lesion compressing the brainstem should be suspected. Down-beat nystagmus may also be positional in a context suggesting a peripheral labyrinthine disorder: vertigo, adaptation, and habituation on repeated testing (Bertholon et al., 2002). Hallpike maneuver may be positive bilaterally in these patients (in classical benign paroxysmal positional vertigo associated with a posterior canalolithiasis, Hallpike maneuver is usually positive on one side only), and nystagmus may be provoked by a straight headhanging procedure, suggesting an anterior semicircular canalolithiasis. A periodic form of downbeat nystagmus due to a metabolic disorder has been reported (Du Pasquier et al., 1998). Up-beat nystagmus is a primary-position nystagmus with the fast phase upwards. It has been reported mainly in drug overdose, midbrain lesions, lesions of the lower brainstem, and midline cerebellar lesions. Up-beat nystagmus is likely due to an imbalance of vertical vestibuloocular reflex tone. Ocular bobbing is a fast movement of the eyes downwards, followed by a slow drift back

Table 3.5 Main extra-cerebellar signs observed in ataxic patients

Clinical sign
Slowing of saccadic movements
Ophthalmoparesis/ophthalmoplegia
Papilledema
Optic neuritis
Concomitant movement disorders (dystonia, rigidity, dyskinesias, rest tremor)
Cognitive deficits
Seizures
Pyramidal signs
Signs of peripheral neuropathy
Dysautonomia

to midposition. It is observed in cerebellar disorders with brainstem compression or may be observed following basilar artery occlusion. Monocular bobbing occurs in patients with contralateral oculomotor palsy. Periodic alternating nystagmus is a spontaneous nystagmus beating in one direction, followed by a silent phase, and then by resurgence of the nystagmus in the opposite direction. It may be congenital or acquired.

Signs of extra-cerebellar disease

Table 3.5 lists the most common neurological signs which are suggestive of an extra-cerebellar involvement. The reader is referred to the specific chapters in the book.

Dysarthria and mutism

Examination of speech

The patient is asked to maintain a sustained vowel phonation ("ah", "ee"), repeat syllables, produce monosyllabic words, repeat a standard sentence, and read aloud a standard text. The clarity, rhythm, and fluency of speech are evaluated. Speed of speech can be estimated by recording on a tape recorder the time taken to pronounce a fixed number of words. Cerebellar disorders are typically associated with slow speech accompanied by slurring. Comprehension is spared. Temporal dysregulation may lead to unintelligible words (Kent et al., 1997). Speech may turn out to be explosive, taking a staccato rhythm and a nasal character. Scanning speech is easily recognizable, made of hesitations, accentuation of some syllables, omission

of some pauses, and addition of inappropriate pauses. Voice tremor may occur also. The disturbed melody of speech is called dysprosody. Dysarthria may even appear more complex because of additional naming difficulties and agrammatism. The superior paravermal segment of the left hemisphere at about lobules VI and VII is one of the cerebellar regions that plays a critical role in speech (Gilman et al., 1981). Cerebellar mutism refers to an absence of speech following posterior fossa surgery in children (Rekate et al., 1985). Mutism usually appears within 12 to 48 hours after surgery and lasts 1.5 to 12 weeks after onset. Dysarthria occurs following resolution of mutism (van Dongen et al., 1994). Focal non-surgically induced cerebellar damage may also cause a mutism (Frassanito et al., 2009). Lesions of the cerebello-thalamocortical pathway after midbrain infarction can present with paroxysmal attacks of dysarthria and limb ataxia (Matsui et al., 2004).

Deficits in limb movements

Clinical examination

For the upper limbs, the patient is seated in a comfortable position. In the finger-to-nose test, the patient is asked to touch his nose with the index finger, with the hand resting initially on the thigh. Each side is tested. During the finger-to-finger test, the examiner moves his index finger in various locations in front of the patient, who has to touch it with his own index finger. To check for a postural tremor, the patient is requested to maintain the upper limbs parallel to the floor, with the elbows extended and hands held in supination. The index-to-index test consists of maintaining the two index fingers medially, pointing at each other at a distance of 1 cm, with the elbows maintained horizontally. For alternate movements, the patient is asked to maintain the forearms vertically and to perform successive pronation/supination hand movements. During the tapping test, the patient places palmar and dorsal surfaces of the hands alternatively on the thigh. To assess muscle tone, the wrists, elbows, and shoulders are passively moved. In addition, the examiner grasps the forearm and shakes the relaxed hand to evaluate the level of hypotonia. To assess difficulties in changing directions of movement, the patient is asked to draw slowly and with accuracy a square in space. The Barany test is performed with the eyes closed. The patient has to extend the arms horizontally, direct them straight over the head, and then come

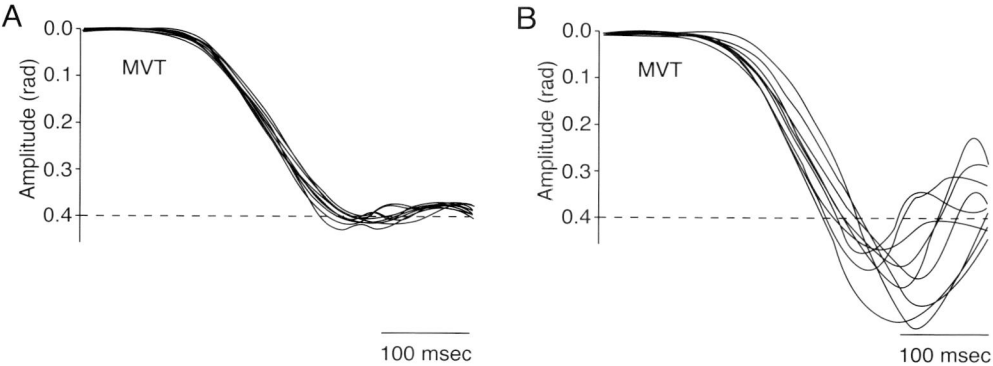

Figure 3.2 Cerebellar hypermetria. Superimposition of nine fast wrist flexion movements in a control subject (A) and a cerebellar patient (B). Movements (MVT) are accurate in A and are hypermetric in B (overshoot of the target). Aimed target (dotted lines) located at 0.4 rad from the start position corresponding to a neutral position of the joint. The target is visually displayed. With permission from: Manto, 2009.

back to the initial position. A similar task is the horizontal pointing maneuver, in which the subject moves quickly one index finger towards a target area delineated by the index finger and thumb contralaterally, keeping the elbows extended. In the Stewart-Holmes test, the patient has to flex the elbow forcefully while the observer attempts to extend the joint by holding the forearm of the patient (Stewart & Holmes, 1904). The forearm is then released abruptly and the examiner notes whether the patient strikes his shoulder or his chest with the hand. For the index-to-wrist maneuver, the examiner holds his wrist horizontally at the height of the patient's shoulder at an approximate distance of 85% of the length of the patient's upper limbs. The patient is asked to touch the wrist with his index finger as fast as possible.

For examination of lower limbs, the patient is in a supine position. The knee-tibia test consists of asking the patient to raise one leg and place the heel on the contralateral knee, which is kept motionless. The patient slides the heel down the tibial surface slowly and regularly up to the ankle. In the heel-to-knee test, the patient is asked to keep the heel motionless on the contralateral knee for several seconds. During the great toe-finger test, the patient touches the index of the examiner with one great toe. To check for a postural tremor in lower limbs, the patient is asked to keep the legs horizontally, with a 90-degree flexion of hips and knees. Muscle tone is again evaluated by passively moving each joint of the lower limbs.

Dysmetria

Dysmetria is a cardinal sign of cerebellar disease. Dysmetria represents an error in trajectory of move-

ment. Hypermetria is usually more evident during fast movements (Figure 3.2 and Figure 3.3). Hypometria is less common. Both forms of dysmetria are usually followed by corrective movements. Dysmetria affects both proximal and distal joints. Patients presenting with chronic cerebellar disease display a worsening of dysmetria when the inertia of the limb is increased mechanically (Manto et al., 1994). Silent cerebellar lesions may be detected with this procedure (Manto et al., 1995). Dysmetria is associated with abnormal patterns of electromyographic activities (Figure 3.4). Kinematics of movement is typically asymmetrical (Figure 3.5).

Kinetic tremor

The terms intention tremor and kinetic tremor refer to oscillations increasing at the end of a voluntary movement. Kinetic tremor is tested during finger-to-nose and knee-tibia tests. It may be present during the whole range of motion, although exaggerated near the goal (Holmes, 1939). Tremor is perpendicular to the main direction of movement and may be predominant in proximal joints (Gilman et al., 1981). Unlike dysmetria, kinetic tremor may be improved with the addition of inertia (Chase et al., 1965). In some patients, kinetic tremor tends to increase in the days or weeks following an initial injury.

Action tremor

Action tremor is observed in tasks requiring precision (Table 3.6): finger-to-finger test, heel-to-knee test, arms maintained outstretched, legs maintained horizontally. Tremor is most evident in the line of gravity (Holmes, 1922). Oscillations during the heel-to-knee

Table 3.6 Postural tremor in cerebellar disorders

Tremor	Anatomical lesion	Precipitants	Frequency (Hz)
Precision tremor	Nuclei Superior cerebellar peduncle	Precision tasks	2–5
Asthenic tremor	Hemisphere	Fatigue	Irregular
Axial postural tremor	?	Posture	2–10
3-Hz leg tremor	Anterior lobe	Posture	2.8–3.3
Midbrain tremor	Outflow tract, nigrostriatal	Posture	2.5–5

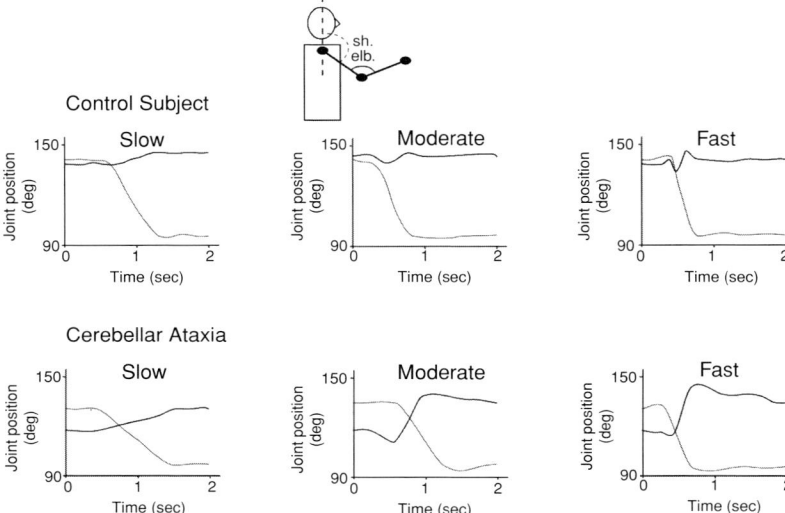

Figure 3.3 Effects of increasing velocities on kinematics of the upper limb pointing movements in a control subject (upper panels) and a cerebellar patient (lower panels). Subjects are seated and comfortably restrained in order to allow only shoulder and elbow movements. They are asked to perform a vertical pointing movement towards a fixed target at various speeds. The target is located in front of the subjects at a distance of 85% of total arm length. In the patient, deficits in angular motion are enhanced with increasing velocities, especially the increased angular motion of elbow resulting in overshoot (hyperextension of the elbow). Black lines: angular position of the elbow; gray lines: angular position of the shoulder. Abbreviations: sh.: shoulder angle; elb.: elbow angle. With permission from: Manto, 2009.

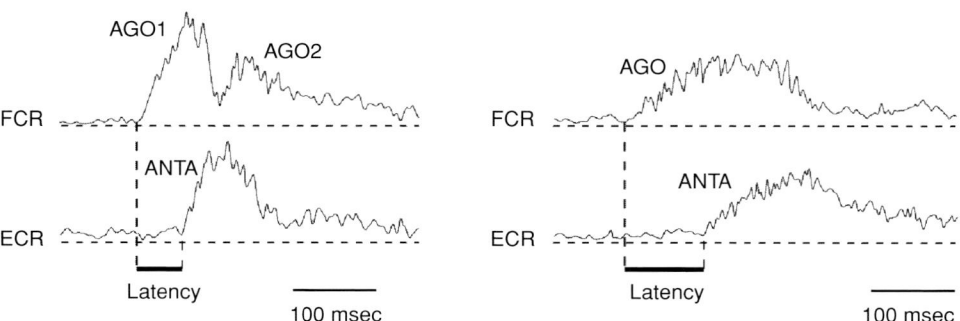

Figure 3.4 Abnormal triphasic pattern of electromyographic (EMG) activities associated with cerebellar ataxia. EMG activities in a control subject (left) and in a cerebellar patient exhibiting hypermetria (right). In the control subject, the first agonist burst (AGO1) is followed by a burst in the antagonist muscle (ANTA), followed by a second burst in the agonist muscle (AGO2). In the cerebellar patient, three EMG deficits are observed: the rate of rise of EMG activities is depressed, the onset latency of the antagonist EMG activity is delayed, and the two agonist bursts are not demarcated. Abbreviations: FCR: flexor carpi radialis; ECR: extensor carpi radialis. EMG traces are full-wave rectified and averaged (n = 10 movements). With permission from: Manto, 2009.

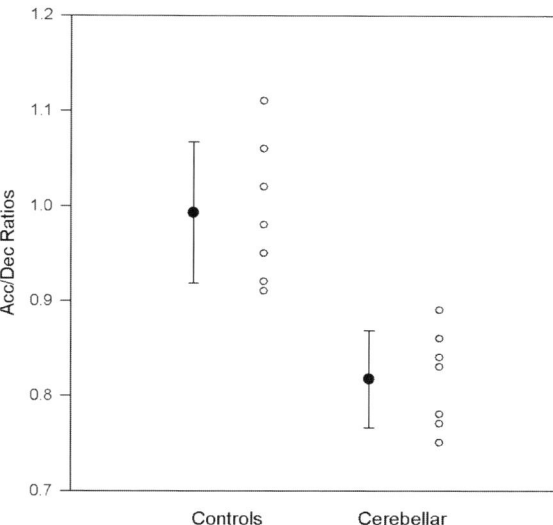

Figure 3.5 Asymmetry in kinematics of fast wrist flexion movements in cerebellar patients exhibiting hypermetria. Values correspond to ratios of Acceleration Peaks divided by Deceleration Peaks (Acc/Dec). Mean ± SD and individual ratios are shown. Data from n = 7 ataxic patients; mean age: 53.2 ± 5.7 years. Control group: n = 7 subjects; mean age: 54.5 ± 6.1 years. Aimed target: 15 degrees; n = 10 movements per subject. With permission from: Manto, 2009.

test evolve in unwanted lateral movements, despite attempts by the patient to block the heel. A typical 3-Hz tremor with a waxing and waning amplitude and taking a spindle-like aspect during a sustained leg elevation while the patient is supine are highly suggestive of a lesion of the anterior lobe (Mauritz et al., 1979; see also Chapter 15). Oscillations may be detected during writing, which is typically irregular. Some patients have abnormally large handwriting with an increase in the height of letters during writing. This macrographia contrasts with the micrographia observed in Parkinson's disease.

Palatal tremor

Palatal tremor is also called rhythmic palatal myoclonus. It may be associated with a hypertrophic contralateral inferior olivary nucleus subsequent to lesions of the so-called "Guillain-Mollaret triangle," at the level of the contralateral dentate nucleus or superior cerebellar peduncle, or at the level of the ipsilateral central tegmental tract (Lapresle, 1979; see also Chapter 14). Frequency of the tremor is between 0.5 and 3 Hz. Palatal tremor may occur in the context of sporadic or familial progressive ataxia

in the so-called progressive ataxia and palatal tremor syndrome (see also Chapter 23) (Samuel et al., 2004).

Essential tremor and orthostatic tremor

Essential tremor is now recognized as a tremor associated with a disorder of cerebellar pathways (see Chapter 19). It affects mainly the upper limbs and the head. Tremor combines postural and kinetic features. Some patients with lesions in the posterior fossa may exhibit an orthostatic tremor of irregular or, exceptionally, of regular frequency (symptomatic orthostatic tremor), which typically affects weight-bearing muscles. Table 3.7 lists the main differential diagnosis of cerebellar tremor.

Disorders of muscle tone

Hypotonia is a decreased resistance to passive manipulation of the limbs. It is classically more intense in children. In adults, it appears early after an extensive cerebellar damage, is usually greater in proximal segments, and tends to disappear quickly. Joints and limbs appear more relaxed (Lechtenberg, 1993). Hypotonia may be associated with pendular reflexes. Differential diagnosis of cerebellar hypotonia includes extensive brainstem lesion, spinal shock, anterior horn cell disease, polyradiculitis/polyneuropathy, and "floppy infant syndrome" in children. Cerebellar fits are spasms associated with intermittent opisthotonos (Stewart & Holmes, 1904). They are associated with posterior fossa tumors, Chiari malformations, and stroke involving the cerebellar cortex but sparing the nuclei. The mechanism is presumably an extensor tone disinhibition. Cerebellar fits are included in the category of "cerebellar seizures," which also includes hemifacial seizures associated with a dysplastic cerebellar tumor in infants (Harvey et al., 1996). In particular, ganglioglioma of the cerebellum may be associated with paroxysmal facial contractions (Chae et al., 2001). Similar symptoms may be observed in children with hamartoma of the floor of the fourth ventricle (Delande et al., 2001).

Decomposition of movement

Cerebellar patients perform compound movements which tend to be decomposed into their elemental components, with a lack of synergy between joints. Typically, the movements of the shoulder and the elbow are asynchronous in maneuvers such as the index-to-wrist test. When the movement is performed slowly, errors in direction and rate of movement

Table 3.7 Differential diagnosis of cerebellar tremor affecting the limbs

Tremor	Type or disease	Features
Postural tremor	Physiological tremor Enhanced physiological tremor Essential tremor	Hands predominantly affected Frequency: 8–13 Hz Drug intake (theophylline, caffeine, steroids, beta-mimetics, epinephrine) Family history Head affected Alcohol reducing tremor Frequency: 5–8 Hz
Rest tremor	Parkinson disease and "Parkinson-plus syndromes" Multiple sclerosis	"Pill-rolling" Rigidity, bradykinesia, impaired postural reflexes Tends to be reduced by movement Frequency: 4–7 Hz
Midbrain tremor	Tumor Trauma Stroke Infection Inflammatory condition	Rest, postural and kinetic Frequency: 2.5–5 Hz
Rhythmic myoclonus		Irregular, shock-like contractions Variable amplitude Regular
Myorhythmias	Paraneoplastic Infectious Immune Genetic CIDP, paraproteinemia	Frequency: 1–3 Hz Postural
Peripheral neuropathy	HSMN Diabetes, uremia	Distal muscles
Psychogenic tremor		Abrupt onset Variable amplitude and frequency Reduced by distraction Favorable effect of placebo

Abbreviations: CIDP: chronic inflammatory demyelinating polyneuropathy; HSMN: hereditary sensorimotor neuropathy.

appear, in absence of detectable rhythmic oscillations. This ataxia of slow movements is thus different from kinetic tremor associated with execution of slow movements. Decomposition of movements is often associated with an inability to generate independent finger movements during successive tapping movements of the index finger against the thumb (index-thumb test). The "sign of the piano" consists of a successive flexion of the third, fourth, and fifth finger followed by a phase of immobility of the fingers during attempts to move the thumb and index finger alone. It is observed early after a cerebellar stroke involving the cerebellar outflow tracts.

Dysdiadochokinesia

Dysdiadochokinesia is characterized by irregular and slow alternate sequential movements. An abnormal sway of the elbow is present in advanced cases.

Dysrhythmokinesia ("arrhythmokinesis")

Dysrhythmokinesia is a disturbed rhythm associated with repetitive sequential movements, such as tapping movements (Wertham, 1929). It is a characteristic of adiadochokinesia.

Check and rebound

Disturbed check consists of a large displacement of the upper limbs when a tap is exerted over the hands while the patient is asked to keep the upper limbs outstretched. The excessive rebound is the overshoot followed by successive oscillations around the initial position. Impaired check is tested during the Stewart-Holmes test.

Isometrataxia

Cerebellar disorders are associated with an inability to generate constant forces, especially during tasks

SPREAD OF FEET IN NATURAL POSITION

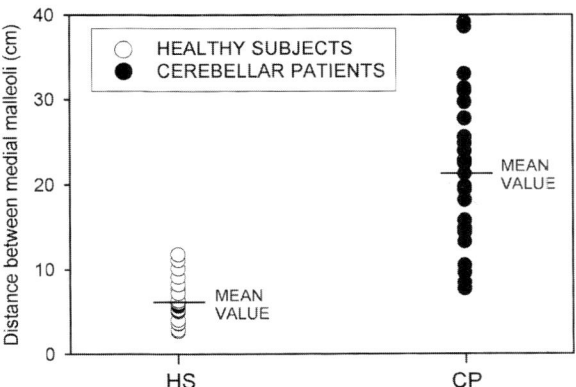

Figure 3.6 Spread of feet in a natural position. Left: healthy subjects (n = 25 subjects, age: 14 to 76 years), right: cerebellar patients (n = 25 patients, age: 13 to 78 years). Distance measured between the internal malleoli using an optoelectronic system. With permission from: Manto, 2002.

requiring hand and finger use (Mai et al., 1989). Isometrataxia is tested by asking the patient to exert a slight and constant pinch force between the lateral parts of the examiner's thumb. An irregular pressure is felt. It may be associated with action tremor. Isometrataxia is usually observed in the first hours following a cerebellar stroke.

Deficits in gait/posture

Gait can be considered as resulting from balance and locomotor tasks. Balance tasks include standing in an upright position, anticipatory adjustments, and postural responses to external forces. Locomotor tasks include the rhythmic character of movement. Both balance and locomotor tasks are defective in cerebellar disorders.

Ataxia of stance

Quiet stance is evaluated with the patient's eyes open and closed. The patient is asked to stand on one foot, then with feet in tandem, and then with feet together. The spread of feet in natural position with the eyes open is a simple and reliable test (Trouillas et al., 1997). The distance between the medial malleoli is measured. Values higher than 12 cm are abnormal (Manto, 2002; Figure 3.6). Eye closure during the Romberg test leads to increased ataxia of stance in the large majority of cerebellar patients. However, the exacerbation induced by eye closure is usually less pronounced than in

proprioceptive ataxia or in the so-called vestibular ataxia (Diener et al, 1984). Ataxia of stance is characterized by unstable body segments. The trunk tends to lurch from side to side. The drift on one side is called lateropulsion, which is usually towards the side of the lesion. Rhythmic extensions–flexions of the feet are common ("dancing feet"). Titubation refers to rhythmic oscillations of the head, trunk, or entire body in an anterior-posterior plane or a lateral plane or which tend to be rotatory. Titubation is often overlooked when oscillations are of small amplitudes (Lou & Jankovic, 1993). The scaling of the amplitude of postural responses is inappropriate, with patients falling in the direction opposite to the one in which a force is applied (Horak & Diener, 1994).

Ataxia of gait

Regular gait is tested in a 10-m test, including the examination of the half-turn. The test is followed by an assessment of walking in a straight line, walking in tandem, and walking backwards. Ataxic gait is irregular and broad-based, with unequal steps and multiple corrections. Rhythm is distorted, with a reduction in speed. Children with a transection of the posterior inferior cerebellar vermis are unable to perform tandem gait, whereas regular gait and standing are relatively preserved (posterior vermian split syndrome; Bastian et al., 1998). Lesions of the flocculonodular lobe are associated with ataxic gait also. "Frontal ataxia" is a form of gait apraxia observed in patients presenting with a frontal lesion. Coordination between trunk and lower limbs is poor, with feet crossing. Crossing the legs is very unusual in cerebellar gait. Cerebellar ataxia of gait needs to be distinguished from sensory ataxia (Table 3.8). Decreased or abolished tendon reflexes and decreased sensation(s) argue for a sensory ataxia. The main causes of sensory ataxia are listed in Table 3.8. Some patients exhibit combinations of cerebellar ataxic gait and sensory ataxia.

Psychogenic gait ataxia

Ataxic gait of psychogenic origin is one of the most common presentations of hysterical gait disorders (Keane, 1989). Suggestive historical clues include an abrupt onset, spontaneous remissions, somatizations, search for a compensation, context of litigations, and previous history of work in health care. Clinical clues include inconsistency of gait, the influence of distraction, self-inflicted injuries, disparities in neurological examination (such as ataxic gait while

Table 3.8 Principal causes of sensory ataxia

Familial sensory neuropathy (autosomal dominant)

Diabetes

Anti-neoplastic drugs (cisplatin, oxaliplatin, paclitaxel)

Immune origin (Miller Fisher syndrome, anti-MAG antibodies, GALOP syndrome)

Paraneoplastic (anti-Hu syndrome)

Intoxication to pyridoxine

Refsum disease

Diphtheria

Abbreviations: GALOP: gait ataxia late-onset polyneuropathy; MAG: myelin-associated glycoprotein.

heel-to-knee test is normal) or discrepancies during repeated neurological examination, uneconomic postures with wastage of energy, remission with placebo, and positive findings during a psychiatric interview. Co-morbidity with a true cerebellar ataxia is not exceptional.

Autonomic signs

Autonomic signs may result from increased intracranial pressure, concomitant brainstem damage, or genuine involvement of the autonomic centers (see also Chapter 18). There is growing evidence that pure cerebellar lesions may affect autonomic control (Haines et al., 1997). These clinical manifestations might be underestimated. Voluntary movements may trigger a vasomotor response, such as face flushing and pupil dilatation. Bradycardia and hyperventilation have been reported.

"Cognitive abnormalities" and emotional disorders

Cerebellar patients may present with cognitive and behavioral changes. Some clinicians still believe that the constellation of cognitive deficits remains very subtle as compared with motor deficits. The concept of cognitive dysmetria has been brought up, by extension to the observations of motor deficits (Andreasen et al., 1996). The terminology of "cerebellar cognitive affective syndrome" (CCAS) encompasses impairment of executive functions, including planning and working memory, deficits in visuospatial skills, linguistic deficiencies such as agrammatism, and inappropriate behavior (Schmahmann & Sherman, 1998). The neuropsychiatric manifestations associated with cerebel-

Table 3.9 Neuropsychiatric symptoms in cerebellar disorders

Domain	Positive symptoms	Negative symptoms
Attention	Distractibility Hyperactivity Compulsive behavior	Perseveration Difficulties for shifting attention Obsessional behavior
Emotion	Impulsiveness, disinhibition Anxiety, agitation Pathological laughing and crying	Anhedonia Depression Dysphoria
Social skill set	Aggression Irritability	Passivity Difficulties with social interactions
Psychosis	Illogical thinking Hallucinations	Lack of empathy Emotional blunting
Autism spectrum	Stereotypes	Avoidant behavior Sensory overload

Adapted from: Schmahmann and Pandya (2008).

Table 3.10 Cerebellar disorders associated with the cerebellar cognitive affective syndrome[a]

Cerebellar stroke

Post-operative period (cerebellar tumor, malformation)

Cerebellar malformation (hypoplasia, agenesis)

Trauma

Superficial siderosis

Hereditary disorders (Gillespie syndrome)

Paraneoplastic cerebellar ataxia

Drugs (topiramate)

[a]See Collinson et al., 2006; Turkel et al., 2006; Baillieux et al., 2008; Mariën et al., 2008; Uttner et al., 2009.

lar disorders are shown in Table 3.9. The conditions associated with CCAS are given in Table 3.10. The main deficits reported in hereditary ataxias (see also Chapter 23) are summarized in Table 3.11. Executive dysfunction is commonly reported. Tasks requiring planning/initiation, sustaining and inhibiting activity, inferring, judging, and shifting set are commonly abnormal in inherited ataxias, but a pre-morbid state might strongly influence their severity and mode of presentation. Some patients with autosomal dominant spinocerebellar ataxia (SCA) exhibit a clear intellectual decline, such as SCA17 or dentatorubral pallidoluysian atrophy (see also Chapter 23). Mood disorders and personality changes are not exceptional.

Table 3.11 Cognitive deficits in hereditary ataxias[a]

Dominant ataxias
  Spinocerebellar ataxias
    Mental deterioration
    Defects in memory
    Defective verbal and non-verbal intelligence
    Impaired executive function
    Restlessness and emotional instability
    Perseverations
    Apathy
    Depression
    Aggressivity
    Psychotic-like behavior

  Episodic ataxias
    Anxiety
    Depression
    Attentional deficits
    Subtle learning deficits

  Gillespie syndrome
    Cerebellar cognitive affective syndrome

  Spastic paraplegia, ataxia, and mental retardation syndrome
    Variable degrees of mental deterioration

Recessive ataxias
  Friedreich ataxia
    Abnormal information processing
    Impaired verbal learning
    Abnormal visuospatial tasks
    Impaired executive function
    Personality changes: irritability, impulsiveness, reduced
      defensiveness, and blunting of affect

  Ataxia with oculomotor apraxia
    Impaired learning and retrieval information
    Impaired executive function

  Ataxia-telangiectasia
    Low verbal IQ

  Joubert syndrome
    Learning deficits (developmental delay, psychomotor
      retardation)

  Congenital disorders of glycosylation syndrome
    Mental deficits

X-linked ataxias
  Fragile X–associated tremor ataxia syndrome
    Impaired executive functions
    Anxiety
    Irritability, agitation
    Psychosis
    Depression
    Frontal-subcortical dementia

[a]See Goldfarb et al., 1989; Spadaro et al., 1992; Dubourg et al., 1995; Zawacki et al., 2002; Bellebaum and Daum, 2007

Lexicosemantic knowledge may be impaired in subjects with advanced SCA, suggesting that language may become affected as the disorder progresses. Reduced speed of processing of visual information and inability to shift attention are encountered in the end stage of the disease. Attentional deficits are congru-ent with the hypothesis of a role of the cerebellum in providing attentional resources allotted in a rapid way. Speech may be characterized by vocal instability, reduced rate, and monotony, complicating dysarthria (Schalling et al., 2008).

The constellation of cognitive/behavioral deficits is suggestive of a disruption of the cerebellar modulation of the neural circuits that link the prefrontal, posterior parietal, superior temporal, and limbic structures, including the amygdala, hippocampus, and septum (Schutter & van Honk, 2009). Actually, nearly all regions of the associative and paralimbic cortices project to the pontine nuclei in a segregated manner, and the pontine nuclei send mossy fibers to the cerebellum. The prefrontal cortex projects to the medial and dorsomedial regions of the pons, the association areas of the temporal lobes project to the lateral pons, the superior regions of the parietal association cortices project to the central pons, the inferior parietal regions send projections to the rostral pons, and the paralimbic regions project to the medial and lateral pontine nuclei. A "limbic cerebellum" has even been suggested (Schmahmann et al., 2007). Impaired performance on the Wisconsin Card Sorting Task points towards damage to the dorsolateral prefrontal cortex and/or its subcortical connections, including the cerebellar circuits (Nagahama et al., 1996). Behavioral changes might be more common in patients presenting with lesions of the posterior cerebellar lobe and the vermis. Attention errors and abnormal visuospatial skills are reported repeatedly in these patients. Visuospatial deficits might be more common in cases of left side cerebellar lesions.

Positive effects of electrical cerebellar stimulation on mood in psychiatric disorders have been reported, suggesting a role of the cerebellum in human emotion (Heath, 1977). Indeed, damage to the vermis has been associated with emotional dysregulation (Levisohn et al., 2000). Which form of the emotional process is handled by cerebellar circuitry remains an open question (Schutter & van Honk, 2005; Koziol & Budding, 2009). The so-called posterior fossa syndrome can be considered as a very acute form of CCAS. The syndrome affects mainly children between the age of 2 and 10 years. Following resection of a midline tumor of the cerebellum, children show mutism, buccal and lingual apraxia, apathy, and poverty of movements (Riva & Giorgi, 2000). Mutism often develops 1 to 5 days after the resection. Post-surgical mutism evolves into speech disorders or language

47

disturbances similar to agrammatism and behavioral disturbances ranging from irritability to behaviors reminiscent of autism, with emotional lability (irritability, emotional reactions, agitation) and regressive personality changes. When the lesion involves the vermis and spares the hemispheres, mutism quickly develops into dysarthria, and dysarthria will improve markedly. When both the vermis and the right cerebellar hemisphere are involved, the recovery of speech is slow, and speech often becomes monotonous and telegraphic, reminiscent of speech deficits found in frontal lobe lesions. Concomitant cognitive deficits are common: impairment in the shifting of attention, perseveration, and difficulties in problem solving.

Some of the behavioral symptoms observed in cerebellar patients are also observed in attention deficit hyperactivity disorder and schizophrenia, two conditions in which the cerebellar circuitry has been implicated via neuroimaging studies and post-mortem investigations (Ashtari et al., 2005; Picard et al., 2008). This is corroborated by the findings of impaired eyeblink conditioning, impaired adaptation of the VOR, deficits in procedural learning tests, the correlation between poor cognitive performance and abnormal cerebellar activations on neuroimaging evaluation, and reports of decreased size of the cerebellar vermis (Okugawa et al., 2003). In addition, diffusion tensor imaging, a technique which detects subtle disruptions of neural connectivity, has shown reduction of fractional anisotropy (a parameter which reflects the integrity and orientation of neural tissue) in the middle and superior cerebellar peduncles of patients with schizophrenia, suggesting a neural disconnectivity between the cerebellum and cerebral cortex (Okugawa et al., 2005; Okugawa et al., 2006). However, the cerebellar contribution might be limited or indirect. Autism spectrum disorders are discussed in Chapter 16.

Lesion–symptom mapping

The introduction of high-resolution structural brain imaging and new analysis methods has led to significant improvements in our understanding of the correlations between the anatomy of cerebellar lesions and the observed clinical deficits (Rorden & Karnath, 2004). Signal-to-noise ratio on MRI increases with increasing field strength and now allows spatial resolution in the submillimeter range (Timmann et al., 2009).

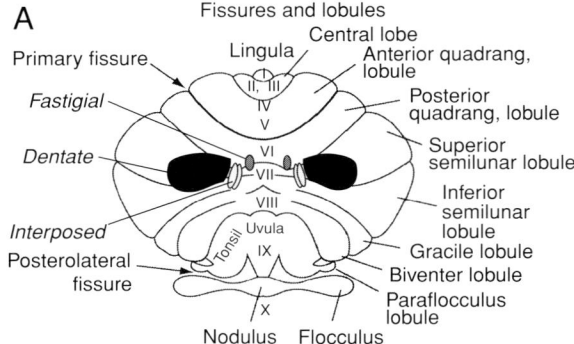

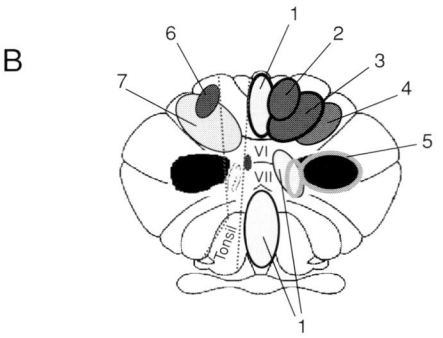

Figure 3.7 Lesion symptom mapping. (A) Cerebellar lobules shown on an unfolded cerebellum. (B) Lesion-symptom mapping. Schematic sketch of findings in patients with focal cerebellar lesions. The figure summarizes the results of lesion-symptom mapping in studies on eyeblink conditioning, cerebellar ataxia rating scores, balance in stance and gait, and upper and lower limb coordination. 1: ataxia of stance/gait; 2: lower limb ataxia; 3: upper limb ataxia; 4: dysarthria; 5: limb ataxia; 6: conditioned eyeblink response (CR) timing; 7: CR acquisition. Adapted from: Timmann et al., 2008. (See color section).

Lesion-based MRI subtraction analysis shows that the fastigial nuclei (and to a lesser degree the interposed nuclei) are more frequently affected in patients with impaired compared with unimpaired dynamic balance control (Timmann et al., 2009; Figure 3.7). Also, the interposed and the adjacent dentate nuclei are more frequently affected in patients with impaired leg placement compared with those with non-impaired leg placement. Patients with impaired leg placement abnormalities exhibit difficulties in the adaptation of locomotion to additional loads. Recent data show that the intermediate zone appears to be of particular importance for multi-joint limb control both in goal-directed leg movements and in locomotion. Lesions of the intermediate zone may lead to impaired leg and trunk coordination.

In cerebellar stroke, a somatotopy of the superior cerebellar cortex is found, in agreement with animal data and functional MRI observations in healthy control subjects (Grodd et al., 2001). Upper limb ataxia is correlated with lesions of cerebellar lobules IV–V and VI. Lower limb ataxia is correlated with lesions of lobules III and IV. Dysarthria is correlated with lesions of lobules V and VI. Limb ataxia is correlated with lesions of the interposed and part of the dentate nuclei, and ataxia of posture and gait is correlated with lesions of the fastigial nuclei, including part of interposed nuclei. Recovery after lesions to the nuclei of the cerebellum is often less complete (Eckmiller & Westheimer, 1983).

In cerebellar cortical degeneration, there is a significant correlation between the cerebellar degeneration and both International Cooperative Ataxia Rating Scale and Scale for Assessment and Rating of Ataxia scores (see Chapter 4). Oculomotor disorders are highly correlated with atrophy of the medial cerebellum. Posture and gait ataxia subscores show the highest correlations with the medial and intermediate cerebellar volume, whereas impairment in limb kinetic functions correlates with atrophy of lateral and intermediate parts of the cerebellum. Atrophy of the intermediate zone is correlated not only with limb ataxia and dysarthria, but also with ataxia of stance and gait.

For classical conditioning of the eyeblink response, a form of motor learning (see Chapter 2), learning rate in healthy subjects is related to the volume of the cortex of the posterior cerebellar lobe (Timmann et al., 2008). In patients with focal cerebellar lesions, acquisition of eyeblink conditioning is significantly decreased in lesions that include the cortex of the superior posterior lobe, but not the inferior posterior lobe. Impaired timing of conditioned eyeblink responses correlates with lesions of the anterior lobe. A meta-analysis of neuroimaging studies supports the following functional topography (Stoodley & Schmahmann, 2009):

- Sensorimotor tasks activate the anterior lobe (lobule V) and adjacent lobule VI, with additional foci in lobule VIII. Motor activation is linked with activation in lobules VIIIA/B, and somatosensory activation is confined to VIIIB.
- The posterior lobe is involved in higher-level tasks. Lobule VI and crus I are activated in language and verbal working memory; lobule VI is activated in spatial tasks; lobules VI, crus I, and lobule VIIB are activated in executive functions;

and lobule VI, crus I, and medial VII are activated during emotional processing. Language is right-lateralized, whereas spatial processing shows a greater left hemisphere activation. Language and executive tasks activate regions of crus I and lobule VII implicated in prefrontal-cerebellar loops. Emotional processing is associated with activation of the vermal lobule VII, participating in cerebellar-limbic circuitry. Functional neuroimaging investigations support the hypothesis that there is an anterior sensorimotor versus posterior cognitive/emotional dichotomy in the human cerebellum (Stoodley & Schmahmann, 2009). Motor tasks are localized to the anterior lobe, with a secondary representation in lobules VIIIA/B; somatosensory tasks also involve the anterior lobe, with a secondary representation in lobule VIIIB. None of the "higher-level" language, working memory, spatial, or executive tasks are associated with activation in the anterior lobe. These observations are in agreement with the hypothesis of a double representation of the body in the cerebellum (Snider & Eldred, 1951).

References

Amarenco P, Chevrie-Muller C, Roullet E, Bousser MG. Paravermal infarct and isolated cerebellar dysarthria. *Ann Neurol* 1991;**30**:211–13.

Andreasen NC, O'Leary DS, Cizadlo T, et al. Schizophrenia and cognitive dysmetria: a positron-emission tomography study of dysfunctional prefrontal-thalamic-cerebellar circuitry. *Proc Natl Acad Sci USA* 1996;**93**:9985–90.

Ashtari M, Kumra S, Bhaskar SL, et al. Attention-deficit/hyperactivity disorder: a preliminary diffusion tensor imaging study. *Biol Psychiatry* 2005;**57**(5):448–55.

Babinski J. De l'asynergie cérébelleuse. *Rev Neurol* 1899;**7**:806–16.

Babinski J. Sur le rôle du cervelet dans les actes volitionnels nécessitant une succession rapide de mouvements (diadococinésie). *Rev Neurol* 1902;**10**:1013–15.

Baier B, Bense S, Dieterich M. Are signs of ocular tilt reaction in patients with cerebellar lesions mediated by the dentate nucleus? *Brain* 2008;**131**(Pt 6): 1445–54.

Baillieux H, Verslegers W, Paquier P, De Deyn PP, Mariën P. Cerebellar cognitive affective syndrome associated with topiramate. *Clin Neurol Neurosurg* 2008;**110**(5):496–9.

Bastian AJ, Mink JW, Kaufman BA, Thach WT. Posterior vermal split syndrome. *Ann Neurol* 1998;**44**:601–10.

Bellebaum C, Daum I. Cerebellar involvement in executive control. *Cerebellum* 2007;**6**:184–92.

Bertholon P, Bronstein AM, Davies RA, Rudge P, Thilo KV. Positional down beating nystagmus in 50 patients: cerebellar disorders and possible anterior semicircular canalithiasis. *J Neurol Neurosurg Psychiatry* 2002;**72**(3):366–72.

Chae JH, Kim SK, Wang KC, et al. Hemifacial seizure of cerebellar ganglioglioma origin: seizure control by tumor resection. *Epilepsia* 2001;**42**(9):1204–7.

Chase RA, Cullen JK, Sullivan SA, Ommaya AK. Modification of intention tremor in man. *Nature* 1965;**206**:485–7.

Cogan DG. Ocular dysmetria, flutter-like oscillations of the eyes, and opsoclonus. *Arch Ophtalmol* 1954;**51**:318–35.

Collinson SL, Anthonisz B, Courtenay D, Winter C. Frontal executive impairment associated with paraneoplastic cerebellar degeneration: a case study. *Neurocase* 2006;**12**(6):350–4.

Delande O, Rodriguez D, Chiron C, Fohlen M. Successful surgical relief of seizures associated with hamartoma of the floor of the fourth ventricle in children: report of two cases. *Neurosurgery* 2001;**49**(3):726–30.

Dichgans J. Clinical symptoms of cerebellar dysfunction and their topogiagnostical significance. *Hum Neurobiol* 1984;**2**:269–79.

Diener HC, Dichgans J, Bacher M, Gompf B. Quantification of postural sway in normals and patients with cerebellar disease. *EEG Clin Neurophysiol* 1984;**57**:134–42.

Dow RS, Moruzzi G. *The Physiology and Pathology of the Cerebellum*. Minneapolis: University of Minnesota Press, 1958.

Dubourg O, Dürr A, Cancel G, et al. Analysis of the SCA1 CAG repeat in a large number of families with dominant ataxia: clinical and molecular correlations. *Ann Neurol* 1995;**37**(2):176–80.

Du Pasquier R, Vingerhoets F, Safran AB, Landis T. Periodic nystagmus. *Neurology* 1998;**51**:1478–80.

Eckmiller R, Westheimer G. Compensation of oculomotor deficits in monkeys with neonatal cerebellar ablations. *Exp Brain Res* 1983;**49**(3):315–26.

Fetter M, Klockgether T, Schultz JB, Koenig E, Dichgans J. Oculomotor abnormalities and MRI findings in idiopathic cerebellar ataxia. *J Neurol* 1994;**241**:234–41.

Frassanito P, Massimi L, Caldarelli M, Di Rocco C. Cerebellar mutism after spontaneous intratumoral

bleeding involving the upper cerebellar vermis: a contribution to the physiopathogenic interpretation. *Childs Nerv Syst* 2009;**25**(1):7–11.

Gilman S, Bloedel JR, Lechtenberg R. *Disorders of the Cerebellum: Contemporary Neurology Series*. Philadelphia: FA Davis, 1981.

Goldfarb LG, Chumakov MP, Petrov PA, Fedorova NI, Gajdusek DC. Olivopontocerebellar atrophy in a large Iakut kinship in eastern Siberia. *Neurology* 1989;**39**(11):1527–30.

Grodd W, Hülsmann E, Lotze M, Wildgruber D, Erb M. Sensorimotor mapping of the human cerebellum: fMRI evidence of somatotopic organization. *Hum Brain Mapp* 2001;**13**(2):55–73.

Haines DE, Dietrichs E, Mihailoff GA, McDonald EF. The cerebellar-hypothalamic axis: basic circuits and clinical observations. In *The Cerebellum and Cognition*, ed. J.D. Schmahmann. San Diego: Academic Press, 1997, pp. 83–107.

Harvey AS, Jayakar P, Duchowny M, et al. Hemifacial seizures and cerebellar ganglioglioma: an epilepsy syndrome of infancy with seizures of cerebellar origin. *Ann Neurol* 1996;**40**:91–8.

Heath RG. Modulation of emotion with a brain pacemaker: treatment for intractable psychiatric illness. *J Nerv Ment Dis* 1977;**165**:300–17.

Holmes G. The cerebellum of man. The Hughlings Jackson memorial lecture. *Brain* 1939;**62**:1–30.

Holmes G. Clinical symptoms of cerebellar disease and their interpretation. The Croonian lecture III. *Lancet* 1922;**2**:59–65.

Holmes G. The symptoms of acute cerebellar injuries from gunshot wounds. *Brain* 1917;**40**:461–535.

Horak FB, Diener HC. Cerebellar control of postural scaling and central set in stance. *J Neurophysiol* 1994;**72**:479–93.

Keane JR. Hysterical gait disorders: 60 cases. *Neurology* 1989;**39**:586–9.

Kent RD, Kent JF, Rosenbek JC, Vorperian HK, Weismer G. A speaking task analysis of the dysarthria in cerebellar disease. *Folia Phoniatr Logop* 1997;**49**:63–82.

Kinsbourne M. Myoclonic encephalopathy in infants. *J Neurol Neurosurg Psychiatry* 1962;**25**:271–9.

Koziol LF, Budding DE. *Subcortical Structures and Cognition: Implications for Neuropsychological Assessment*. New York: Springer, 2009.

Lapresle J. Rhythmic palatal myoclonus and the dentato-olivary pathway. *J Neurol* 1979;**220**; 223–30.

Lechtenberg R. Signs and symptoms of cerebellar disease. In *Handbook of Cerebellar Diseases*, ed. R. Lechtenberg. New York: Marcel Dekker, 1993, pp. 31–43.

Levisohn L, Cronin-Golomb A, Schmahmann JD. Neuropsychological consequences of cerebellar tumour resection in children: cerebellar cognitive affective syndrome in a paediatric population. *Brain* 2000;**123**:1041–50.

Lewis RF, Zee DS. Ocular motor disorders associated with cerebellar lesions: pathophysiology and topical localization. *Rev Neurol (Paris)* 1993;**149**:665–77.

Lou JS, Jankovic J. Origin and treatment of tremor in cerebellar disease. In *Handbook of Cerebellar Diseases*, ed. R. Lechtenberg. New York: Marcel Dekker, 1993, pp. 45–63.

Mai N, Diener HC, Dichgans J. On the role of feedback in maintaining constant grip force in patients with cerebellar disease. *Neurosci Lett* 1989;**99**:340–4.

Manto M. Clinical signs of cerebellar disorders. In *The Cerebellum and its Disorders*, ed. M. Manto and M. Pandolfo. Cambridge, UK: Cambridge University Press, 2002, pp. 97–120.

Manto M. Mechanisms of human cerebellar dysmetria: experimental evidence and current conceptual bases. *J Neuroeng Rehabil* 2009;**6**:10.

Manto M, Godaux E, Jacquy J. Cerebellar hypermetria is larger when the inertial load os artificially increased. *Ann Neurol* 1994;**35**:45–52.

Manto M, Godaux E, Jacquy J. Detection of silent cerebellar lesions by increasing the inertial load of the moving hand. *Ann Neurol* 1995;**37**:344–50.

Mariën P, Brouns R, Engelborghs S, et al. Cerebellar cognitive affective syndrome without global mental retardation in two relatives with Gillespie syndrome. *Cortex* 2008;**44**(1):54–67.

Matsui M, Tomimoto H, Sano K, et al. Paroxysmal dysarthria and ataxia after midbrain infarction. *Neurology* 2004;**63**(2):345–7.

Mauritz KH, Dichgans J, Hufschmidt A. Quantitative analysis of stance in late cortical cerebellar atrophy of the anterior lobe and other forms of cerebellar ataxia. *Brain* 1979;**102**:461–82.

Mossman S, Halmagyi GM. Partial ocular tilt reaction due to unilateral cerebellar lesion. *Neurology* 1997;**49**:491–3.

Nagahama Y, Fukuyama H, Yamauchi H, et al. Cerebral activation during performance of a card sorting test. *Brain* 1996;**119**(Pt 5):1667–75.

Okugawa G, Nobuhara K, Minami T, et al. Neural disorganization in the superior cerebellar peduncle and cognitive abnormality in patients with schizophrenia a diffusion tensor imaging study. *Prog Neuropsychopharmacol Biol Psychiatry* 2006;**30**(8):1408–12.

Okugawa G, Nobuhara K, Sugimoto T, Kinoshita T. Diffusion tensor imaging study of the middle cerebellar peduncles in patients with schizophrenia. *Cerebellum* 2005;**4**(2):123–7.

Okugawa G, Sedvall GC, Agartz I. Smaller cerebellar vermis but not hemisphere volumes in patients with chronic schizophrenia. *Am J Psychiatry* 2003;**160**(9):1614–7.

Orzechowski K. De l'ataxie dysmétrique des yeux: remarques sur l'ataxie des yeux dite myoclonique (opsoclonie, opsochorie). *J Psychol Neurol* 1927;**35**:1–18.

Picard H, Amado I, Mouchet-Mages S, Olié JP, Krebs MO. The role of the cerebellum in schizophrenia: an update of clinical, cognitive, and functional evidences. *Schizophr Bull* 2008;**34**(1):155–72.

Rekate HL, Grubb RL, Aram DL, Hahn JF, Ratcheson RA. Muteness of cerebellar origin. *Arch Neurol* 1985;**42**:697–8.

Riva D, Giorgi C. The cerebellum contributes to higher functions during development: evidence from a series of children surgically treated for posterior fossa tumours. *Brain* 2000;**123**(Pt 5):1051–61.

Rorden C, Karnath HO. Using human brain lesions to infer function: a relic from a past era in the fMRI age? *Nat Rev Neurosci* 2004;**5**:813–19.

Samuel M, Torun N, Tuite PJ, Sharpe JA, Lang AE. Progressive ataxia and palatal tremor (PAPT): clinical and MRI assessment with review of palatal tremors. *Brain* 2004;**127**(Pt 6):1252–68.

Schalling E, Hammarberg B, Hartelius L. A longitudinal study of dysarthria in spinocerebellar ataxia: aspects of articulation, prosody and voice. *J Med Speech Lang Pathol* 2008;**16**(2):103–17.

Schmahmann JD, Pandya DN. Disconnection syndromes of basal ganglia, thalamus, and cerebrocerebellar systems. *Cortex* 2008;**44**(8):1037–66.

Schmahmann JD, Sherman JC. The cerebellar cognitive affective syndrome. *Brain* 1998;**121**:561–79.

Schmahmann JD, Weilburg JB, Sherman JC. The neuropsychiatry of the cerebellum: insights from the clinic. *Cerebellum* 2007;**6**(3):254–67.

Schutter DJ, van Honk J. The cerebellum in emotion regulation: a repetitive transcranial magnetic stimulation study. *Cerebellum* 2009;**8**(1):28–34.

Schutter DJ, van Honk J. The cerebellum on the rise of human emotion. *Cerebellum* 2005;**4**:290–4.

Selhorst JB, Stark L, Ochs AL, Hoyt WF. Disorders in cerebellar ocular motor control: I. Saccadic overshoot dysmetria. An oculographic, control system and clinico-anatomical analysis. *Brain* 1976;**99**:497–508.

Snider R, Eldred E. Electro-anatomical studies on cerebro-cerebellar connections in the cat. *J Comp Neurol* 1951;**95**:1–16.

Spadaro M, Giunti P, Lulli P, et al. HLA-linked spinocerebellar ataxia: a clinical and genetic study of large Italian kindreds. *Acta Neurol Scand* 1992;**85**(4):257–65.

Stewart TG, Holmes G. Symptomatology of cerebellar tumors: a study of forty cases. *Brain* 1904;**27**: 522–91.

Stoodley CJ, Schmahmann JD. Functional topography in the human cerebellum: a meta-analysis of neuroimaging studies. *NeuroImage* 2009;**44**:489–501.

Timmann D, Brandauer B, Hermsdörfer J, et al. Lesion-symptom mapping of the human cerebellum. *Cerebellum* 2008;**7**(4):602–6.

Timmann D, Konczak J, Ilg W, et al. Current advances in lesion-symptom mapping of the human cerebellum. *Neuroscience* 2009;**162**:836–51.

Trouillas P, Takayanagi T, Hallett M, et al. International cooperative ataxia rating scale for pharmacological assessment of the cerebellar syndrome. *J Neurol Sci* 1997;**145**:205–11.

Turkel SB, Brumm VL, Mitchell WG, Tavare CJ. Mood and behavioral dysfunction with opsoclonus-myoclonus ataxia. *J Neuropsychiatry Clin Neurosci* 2006;**18**(2):239–41.

Uttner I, Tumani H, Arnim C, Brettschneider J. Cognitive impairment in superficial siderosis of the central nervous system: a case report. *Cerebellum* 2009;**8**(1):61–3.

Van Dongen HR, Catsman-Berrevoets CE, van Mourik M. The syndrome of 'cerebellar' mutism and subsequent dysarthria. *Neurology* 1994;**44**:2040–6.

Wertham FI. A new sign of cerebellar disease. *J Nerv Ment Dis* 1929;**69**:486–93.

Yee RD, Baloh RW, Honrubia V. Episodic vertical oscillopsia and nystagmus in a Chiari malformation. *Arch Ophtalmol* 1984;**102**:723–5.

Zawacki T, Grace J, Friedman J, Sudarsky L. Executive and emotional dysfunction in Machado-Joseph disease. *Mov Disord* 2002;**17**(5):1004–10.

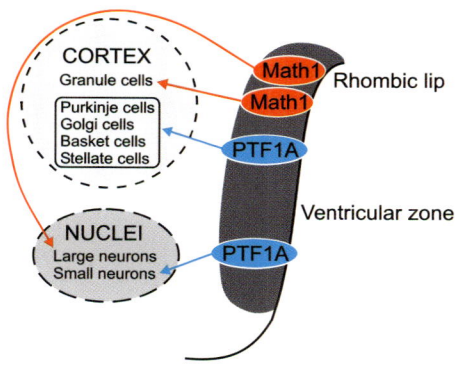

Figure 1.4 Cerebellar neurons are generated from two anatomically distinct progenitor zones within the primordia. Math-1 expressing neuroepithelium (rhombic lip) generates glutamatergic neurons (red arrows). PTF1A-expressing neuroepithelium (ventricular zone) generates GABAergic neurons (blue arrows). Cells leaving the rhombic lip migrate over the anlage and form an external layer of cells which continue to proliferate. Granule neuron progenitors form the external granular layer (EGL). Inward radial migration of EGL generates the internal granular layer (IGL). Cerebellar Purkinje neurons are post-mitotic as they leave the ventricular zone. Adapted from: Hoshino, 2006.

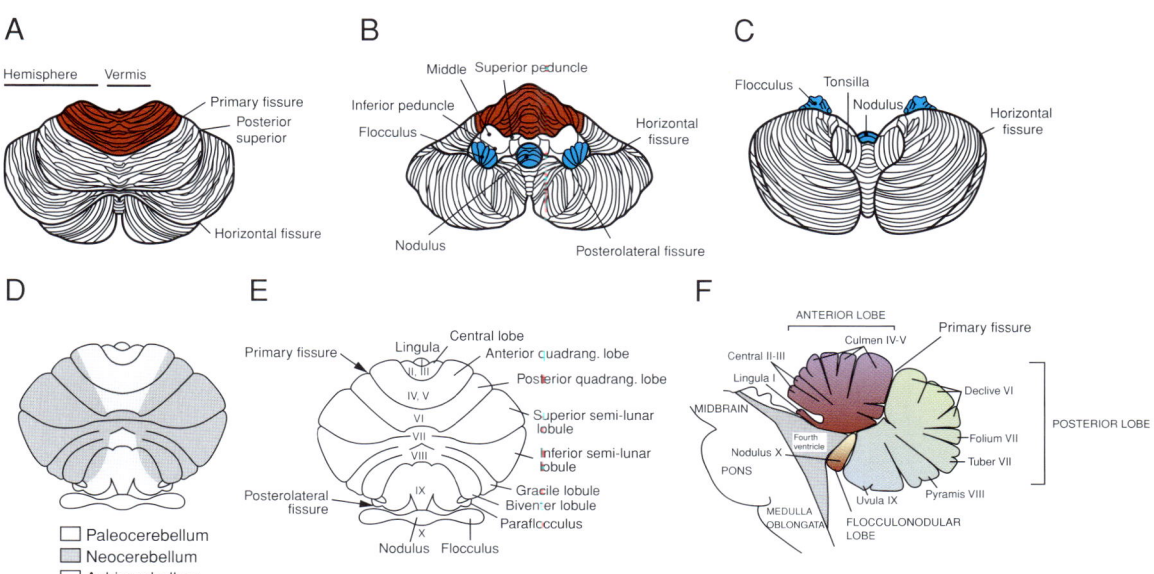

Figure 1.6 Illustration of the human cerebellum. (A) Superior view. The anterior lobe is demarcated from the posterior lobe by the primary fissure. (B) Anterior-inferior view showing the cerebellar peduncles. The flocculonodular lobe, delineated by the posterolateral fissure, is visible. (C) Inferior view showing the posterior part of the posterior lobe and the flocculonodular lobe. (D) Phylogenetic division of the cerebellum in paleocerebellum (medially), neocerebellum (laterally), and archicerebellum (flocculonodular lobe) represented on an unfolded cerebellum. (E) Division in 10 lobules. (F) Components of the vermis. From: Colin et al., 2002. With permission.

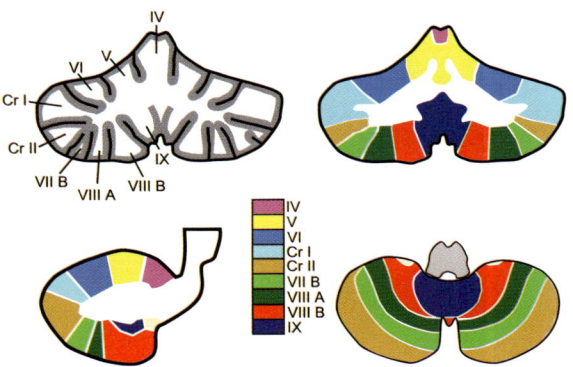

Figure 1.7 Parcellation of the cerebellum in individual lobules. Upper panels, coronal sections; lower left, parasagittal section; lower right, inferior view of the cerebellum.

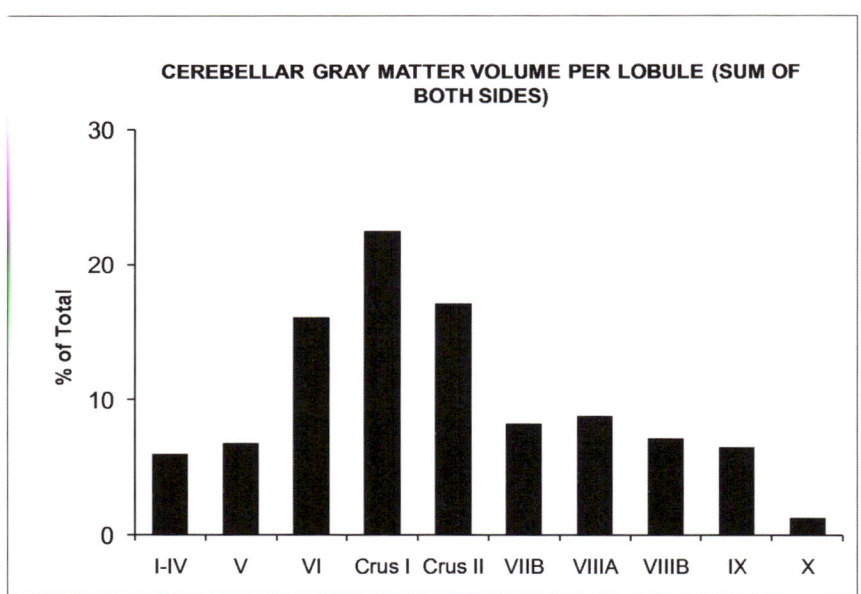

Figure 1.9 Volume of lobules in percentage of the total estimated cerebellar gray matter volume in healthy adults (total = 100%). Volumes of left and right side are considered together. Adapted from: Diedrichsen et al., 2009.

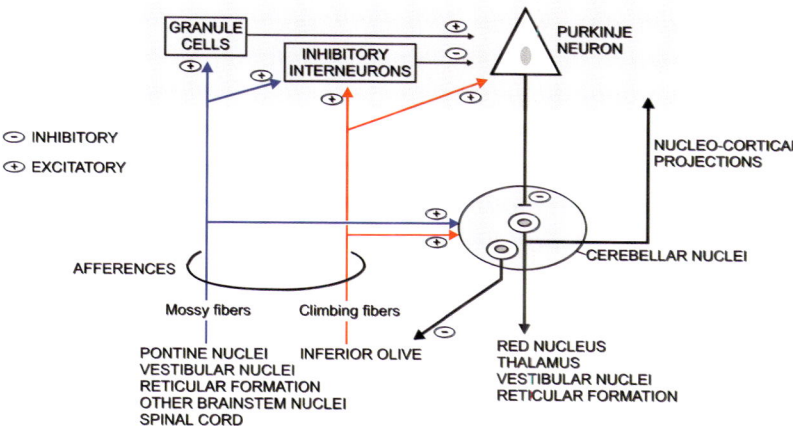

A

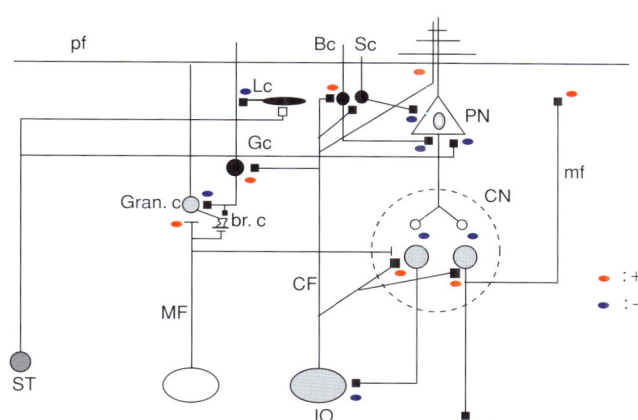

B

Figure 1.10 Wiring and connections of the cerebellar circuitry. (A) Mossy fibers (blue) and climbing fibers (red) project to cerebellar cortex (grey area) and cerebellar nuclei. The Purkinje neuron interacts with granule cells and inhibitory interneurons of the cerebellar cortex. Purkinje cells represent the output of the cerebellar cortex. Purkinje neurons inhibit cerebellar nuclei, which are the origin of the output emerging from the cerebellum. (B) Neurons of cerebellar circuitry. Abbreviations: MF: mossy fiber; CF: climbing fiber; IO: inferior olive; Gran. c: granule cell; br. C: brush cell; Gc: Golgi cell; Lc: Lugaro cell; Bc: basket cell; Sc: stellate cell; pf: parallel fiber; PN: Purkinje neuron; CN: cerebellar nuclei. +: excitatory; – : inhibitory.

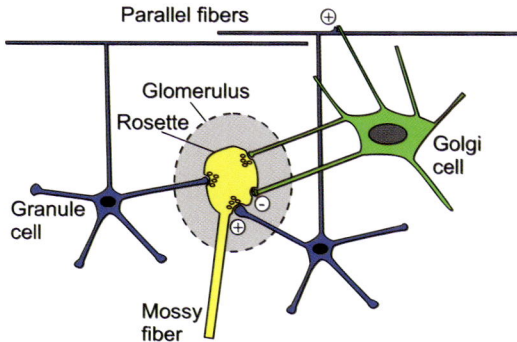

Figure 1.11 The glomerulus. The enlarged extremity of a mossy fiber (represented in yellow), called "rosette," is connected with dendrites of the granule cells (shown in blue) and a Golgi cell (illustrated in green). It also receives an axonal projection from the latter. Therefore, Golgi cells regulate mossy fiber inputs. Golgi cells are themselves excited by parallel fibers emerging from the granule cells.

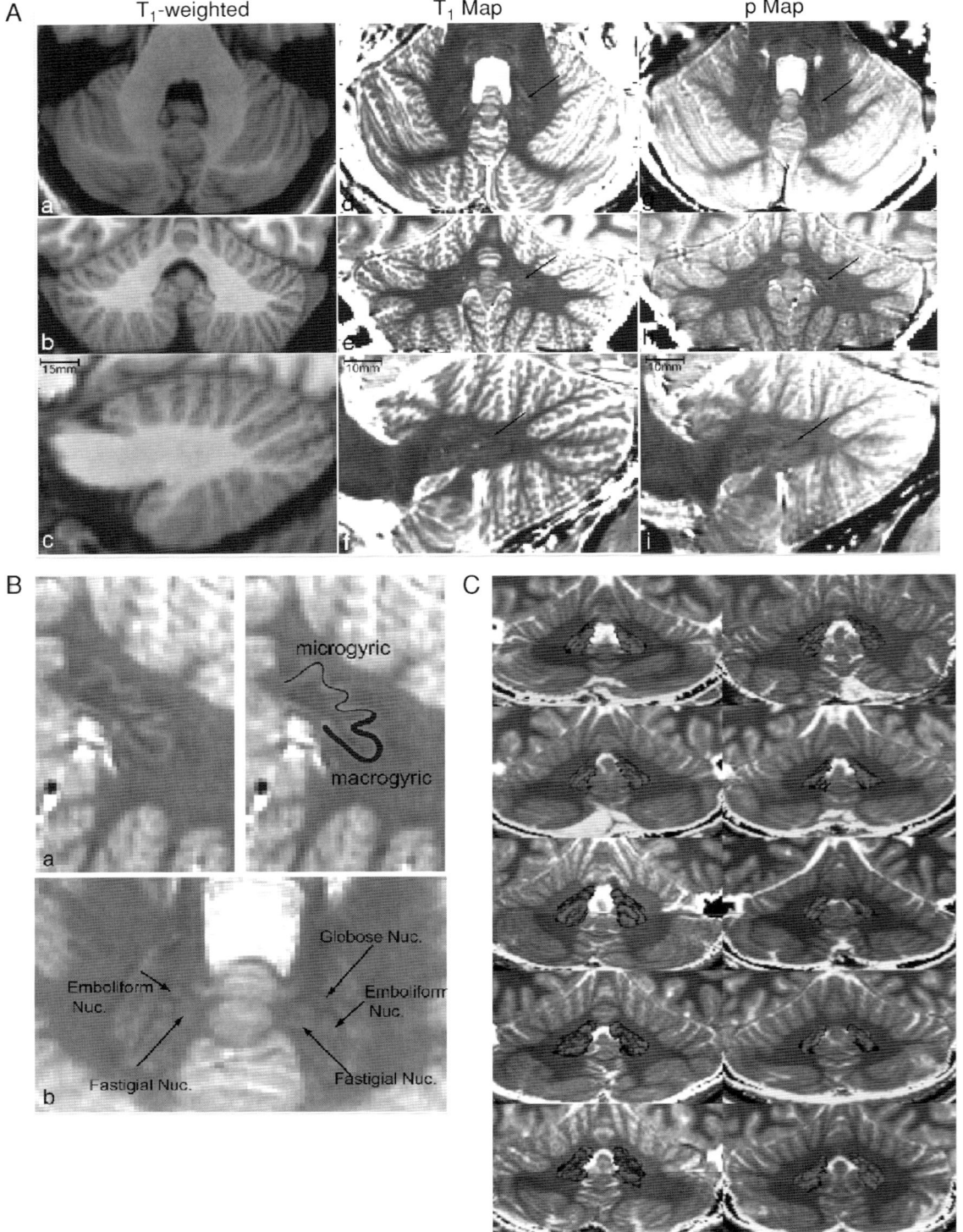

Figure 1.12 Imaging of cerebellar nuclei in adults using high-resolution MRI. (A) (a–c) Axial, coronal, and sagittal slices of the human cerebellum and corresponding slices through the high resolution (0.7 × 0.7 × 0.7 mm 3 voxels) ρ (d–f) and T1 (g–i) maps calculated from multi-averaged data requiring 40 min of scan time. The dentate, as well as globose and emboliform nuclei of the interposed nucleus, can be clearly delineated on both the T1 and ρ maps, allowing their anatomy to be fully appreciated. Arrows indicate the dentate nucleus on each image. (B) Anatomy of the deep cerebellar nuclei. Upper row, the dentate nucleus is composed of two parts: a dorsomedial and rostral region with narrow dentations (microgyric dentate) and a ventrolateral and caudal portion with wide and subdivided gyrations (macrogyric dentate). Lower picture: identification of the fastigial, globose and emboliform nuclei. (C) Volume renderings of the dentate nuclei of each of 10 adults, superimposed on their corresponding T1 maps. The images are taken from the superior-anterior viewpoint. From: Deoni and Catani, 2007. With permission.

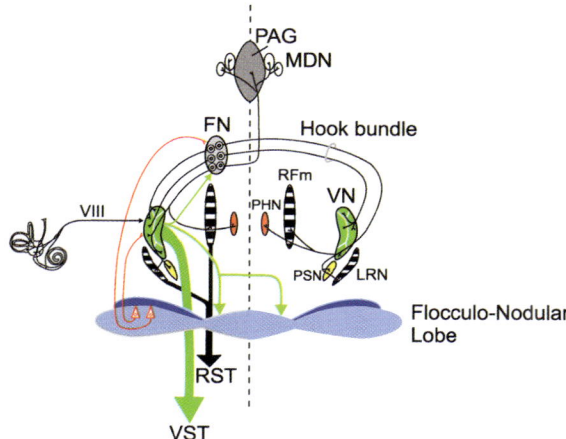

Figure 1.13 Connections of the fastigial nucleus (FN). FN projects bilaterally to vestibular nuclei (VN) and projects to the periaqueductal gray (PAG) and the mesodiencephalic nuclei (MDN: interstitial and Darkschewitsch nuclei). FN also projects to bulbar reticular formation: medial bulbar reticular formation (RFm) and lateral reticular nuclei (LRN), at the origin of the reticulospinal tract (RST). Reticular nuclei project back to cerebellar nuclei (cerebello-reticulocerebellar loops, not illustrated) and receives afferents from the spinal cord. FN is also connected with the parasolitarius nuclei (PSN) and the perihypoglossal nuclei (PHN) VN projects to the spinal cord via the vestibulospinal tract (VST) and projects back to the FN and the flocculonodular lobe. Interrupted line: midline.

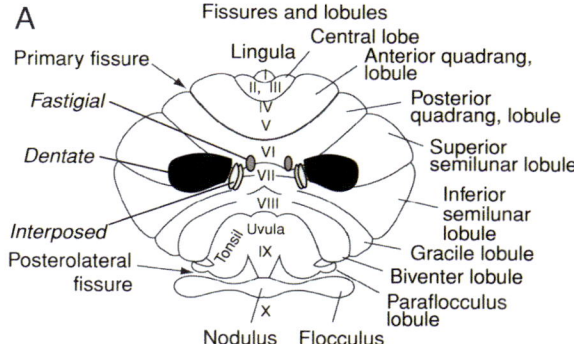

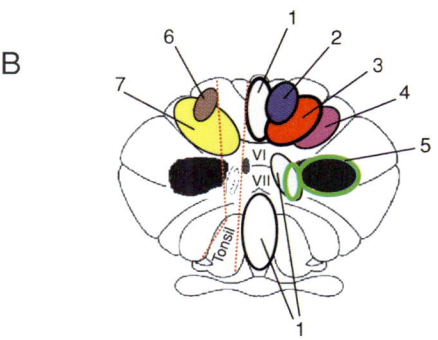

Figure 3.7 Lesion symptom mapping. (A) Cerebellar lobules shown on an unfolded cerebellum. (B) Lesion-symptom mapping. Schematic sketch of findings in patients with focal cerebellar lesions. The figure summarizes the results of lesion-symptom mapping in studies on eyeblink conditioning, cerebellar ataxia rating scores, balance in stance and gait, and upper and lower limb coordination. 1: ataxia of stance/gait; 2: lower limb ataxia; 3: upper limb ataxia; 4: dysarthria; 5: limb ataxia; 6: conditioned eyeblink response (CR) timing; 7: CR acquisition. Adapted from: Timmann et al., 2008.

OUTPUT CHANNELS OF THE DENTATE NUCLEUS

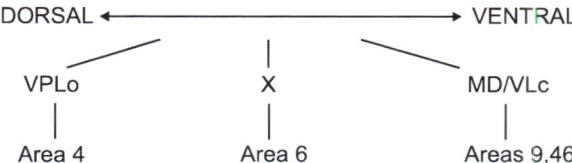

Figure 1.14 Output channels of the dentate nucleus. Distinct areas of the dentate nucleus project predominantly upon different regions of the contralateral cerebral cortex, via thalamic nuclei (MD/VLc: medial dorsal/ventralis lateral pars caudalis nuclei; area X, VPLo: nucleus ventralis posterior lateralis pars oralis). Dorsal portions of the dentate nucleus project mainly upon area 4. With permission from: Manto, 2009.

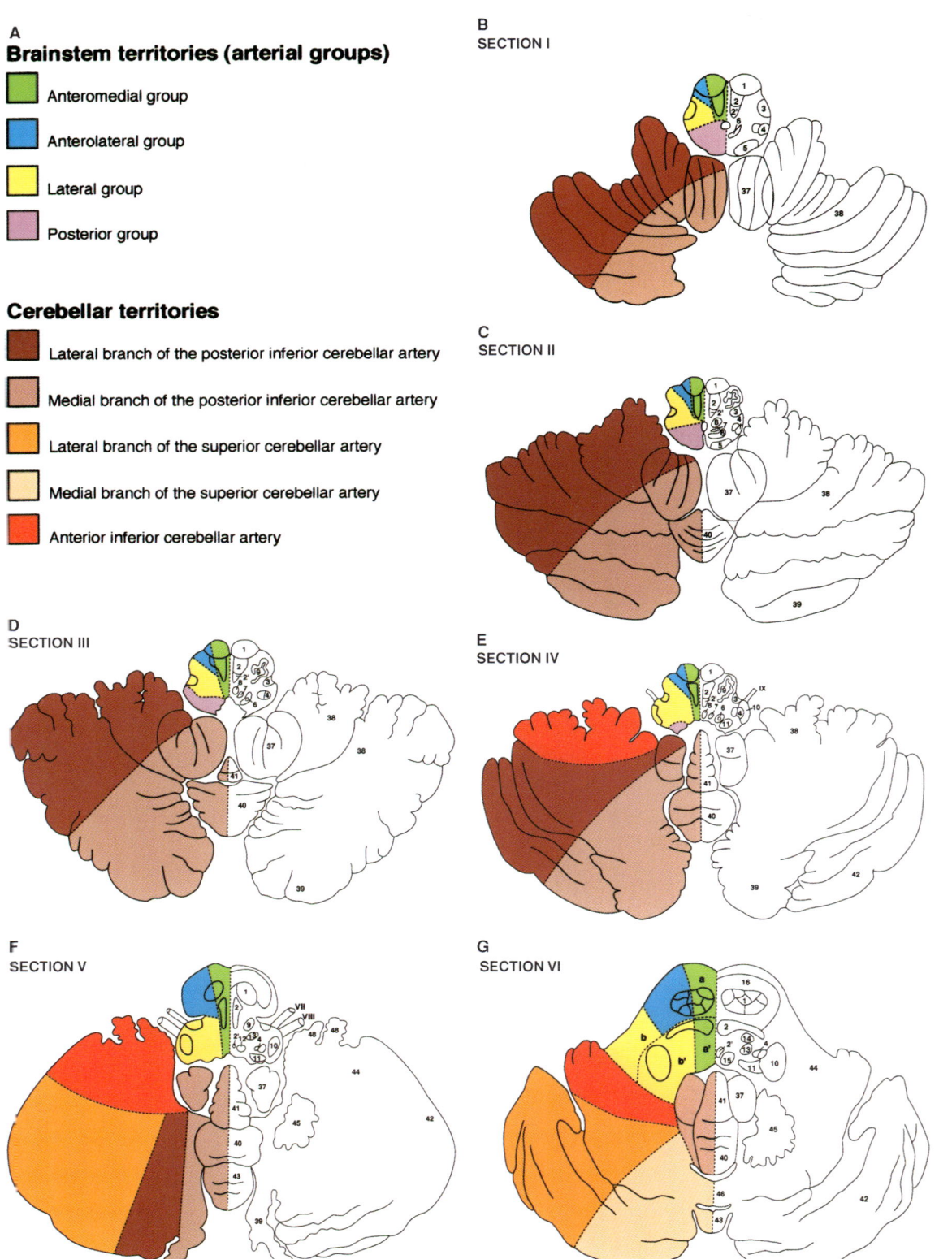

A
Brainstem territories (arterial groups)

- 🟩 Anteromedial group
- 🟦 Anterolateral group
- 🟨 Lateral group
- 🟪 Posterior group

Cerebellar territories

- 🟫 Lateral branch of the posterior inferior cerebellar artery
- 🟫 Medial branch of the posterior inferior cerebellar artery
- 🟧 Lateral branch of the superior cerebellar artery
- ⬜ Medial branch of the superior cerebellar artery
- 🟥 Anterior inferior cerebellar artery

B
SECTION I

C
SECTION II

D
SECTION III

E
SECTION IV

F
SECTION V

G
SECTION VI

Figure 8.2 Arterial groups and cerebellar territories supplied by the main cerebellar arteries. Illustration of serial sections (4-mm thick) based on a bicommissural plane passing through the anterior and posterior commissures. From: Tatu et al., 1996. With permission. (See color section.)

Ar atomic structures of sections I to XII

1 Corticospinal tract; 2 Medial lemniscus; 2' Medial longitudinal fasciculus; 3 Spinothalamic tract; 4 Spinal trigeminal tract/nuclei; 5 Gracile and cuneate nuclei; 6 Nucleus of solitary tract; 7 Dorsal motor vagal nucleus; 8 Hypoglossal nucleus; 9 Inferior olivary nucleus; 10 Inferior

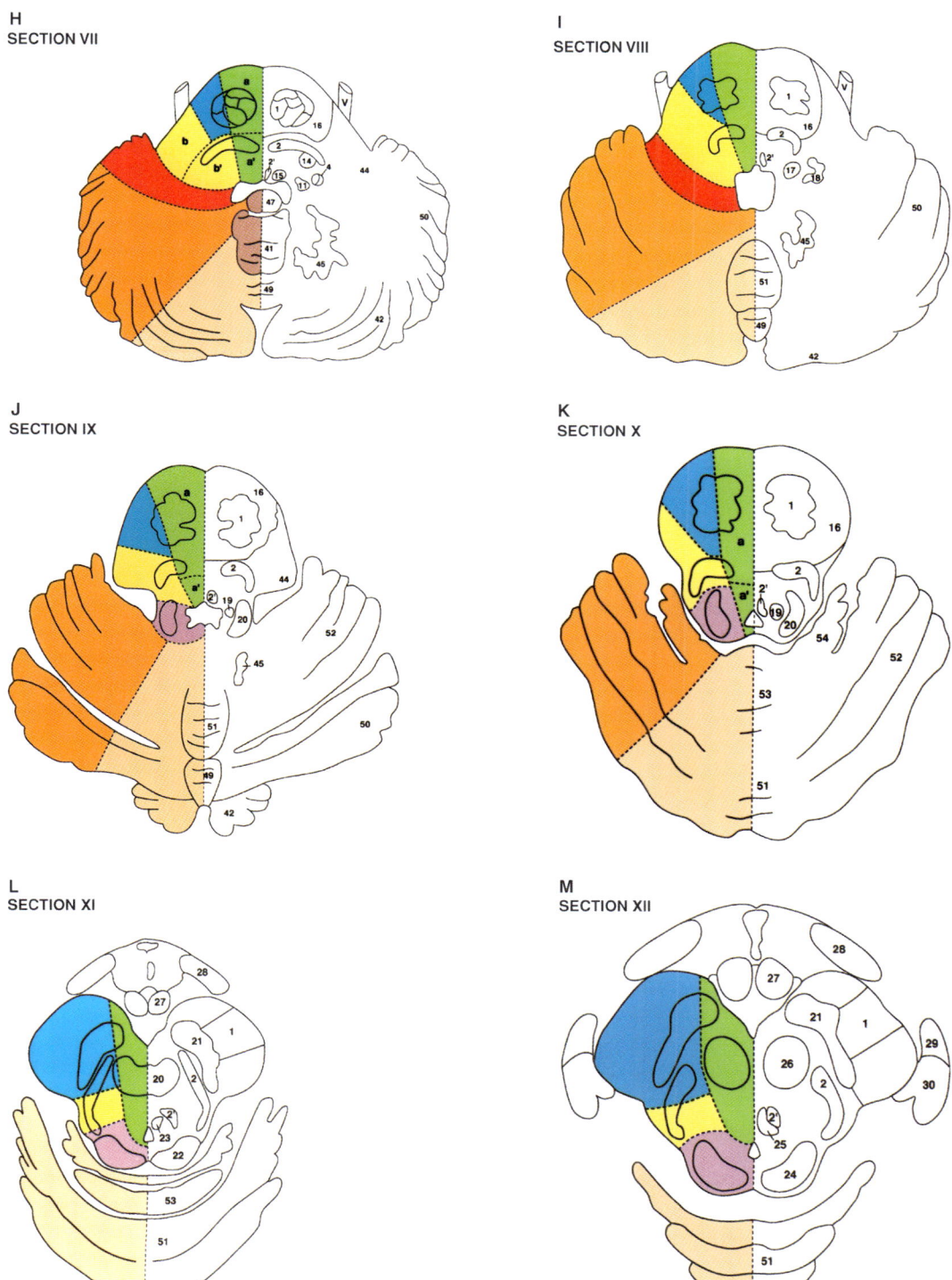

Figure 8.2 (*cont.*) cerebellar peduncle; 11 Vestibular nucleus; 12 Nucleus prepositus; 13 Facial nucleus; 14 Superior olivary nucleus; 15 Abducens nucleus; 16 Pontine nuclei; 17 Motor trigeminal nucleus; 18 Principal sensory trigeminal nucleus; 19 Nucleus ceruleus; 20 Superior cerebellar peduncle; 21 Substantia nigra; 22 Inferior colliculus; 23 Trochlear nucleus; 24 Superior colliculus; 25 Oculomotor nucleus; 26 Red nucleus; 27 Mammillary body; 28 Optic tract; 29 Lateral geniculate nucleus; 30 Medial geniculate body; 31 Pulvinar; 32 Mamillothalamic tract; 33 Column of fornix; 34 Caudate nucleus; 35 Putamen; 36 Anterior commissure; 37 Tonsil; 38 Biventer lobule; 39 Inferior semilunar lobule; 40 Pyramid of vermis; 41 Uvula; 42 Superior semilunar lobule; 43 Tuber of vermis; 44 Middle cerebellar peduncle; 45 Dentate nucleus; 46 Folium of vermis; 47 Nodulus; 48 Flocculus; 49 Declive; 50 Simple lobule; 51 Culmen; 52 Quadrangular lobule; 53 Central lobule; 54 Ala of the central lobule, V Trigeminal nerve, VII Facial nerve, VIII Vestibulocochlear nerve, IX Glossopharyngeal nerve.

LATERAL MEDULLARY INFARCTION (Wallenberg syndrome)

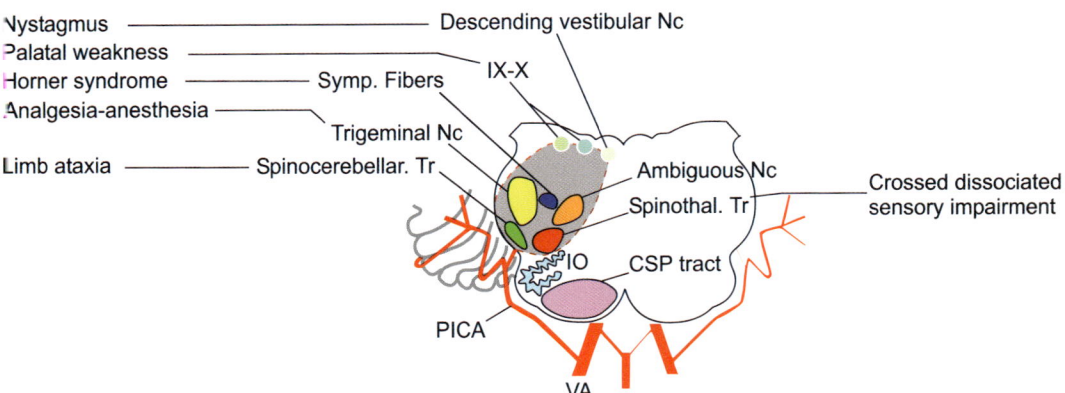

Figure 8.4 Anatomical basis of the symptoms in lateral medullary infarction. The lateral region of the medulla (grey zone) is supplied by small perforating branches. Abbreviations: Ambiguous Nc: ambiguous nucleus; Spinothal. Tr: spinothalamic tract; CSP tract: corticospinal tract; VA: vertebral artery; PICA: posterior inferior cerebellar artery; Trigeminal Nc: trigeminal nucleus; Symp. Fibers: sympathetic fibers; IX–X: cranial nerves IX–X.

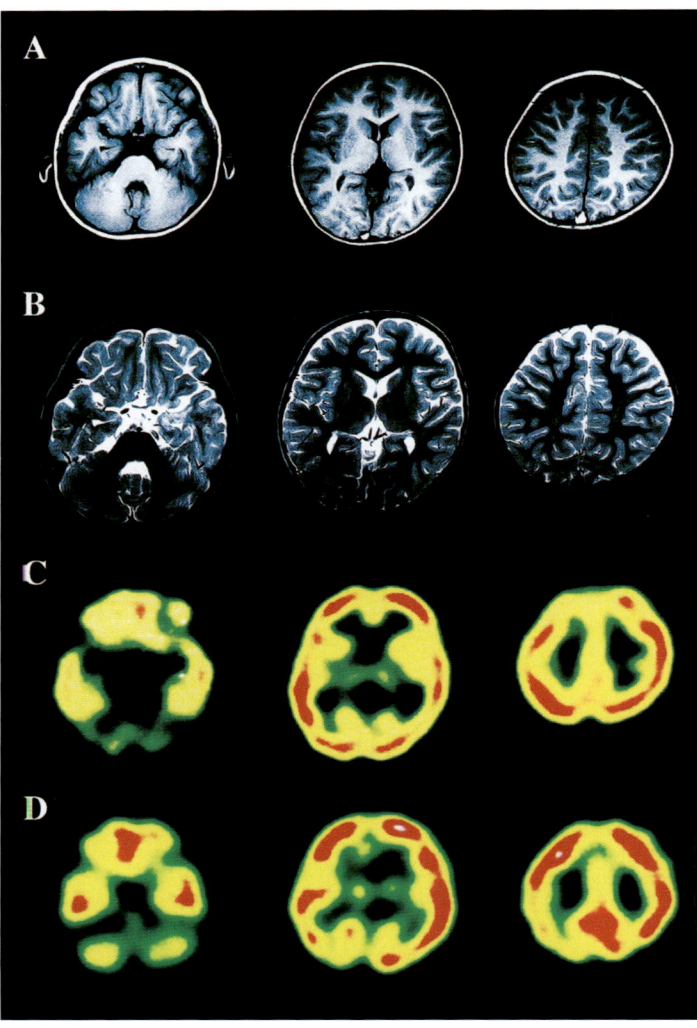

Figure 11.1 Post-infectious cerebellitis. (A,B) T1- and T2-weighted images show no abnormality. (C) By contrast, ^{123}I-SPECT demonstrates a decreased regional cerebral blood flow (rCBF) in the cerebellum. (D) SPECT in a control subject. From: Nagamitsu et al., 1999. With permission.

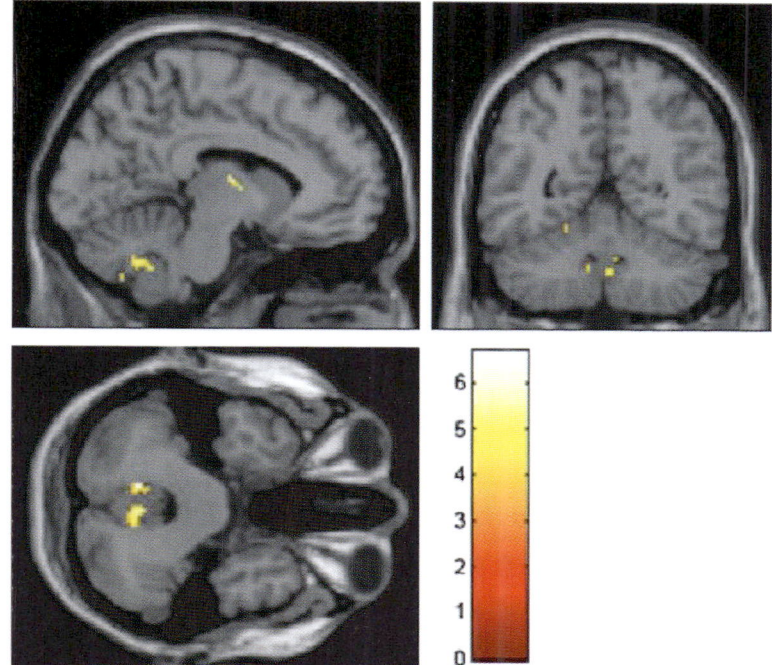

A

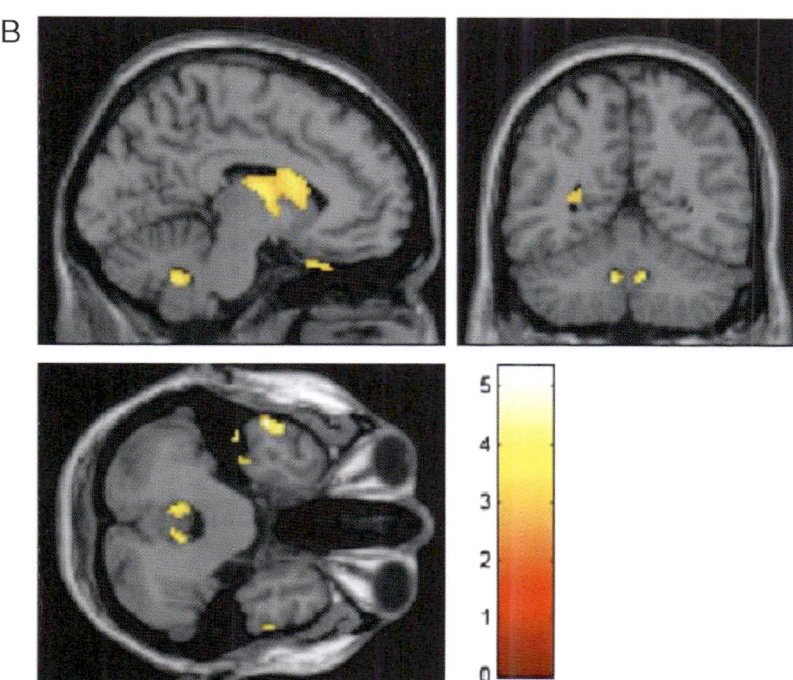

B

Figure 11.2 Cerebellar involvement in Creutzfeldt-Jakob disease. The larger cerebellar loci of significantly elevated apparent diffusion coefficient (ADC) and CSF volume (respectively in A and B) are found bilaterally in the cerebellar nodule, shown here in three orthogonal projections. Focal atrophy cannot be detected on clinical reading of standard MRI sequences but is highly significant on statistical group analysis. Degenerative changes are reflected in elevated diffusion in the cerebellum, presumably due to tissue destruction and replacement by CSF. From: Cohen et al., 2009. With permission.

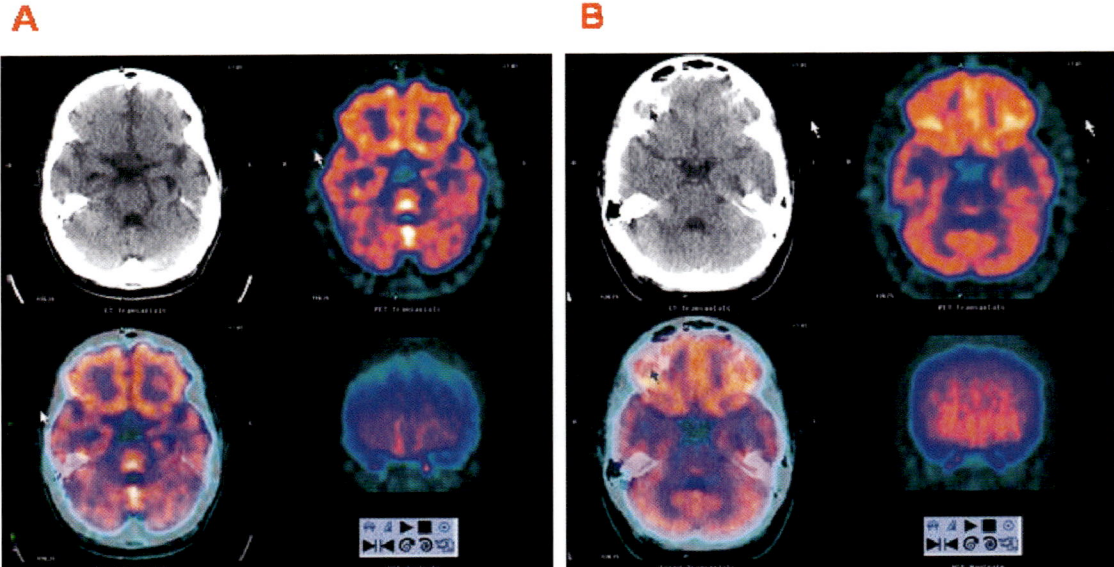

Figure 14.6 (A) Relative hypermetabolism of the cerebellar vermis and pons in a patient with post-anoxic coma. (B) Control case. From: Lupi e⁻ al., 2007. With permission.

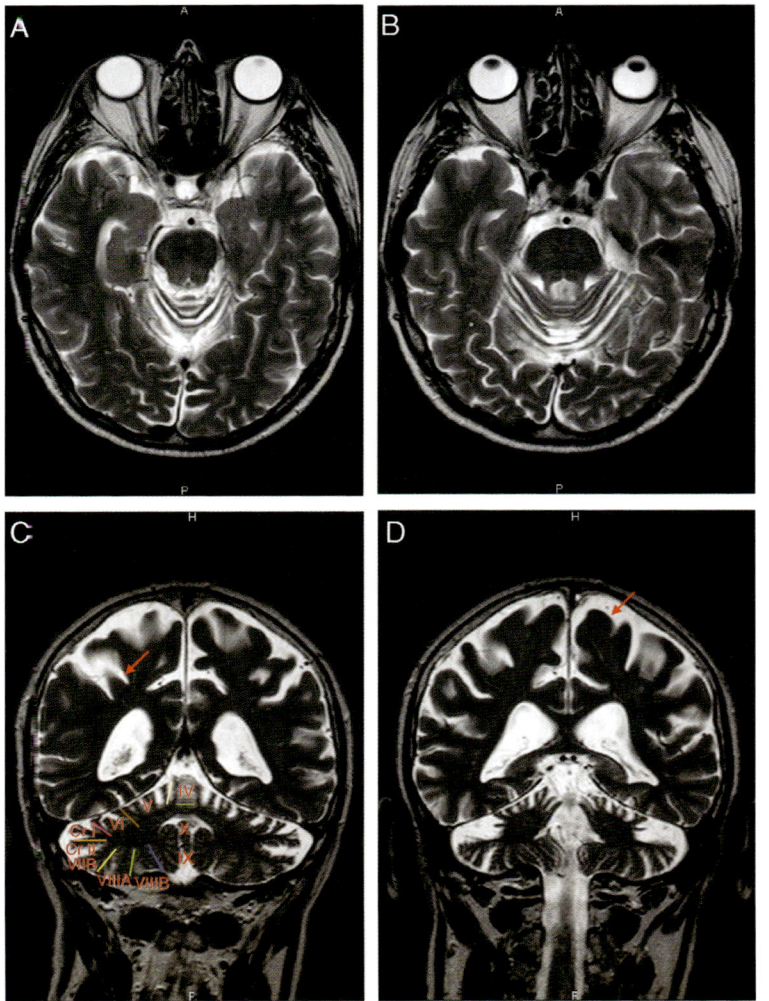

Figure 15.1 Cerebral atrophy in a patient with a history of chronic alcohol abuse. (A, B) Axial T2-weighted images show widening of cerebellar sulci of the anterior lobe. (C, D) Coronal images show atrophy of the cerebellar cortex in different lobules, as well as cerebral cortical atrophy (arrows).

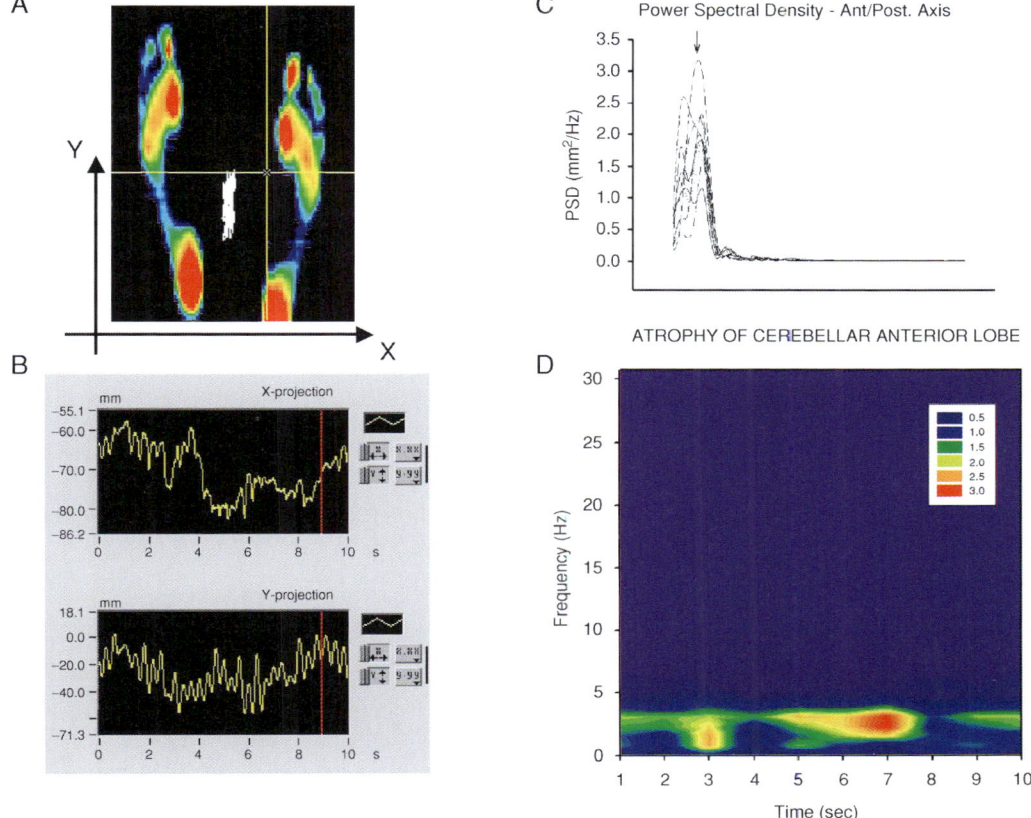

Figure 15.2 A 3-Hz body sway in chronic alcoholic cerebellar degeneration. (A) Representation of the center of pressure during a Romberg test using a pressure platform. (B) Displacements of the center of pressure in orthogonal axis X–Y. (C) Superimposition of power spectral density curves in the anterior-posterior axis. A 3-Hz tremor is found (arrow). (D) Time frequency representation of the oscillations.

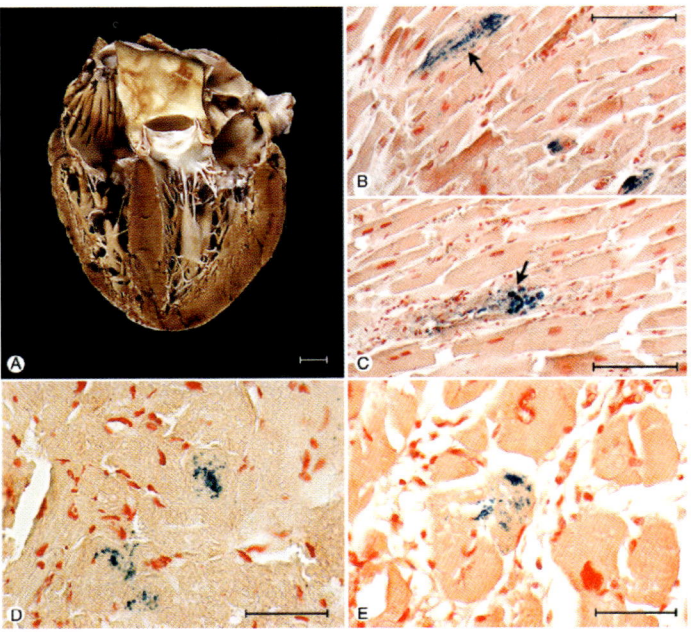

Figure 20.2 Gross pathology of a Friedreich (FRDA) heart and light microscopy of iron-reactive granules in sarcoplasm and endomysium. (A) Gross specimen. Left and right ventricular walls are greatly thickened. The myocardium is discolored, lacking the normal dark and homogeneous appearance of normal heart. (B–E) Iron histochemistry. The stain shows finely granular reaction products that lie parallel to the long axis of cardiomyocytes (arrow in B). A cluster of much larger iron-positive granules lies adjacent to or within a necrotic muscle fiber (arrow in C). (D, E) Iron histochemistry of an endocardial biopsy of an FRDA patient at the age of 9 years (D) and a section of the autopsy specimens at the age of 26 years (E). Both sections display iron-positive granules in cardiac muscle fibers, and the frequency of iron-reactive fibers among all cardiomyocytes is similar. Sections illustrated in B–E are counterstained with Brazilin. Markers: A, 1 cm; B, C, 100 mm. D, E, 50 mm. From: Michael et al., 2006. With permission.

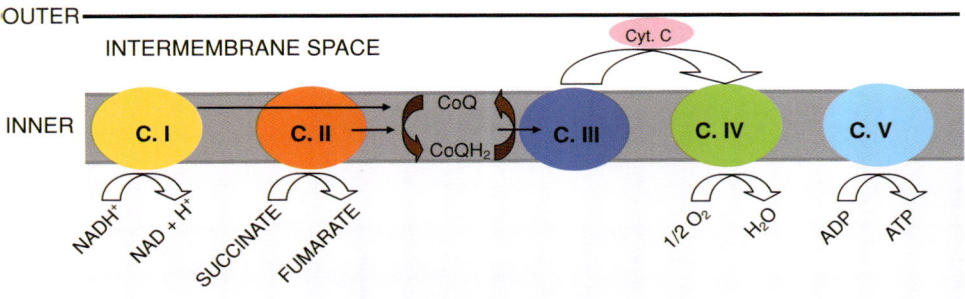

OUTER
INTERMEMBRANE SPACE
INNER

C. I   C. II   CoQ   CoQH$_2$ C. III   C. IV   C. V   Cyt. C

NADH$^+$ NAD + H$^+$ SUCCINATE   FUMARATE   1/2 O$_2$ H$_2$O   ADP   ATP

MITOCHONDRIAL MATRIX

Figure 20.4 Illustration of the mitochondrial respiratory chain. Electrons are transferred from complex I (C. I) and II (C. II) to the oxidized form of coenzyme Q10 (CoQ). CoQ is reduced to CoQH$_2$, which transfers the electrons to Complex III (C. III). Other abbreviations: C. IV: complex IV; C. V: complex V; Cyt. C: cytochrome C.

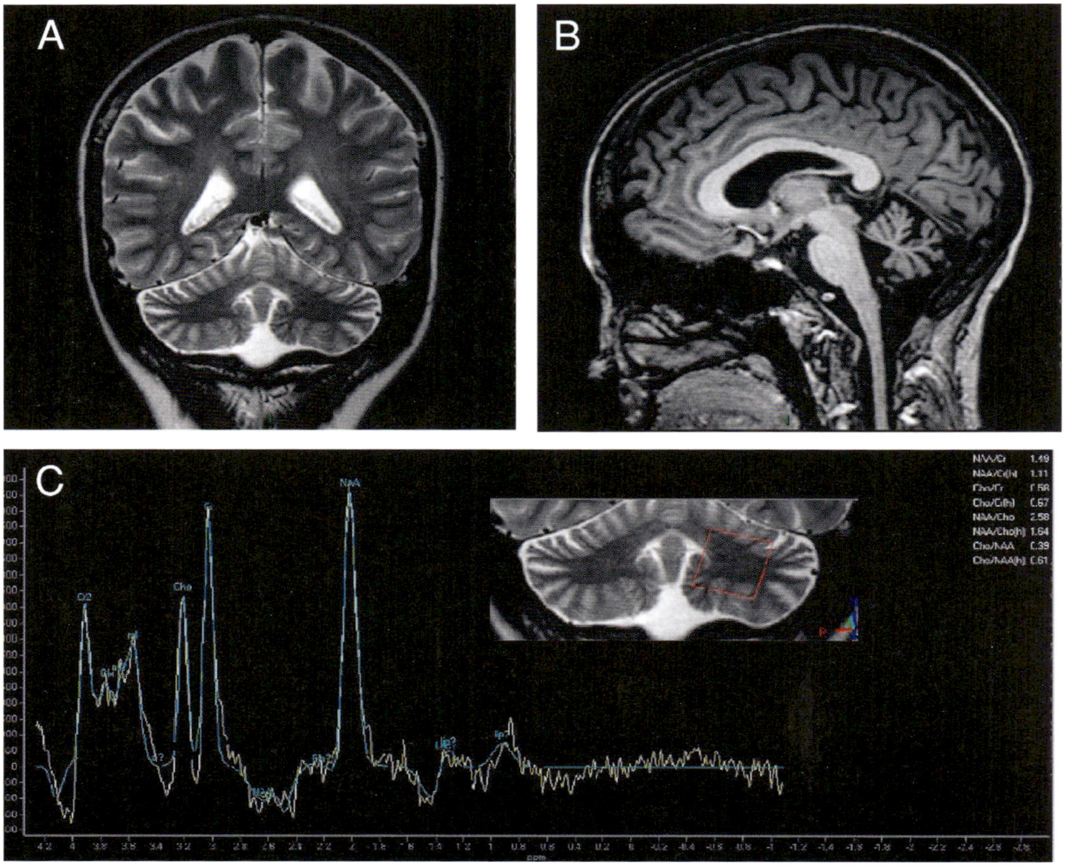

Figure 21.4 Brain MRI and magnetic resonance spectroscopy (MRS) in a patient with a mitochondrial disease. (A) Coronal T2-weighted sequence; (B) sagittal T1-weighted image demonstrating atrophy of the vermis; (C) a peak of lactate in the cerebellar parenchyma is detected on MRS.

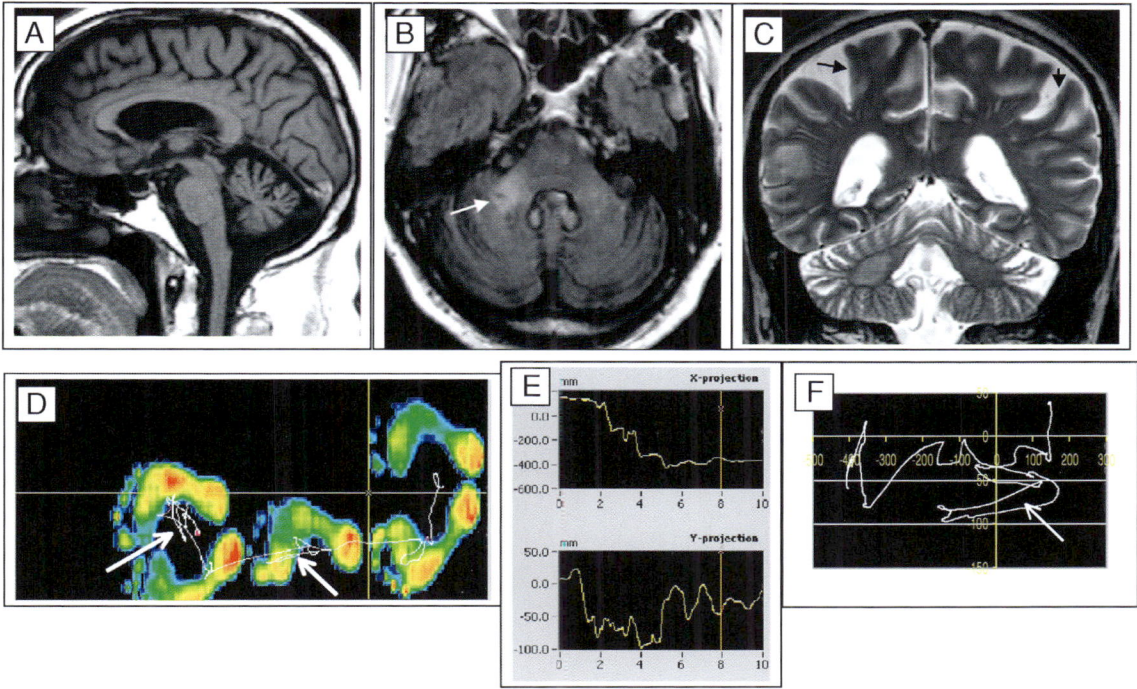

Figure 22.1 Brain MRI and gait analysis in a patient with fragile X tremor ataxia syndrome (FXTAS). (A) Sagittal T1-weighted image showing a moderate atrophy of the vermis; (B) hyperintense signals in the middle cerebellar peduncles on a T1-weighted axial image; (C) atrophy of the cerebellar cortex and cerebral sulci (arrows; T2-weighted image). (D–F) Analysis of tandem gait. The path of the center of pressure is dysmetric (arrows in D and F). (E) Representation of the displacements of the center of pressure in orthogonal planes X and Y. Reproduced in part from: Manto and Jissendi, 2009. With permission.

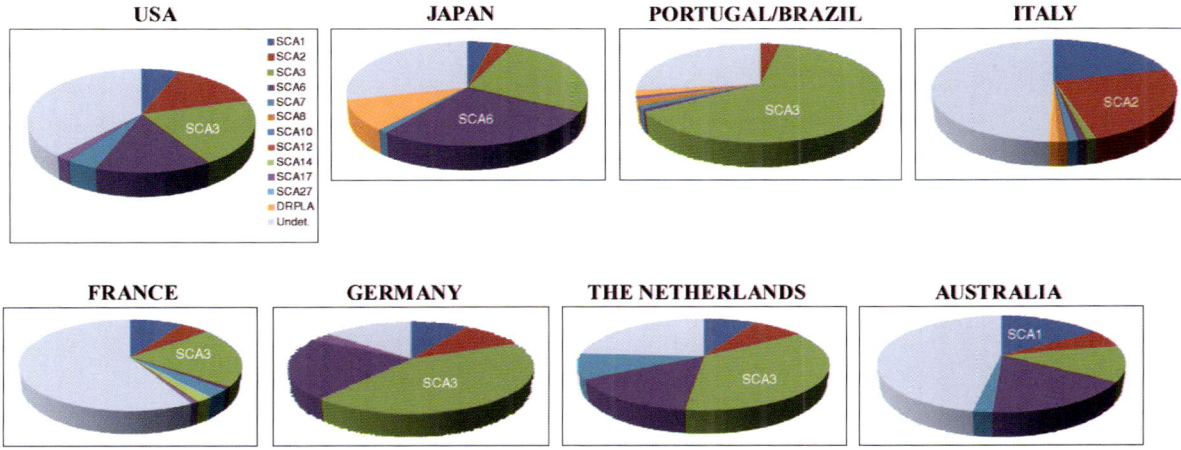

Figure 23.1 Relative frequencies of spinocerebellar ataxias (SCAs). The SCA with highest frequency is indicated in each pie.

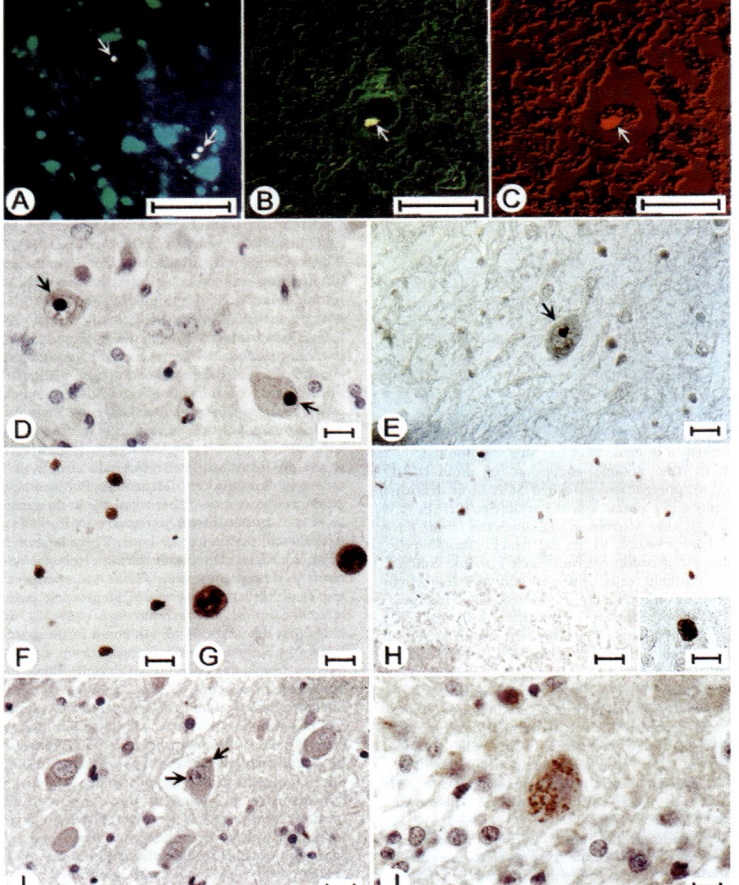

Figure 23.2 Inclusions in spinocerebellar ataxias (SCAs). Inclusion bodies in selected SCAs. (A–C) SCA-3/Machado-Joseph disease (MJD), anti-ataxin-3 (A and B), anti-ubiquitin (C): confocal fluorescence microscopy shows multiple small nucleoliform ataxin-3-reactive intranuclear inclusions in neurons of the basis pontis (arrows in A; fluorescein isothiocyanate [FITC]). Ataxin-3 reaction product in B (FITC) colocalizes with ubiquitin in C (Quantum Red) (arrows). The images were processed to reduce lipofuscin fluorescence. (D) SCA1, anti-polyglutamine: Positive-contrast reaction product is present in large intranuclear inclusions (arrows). (E) SCA-2, anti-polyglutamine: the intranuclear inclusion body (arrow) is relatively small compared with those in SCA-1 (D). (F–H) SCA-17, anti-polyglutamine (F and H), TATA-binding protein (G): Neurons of the basis pontis reveal pan-nuclear reaction product (F, G). In the cerebellar cortex, pan-nuclear inclusions are present in the basket and stellate cells (H). The inset shows an intranuclear inclusion in a surviving Purkinje cell. (I, J) SCA-6, anti-polyglutamine: Pontine neurons show small intracytoplasmic inclusions (I, arrows). A Purkinje cell contains multiple cytoplasmic inclusion bodies (J). Magnification markers: A–C, F, and H, 25 mm; D–E, G, J, and inset in H, 10 mm; I, 15.9 mm. From: Koeppen, 2005. With permission.

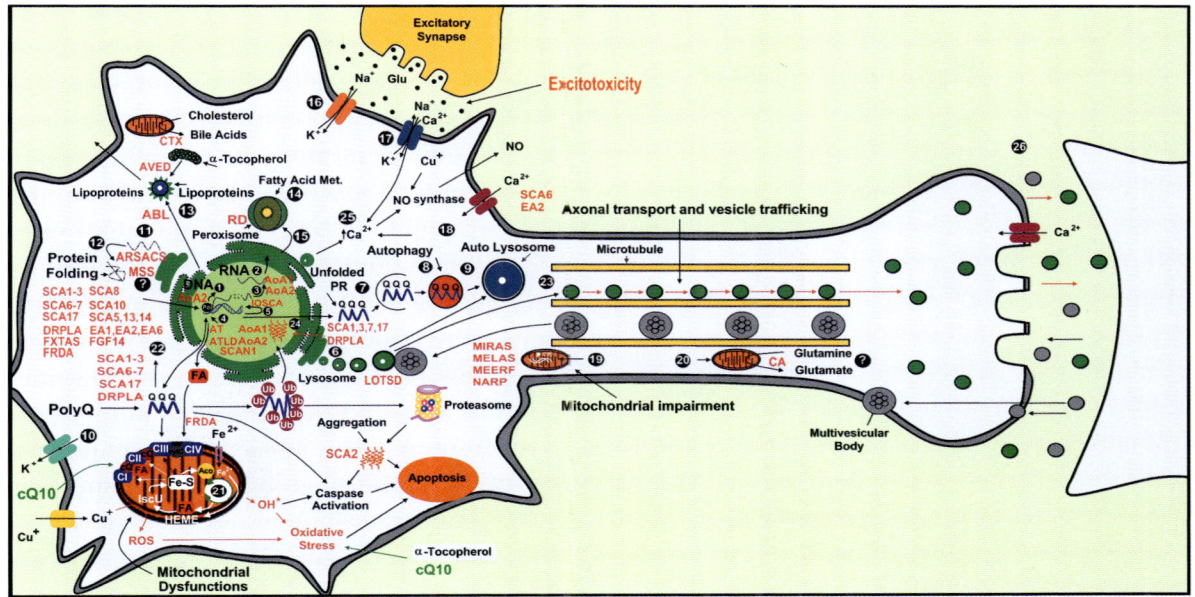

Figure 23.4 Illustration of the mechanisms of cerebellar ataxias at the cellular level. 1, transcription; 2, DNA repair; 3, transport; 4, processing; 5, replication; 6, glycosphingolipid metabolism; 7, isolation membrane; 8, autophagy; 9, autolysosome; 10, Ca2+ activated voltage-gated K+ channel; 11, translation; 12, protein folding; 13, lipoprotein assembly; 14, fatty acid metabolism; 15, protein import; 16, non-NMDA receptor; 17, NMDA receptor; 18, voltage-gated Ca2+ channels; 19, DNA repair/replication; 20, mitochondrial impairment; 21, Krebs cycle; 22, chaperones; 23, axonal transport and vesicle trafficking; 24, aggregation; 25 Ca2+ homeostasis; 26, synaptic function. Abbreviations: Ca2+: Calcium Ions; ER: endoplasmic reticulum; Glu: glutamate; K+: potassium ions; Na+: sodium ions; Q: glutamine; Ub: ubiquitin; CI: respiratory chain complex I; CII: respiratory chain complex II; CIII: respiratory chain complex III; CIV: respiratory chain complex IV; cQ: coenzyme Q; cytC: cytochrome C; ACO: aconitase; HEME; Fe2+: ferrous iron; IscU: iron-sulphur cluster scaffold protein; ROS: reactive oxygen species; RNA: ribonucleic acid; OH*: hydroxyl radical; Fe-S: iron-sulfur cluster; Vitamin E; cQ10: coenzyme Q10; Cu+: copper; SCA (1–17): spinocerebellar ataxia (Type 1–17); DRPLA: dentatorubral-pallidoluysian atrophy; EA (Type 1–6): episodic ataxia (Type 1–6); FGF14: fibroblast growth factor 14; FXTAS: Fragile X tremor/ataxia syndrome; FA: Friedreich ataxia; AOA (type 1–2): ataxia with oculomotor apraxia (Type 1–2); IOSCA: infantile-onset spinocerebellar ataxia; AT: ataxia telangiectasia; SCAN1: spinocerebellar ataxia with axonal neuropathy; LOTSD: late-onset Tay-Sachs disease; RD: Refsum disease; ARSACS: autosomal recessive ataxia of Charlevoix-Saguenay; MSS: Marinesco-Sjögren syndrome; ABL: abetalipoproteinemia; CTX: cerebrotendinous xanthomatosis; AVED: ataxia with vitamin E deficiency; CA: Cayman ataxia; MIRAS: mitochondrial recessive ataxia syndrome; MELAS: mitochondrial myopathy, encephalopathy, lactic acidosis, and stroke; MERRF: myoclonus epilepsy associated with ragged-red fibers; NARP: neuropathy, ataxia, and retinitis pigmentosa. From: Manto and Marmolino, 2009. With permission.

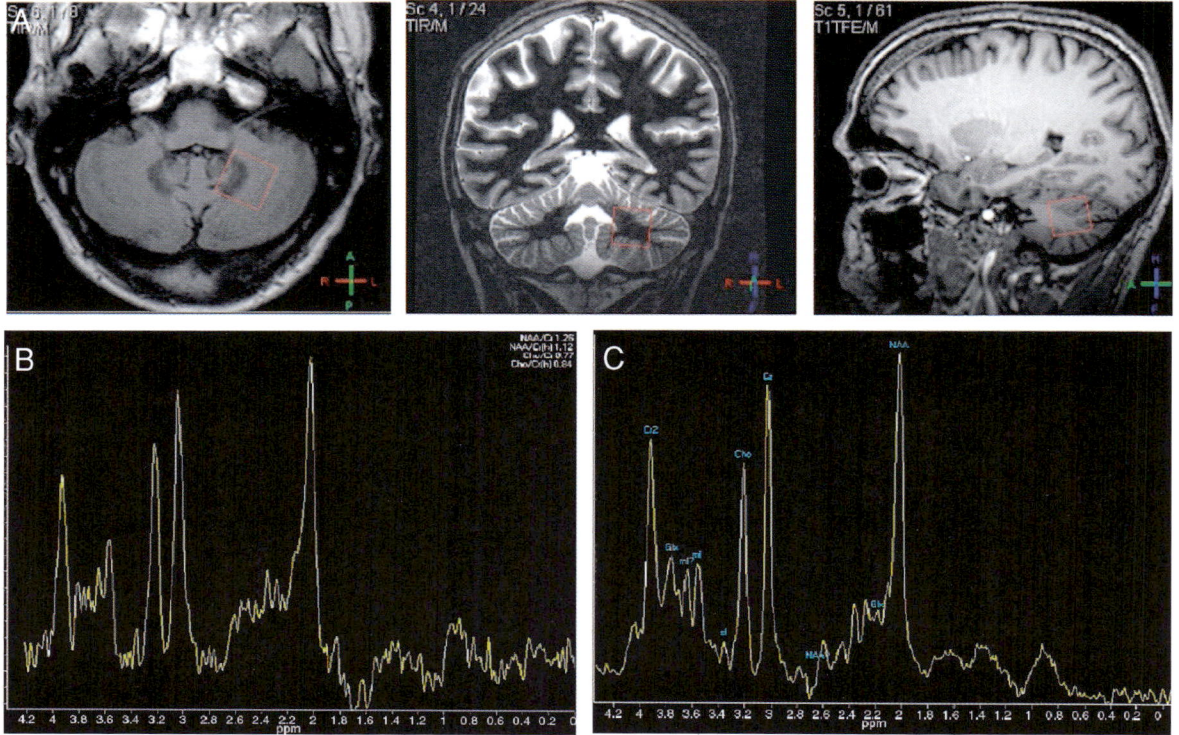

Figure 23.7 Brain MRI and H1 magnetic resonance spectroscopy of a patient with SCA2 exhibiting a slight cerebellar syndrome: (A) MRI used to plan the single voxel acquisition; (B) spectrum acquired in the deep left cerebellum of patient; (C) spectrum acquired in the deep left cerebellum of age- and sex-matched control. The images in (A), axial fluid-attenuated inversion recovery, coronal T2-weighted, and sagittal T1-weighted (from left to right), show global atrophy in the posterior fossa as well as in the supratentorium. The spectrum in (B) shows a decrease of the N-acetyl-aspartate/creatine ratio (1.26) compared with the control (1.53). From: Manto and Jissendi, 2009. With permission.

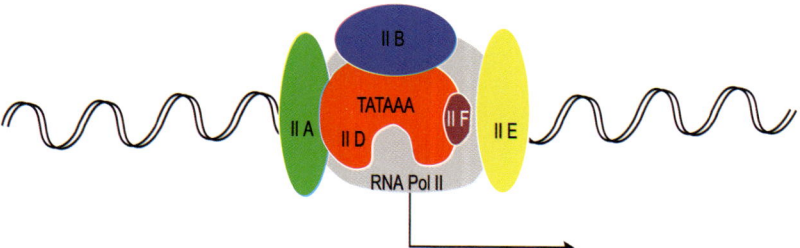

Figure 23.10 The transcription initiation complex. The initiation of the RNA synthesis by RNA polymerase II requires the transcription factors TFIIA, B, D, E and F. TFIID (TBP: TATA-box binding protein) binds to the TATA-box (TATAAA). TBP has a variable size depending on the number of glutamine residues (25–42 in normal condition). Arrow corresponds to the transcription start site. Adapted from: Zühlke and Bürk, 2007.

Clinical scales

Several scales are used to quantify cerebellar ataxia according to the severity of symptoms (Trouillas et al., 1997). The need for standardized scales is obvious for the assessment of patients, not only for the follow-up of patients, but also during clinical trials or pharmacological studies.

ICARS

The International Cooperative Ataxia Rating Scale (ICARS) (Trouillas et al., 1997) is a 100-point semi-quantitative scale. It is divided into four parts, on the basis of the compartmentalization of cerebellar symptoms (Babinski & Tournay, 1913):

1. Postural and stance disturbances (subscore: /34)
2. Limb movement disturbances (subscore: /52)
3. Speech disorders (subscore: /8)
4. Oculomotor deficits (subscore: /6)

Posture and Gait Score (total of scores A to G)

A. Walking capacities: 10-m test including half-turn, near a wall

   0 Normal
   1 Almost normal naturally, unable to walk with feet in tandem
   2 Walking without support, but abnormal and irregular
   3 Walking without support but with considerable staggering; difficulties in half-turn
   4 Walking with autonomous support impossible; episodic support of the wall for a 10-m test
   5 Walking only possible with one stick
   6 Walking only possible with two special sticks or with a stroller
   7 Walking only with accompanying person

   8 Walking impossible, even with accompanying person (wheelchair)

   SCORE . . . .

B. Gait speed: a preceding score of 4 or more gives directly a score of 4 in this test

   0 Normal
   1 Slightly reduced
   2 Markedly reduced
   3 Extremely slow
   4 Walking with autonomous support no longer possible

   SCORE . . . .

C. Standing capacities, eyes open

   0 Normal, able to stand on 1 foot more than 10 sec
   1 Cannot stand on 1 foot more than 10 sec, but can stand with feet together
   2 Able to stand with feet together, but cannot stand with feet in tandem position
   3 Able to stand in natural position without support, with no or moderate sway. Cannot stand with feet together
   4 Standing in natural position without support, with considerable sway and corrections
   5 Unable to stand in natural position without strong support of one arm
   6 Unable to stand at all, even with strong support of two arms

   SCORE . . . .

D. Spread of feet in natural position without support, eyes open: patient is asked to find a comfortable position, and the distance between the medial malleoli is measured.

   0 Normal (<10 cm)
   1 Slightly enlarged (>10 cm)

2 Clearly enlarged (between 25 and 35 cm)
3 Severely enlarged (>35 cm)
4 Standing in natural position impossible

SCORE ....

E. Body sway with feet together, eyes open

0 Normal
1 Slight oscillations
2 Moderate oscillations (<10 cm at the level of head)
3 Severe oscillations with risk of fall (>10 cm at the level of head)
4 Immediate falling

SCORE ....

F. Body sway with feet together, eyes closed

0 Normal
1 Slight oscillations
2 Moderate oscillations (<10 cm at the level of head)
3 Severe oscillations with risk of fall (>10 cm at the level of head)
4 Immediate falling

SCORE ....

G. Quality of sitting position: on a hard surface, thighs together, arms folded

0 Normal
1 Slight trunk oscillations
2 Moderate oscillations of trunk/legs
3 Severe dysequilibrium
4 Impossible

SCORE ....

Kinetic functions (total of scores H to N)

H. Knee-tibia test: patient in a supine position, head tilted. Patient asked to raise one leg and place the heel on the knee and then slide the heel down the anterior tibial surface of the resting leg towards the ankle. On reaching the ankle joint, the leg is again raised in the air to a height of about 40 cm, and the action is repeated. At least three movements of each limb. Under visual guidance.

0 Normal

1 Lowering of heel in continuous axis, movement decomposed in several phases, without real jerks, or abnormally slow
2 Lowering jerkily in the axis
3 Lowering jerkily with lateral movements
4 Lowering jerkily with extremely strong lateral movements or test impossible

SCORE Right ....
SCORE Left ....

I. Heel-to-knee test: the action tremor of the heel-to-knee test is specifically observed when the patient holds the heel on the knee for a few seconds before sliding down the anterior tibial surface under visual control.

0 No trouble
1 Tremor stopping immediately when the heel reaches the knee
2 Tremor stopping in less than 10 sec after reaching the knee
3 Tremor continuing for more than 10 sec after reaching the knee
4 Uninterrupted tremor or test impossible

SCORE Right ....
SCORE Left ....

J. Finger-to-nose test: subject sitting on a chair. Hand is resting on the knee before the beginning of the movement. Three movements of each limb are performed under visual guidance.

0 Normal
1 Oscillating movement without decomposition
2 Segmented movement in two phases and/or moderate dysmetria in reaching the nose
3 Movement segmented in more than two phases and/or considerable dysmetria in reaching the nose
4 Patient unable to reach the nose

SCORE Right ....
SCORE Left ....

K. Finger-to-nose test: the "intention" tremor is specifically looked for. Tremor appearing during the "ballistic" phase of the movement is assessed. See previous task.

0 Normal
1 Simple swerve of the movement

2 Moderate tremor with estimated amplitude <10 cm

3 Amplitude of tremor between 10 cm and 40 cm

4 Amplitude of tremor >40 cm

SCORE Right . . . .
SCORE Left . . . .

L. Finger-finger test: the sitting patient is asked to maintain medially the two fingers pointing at each other for about 10 sec at a distance of about 1 cm, at the level of the thorax, under visual guidance. Action tremor is specifically looked for.

0 Normal

1 Mild instability

2 Moderate oscillations of fingers with estimated amplitude <10 cm

3 Oscillations of the fingers between 10 and 40 cm

4 Jerky movements >40 cm of amplitude

SCORE Right . . . .
SCORE Left . . . .

M. Pronation-supination alternating movements: the subject is sitting on a chair. Forearms are raised vertically, and alternative movements of the hands are performed. Each side is assessed separately.

0 Normal

1 Slightly irregular and slowed

2 Clearly irregular and slowed, with no sway of the elbow

3 Extremely irregular and slowed movement, with sway of the elbow

4 Movement completely disorganized or impossible

SCORE Right . . . .
SCORE Left . . . .

N. Drawing of the Archimedes spiral on a pre-drawn pattern: subject comfortably settled in front of a table. The sheet of paper is fixed on the table. No timing requirement. Dominant hand examined.

0 Normal

1 Impairment and decomposition, the line quitting the pattern slightly, but without hypermetric swerve

2 Line completely out of the pattern with recrossings and/or hypermetric swerves

3 Major disturbance due to hypermetria and decomposition

4 Drawing completely disorganized or impossible

SCORE . . . .

Speech assessment (total of scores O to P)

O. Fluency of speech: the patient is requested to repeat several times a standard sentence, for instance: "A mischievous spectacle in Czechoslovakia"

0 Normal

1 Mild modification of fluency

2 Moderate modification of fluency

3 Considerably slow and dysarthric speech

4 No speech

SCORE . . . .

P. Clarity of speech

0 Normal

1 Suggestion of slurring

2 Definite slurring, most words understandable

3 Severe slurring, speech not understandable

4 No speech

SCORE . . . .

Oculomotor deficits (total of scores Q to S)

Q. Gaze-evoked nystagmus: the subject is asked to look laterally at the finger of the examiner: the movements assessed are mainly horizontal, but may be oblique, rotatory, or vertical.

0 Normal

1 Transient

2 Persistent but moderate

3 Persistent and severe

SCORE . . . .

R. Abnormalities of the ocular pursuit: the subject is asked to follow the slow lateral movement performed by the finger of the examiner

0 Normal

1 Slightly saccadic

2 Clearly saccadic

SCORE . . . .

S. Dysmetria of saccades: the index fingers of the examiners are placed in each temporal visual field of the patient, whose eyes are in the primary position. The patient is asked to look laterally at the finger on the right and on the left. The average overshoot or undershoot of the two sides is estimated.

   0 Absence of dysmetria

   1 Bilateral clear overshoot or undershoot of the saccade

SCORE ....

The ICARS is a reliable scale satisfying accepted criteria for inter-rater reliability, test–retest reliability, and internal consistency (Schmitz-Hubsch et al., 2006a). Inter-rater correlation is very high for the total score, and high to very high for each component subscore (Storey et al., 2004). The scale is sensitive to a range of ataxia severities from mild to severe. Some authors argue that the ICARS might show some redundancies of several items and that the different factors extracted by a factorial analysis do not coincide with the ICARS subscores, questioning its usefulness (see section Comparison between scales).

The ICARS is also useful to extract and rate the severity of cerebellar signs in multiple system atrophy, although it is contaminated by parkinsonian features (Tison et al., 2002).

BARS (Brief Ataxia Rating Scale)

The Brief Ataxia Rating Scale (BARS) evaluates gait (score from 0 to 8), knee-tibia test (score from 0 to 4 on each side), finger-to-nose test (score from 0 to 4 on each side), dysarthria (score from 0 to 4) and oculomotor deficits (score from 0 to 2), with a maximal total score of 30 (Schmahmann et al., 2009). BARS provides a quick and easy to perform estimation of the overall cerebellar function.

AS20 (Ataxia Scale on 20 points)

This rapid scale has three parts: a first allowing a very quick evaluation of the severity of ataxia, a second estimating globally the disability, and a third characterizing the quality of life by a visual analog rating scale. The scores are combined. The scale is highly correlated with the speed and accuracy of three-dimensional movements in upper limbs.

Part I

Body sway

0 Normal

1 Cannot stand with feet joined, but can stand with feet apart; minor oscillations of the trunk or the body

2 Marked body sway despite feet apart; however, no external support required

3 Requires a support or assistance. Falls without assistance

4 Impossible

Score ....

Gait (10 m go/return)

0 Normal

1 Mild ataxia

2 Walks with a cane or needs a support (intermittently puts his hands on a wall to avoid falling)

3 Gait with assistance or with a walker. Cannot walk with a cane

4 Unable to walk with aid or support

Score ....

Upper limb ataxia during self-paced finger-to-nose test

0 Normal

1 Errors near the target, the trajectory of the movement is curved, immediate corrections

2 Ataxia at the end of movement, presence of a discernible kinetic tremor, but the patient can stop the finger at the target. Fewer than 2 cycles of movement

3 Tremor is marked. The patient exhibits difficulties to stop the hand at the target. At least three cycles of oscillations

4 Unable to stop tremor

Score ....

Dysarthria: the patient repeats "mi-mi," "la-la," "ga-ga," "AhAhAhAh," "Pataka"

0 Normal

1 Mildly irregular voice. All words understandable. No need to repeat statements

2 Speech is slow, slurred, and/or scanned. Has to repeat some statements to make them understandable

3 Some words are not understandable

4 Unintelligible

Score . . . .

Ocular movements

1 Presence of a transient nystagmus on vertical and/or lateral gaze
2 Presence of a sustained nystagmus on vertical and/or lateral gaze
3 Square wave jerks
4 Hypometric or hypermetric saccades
5 Slow saccades
6 Absence of saccades

Score . . . .
TOTAL . . . ./20

Part II

Global disability score

A. Patient remaining fully independent in daily life
B. Patient requiring some help, but most tasks are performed alone
C. External aid is required most of the time
D. Totally dependent

Part III

Visual analog scale
A card with a vertical scale ranging from 0 to +100, with unit marks and numbers appearing every five scores, is presented to the subject. The respondent is told that 0 signifies death and 100 is associated with perfect health. The subject is asked to report verbally the number on the above scale. This number represents the general quality of life during the month preceding the visit.

SARA (Scale for Assessment and Rating of Ataxia)

The scale is based on a semiquantitative assessment of cerebellar ataxia on an impairment level (Schmitz-Hübsch et al., 2006b). SARA rates only ataxia-related symptoms and does not take into account extra-cerebellar symptoms which may be found. The scale has 8 items yielding a total score of 0 (no ataxia) to 40 (most severe ataxia):

1. Gait (subscore: /8)
2. Stance (subscore: /6)
3. Sitting (subscore: /4)
4. Speech deficits (subscore: /6)
5. Finger chase (subscore: /4)
6. Nose-finger test (subscore: /4)
7. Fast alternating movements (subscore: /4)
8. Heel-shin slide (subscore: /4)

Items 5 to 8 are rated for each side. The arithmetic mean of both sides is included in the total score.

I. Gait: the subject is asked to walk at a safe distance parallel to a wall including a half-turn and to walk in tandem without support

0 Normal
1 Slight difficulties, only visible when walking 10 consecutive steps in tandem
2 Clearly abnormal, tandem walking >10 steps impossible
3 Considerable staggering, difficulties in half-turn, but without support
4 Marked staggering, intermittent support of the wall required
5 Severe staggering, permanent support of one stick or light support by one arm required
6 Walking >10 m only with strong support (2 special sticks or stroller or accompanying person)
7 Walking <10 m only with strong support (2 special sticks or stroller or accompanying person)
8 Unable to walk, even support

SCORE . . . .

II. Stance: the subject is asked to stand first in a natural position, second with feet together in parallel (big toes touching each other), and finally in tandem (no space between heel and toe, feet on one line). The subject keeps eyes open and cannot wear shoes. For each of the three conditions, three trials are allowed and the best of them is rated.

0 Normal, can stand in tandem for >10 sec
1 Can stay with feet together without sway, but not in tandem for >10 sec
2 Able to stand with feet together for >10 sec, but only with sway
3 Able to stand for >10 sec without support in natural position, cannot stand with feet together
4 Able to stand for >10 sec in natural position only with intermittent support

57

5   Able to stand >10 sec in natural position only with constant support of 1 arm

6   Unable to stand for >10 sec even with constant support of 1 arm

SCORE . . . .

III. Sitting: the subject is sitting on an examination bed. No support of feet. Eyes open and arms outstretched to the front.

0   Normal, no difficulties to sit for >10 sec

1   Slight difficulties, intermittent sway

2   Constant sway, able to sit for >10 sec without support

3   Can sit for >10 sec only with intermittent support

4   Unable to sit for >10 sec without continuous support

SCORE . . . .

IV. Speech deficits: assessment during normal conversation.

0   Normal

1   Suggestive of a speech disturbance

2   Impaired speech, but easy to understand

3   Words occasionally difficult to understand

4   Many words difficult to understand

5   Only single words understandable

6   Speech is unintelligible/anarthria

SCORE . . . .

V. Finger chase: rating for each side. Subject is sitting comfortably. Support of feet and trunk allowed if required. The examiner is in front of the subject and performs five consecutive sudden and fast pointing movements in unpredictable directions in a frontal plane at about 50% of the proband's reach. Movements have an amplitude of 30 cm and a frequency of 1 movement every 2 sec. The subject is asked to follow the movements with his index finger as fast/accurately as possible. The average performance of last three movements is rated.

0   No dysmetria

1   Dysmetria, under/overshooting target <5 cm

2   Dysmetria, under/overshooting target <15 cm

3   Dysmetria, under/overshooting target >15 cm

4   Unable to perform five pointing movements

SCORE Right . . . .
SCORE Left . . . .
Mean of Right/Left . . . .

VI. Nose-finger test: rating for each side. The subject is sitting comfortably. Support of feet and trunk allowed if required. The subject is asked to point repeatedly with his index finger from his nose to examiner's finger which is in front of the proband at about 90% of the proband's reach. Speed of movement is moderate. The average performance of movements is rated according to the amplitude of the kinetic tremor.

0   No tremor

1   Tremor with an amplitude <2 cm

2   Tremor with an amplitude <5 cm

3   Tremor with an amplitude >5 cm

4   Unable to perform five pointing movements

SCORE Right . . . .
SCORE Left . . . .
Mean of Right/Left . . . .

VII. Fast alternating hand movements: rating for each side. Support of feet and trunk allowed if required. The subject is asked to perform 10 cycles of repetitive alternation of pronations and supinations of the hand on his/her thigh as fast/accurately as possible. Movement is demonstrated by the examiner at a speed of about 10 cycles within 7 sec. Exact times for movement execution have to be taken.

0   Normal, no irregularities (performs in <10 sec)

1   Slightly irregular (performs in <10 sec)

2   Clearly irregular, single movements difficult to distinguish or relevant interruptions, performs in <10 sec

3   Very irregular, single movements difficult to distinguish or relevant interruptions, performs in >10 sec

4   Cannot complete 10 cycles

SCORE Right . . . .
SCORE Left . . . .
Mean of Right/Left . . . .

VIII. Heel-shin slide: each side is rated. The subject is lying on the examination bed, without sight of his legs. The subject is asked to lift one leg, point with the heel to the opposite knee, slide down along the shin to the ankle, and lay the leg back on the examination bed. The task is performed three times. Slide-down movements should be performed within 1 sec. If the subject slides down without contact to shin in all three trials, rating is 4.

0   Normal
1   Slightly abnormal, contact to shin maintained
2   Clearly abnormal, goes off shin up to three times during three cycles
3   Severely abnormal, goes off shin four or more times during three cycles
4   Unable to perform the task

SCORE Right ....
SCORE Left ....
Mean of Right/Left ....

SARA score is closely correlated with the Barthel Index, which is widely used to estimate activities of daily living. The score correlates poorly with duration of the disease, and the scale presents some difficulties in detecting the beginning stage of cerebellar ataxias.

Comparison between scales

Inter-rater reliability and test–retest reliability are high for total ICARS and all but one of its subscales (Schmitz-Hübsch et al., 2006a). Internal consistency is good (Schoch et al., 2007). However, the score on certain items determines the score on other items, and internal validity might be problematic in degenerative ataxias. Ideally, the rating results of the ICARS should be determined by four factors that correspond to the four subscales in a factorial analysis. Principal-component analysis reveals five distinct and clinically meaningful factors in patients with focal cerebellar lesions (Schoch et al., 2007). These correspond to the four ICARS subscales and the laterality of kinetic functions. Inter-rater reliability is high for total SARA and single items except for nose-to-finger left and heel-to-shin left. Test–retest reliability is high. Factorial analysis shows that results on each item are determined by a single factor, suggesting that SARA measures a common underlying construct: ataxia. Advantageously, SARA is easier to administer and requires

less time (less than 10 min). However, SARA contains redundancies and excludes oculomotor assessment (Schmahmann et al., 2009).

Use of total ICARS is justified for both focal and degenerative disorders, and use of ICARS subscores remains justified in patients with focal lesions. The ICARS is probably more sensitive than the SARA scale for mild cerebellar dysfunction.

The AS20 is very quick and includes a global estimation of the disability and an estimation of the quality of life. However, it is less sensitive than the ICARS or the SARA scale. The BARS scale is easy to perform and sufficiently accurate for clinical purposes.

Quantitative tests

Timed tests are a good complement to clinical scales. They provide quantitative data, which are used for parametric testings.

The SCA Functional Index (SCAFI) has been proposed for autosomal dominant spinocerebellar ataxias (SCAs), taking into account three functional measures: 8-m walking time (8MW), 9-hole peg test (9HPT), and PATA repetition rate (Schmitz-Hübsch et al., 2008). Z-scores are correlated with SARA ratings.

The Composite Cerebellar Functional Severity (CCFS) score takes into account the 9-hole peg test (9HPT) and the click test performed with two mechanical counters located 39 cm apart (du Montcel et al., 2008). This distance is based on kinematic and kinetic analysis showing that it is the optimal inter-counter distance to evaluate the metrics of goal-directed multi-joint movements under visual guidance in the upper limbs. The subject presses buttons alternatively 10 times. CCFS is calculated as follows:

$$CCFS = \log_{10}[7 + Z1 + 4 \times Z2]$$

Where: $Z1 = Z$ pegboard dominant hand/10, and $Z2 = Z$ click dominant hand/10

The CCFS score is significantly higher in autosomal dominant SCAs as compared with controls and autosomal dominant spastic paraplegias. CCFS rating is correlated with disease duration. It is anticipated that the CCFS might be particularly useful for the discrimination of paucisymptomatic carriers and to monitor disease progression.

FARS (Friedreich Ataxia Rating Scale)

This scale was designed as a disease-specific scale for rating of Friedreich ataxia (Subramony et al., 2005).

It takes into account extra-cerebellar symptoms. The authors aimed to give a greater weight to gait. The examination assessed bulbar, upper limb, lower limb, peripheral nerve, and upright stability/gait functions. Timed activities tested included the timed walk of 50 feet, the number of repetitions of "PATA" in a 10-sec interval for speech assessment, and time taken to retrieve pegs in a 9-hole pegboard test. The scale starts with a functional staging and an evaluation of daily living.

Functional staging for ataxia

Increment by 0.5 may be used if the status is about the middle between two stages.

STAGE 0	Normal.
STAGE 1.0	Minimal signs detected by physician during screening. Can run or jump without loss of balance. No disability.
STAGE 2.0	Symptoms present, recognized by patient, but still mild. Cannot run or jump without losing balance. The patient is physically capable of leading an independent life, but daily activities may be somewhat restricted. Minimal disability.
STAGE 3.0	Symptoms are overt and significant. Requires regular or periodic holding onto wall/furniture or use of a cane for stability and walking. Mild disability. (Note: many patients postpone obtaining a cane by avoiding open spaces and walking with the aid of walls/people etc. These patients are graded as stage 3.0.)
STAGE 4.0	Walking requires a walker, Canadian crutches, or two canes. Or other aids such as walking dogs. Can perform several activities of daily living. Moderate disability.
STAGE 5.0	Confined but can navigate a wheelchair. Can perform some activities of daily living that do not require standing or walking. Severe disability.
STAGE 6.0	Confined to wheelchair or bed with total dependency for all activities of daily living. Total disability.

Activities of daily living

Increments of 0.5 may be used if strongly felt that a task falls between two scores.

1. Speech

   0 Normal.
   1 Mildly affected. No difficulty being understood.
   2 Moderately affected. Sometimes asked to repeat statements.
   3 Severely affected. Frequently asked to repeat statements.
   4 Unintelligible most of the time.

2. Swallowing

   0 Normal.
   1 Rare choking (<once a month).
   2 Frequent choking (<once a week, >once a month).
   3 Requires modified food or chokes multiple times a week, or patient avoids certain foods.
   4 Requires nasogastric tube or gastrostomy feedings.

3. Cutting Food and Handling Utensils

   0 Normal.
   1 Somewhat slow and clumsy, but no help needed.
   2 Clumsy and slow, but can cut most foods with some help needed. Or needs assistance when in a hurry.
   3 Food must be cut by someone, but can still feed self slowly.
   4 Needs to be fed.

4. Dressing

   0 Normal.
   1 Somewhat slow, but no help needed.
   2 Occasional assistance with buttoning, getting arms in sleeves, etc., or has to modify activity in some way (e.g. having to sit to get dressed; use velcro for shoes, stop wearing ties, etc.).
   3 Considerable help required, but can do some things alone.
   4 Helpless.

5. Personal Hygiene

   0 Normal.
   1 Somewhat slow, but no help needed.

2 Very slow hygienic care or has need for devices such as special grab bars, tub bench, shower chair, etc.

3 Requires personal help with washing, brushing teeth, combing hair, or using toilet.

4 Fully dependent.

6. Falling (assistive device = score 3)

   0 Normal.
   1 Rare falling (<once a month).
   2 Occasional falls (once a week to once a month).
   3 Falls multiple times a week or requires device to prevent falls.
   4 Unable to stand or walk.

7. Walking (assistive device = score 3)

   0 Normal.
   1 Mild difficulty, perception of imbalance.
   2 Moderate difficulty, but requires little or no assistance.
   3 Severe disturbance of walking, requires assistance or walking aids.
   4 Cannot walk at all even with assistance (wheelchair bound).

8. Quality of Sitting Position

   0 Normal.
   1 Slight imbalance of the trunk, but needs no back support.
   2 Unable to sit without back support.
   3 Can sit only with extensive support (geriatric chair, posy, etc.).
   4 Unable to sit.

9. Bladder Function (if using drugs for bladder, automatic score of 3)

   0 Normal.
   1 Mild urinary hesitance, urgency, or retention (<once a month).
   2 Moderate hesitance, urgency, rare retention/incontinence (>once a month, but <once a week).
   3 Frequent urinary incontinence (>once a week).
   4 Loss of bladder function requiring intermittent catheterization/indwelling catheter.

Total activities of daily living score:

Neurological examination

Each item is scored on the basis of the patient status during examination. Increments of 0.5 may be used if examiner feels an item falls between two defined severities.

A. Bulbar

   1. Facial Atrophy, Fasciculation, Action Myoclonus, and Weakness:

      0 None.
      1 Fasciculations or action myoclonus, but no atrophy.
      2 Atrophy present but not profound or complete.
      3 Profound atrophy and weakness.

   2. Tongue Atrophy, Fasciculation, Action Myoclonus, and Weakness:

      0 None.
      1 Fasciculations or action myoclonus, but no atrophy.
      2 Atrophy present but not profound or complete.
      3 Profound atrophy and weakness.

   3. Cough (patient asked to cough forcefully three times):

      0 Normal.
      1 Depressed.
      2 Totally or nearly absent.

   4. Spontaneous Speech (ask the patient to read or repeat the sentence "The President lives in the White House" or "The traffic is heavy today"):

      0 Normal.
      1 Mild (all or most words understandable).
      2 Moderate (most words not understandable).
      3 Severe (no or almost no useful speech).

Total bulbar score:

Upper limb coordination

Each limb is assessed and scored.

1. Finger-to-Finger Test (The index fingers are placed in front of each other with flexion at the elbow about 25 cm from the sternum. Observe for 10 sec. Score amplitude of oscillations.):

0 Normal.
1 Mild oscillations of finger (<2 cm).
2 Moderate oscillations of finger (2–6 cm).
3 Severe oscillations of finger (>6 cm).

2. Nose-Finger Test (Assess kinetic or intention tremor during and towards the end of movement: examiner holds index finger at 90% reach of patient; test at least three nose-finger-nose trials; movement slow >3 sec.):

0 None.
1 Mild (<2 cm amplitude).
2 Moderate (2–4 cm amplitude or persisting through movement).
3 Severe (>6 cm and persisting through movement).
4 Too poorly coordinated to perform task.

3. Dysmetria (Fast Nose-Finger) Test (Assess dysmetria: The patient touches tip of examiner's finger eight times as rapidly as possible while the examiner moves his finger and stops at different locations at about 90% reach of the patient. Assess dysmetria – i.e. inaccuracy of reaching the target – at examiner's finger.):

0 None.
1 Mild (misses 2 or fewer times).
2 Moderate (misses 3–5 times).
3 Severe (misses 6–8 times).
4 Too poorly coordinated to perform task.

4. Rapid Alternating Movements of Hands (Forearm pronation/supination 15 cm above thigh; 10 full cycles as fast as possible; assess rate, rhythm, accuracy; practice 10 cycles before rating, if time >7 sec, add 1 to score. Use stopwatch.):

0 Normal.
1 Mild (slightly irregular or slowed).
2 Moderate (irregular and slowed).
3 Too poorly coordinated to perform task.

5. Finger Taps (Index fingertip-to-thumb crease; 15 reps as fast as possible; practice 15 reps once before rating; if time >6 sec, add 1 to rating. Use stopwatch.):

0 Normal.
1 Mild (misses 1–3 times).
2 Moderate (misses 4–9 times).

3 Severe (misses 10–15 times).
4 Cannot perform the task.

Total upper limb coordination score:

Lower limb coordination

Each limb is assessed.

1. Heel Along Shin Slide (Under visual control, slide heel on the contralateral tibia from the patella to the ankle up and down, three cycles at moderate speed, 2 sec/cycle, one at a time. May be seated with contralateral leg extended or supine, but perform same way each time. Circle which: supine seated.):

0 Normal (stay on shin).
1 Mild (abnormally slow, tremulous but contact maintained).
2 Moderate (goes off shin a total of 3 or fewer times during 3 cycles).
3 Severe (goes off shin 4 or more times during 3 cycles).
4 Too poorly coordinated to attempt the task.

2. Heel-to-Shin Tap (Patient taps heel on midpoint of contralateral shin 8 times on each side from about 6–10 in, one at a time. May be seated with contralateral leg extended or supine but perform the same way each time. Circle which: supine seated.):

0 Normal (stays on target).
1 Mild (misses shin 2 or fewer times).
2 Moderate (misses shin 3–5 times).
3 Severe (misses shin 4 or more times).
4 Too poorly coordinated to perform task.

Total lower limb coordination score:

Peripheral nervous system

1. Muscle Atrophy (Score most severe atrophy in either upper or lower limb.):

0 None.
1 Present – mild/moderate.
2 Severe/total wasting.

2. Muscle Weakness (Test deltoids, interossei, iliopsoas, and tibialis anterior. Score most severe weakness in either upper or lower limb.):

0 Normal (5/5).

1 Mild (movement against resistance but not full power; 4/5).
2 Moderate (movement against gravity but not with added resistance; 3/5)
3 Severe (movement of joint but not against gravity; 2/5).
4 Near paralysis (muscular activity without movement; 1/5).
5 Total paralysis (0/5).

3. Vibratory Sense (Educate patient regarding the sensation. Test with 128-cps tuning fork set to near-full vibration; eyes closed; test over index finger and great toe. Abnormal <15 sec for toes and <25 sec for hands.):

Time felt for toes and fingers is noted for each side.

0 Normal.
1 Impaired at toes.
2 Impaired at toes or fingers.

4. Position Sense (Test using minimal random movement of distal interphalangeal joints of index finger and big toe.):

0 Normal.
1 Impaired at toes or fingers.
2 Impaired at toes and fingers.

5. Deep Tendon Reflexes (0 – absent; 1 – hyporeflexia; 2 – normal; 3 – hyperreflexia; 4 – pathologic hyperreflexia):

Right:

BJ___   BrJ___   KJ___   AJ___

Left:

BJ___   BrJ___   KJ___   AJ___

0 No areflexia.
1 Areflexia in either upper or lower limbs.
2 Generalized areflexia.

Total peripheral nervous system score:

Upright stability

For sitting posture, patient can sit in a chair or on an examination table. For standing and walking assessment, instruct patient to wear best walking shoes and record below if barefoot, footwear, or ankle-foot orthoses (AFOs) used. Stance assessment begins with feet 20 cm apart. Place marker tapes in the exam room 20 cm apart, and the insides of the feet are lined up against these. Subsequent stance tests get more difficult. For feet together, the entire inside of the feet should be close together as much as possible. For tandem stance, the dominant foot is in the back and the heel of the other foot is lined with the toes of the dominant foot but not in front of the toes (because this makes it even more difficult). For one-foot stance, the patient is asked to stand on the dominant foot and the other leg is elevated by bringing it forward with knee extended; this gives some advantage to the patient. If a patient can stand in a particular position for 1 minute or longer in trial 1, then trials 2 and 3 are abandoned. Otherwise, each of three trials is timed and then averaged. Grading scores are then given as noted. Tandem walk and gait are performed in a hallway, preferably with no carpet, but at least serial examinations should be done on the same surface. For gait, place markers 25 feet apart. The patient walks the distance, turns around, and comes back, and the activity is timed. Note if the gait was achieved with or without device, and serial examinations should be done with the same device as in the first examination.

Stance and gait tests may be done barefoot if the patient does have appropriate footwear; however, they should be done the same way for serial measurement.

Circle which:	Barefoot	Footwear
Also, indicate if AFOs are used:	Yes	No

1. Sitting Posture (Patient seated in chair with thighs together, arms folded, back unsupported; observe for 30 sec.):

0 Normal.
1 Mild oscillations of head/trunk without touching chair back or side.
2 Moderate oscillations of head/trunk; needs contact with chair back or side for stability.
3 Severe oscillations of head/trunk; needs contact with chair back or side for stability.
4 Support on all four sides for stability.

2. Stance – Feet Apart (Inside of feet 20 cm apart marked on floor. Use stopwatch; three attempts;

time in seconds. Three trials are performed and the averaged is noted.):

0   1 min or longer.
1   <1 min, >45 sec.
2   <45 sec, >30 sec.
3   <30 sec, >15 sec.
4   <15 sec or needs hands held by assistant/device.

3. Stance – Feet Together (Use stopwatch; three attempts; time in seconds. Three trials are performed and the averaged is noted.):

0   1 min or longer.
1   <1 min, >45 sec.
2   <45 sec, >30 sec.
3   <30 sec, >15 sec.
4   <15 sec.

4. Tandem Stance (Use stopwatch; three attempts, dominant foot in front; time in seconds. Three trials are performed and the averaged is noted.)

0   1 min or longer.
1   <1 min, >45 sec.
2   <45 sec, >30 sec.
3   <30 sec, >15 sec.
4   <15 sec.

5. Stance on Dominant Foot (Use stopwatch; three attempts; time in seconds. Three trials are performed and the averaged is noted.):

0   **1 min or longer.**
1   <1 min, >45 sec.
2   <45 sec, >30 sec.
3   <30 sec, >15 sec.
4   <15 sec.

6. Tandem Walk (Tandem walk 10 steps in straight line; performed in hallway with no furniture within reach of 1 m/3 ft and no loose carpet.):

0   Normal (able to tandem walk >8 sequential steps).
1   Able to tandem walk in less than perfect manner/can tandem walk >4 sequential steps, but <8.
2   Can tandem walk, but <4 steps before losing balance.
3   Too poorly coordinated to attempt task.

7. Gait (Use stopwatch; walk 8 m/25 ft at normal pace, turn around using single-step pivot and return to start; performed in hallway with no furniture within reach of 1 m/3 ft and no loose carpet.):

Device, if any:_____
Time in seconds:_____

0   Normal.
1   Mild ataxia/veering/difficulty in turning; no cane/other support needed to be safe.
2   Walks with definite ataxia; may need intermittent support or examiner needs to walk with patient for safety sake.
3   Moderate ataxia/veering/difficulty in turning; walking requires cane/holding onto examiner with one hand to be safe.
4   Severe ataxia/veering; walker or both hands of examiner needed.
5   Cannot walk even with assistance (wheelchair bound).

Total upright stability score:
Total neurologic examination score:

Instrumental testing

1. PATA Rate
2. Nine-Hole Pegboard Test

Scores correlate significantly with functional disability, activities of daily living scores, and disease duration. The scale is well correlated with the Functional Independence Measure (FIM, an 18-item scale evaluating the functional abilities) and the Modified Barthel Index, and is well suited for clinical trials (Fahey et al., 2007).

Unified Multiple System Atrophy Rating Scale (UMSARS)

The scale includes the following components (Wenning et al., 2004):

*   Part I: historical (12 items)
*   Part II: motor examination (14 items)
*   Part III: autonomic examination
*   Part IV: global disability scale

Part I. Historical review. The average functional situation for the past 2 weeks (unless specified) is rated, according to the patient and caregiver interview.

1. **Speech–**
   0   Not affected.
   1   Mildly affected. No difficulties being understood.
   2   Moderately affected. Sometimes (less than half of the time) asked to repeat statements.
   3   Severely affected. Frequently (more than half of the time) asked to repeat statements.
   4   Unintelligible most of the time.

2. **Swallowing–**
   0   Normal.
   1   Mild impairment. Choking less than once a week.
   2   Moderate impairment. Occasional food aspiration with choking more than once a week.
   3   Marked impairment. Frequent food aspiration.
   4   Nasogastric tube or gastrostomy feeding.

3. **Handwriting–**
   0   Normal.
   1   Mildly impaired, all words are legible.
   2   Moderately impaired, up to half of the words are not legible.
   3   Markedly impaired, the majority of words are not legible.
   4   Unable to write.

4. **Cutting food and handling utensils–**
   0   Normal.
   1   Somewhat slow and/or clumsy, but no help needed.
   2   Can cut most foods, although clumsy and slow; some help needed.
   3   Food must be cut by someone, but can still feed slowly.
   4   Needs to be fed.

5. **Dressing–**
   0   Normal.
   1   Somewhat slow and/or clumsy, but no help needed.
   2   Occasional assistance with buttoning, getting arms in sleeves.
   3   Considerable help required, but can do some things alone.
   4   Completely helpless.

6. **Hygiene–**
   0   Normal.
   1   Somewhat slow and/or clumsy, but no help needed.
   2   Needs help to shower or bathe, or very slow in hygienic care.
   3   Requires assistance for washing, brushing teeth, combing hair, using the toilet.
   4   Completely helpless.

7. **Walking–**
   0   Normal.
   1   Mildly impaired. No assistance needed. No walking aid required (except for unrelated disorders).
   2   Moderately impaired. Assistance and/or walking aid needed occasionally.
   3   Severely impaired. Assistance and/or walking aid needed frequently.
   4   Cannot walk at all even with assistance.

8. **Falling (rate the past month)–**
   0   None.
   1   Rare falling (less than once a month).
   2   Occasional falling (less than once a week).
   3   Falls more than once a week.
   4   Falls at least once a day (if the patient cannot walk at all, rate 4).

9. **Orthostatic symptoms–**
   0   No orthostatic symptoms.[a]
   1   Orthostatic symptoms are infrequent and do not restrict activities of daily living.
   2   Frequent orthostatic symptoms developing at least once a week. Some limitation in activities of daily living.
   3   Orthostatic symptoms develop on most occasions. Able to stand >1 min on most occasions. Limitation in most of activities of daily living.
   4   Symptoms consistently develop on orthostasis. Able to stand <1 min on most occasions. Syncope/presyncope is common if patient attempts to stand.

10. **Urinary function[b]–**
   0   Normal.
   1   Urgency and/or frequency, no drug treatment required.
   2   Urgency and/or frequency, drug treatment required.
   3   Urge incontinence and/or incomplete bladder emptying needing intermittent catheterization.
   4   Incontinence needing indwelling catheter.

11. **Sexual function–**
   0   No problems.
   1   Minor impairment compared with healthy days.
   2   Moderate impairment compared with healthy days.
   3   Severe impairment compared with healthy days.
   4   No sexual activity possible.

12. **Bowel function–**
   0   No change in pattern of bowel function from previous pattern.
   1   Occasional constipation but no medication needed.
   2   Frequent constipation requiring use of laxatives.
   3   Chronic constipation requiring use of laxatives and enemas.
   4   Cannot have a spontaneous bowel movement.

Total score Part I:

[a]Syncope, dizziness, visual disturbances or neck pain, relieved on lying flat.
[b]Urinary symptoms should not be due to other causes.

Part II. Motor examination. The worst affected limb is rated.

1. **Facial expression–**
   0   Normal.
   1   Minimal hypomimia, could be normal (Poker face).
   2   Slight but definitely abnormal diminution of facial expression.

3   Moderate hypomimia; lips parted some of the time.
4   Masked or fixed facies with severe or complete loss of facial expression, lips parted 0.25 in or more.

2. Speech–
The patient is asked to repeat several times a standard sentence.
0   Normal.
1   Mildly slow, slurred, and/or dysphonic. No need to repeat statements.
2   Moderately slow, slurred, and/or dysphonic. Sometimes asked to repeat statements.
3   Severely slow, slurred, and/or dysphonic. Frequently asked to repeat statements.
4   Unintelligible.

3. Ocular motor dysfunction–
Eye movements are examined by asking the subject to follow slow horizontal finger movements of the examiner, to look laterally at the finger at different positions, and to perform saccades between two fingers, each held at an eccentric position of approximately 30 °. The examiner assesses the following abnormal signs: (1) broken-up smooth pursuit, (2) gaze-evoked nystagmus at an eye position of more than 45 degrees, (3) gaze-evoked nystagmus at an eye position of less than 45 degrees, and (4) saccadic hypermetria. Sign 3 suggests that there are at least two abnormal ocular motor signs, because Sign 2 is also present.
0   None.
1   One abnormal ocular motor sign.
2   Two abnormal ocular motor signs.
3   Three abnormal ocular motor signs.
4   Four abnormal ocular motor signs.

4. Tremor at rest (rate the most affected limb)–
0   Absent.
1   Slight and infrequently present.
2   Mild in amplitude and persistent. Or moderate in amplitude, but only intermittently present.
3   Moderate in amplitude and present most of the time.
4   Marked in amplitude and present most of the time.

5. Action tremor–
Postural tremor of outstretched arms (A) and action tremor on finger pointing (B) are assessed. Maximal tremor severity in Task A and/or B (whichever is worse) is rated for the most affected limb.
0   Absent.
1   Slight tremor of small amplitude (A). No interference with finger pointing (B).
2   Moderate amplitude (A). Some interference with finger pointing (B).
3   Marked amplitude (A). Marked interference with finger pointing (B).
4   Severe amplitude (A). Finger pointing impossible (B).

6. Increased tone (rate the most affected limb)–
Judged on passive movement of major joints with patient relaxed in sitting position; ignore cogwheeling.
0   Absent.
1   Slight or detectable only when activated by mirror or other movements.

2   Mild to moderate.
3   Marked, but full range of motion easily achieved.
4   Severe, range of motion achieved with difficulty.

7. Rapid alternating movements of hands–
Pronation–supination movements of hands, vertically or horizontally, with as large an amplitude as possible, each hand separately, rate the worst affected limb. Note that impaired performance on this task can be caused by bradykinesia and/or cerebellar incoordination. Rate functional performance regardless of underlying motor disorder.
0   Normal.
1   Mildly impaired.
2   Moderately impaired.
3   Severely impaired.
4   Can barely perform the task.

8. Finger taps–
Patient taps thumb with index finger in rapid succession with widest amplitude possible, each hand at least 15 to 20 sec. Rate the worst affected limb. Note that impaired performance on this task can be caused by bradykinesia and/or cerebellar incoordination. Rate functional performance regardless of underlying motor disorder.
0   Normal.
1   Mildly impaired.
2   Moderately impaired.
3   Severely impaired.
4   Can barely perform the task.

9. Leg agility–
Patient is sitting and taps heel on ground in rapid succession, picking up entire leg. Amplitude should be approximately 10 cm, rate the worst affected leg. Note that impaired performance on this task can be caused by bradykinesia and/or cerebellar incoordination. Rate functional performance, regardless of underlying motor disorder.
0   Normal.
1   Mildly impaired.
2   Moderately impaired.
3   Severely impaired.
4   Can barely perform the task.

10. Heel-knee-shin test–
The patient is requested to raise one leg and place the heel on the knee, and then slide the heel down the anterior tibial surface of the resting leg toward the ankle. On reaching the ankle joint, the leg is again raised in the air to a height of approximately 40 cm and the action is repeated. At least three movements of each limb must be performed for proper assessment. Rate the worst affected limb.
0   Normal.
1   Mildly dysmetric and ataxic.
2   Moderately dysmetric and ataxic.
3   Severely dysmetric and ataxic.
4   Can barely perform the task.

11. **Arising from chair–**
Patient attempts to arise from a straight-back wood or metal chair with arms folded across chest.
0   Normal.
1   Clumsy, or may need more than one attempt.
2   Pushes self up from arms of seat.
3   Tends to fall back and may have to try more than once but can get up without help.
4   Unable to arise without help.

12. **Posture–**
0   Normal.
1   Not quite erect, slightly stooped posture; could be normal for older person.
2   Moderately stooped posture, definitely abnormal; can be slightly leaning to one side.
3   Severely stooped posture with kyphosis; can be moderately leaning to one side.
4   Marked flexion with extreme abnormality of posture.

13. **Body sway–**
Rate spontaneous body sway and response to sudden, strong posterior displacement produced by pull on shoulder while patient erect with eyes open and feet slightly apart. Patient has to be warned.
0   Normal.
1   Slight body sway and/or retropulsion with unaided recovery.
2   Moderate body sway and/or deficient postural response; might fall if not caught by examiner.
3   Severe body sway. Very unstable. Tends to lose balance spontaneously.
4   Unable to stand without assistance.

14. **Gait–**
0   Normal.
1   Mildly impaired.
2   Moderately impaired. Walks with difficulty, but requires little or no assistance.
3   Severely impaired. Requires assistance.
4   Cannot walk at all, even with assistance.

Total score Part II:

Part III. Autonomic examination. Supine blood pressure and heart rate are measured after 2 min of rest and again after 2 min of standing. Orthostatic symptoms may include lightheadedness, dizziness, blurred vision, weakness, fatigue, cognitive impairment, nausea, palpitations, tremulousness, headache, neck and coat-hanger ache.

Systolic blood pressure

Supine
Standing (2 min)
Unable to record

Diastolic blood pressure

Supine
Standing (2 min)
Unable to record

Heart rate

Supine
Standing (2 min)
Unable to record

Orthostatic symptoms

Yes
No

Part IV. Global disability scale.

1. Completely independent. Able to do all chores with minimal difficulty or impairment. Essentially normal. Unaware of any difficulty.

2. Not completely independent. Needs help with some chores.

3. More dependent. Help with half of chores. Spends a large part of the day with chores.

4. Very dependent. Now and then does a few chores alone or begins alone. Much help needed.

5. Totally dependent and helpless. Bedridden.

References

Babinski J, Tournay A. Symptômes des maladies du cervelet. *Rev Neurol* 1913;**18**:306–22.

du Montcel ST, Charles P, Ribai P, et al. Composite cerebellar functional severity score: validation of a quantitative score of cerebellar impairment. *Brain* 2008;**131**(Pt 5):1352–61.

Fahey MC, Corben L, Collins V, Churchyard AJ, Delatycki MB. How is disease progress in Friedreich's ataxia best measured? A study of four rating scales. *J Neurol Neurosurg Psychiatry* 2007;**78**(4):411–3.

Schmahmann JD, Gardner R, MacMore J, Vangel MG. Development of a brief ataxia rating scale (BARS) based on a modified form of the ICARS. *Mov Disord* 2009;**24**:1820–1828.

Schmitz-Hübsch T, Giunti P, Stephenson DA, et al. SCA Functional Index: a useful compound performance measure for spinocerebellar ataxia. *Neurology* 2008;**71**(7):486–92.

Schmitz-Hübsch T, Tezenas du Montcel S, Baliko L, et al. Reliability and validity of the International Cooperative Ataxia Rating Scale: a study in 156 spinocerebellar ataxia patients. *Mov Disord* 2006a;**21**:699–704.

Schmitz-Hübsch T, Tezenas du Montcel S, Baliko L, et al. Scale for the assessment and rating of ataxia. Development of a new clinical scale. *Neurology* 2006b;**66**:1717–1720.

Schoch B, Regel JP, Frings M, et al. Reliability and validity of ICARS in focal cerebellar lesions. *Mov Disord* 2007;**22**(15):2162–9.

Storey E, Tuck K, Hester R, et al. Inter-rater reliability of the International Cooperative Ataxia Rating Scale (ICARS). *Mov Disord* 2004;**19**:190–2.

Subramony SH, May W, Lynch D, et al. Measuring Friedreich ataxia: interrater reliability of a neurologic rating scale. *Neurology* 2005;**64**: 1261–2.

Tison F, Yekhlef F, Balestre E, et al. Application of the International Cooperative Ataxia Scale rating in multiple system atrophy. *Mov Disord* 2002;**17**: 1248–54.

Trouillas P, Takayanagi T, Hallett M, et al. International cooperative ataxia rating scale for pharmacological assessment of the cerebellar syndrome. *J Neurol Sci* 1997;**145**:205–11.

Wenning GK, Tison F, Seppi K, et al. Development and validation of the Unified Multiple System Atrophy Rating Scale (UMSARS). *Mov Disord* 2004;**19**:1391–1402.

Wright J. The FIM(TM). The Center for Outcome Measurement in Brain Injury. Available at http://www.tbims.org/combi/FIM (accessed August 25, 2009).

Diagnosis of cerebellar disorders as a function of age

The importance of obtaining a detailed genealogy

Ataxias can be divided into sporadic forms and hereditary ataxias. These latter include autosomal recessive forms, autosomal dominant ataxias (spinocerebellar ataxias [SCAs]), X-linked disorders, and mitochondrial diseases. The reader is also referred to Chapters 20, 21, 22, and 23.

Family history and detailed clinical examination provide major information for the work-up of cerebellar ataxias. Obtaining a detailed description of the onset and progression of symptoms is an important step (Fogel & Perlman, 2006). Concomitant symptoms such as dementia, seizures, parkinsonian features, or peripheral neuropathy can be useful for differentiating ataxias.

Detailed genealogy often reveals an apparent mode of inheritance (Brusse et al., 2007):

- Multiple affected siblings in a family or consanguinity indicates a possible autosomal recessive transmission.
- Ataxia in consecutive generations suggests an autosomal dominant inheritance.
- X-linked transmission is characterized by affected males in the maternal line.
- Mitochondrial ataxias may be difficult to suspect, because mutations may occur in nuclear or mitochondrial DNA. These latter may present like autosomal dominant or recessive diseases due to mechanisms such as heteroplasmy. In addition, mitochondrial deletions/insertions are often sporadic (Finsterer, 2004).

Anticipation and reduced penetrance should be kept in mind when facing ataxic patients. There is a clear correlation between the age of onset/severity of disease and the size of the triplet expansion in SCAs. Moreover, de novo mutations may occur, and therefore the absence of family history does not rule out hereditary ataxia. Autosomal dominant ataxias include SCA, dentatorubral-pallidoluysian atrophy (DRPLA), episodic ataxias (where the episodic occurrence of symptoms is suggestive), hereditary spastic ataxias, sensorimotor neuropathies with ataxias, and several leukodystrophies (Schöls et al., 2004; Brusse et al., 2007). The most common recessive ataxias are Friedreich ataxia (FRDA), ataxia telangiectasia (AT), and ataxia and oculomotor apraxia type 1 (more frequent in Portugal and Japan). Although there are exceptions, most recessive ataxias are symptomatic before the age of 25 years, unlike dominant ataxias, which tend to appear later.

Because more and more new genetic tests are becoming available, patients who are suspected to present with a hereditary cerebellar ataxia should be re-evaluated regularly with updated tests. Acquired and hereditary causes may coexist and a multifactorial disease is not exceptional, especially in the elderly (Fogel & Perlman, 2006).

The role of brain imaging

Brain imaging, in particular MRI and to a lesser extent CT scan, immediately identifies structural lesions in the posterior fossa. Cerebellar atrophy itself is a relatively aspecific finding. The atrophy may be asymmetrical (Figure 5.1). However, the topography of the atrophy or concomitant lesions may point towards a diagnosis. For instance, atrophy of the anterior lobe in adults may suggest a toxic cause (see Chapter 15), white matter lesions in the middle cerebellar peduncles may point towards a fragile X-associated tremor/ataxia syndrome (FXTAS) (see Chapter 22), adult-onset hemicerebellar atrophy suggests a post-infectious origin (see Chapter 11), and calcifications in dentate nuclei are found in SCA20 (see Chapter 23; Storey et al., 2005). Atrophy of the brainstem or spinal cord may be observed in several diseases, such as FRDA.

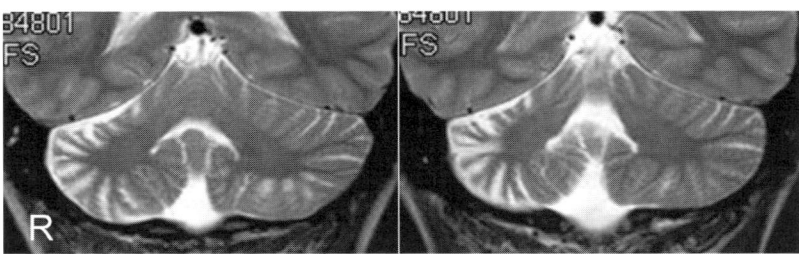

Figure 5.1 Illustration with MRI of hemiatrophy of the cerebellum, with widening of the cerebellar sulci on the right side (R). T2-weighted coronal section.

Blood studies

Biochemical/blood studies and genetic tests may confirm the diagnosis of a cerebellar ataxia. Examples are decreased levels of vitamin E in ataxia associated with vitamin E deficiency (AVED), elevated plasma levels of cholestanol in cerebrotendinous xanthomatosis (CTX, see Chapter 20), impaired copper metabolism in Wilson disease, and mutation in a given locus in a genetically determined form of ataxia (see Chapter 20).

Which cutoff for age?

Cutoff points for age of onset need a flexible interpretation. The following classification considers congenital and childhood disorders (until adolescence), ataxia in young adults, and ataxia in the elderly. Local factors (environment, etc.) and regional prevalence of diseases need to be taken into account. The origin of a family needs special attention.

Congenital and childhood disorders

There is an overlap between congenital and childhood ataxias. Ataxias are most often related to:

- developmental disorders (see Chapter 7)
- infections and para-infectious manifestations (see Chapter 11)
- X-linked disorders
- autosomal dominant ataxias (especially SCA1, SCA2, SCA7, SCA8, SCA13, SCA25, SCA27, DRPLA, and episodic ataxias)
- autosomal recessive diseases (see Table 5.1. for laboratory investigations): the most common are FRDA, AT, ataxia with oculomotor apraxia (AOA), AVED, abetalipoproteinemia, Refsum disease, GM2 gangliosidosis, Krabbe disease, Niemann-Pick (type C) disease, adrenoleukodystrophy, CTX, spastic ataxia of Charlevoix-Saguenay, and Marinesco-Sjögren

Table 5.1 Laboratory investigations in autosomal recessive ataxias

Genetic tests

Blood studies
  Vitamin E
  Acanthocytes
  Lipids (cholesterol, triglycerides, LDL, VLDL)
  Lactate/pyruvate
  Albumin
  Immunoglobulins
  Alpha-fetoprotein
  Folic acid
  Vitamin B12
  Phytanic acid
  Copper/ceruloplasmin
  Enzymes (hexosaminidase, arylsulfatase, alpha/beta-galactosidase, beta-galactocerebrosidase, neuraminidase)
  VLCFA (very long chain fatty acids)
  Organic acids

Urine studies
  Metabolic screening
  Bile alcohols

Skin biopsy

syndrome. Some diseases are very rare, such as L-2-hydroxyglutaric aciduria.

Symptoms of FRDA usually start at the end of the first decade or the beginning of the second. Phenotype includes tendon areflexia, sensory deficits, pyramidal signs, cardiomyopathy, scoliosis, diabetes, and sensorimotor deafness. The clinical spectrum of AT includes oculocutaneous telangiectasias, choreoathetosis, and dystonic posture. Patients develop immunodeficiencies and are at risk for malignancies. AT usually starts in early childhood. AOA starts in childhood or in early teenage years in most cases. Blood levels of alpha-fetoprotein are raised in AT and AOA2 (Date et al., 2001). AVED shares with FRDA the tendon areflexia, loss of vibration sense in lower limbs (as a result of a polyneuropathy), and pyramidal signs. However, cardiac involvement and diabetes are uncommon in AVED. Age of onset ranges between 2 and 50 years, being usually before

18 years. Evidence of peripheral nerve disease is also observed in abetalipoproteinemia, which usually starts between 4 and 15 years of age by digestive symptoms. A retinopathy should be searched for. Blood studies show acanthocytes (on fresh blood smears) and evidence of malabsorption. Vitamin A and vitamin E levels may be decreased. Refsum disease starts before the age of 26 years in most patients. The syndrome includes retinitis pigmentosa, anosmia, polyneuropathy, deafness, and ichthyosis. L-2-hydroxyglutaric aciduria presents with cerebellar ataxia associated with pyramidal signs, mental decline, seizures, and macrocephaly. Cerebral folate deficiency is associated with low cerebrospinal fluid (CSF) 5-methyltetrahydrofolate (the active folate metabolite), in the presence of normal folate metabolism outside the nervous system (Ramaekers & Blau, 2004). Typical features are manifest from the age of 4 months: marked unrest, irritability, and sleep disturbances followed by psychomotor retardation, cerebellar ataxia, spastic paraplegia, dyskinesias, and seizures. Most children show deceleration of head growth from the age of 4 to 6 months, and visual deficits start around the age of 3 years. Neuroimaging shows atrophy of frontotemporal regions, periventricular demyelination, and slowly progressive supra- and infratentorial atrophy. Disorders of folate metabolism may cause elevated plasma homocysteine levels and homocystinuria presenting clinically as a subacute syndrome comprising progressive ataxia, dysarthria, tremor, and mental deficits (Bishop et al., 2008). Another metabolic disorder which should not be overlooked in early infancy is the Glut1 deficiency syndrome, a potentially treatable disorder. Clinical features usually comprise motor and mental developmental delay, seizures, deceleration of head growth, and movement disorders with ataxia, dystonia, and spasticity (Brockmann, 2009). Symptoms may be carbohydrate-responsive. A laboratory hallmark is the reduced glucose level in CSF with decreased CSF-to-blood glucose ratio. Ataxia may be intermittent (Joshi et al., 2008). Trauma and its complications should not be underestimated in infants.

Ataxias in young adults

The principal causes of ataxias in young adults are listed in Table 5.2. Mean age of onset of SCAs is in the third and fourth decade, but there is considerable variation among the various SCAs (see Chapter 23).

Severe anticipation is usually indicative of SCA7, SCA17, and SCA2. Childhood or early adult onset of tremor points to SCA27.

Late-onset Friedreich ataxia presents between the ages of 25 and 50 years. The phenotype is usually milder as compared with classical FRDA. Cardiomyopathy is often absent (Bhidayasiri et al., 2005).

Copper metabolism disorders include Wilson disease, hypo- or aceruloplasminemia, and hypercupremia with ataxia. Eye examination shows Kayser-Fleischer ring in Wilson disease and retinal degeneration in aceruloplasminemia. Partial ceruloplasmin deficiency may present with a moderate cerebellar syndrome starting in the fourth decade (Miyajima et al., 2001). Brain MRI shows cerebellar atrophy.

Cataract in young adults presenting with cerebellar ataxia, pyramidal signs, mental deterioration, and polyneuropathy and in whom white matter lesions are observed on brain MRI should point to a possible CTX. Other findings are tendon xanthomas and diarrhea. White matter lesions are also found in various adult-onset leukodystrophies.

Table 5.3 shows the laboratory investigations and Table 5.4 lists the secondary investigations facing a young adult presenting with cerebellar ataxia.

Ataxia in the elderly

The most common causes of ataxia in the elderly are stroke, trauma, infections, cerebellar multiple system atrophy, SCAs, FXTAS, metastases, and paraneoplastic diseases.

Multiple system atrophy (MSA) is discussed in Chapter 18. The cerebellar presentation is increasingly recognized as one of the most common causes of ataxia starting in the elderly. Clinical hallmarks are autonomic dysfunction, cerebellar ataxia, parkinsonism, and pyramidal signs. The following studies can be helpful to distinguish MSA from other neurodegenerative diseases: brain MRI, functional imaging, sphincter electromyography, and investigations of the autonomous system.

FXTAS combines cerebellar ataxia and tremor, parkinsonism, cognitive decline, and autonomic dysfunction. Patients may present with a peripheral neuropathy. Brain MRI is suggestive (see Chapter 22). In the older male without overt family history, the late-onset phenotype of FXTAS can be misdiagnosed as dementia, essential tremor, stroke, or Parkinson disease (Fogel & Perlman, 2006).

Table 5.2 Differential diagnosis of cerebellar ataxias in young adults[a]

Disease	Clues
Spinocerebellar ataxia (SCA)	Dominantly inherited Predominant cerebellar syndrome Extra-cerebellar signs present in various SCAs (mainly ophthalmoplegia, movement disorders, pyramidal deficits, cognitive/behavioral symptoms, seizures, peripheral neuropathy)
Episodic ataxia (EA)	Dominantly inherited Attacks of ataxia History of migraine in EA2 Interictal myokymia, kinesigenic ataxia, and brief attacks in EA1
Friedreich ataxia (FRDA)/Late-onset Friedreich ataxia (LOFA)	Tendon areflexia Babinski sign
Other recessive ataxias (see Table 5.1)	
Fragile X tremor–associated ataxia (FXTAS)	X-linked ataxia Family history of infertility, early menopause, or mental retardation Cognitive deficits Parkinsonian syndrome
Wilson disease	Chorea, dystonia Kayser-Fleischer ring Liver dysfunction
Primary tumor	
Paraneoplastic ataxia	Subacute course Symptoms of general cancer
Infectious/parainfectious	History of infection Immunoglobulin M/immunoglobulin G antibodies in serum CSF studies
Immune Multiple sclerosis	Optic neuritis
Celiac ataxia	History of relapses CSF studies, brain MRI, and evoked potentials suggestive Anti-gliadin antibodies
Toxics	
Endocrine diseases	Hypothyroidism Thyroiditis (Hashimoto)

Leukodystrophies
    Metachromatic leukodystrophy
    X-linked adrenoleukodystrophy
    Krabbe disease
    Niemann-Pick disease
	Dementia
	Psychiatric manifestations

Mitochondrial disorders	
Kearns-Sayre syndrome	Ophthalmoplegia, pigmentary retinopathy, cardiac conduction defects
MELAS	Myopathy, encephalopathy, lactic acidosis, stroke-like episodes
MERRF	Myoclonic epilepsy, myopathy, dementia, ophthalmoplegia, deafness, seizures
NARP	Peripheral neuropathy, retinitis pigmentosa
May-White syndrome IOSCA (Finland mainly) MIRAS[b] SANDO[b]	Myoclonus, deafness Polyneuropathy, ophthalmoplegia, optic atrophy, seizures Migraine, epilepsy, myoclonus, ophthalmoplegia, polyneuropathy Sensory ataxic neuropathy, dysarthria/dysphagia, ophthalmoparesis

Abbreviations: IOSCA: infantile onset spinocerebellar ataxia; MELAS: mitochondrial encephalomyopathy, lactic acidosis, and stroke-like episodes; MERRF: myoclonic epilepsy with ragged-red fibers; MIRAS: mitochondrial recessive ataxia syndrome; NARP: neuropathy, ataxia, and retinitis pigmentosa; SANDO: sensory ataxic neuropathy, dysarthria, and ophthalmoparesis.
[a]Readers are referred to corresponding chapters in the book for a detailed description of the disorders. The main features are indicated in this table.
[b]Associated with mutations of the DNA polymerase gamma (gene locus 15q24–15q26).

Table 5.3 Laboratory investigations in adult-onset cerebellar ataxia

Genetic tests

Blood studies
   Sedimentation rate, C-reactive protein
   Complete blood cell count
   Renal and liver function tests
   Serum electrolytes
   Glucose, glucose tolerance test, glycated hemoglobin
   Antinuclear antibodies
   Thyroid-stimulating hormone, anti-TPO antibodies
   Protein electrophoresis
   Angiotensin-converting enzyme
   Vitamin E
   Vitamin B12, homocysteine, folate
   Acanthocytes
   Lipids (cholesterol, triglycerides, LDL, VLDL)
   Lactate/pyruvate
   Copper/ceruloplasmin
   Antigliadin antibodies
   Anti-GAD antibodies
   Anti-cerebellar antibodies (Yo, Ri, Hu, CV2, Tr, Ma1, mGluR1, Amphiphysin)

CSF studies
   Cell count, protein, glucose, lactate
   Cytology
   Cultures
   IgG index, oligoclonal bands
   14–3–3 protein
   Paraneoplastic antibodies

Urine studies
   Protein electrophoresis
   Metabolic screening
   Bile alcohols
   Heavy metals

Abbreviations: GAD: glutamic acid decarboxylase; LDL: low-density lipoprotein; TPO: thyroid peroxidase; VLDL: very low density lipoprotein.

Table 5.4 Secondary investigations in adult-onset cerebellar ataxia

Diagnosis suspected	Investigation
Prion disease	Electroencephalography, genetic tests
Neuropathy	Electromyography/nerve conduction velocities Nerve biopsy
Demyelinating disease	Evoked potentials MRI of spine
Multiple systemic atrophy (MSA)	Autonomic tests, FDopa/fluorodeoxyglucose-positron emission tomography (FDG-PET) scan
Paraneoplastic ataxia	CT scan/FDG-PET scan of whole body
Mitochondrial disease	Muscle biopsy, MR spectroscopy (MRS) Genetic tests
Metabolic disorder	MRS
Lysosomal storage disease	Bone marrow biopsy Genetic tests
Peroxisomal disease	Conjunctival/skin biopsy Genetic tests

Prion disorders usually manifest with prominent dementia, but patients may present with an ataxic syndrome, particularly for sporadic Creutzfeldt-Jakob disease or familial Gerstmann-Sträussler-Scheinker disease. Electroencephalography, CSF studies, and MRI are informative, but neuropathology remains a cornerstone for a definitive diagnosis.

The acronym of ILOCA refers to an idiopathic late-onset cerebellar ataxia associated with cerebellar atrophy on MRI. The diagnosis is retained when the other causes of cerebellar atrophy have been excluded.

Genetic testing

Genetic testing can be used not only for diagnosis, but also for pre-natal evaluation, predictive testing, and carrier testing (for relatives of patients with X-linked or autosomal recessive ataxia).

Pre-natal testing requires tissue obtained by amniocentesis or chorionic villous biopsy. Such procedures require a clear understanding of the risks and outcomes of the tests. The decision to terminate the pregnancy as a result of these tests should be provided by a genetic counselor and an obstetrician or gynecologist. Preimplantation testing with subsequent implantation of embryos free of any mutation should be carefully discussed with the family.

Although presymptomatic patients may have a psychosocial benefit, there are potential negative consequences, such as loss of insurability, problems of employability, and impact on self-perception and familial social interactions. Predictive testing should be avoided in non-consenting adults. In addition, disorders characterized by a high variability in expression should be considered very cautiously regarding predictive evaluation. Indeed, some patients with mild deficits may consider that they are not affected. In addition, the disease may progress so slowly that a patient may die of another disease.

References

Bhidayasiri R, Perlman SL, Pulst SM, et al. Late-onset Friedreich ataxia: phenotypic analysis, magnetic resonance imaging findings and review of the literature. *Arch Neurol* 2005;**62**:1865–9.

Bishop L, Kanoff R, Charnas L, et al. Severe methylenetetrahydrofolate reductase (MTHFR) deficiency: a case report of nonclassical homocystinuria. *J Child Neurol* 2008;**23**(7):823–8.

Brockmann K. The expanding phenotype of GLUT1-deficiency syndrome. *Brain Dev* 2009;**31**(7):545–52.

Brusse E, Maat-Kievit JA, van Swieten JC. Diagnosis and management of early- and late-onset cerebellar ataxia. *Clin Genet* 2007;**71**:12–24.

Date H, Onodera O, Tanaka H, et al. Early-onset ataxia with oculomotor apraxia and hypoalbuminemia is caused by mutations in a new HIT superfamily gene. *Nat Genet* 2001;**21**:184–8.

Finsterer J. Mitochondriopathies. *Eur J Neurol* 2004;**11**:163–86.

Fogel BL, Perlman S. An approach to the patient with late-onset cerebellar ataxia. *Nat Clin Pract Neurol* 2006;**2**:629–35.

Joshi C, Greenberg CR, De Vivo D, et al. GLUT1 deficiency without epilepsy: yet another case. *J Child Neurol* 2008;**23**(7):832–4.

Miyajima H, Kono S, Takahashi Y, et al. Cerebellar ataxia associated with heteroallelic ceruloplasmin gene mutation. *Neurology* 2001;**26**:2205–10.

Ramaekers VT, Blau N. Cerebral folate deficiency. *Dev Med Child Neurol* 2004;**46**(12):843–51.

Schöls L, Bauer P, Schmidt T, et al. Autosomal dominant cerebellar ataxias: clinical features, genetics and pathogenesis. *Lancet Neurol* 2004;**3**:291–304.

Storey E, Knight MA, Forrest SM, McKinlay Gardner RJ. Spinocerebellar ataxia type 20. *Cerebellum* 2005;**4**: 55–57.

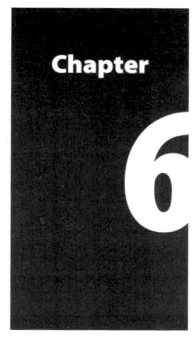

Chapter

6

Overview of the general management of cerebellar disorders

This chapter summarizes the main treatments in the various causes of cerebellar ataxias. Readers are also referred to the corresponding chapters for more details regarding the specific management of a given disorder.

Medical treatment

An overview of the sites of action of drugs is provided in Figure 6.1. The first line is to treat the underlying disorder in symptomatic ataxias:

- Cerebellar ataxia due to intoxication is potentially treatable in most cases.
- Cerebellar stroke requires management of risk factors, prevention of secondary lesions (see also Chapter 8 for antiplatelets agents and anticoagulants).
- Patients presenting with a paraneoplastic ataxia should be treated as soon as possible for the underlying cancer.
- Patients with gluten ataxia should be put on gluten-free diet.
- Specific deficiencies in vitamins require immediate supplementation. Vitamin E deficiency is discussed in Chapter 20. In cerebral folate deficiency, oral treatment with 5-formyltetrahydrofolate (folinic acid; 5MTHF) should be started in low doses at 0.5 to 1 mg/kg/day (Ramaekers & Blau, 2004). In some patients, higher daily doses of folinic acid at 2 to 3 mg/kg/day are required to normalize CSF 5MTHF values. Careful clinical follow-up is mandatory. After 4 to 6 months of folinic acid treatment, CSF analysis should be repeated in order to prevent over- or underdosage.
- Glut-1 deficiency syndrome responds to ketogenic diet (Brockmann, 2009).

- Copper overload in Wilson disease can be treated with zinc supplements (see Chapter 20).
- Restriction of phytanic acid intake may slow down symptoms in Refsum disease. Chenodeoxycholic acid is recommended in cerebrotendinous xanthomatosis.
- Endocrine diseases require a specific treatment.

Several drugs need to be used cautiously in cerebellar patients, due to their potential cerebellar toxicity (Table 6.1; see also Chapter 15). Various drugs have been suggested to improve cerebellar ataxia, cerebellar tremor, and nystagmus (Table 6.2; Fogel & Perlman, 2006). Regarding tremor, propranolol provides only a little benefit in most cases. Valproate may exacerbate postural tremor. Clonazepam has been proposed in kinetic tremor associated with multiple sclerosis or olivopontocerebellar atrophy (Trelles et al., 1984). Stimulation of the Vim nucleus may improve significantly postural/kinetic tremor in selected cases. Aminopyridines (3,4-diaminopyridine and 4-aminopyridine) are non-selective blockers of the Kv family of voltage-gated potassium channels, which increase Purkinje cell excitability. Aminopyridine may significantly reduce the intensity of downbeat nystagmus and restore gaze-holding capacities (Strupp et al., 2008). However, in many cases, treatments currently available are only symptomatic and provide little or moderate benefits at most. So far, no treatment has been shown to stop or reverse the progression of neurodegeneration.

In spinocerebellar ataxias, medical treatment remains limited, but several drugs targeting deleterious pathways are under investigation (see Chapter 23). In episodic ataxias, acetazolamide may be very effective to prevent attacks and stabilize ataxia.

Management of seizures in progressive myoclonic epilepsies with drugs is discussed in Chapter 17. Modified diet and percutaneous gastrostomy may be

Table 6.1 Drugs which might exacerbate cerebellar ataxia

Lithium salts

Phenytoin

Valproate

Amiodarone

Metronidazole[a]

Procainamide

Calcineurin inhibitors

Mefloquine

Isoniazid

Lindane

Perhexiline maleate

Cimetidine

[a]Toxicity predominating for cerebellar nuclei and perinuclear areas.

required for dysphagia. Psychological support should be provided in chronic disorders.

Surgery

In children, developmental malformations may require surgical procedures. The principal indications of surgery in adults are tumors and space-occupying lesions in the posterior fossa (trauma, infections, etc.), to relieve increased intracranial pressure and prevent life-threatening herniation. Deep brain stimulation (Vim) may improve postural/kinetic tremor in selected cases (see also Chapters 19 and 23).

Rehabilitation and assistive therapy

Maintaining a safe deambulation and autonomy in activities of daily life are main objectives for chronic cerebellar disorders. Occupational therapy is valuable for improving activities of daily life.

Rehabilitation with postural training, if possible on a daily basis, is recommended in ataxic patients, although we are still missing large studies confirming a beneficial effect. Nevertheless, patients participating in daily motor rehabilitation show a less abrupt deterioration in progressive degenerative disorders. Physical and occupational therapies should attempt to reinforce muscle activity and maximize functional capacities. Passive movements under various conditions of inertia might improve coordination.

Patients who are wheelchair-bound or confined to beds should receive specific care to prevent complications such as pressure sores.

Assistive therapy improves the autonomy of patients. Orthotic devices are used to stabilize joints. A wearable orthosis may be used for short periods.

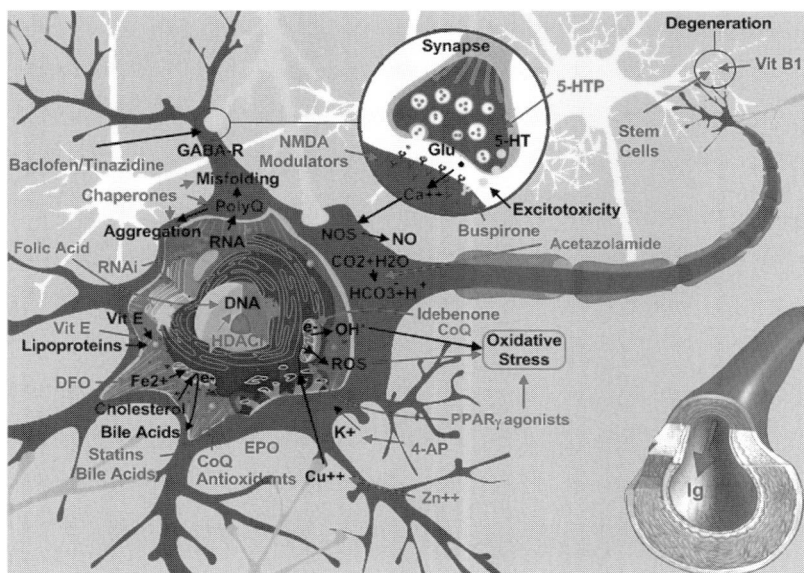

Figure 6.1 Overview of the sites of action of therapies in cerebellar disorders. A neuron is represented (insert: the circle corresponds to a synapse). Drugs and other alternatives are shown in green. Abbreviations: 5-HTP: 5 hydroxytryptophan; Co-Q: coenzyme Q; 4-AP: 4-aminopyridine; PPARγ agonists: peroxisome proliferator–activated receptor agonists; Zn^{++}: zinc; DFO: deferiprone; FE2+: iron; Vit E: vitamin E; RNAi: RNA inhibitors; ROS: reactive oxygen species; NOS: NO synthase; NO: nitric oxide; PolyQ: polyglutamine; GABA-R: gamma-aminobutyric acid receptor; HDACi: histone deacetylase inhibitors; K^+: potassium; Cu^{++}: copper; NMDA: N-methyl-D-aspartate; Ig: immunoglobulins. Courtesy of D. Marmolino. Adapted from http://commons.wikimedia.org/wiki.

Table 6.2 Principal drugs which have been suggested for cerebellar symptoms in adults

Symptom	Drug
Cerebellar ataxia	Amantadine (release of dopamine and modulation of NMDA pathway) 50–300 g/day
	Buspirone (5-HT1A agonist) 10–60 mg/day
	Tandospirone (5-HT1A agonist) 15–30 mg/day
	D-cycloserine (partial NMDA receptor allosteric agonist) 50 mg/day
	L-tryptophan (precursor of 5-HT) 600–1000 mg/day
Tremor	Propranolol (beta-blocker) 80–240 mg/day
	Clonazepam (benzodiazepine derivative) 2–8 mg/day
	Ondansetron (5-HT3 antagonist) 4–16 mg/day
	Primidone (interactions with voltage-gated sodium channels) 250–500 mg/day
	Pregabalin (acting on $\alpha 2\delta$ subunit of the voltage-dependent calcium channel) 75–300 mg/day
Nystagmus	Gabapentin (GABA analog) 900–4200 mg/day
	Clonazepam 0.5–3 mg/day
	3,4-diaminopyridine 40–80 mg/day
	Baclofen (GABA-B receptor agonist) 20–80 mg/day
	Memantine (uncompetitive NMDA antagonist) 5–20 mg/day

Abbreviations: GABA: gamma-aminobutyric acid; NMDA: N-methyl-D-aspartic acid.
Adapted from: Fogel and Perlman (2006).

Although about one-third of patients feel improvements in daily life with wearable orthoses, comfort and aesthetics often limit their use. Wearable dynamic assistive devices (gait, limb movements) are under development.

Speech therapy is useful for dysarthria and dysphagia. Neuropsychological rehabilitation should be promoted. Social workers and psychologists should be integrated in the discussion on therapeutic procedures, especially in chronic disorders of the cerebellum.

Treatments under investigation

Several treatments are currently under investigation (inhibitors of histone deacetylase in animal models of Friedreich ataxia and spinocerebellar ataxias, RNA interference, grafting procedures). They are discussed in Chapter 23.

References

Brockmann K. The expanding phenotype of GLUT1-deficiency syndrome. *Brain Dev* 2009;**31**(7):545–52.

Fogel BL, Perlman S. An approach to the patient with late-onset cerebellar ataxia. *Nat Clin Pract Neurol* 2006;**2**:629–35.

Ramaekers VT, Blau N. Cerebral folate deficiency. *Dev Med Child Neurol* 2004;**46**(12):843–51.

Ramaekers VT, Heimann G, Reul J, Thron A, Jaeken J. Genetic disorders and cerebellar structural abnormalities in childhood. *Brain* 1997;**120**:1739–51.

Strupp M, Kalla R, Glasauer S, et al. Aminopyridines for the treatment of cerebellar and ocular motor disorders. *Prog Brain Res* 2008;**171**:535–41.

Trelles L, Trelles JO, Castro C, Altamirano J, Benzaquen M. Successful treatment of two cases of intention tremor with clonazepam. *Ann Neurol* 1984; **16**(5):621.

Classification of cerebellar malformations

The embryologic development of the posterior fossa structures begins at about 3 weeks of gestation and continues until 20 months of post-natal life for cellular differentiation and neuronal arborization in humans (Parisi & Dobyns, 2003). The cerebellum is a derivative of the most rostral segment of the primitive hindbrain or rhombencephalon (rhombomere 1), the pons emerges from the rostral half of the hindbrain (metencephalon), and the medulla emerges from the lower half of the hindbrain (myelencephalon; see also Chapter 1).

Our understanding of the morphology of posterior fossa malformations is growing (Patel & Barkovich, 2002). Several classifications have been proposed (Ramaekers et al., 1997; Patel & Barkovich, 2002). The classification suggested by Parisi and Dobyns (2003) is based upon the embryological structures involved (Table 7.1).

Advances in imaging (sonography, CT, MRI) have led to the identification of a growing number of subtle abnormalities in fetuses and in neonates (Forzano et al., 2007). A crucial element for accurate diagnosis is the quality of imaging, especially MRI scans. Serial imaging may be necessary to confirm the diagnosis of a malformation. Ultrasonography is useful for fetal and neonatal screening, especially for any unstable infant who cannot be examined in the radiology department (Madsen et al., 2002). Transcranial Doppler can provide useful information for identifying infants and newborns with increased intracranial pressure. CT is the primary imaging modality when the acoustic window is no longer available for ultrasonography. It is of particular interest in detecting gross anomalies, for acute presentations, when an increased intra-cranial pressure is suspected, and to rule out a shunt malfunction or a post-operative complication (Madsen et al., 2002). MRI provides a more detailed delineation of complex anomalies for diagnosis, treatment, and genetic counseling. MRI is a powerful tool for assessing subtle malformations. Cerebrospinal fluid (CSF) dynamics can be evaluated with motion-sensitive MRI techniques.

Ataxia related to autism spectrum disorders is discussed in Chapter 16.

Table 7.2 lists the main clinical features and the loci/genes associated with the four major groups of malformations.

Malformations of both midbrain and hindbrain

The group of brainstem-cerebellar hypoplasia-dysplasia includes a spectrum of developmental disorders from the very rare complete cerebellar agenesis to more common forms of hypoplasia with diffuse brainstem involvement. Figure 7.1 illustrates an example of nearly complete cerebellar agenesis. Hypoplasias can affect different cerebellar regions. In addition to motor deficits, children may exhibit diminished levels of intelligence with decreased or borderline IQ values, impairments in executive functioning, language deficits, and psychoaffective disturbances, including autistic-like behavior and obsessive rituals (Courchesne et al., 1994). Cerebellar hypoplasia with endosteal sclerosis is a rare disorder with a probable autosomal recessive transmission (Ozgen et al., 2005). Patients exhibit cerebellar ataxia associated with cerebellar hypoplasia, hypotonia, developmental delay, microcephaly, growth retardation, endosteal sclerosis, tooth eruption disturbances, and hip dislocations.

Chiari malformations represent the most common posterior fossa malformations. They are characterized by a downwards displacement of brainstem and cerebellar tonsils through the foramen magnum (Chiari, 1891). Type II Chiari malformations are complex malformations of the entire neuraxis. Almost all

Table 7.1 Classification of mid-hindbrain developmental disorders

Malformations of both midbrain and hindbrain	Brainstem-cerebellar hypoplasia/dysplasia Chiari type II Cobblestone lissencephaly Molar tooth sign–associated malformations (Joubert syndrome and associated disorders) Rhombencephalosynapsis
Malformations affecting mainly the cerebellum and derivatives (Rhombomere 1)	Focal or hemispheric hypoplasia Paleocerebellar hypoplasia (affecting mainly the vermis; including Dandy-Walker malformation and cerebellar vermis hypoplasias) Neocerebellar hypoplasia
Malformations affecting mainly the lower hindbrain (Rhombomeres 2–8)	Chiari type I Cranial nerve and nuclear aplasias
Developmental abnormalities of posterior fossa	Abnormal fluid collections Abnormal bone and brain structure
Pre-natal onset degeneration	Pontocerebellar hypoplasia Congenital disorders of glycosylation

Adapted from: Parisi and Dobyns (2003).

patients have an associated meningomyelocele, most often in the lumbar region (Arnold-Chiari malformation). Clinically, the spectrum of symptoms is large. Patients may be nearly asymptomatic or exhibit severe disabilities. Respiratory failure, swallowing difficulties, and vocal cord dysfunction due to brainstem involvement are causes of death. While neonates typically show a rapid neurological deterioration over a period of several days, older patients experience an insidious progression of symptoms. Cerebellar dysplasia may be associated, and there may be a dorsal angulation of the cerebellar fissures (Madsen et al., 2002). The cerebellum and brainstem are inferiorly displaced through a wide foramen magnum, leading to compression and impaction of pyramis, uvula, and nodulus. Axial views show an "angel wing" aspect of the brainstem due to prepontine migration of the cerebellum at the level of the middle cerebellar peduncles. Inferior vermian pegs posterior to the medulla is a constant observation (Wolpert et al., 1987). The fourth ventricle is usually collapsed, but may be dilated if trapped. Mesencephalic abnormalities involving the aqueduct and colliculi are common (Naidich et al., 1980). The tectum may be bulbous or beaked. Aplasia/hypoplasia of cranial nerve nuclei may be found. Defects of the corpus callosum are observed in up to 80% of patients (Barkovich, 1995). Complete agenesis occurs in one-third of patients. Supratentorial CSF spaces are commonly prominent. A majority of patients before 6 months of age present a marked thinning of the occipital and parietal bones (craniofenestria). Surgery for the Chiari II malformation is often difficult. Suboc-cipital craniectomy may be dangerous due to the low position of the torcular. Possible hydrocephalus following surgical closure of the myelomeningocele and complications of ventricular shunting such as isolation of the fourth ventricle must be kept in mind. Chiari type III malformation is characterized by a cervico-occipital cephalocele with hindbrain dysplasia. Stigmata of Chiari type II are commonly found.

Cobblestone lissencephaly with mid-hindbrain abnormalities and cerebellar hypoplasia may be associated with congenital muscular dystrophy and ocular deficits, including muscle-eye-brain disease and Fukuyama congenital muscular dystrophy (Dobyns & Truwit, 1995).

Molar tooth sign–associated malformations include Joubert syndrome and Joubert syndrome–related disorders. The estimated prevalence is about 1 per 100 000. Joubert syndrome is characterized by both intrafamilial and interfamilial phenotypic variability, including in monozygotic twins (Raynes et al., 1999). Joubert syndrome has been defined on the basis of clinical findings, including hypotonia, developmental delay and mental retardation, abnormal ocular movements, and abnormal breathing with episodes of hyperpnea or apnea, and the presence of the molar tooth sign on cranial MRI (Maria et al., 1999). This sign includes a deepened interpeduncular fossa, hypoplastic cerebellar vermis, and prominent superior cerebellar peduncles. The molar tooth aspect is consecutive to an axonal migration defect (Millen & Gleeson, 2008). The cerebellar vermis often has a "kinked" appearance, with enlargement of the fourth ventricle.

Table 7.2 Clinical features and genetic basis

Disorders	Clinical signs	Loci/genes (mode of inheritance)
Molar tooth sign and associated disorders		
Classic Joubert syndrome	Hypotonia, DD, MR	9q34 (AR)
	Oculomotor apraxia	
	Apnea/tachypnea	
Joubert syndrome–Leber congenital amaurosis-like	Retinal dystrophy with severe visual impairment	? (AR)
Coach syndrome	Ocular coloboma	? (AR)
(cerebellar vermis hypoplasia, oligophrenia, ataxia, coloboma, hepatic fibrosis)	Hepatic fibrosis, liver failure	
Senior-Løken syndrome	Retinal dystrophy, nephronophthisis	2q13; 3q22;
(retinopathy with nephronophthisis)		1p36 (AR)
Dandy-Walker malformation		
Classic form	Cerebellar vermis hypoplasia	3q24
	Dilatation of fourth ventricle	Sporadic?
	Elevated torcula	Multiple
Other forms	Other structural malformations associated	(chromosomal, syndromic)
Cerebellar vermis hypoplasia		
X-linked	Cerebellar vermis hypoplasia Xq12	
	Retrocerebellar cyst, hypotonia,	(X-linked)
	spasticity, seizures	
Other		(AR?)
Posterior fossa collections	Non-communicating membrane–	(?)
	enclosed cyst; ataxia; hydrocephalus	
Pontocerebellar hypoplasia		(AR)
Type 1	Spinal muscular atrophy	
	Respiratory insufficiency	?
	Contractures	(AR)
Type 2	Microcephaly	
	Dyskinesia	
	Poor feeding	7q11–21 (AR)
	Seizures	
Type 3	Microcephaly	
	Seizures, spasticity	
Congenital disorders of glycosylation	Pontocerebellar hypoplasia	Ia: 16p13
	Hypotonia	Ib: 15q22
	Stroke-like deficits	Ic: 1p22.3
	Seizures	Id: 3q27
	Dysmorphic facies	(AR)
	Failure to thrive	
	Strabismus	
	Lipodystrophy	
	Inverted nipples	
	Vomiting, diarrhea, liver dysfunction	
	Kyphoscoliosis	

Abbreviations. AR: autosomal recessive; DD: developmental delay; MR: mental retardation.
Adapted from: Parisi and Dobyns (2003).

CEREBELLAR AGENESIS

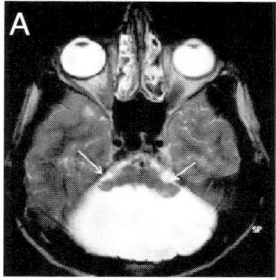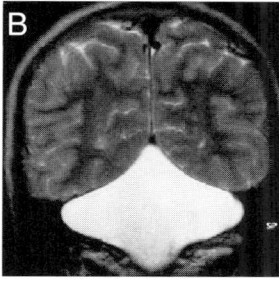

Figure 7.1 Cerebellar agenesis. Top panels: Magnetic resonance axial (A) and coronal (B) T2-weighted imaging in a patient with ataxia and nystagmus. A near-complete cerebellar agenesis is observed. The cerebellar remnant comprises anterior quadrangular lobes (arrows). From: Alkan et al., 2009. With permission.

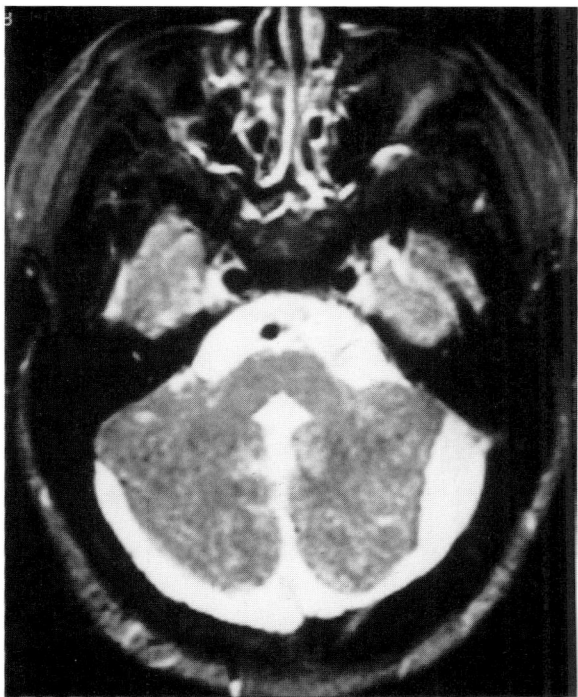

Figure 7.2 Joubert syndrome. Axial T2-weighted image showing an absence of cerebellar vermis and dysplasia of the brainstem. From: Madsen et al., 2002. With permission.

Dysplasia of cerebellar nuclei and brainstem is very common (Figure 7.2). Breathing deficits may improve with age and even completely disappear. Seizures and autistic behavior have been described. Other abnormalities include a pigmentary retinopathy, pendular nystagmus, colobomas, cystic dysplasia of the kidneys, and nephronophthisis. Retinal dystrophy and

nephronophthisis are related to defective functions of primary cilia, appendages composed of a membrane with a microtubule structure and a centrosome at the base. Several diseases sharing clinical features and the molar tooth sign with Joubert syndrome are categorized in the group of Joubert syndrome and related disorders, such as the orofacial-digital syndrome type VI, with vermal hypoplasia, tongue hamartomas, midline cleft lip, and polydactyly. Recommendations for the work-up in all children suspected to present with Joubert syndrome or a related disease are the following: genetics referral to evaluate for consanguinity, physical examination, peripheral blood karyotype to exclude a chromosomal disorder, polysomnogram to identify possible apnea, swallowing studies, EEG monitoring, developmental testing, ophthalmological evaluation including electroretinogram if necessary, yearly kidney ultrasound examination, renal and liver function tests, and brain MRI. Children with Joubert syndrome are very sensitive to the respiratory depressant effects of drugs. Complications of end-stage renal disease resulting from cystic kidney disease or nephronophthisis often require specific treatments, including dialysis and/or kidney transplantation. Individuals with liver failure and/or fibrosis may be candidates for portal shunting or orthotopic liver transplantation. Polydactyly may require surgery.

Rhombencephalosynapsis is characterized by an absence of the vermis or a severe dysgenesis of midline cerebellar structures. There is a fusion of the cerebellar hemispheres, peduncles, and dentate nuclei (Truwit et al., 1991). Fusion of dentate nuclei and inferior colliculi may be associated with a peculiar diamond-shaped fourth ventricle (Utsunomiya et al., 1998). Coronal MRI typically shows horizontally oriented folia and fissures. The thalami may also be fused. Other findings include hydrocephalus and absence of a corpus callosum (Toelle et al., 2002). Partial rhombencephalosynapsis is characterized by a relatively normal anterior vermis and nodulus, with a deficient posterior vermis and a partial fusion of cerebellar hemispheres (Figure 7.3). This latter malformation can occur in combination with Chiari type II malformation (Wan et al., 2005). Clinical deficits depend on the extent of the cerebellar involvement and the coexistence of supra-tentorial lesions, ranging from mild ataxia to a syndrome of cerebral palsy (Toelle et al., 2002). Rhombencephalosynapsis is considered to be due to a defect of vermian differentiation occurring between 28 and 40 days of gestation, as a result of impaired

PARTIAL RHOMBENCEPHALOSYNAPSIS

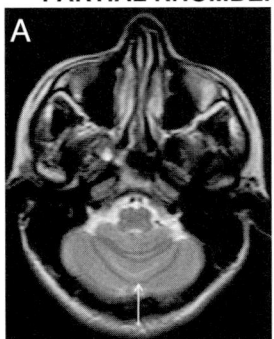 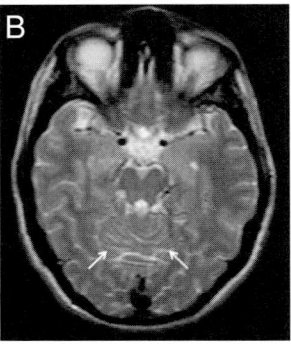

Figure 7.3 Rhombencephalosynapsis. Magnetic resonance axial T2-weighted imaging in a patient with partial rhombencephalosynapsis. Inferior vermian agenesis, fusion of the inferoposterior parts of the cerebellar hemispheres (arrow in left panel), and dysplasia of the superior vermis (short arrows in right panels). From: Alkan et al., 2009. With permission.

expression of a dorsalizing organizer gene (Sarnat et al., 2000).

Malformations predominantly affecting the cerebellum and derivatives

Focal cerebellar hypoplasias are a heterogeneous group characterized by hypoplastic cerebellar structures observed focally. Paleocerebellar hypoplasias include Dandy-Walker malformations, isolated cerebellar vermis hypoplasia, and cerebellar vermis hypoplasias associated with other malformations, such as periventricular nodular heterotopia, lissencephaly, and polymicrogyria (Ross et al., 2001). Dandy-Walker malformation presents clinically with nystagmus, truncal ataxia, and variable combinations of extra-cerebellar deficits. Elemental features of Dandy-Walker malformations are the hypoplastic cerebellar vermis and the cystic dilatation of the fourth ventricle (Figure 7.4; Dandy & Blackfan, 1914; Taggart & Walker, 1942). The fourth ventricle communicates with a retrocerebellar cyst which may enlarge the posterior fossa. The roof of the posterior torcula appears elevated on MRI. Falx cerebelli is absent. A communicating hydrocephalus, leading to macro-cephaly, with enlarged lateral ventricles is variably present. Dandy-Walker malformations would represent about 4% of cases of hydrocephalus, with an incidence of about 1/3500 births (Kaiser et al., 1977). Associated malformations including occipital

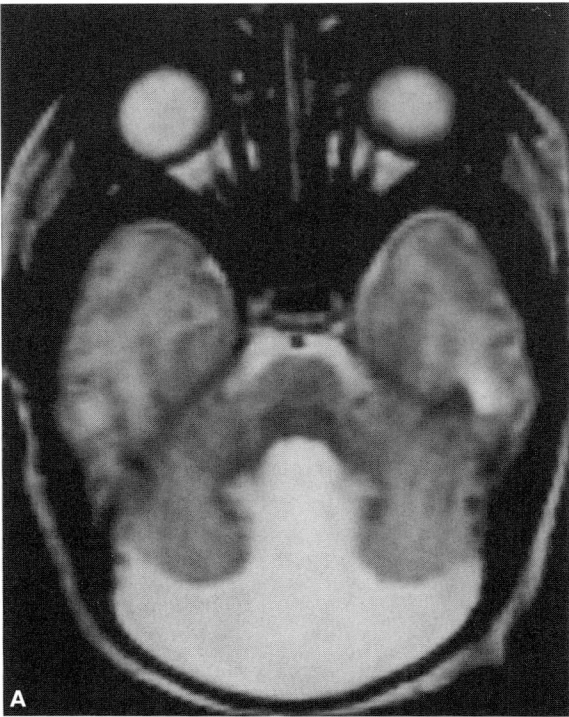

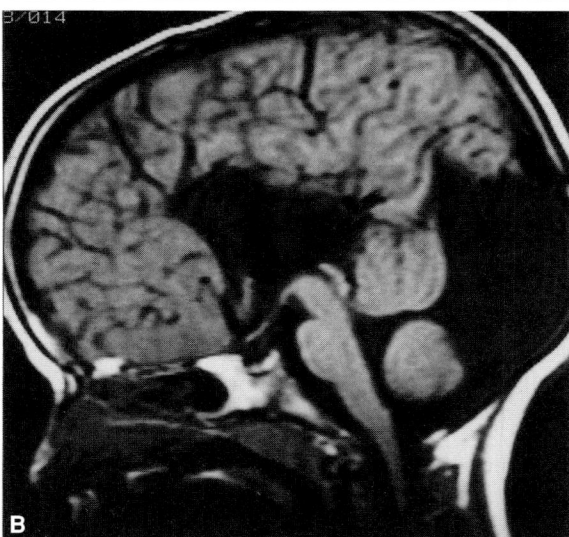

Figure 7.4 Dandy-Walker malformation. (A) Axial T2-weighted image showing an absence of cerebellar vermis with dilatation of the fourth ventricle. (B) A concomitant callosal dysgenesis is shown. From: Madsen et al., 2002. With permission.

encephalocele, polymicrogyria, and heterotopia are observed in about one-third of patients. About 1 child in 10 has a concomitant agenesis or dysgenesis of the corpus callosum. The heterogeneity in Dandy-Walker malformation is reinforced by the presence of other anomalies, such as congenital heart disease and facial hemangiomas in the so-called PHACE syndrome (posterior fossa malformation, hemangiomas, arterial anomalies, coarctation of the aorta, eye defects) (Metry et al., 2001). Moreover, Dandy-Walker malformation has been reported in a wide variety of chromosomal abnormalities and has been described in many genetic syndromes. Parisi and Dobyns (2003) have suggested to distinguish four groups of malformations: (1) "true" Dandy-Walker malformation, which features cerebellar vermis hypoplasia with upward vermis rotation and elevation of the torcula, enlarged fourth ventricle extending posteriorly as a retrocerebellar cyst, and hydrocephalus present in about 50% to 80% of subjects; (2) Dandy-Walker variants, made of malformations with less severe cerebellar vermis hypoplasia, less notable or absent upward rotation of the vermis, and relatively smaller fluid collections; (3) diffuse cerebellar hypoplasia involving the vermis and the hemispheres, usually associated with brainstem hypoplasia; and (4) patients with posterior fossa fluid collections (see section Developmental abnormalities with fluid collections). The first group often presents in the neonatal period with macrocephaly, occipital cephaloceles, and/or hydrocephalus (Hirsch et al., 1984). Apnea and seizures are not uncommon. Intellectual capacities are normal in up to 80% of children. From a genetic point of view, deletions on chromosome 3q24 have been identified in several patients. This region encompasses the adjacent ZIC1 and ZIC4 genes involved in granule neuron progenitor proliferation (see discussion of SHH pathway in Chapter 1).

Cerebellar vermis hypoplasia/dysplasia is associated with normal position of the cerebellar vermis. Due to its craniocaudal pattern of formation, cerebellar hypoplasia always involves the caudal rather than the rostral part. The fourth ventricle may be enlarged. The tentorium cerebelli is not elevated. The retrocerebellar fluid collection is generally small as compared with a true Dandy-Walker malformation. In several families, cerebellar vermis hypoplasia has an X-linked inheritance. Nevertheless, many disorders sharing features with cerebellar vermis hypoplasia/dysplasia appear sporadic in inheritance. The following syndromes with primary vermis hypoplasia have been described: Cogan syndrome, combining oculomotor apraxia with motor impairment; otopalatodigital syndromes; and hypoplasia

with lissencephaly (Barth, 1993; Ross et al., 2001). Malformation of the cerebral cortex is generally the most striking finding in these disorders.

Pre-natal diagnosis of Dandy-Walker malformation and cerebellar vermis hypoplasia/dysplasia may be problematic. Indeed, it may be difficult to identify the type of malformation with pre-natal imaging. The cisterna magna is detectable visually between weeks 15 and 25 of gestation, and a mild dilatation may be hard to diagnose (see also Chapter 1). Concerns have been raised in the last few years about early diagnosis that would have led to the termination of pregnancies of children who would have had normal cognitive or motor development. Paradoxically, a milder dilatation may be associated with a worse prognosis than a classic Dandy-Walker malformation associated with a large dilatation. Recurrence risks in Dandy-Walker malformation and cerebellar vermal hypoplasias are variable, estimated at between 0.5% and 5% in subsequent pregnancies for the former. Surgical treatment of Dandy-Walker malformation involves diversion of the CSF from the ventricular space or the cystic space to another site, such as the peritoneal cavity.

Tectocerebellar dysraphia has features overlapping those of Dandy-Walker malformation, Chiari II malformation, and ventriculocele of the posterior fossa. It is characterized by vermian hypoplasia/aplasia and dorsal traction of the brainstem. Cerebellar hemispheres are displaced ventrolaterally. The tectum appears fused.

Neocerebellar hypoplasias, aplasias, and dysplasias are grouped under the terminology of dysgenesis of the neocerebellum. The vermis may appear moderately atrophic, but is relatively spared. Neocerebellar dysgenesis may occur at any time between week 7 of gestation and the first post-natal year (Madsen et al., 2002).

Very low birth weight infants born between 24 and 32 weeks of gestation are at risk for developing a smaller cerebellum (Messerschmidt et al., 2008). Additional supra-tentorial hemorrhagic brain injury followed by hydrocephalus, neurosurgical interventions, and hemosiderin deposits on the cerebellar surface are significantly related to disruptive cerebellar development.

Malformations predominantly affecting the lower hindbrain

Chiari type I malformation consists of a hindbrain herniation through the foramen magnum. It occurs more commonly in adults. The extension of cerebellar tonsils below the foramen magnum is at least 3 to 5 mm. Tonsils are characteristically pointed inferiorly. Patients complain of headache and neck pain and may develop paroxysmal dizziness, vertigo, or vomiting. Neurological examination may show a nystagmus and symmetrical or asymmetrical cranial nerve palsies. Craniocervical dysgenesis, Klippel-Feil syndrome, and basilar invagination may be associated. Positional changes and coughing may exacerbate or precipitate symptoms. In about 60% of patients, the tonsils extend to C1 (Madsen et al., 2002). Unlike Chiari type II, supratentorial anomalies are usually lacking. Hydrocephalus is observed in one-fourth of patients. Possible associated findings include hydrosyringomyelia, possibly due to transmission of increased pressure into the spinal cord, and a progressive scoliosis (Oldfield et al., 1994). Surgical intervention aims at decompressing the structures of posterior fossa (Madsen et al., 2002).

Möbius syndrome belongs to the group of cranial nerve and nuclear aplasias. Aplasias of cranial nerves VI and VII are associated with lateral gaze deficits and facial nerve palsy.

Developmental abnormalities with fluid collections

Arachnoid cysts represent collections of CSF surrounded by a pia-arachnoid layer. Mega-cisterna magna is a retrocerebellar fluid collection with normal positioning of the cerebellum and a normal shape of the fourth ventricle. It can be found incidentally or it may be associated with hydrocephalus and mental retardation (Niesen, 2002). It is sometimes difficult to distinguish mega-cisterna magna from cerebellar vermis hypoplasia (Parisi & Dobyns, 2003). There is no significant mass effect appearance in the large majority of cases, although the cerebellum may sometimes take a scalloped aspect.

Mega-cisterna magna is diagnosed pre-natally using ultrasound when the enlargement is greater than 10 mm at 18 to 23 weeks of gestation (Forzano et al., 2007). In a recent series of posterior fossa malformations detected pre-natally, it accounted for 40% of all the posterior fossa malformations detected. An isolated finding of mega-cisterna magna on pre-natal ultrasound with a normal fetal karyotype carries a good prognosis. When additional abnormalities are found, the risk of poor outcome increases significantly.

Blake pouch cyst (retrocerebellar arachnoid cyst) is a malformation closely related to Dandy-Walker malformation, lined by ependyma or astroglial membrane. Mass effect on the cerebellum is common, with the cerebellum taking a compressed aspect. The tentorium may bulge. CT cystogram or CSF MRI flow study may be necessary to distinguish the cyst from mega-cisterna magna. Shunting may be necessary. The cyst is presumably due to a maldevelopment occurring around the fifth week of gestation (Barkovich et al., 1989).

Prenatal–onset degeneration

Pontocerebellar hypoplasias, or atrophies, are characterized by progressive neuronal loss on serial brain imaging studies (Barth, 1993). Typically, repeated MRI will demonstrate a progressive atrophy of the ventral pons and the inferior olivary nuclei, vermis, and cerebellar hemispheres. Enlargement of lateral ventricles and widened cerebral sulci with a thinning of the corpus callosum may be observed (Zelnik et al., 1996). Children exhibit post-natal marked developmental delay and mental retardation, usually with a poor outcome. Several forms of pontocerebellar hypoplasias are distinguished. Pontocerebellar hypoplasia with spinal muscular atrophy (type I) is characterized by respiratory insufficiency in the neonatal period and arthrogryposis. Feeding and respiratory complications result in death in the first year of life. MRI shows hypoplasia of the cerebellum and the brainstem, as well as degeneration of the anterior horns in the spinal cord similar to Werdnig-Hoffman disease. Pontocerebellar hypoplasia with dyskinesia (type II) presents clinically with a marked microcephaly in the neonatal period. Generalized seizures, chorea, and dystonia appear after (Barth et al., 1995). The anterior horn of the spinal cord is spared. Most children die within the first 10 years of life. Pontocerebellar hypoplasia without dyskinesia (type III) has been reported in consanguineous families. Children develop mental retardation, a progressive microcephaly, spasticity, and generalized epilepsy. Extra-pyramidal signs are lacking. Congenital disorders of glycosylation (CDG; also called carbohydrate-deficient glycoprotein syndromes) are autosomal recessive conditions presenting clinically with severe feeding difficulties, failure to thrive in early infancy, mental retardation, hypotonia, ataxia, and peripheral neuropathy due to defective synthesis of N-linked oligosaccharides (Jaeken et al., 1980). Febrile and afebrile seizures are relatively common. Stroke-like deficits (hemiparesis, coma) are variably present. Dysmorphic face with strabismus, inverted nipples, and lipodystrophy (fat pads) are suggestive. Pericardial effusions occur in up to 50% of cases. Absence of puberty and hypergonadotropic hypogonadism are reported repeatedly in girls with CDG-Ia, one of the most common types of CDG syndrome. MRI shows in most cases a cerebellar hypoplasia or a pontocerebellar atrophy, ending in global cerebral atrophy. Cerebellar atrophy often runs a progressive course, with some patients having an apparently normal size of the cerebellum in the first months of life. The number of adults with CDG-Ia syndrome is growing (Krasnewich et al., 2007). They exhibit a moderate mental retardation, cerebellar ataxia, seizures, retinitis pigmentosa, peripheral neuropathy, kyphoscoliosis, and endocrinopathies. Abnormal liver function tests are usually found (Kjaergaard et al., 2001). Isoelectric focusing of serum sialotransferrin shows an abnormal glycosylation of this glycoprotein in type I CDG (Stibler et al., 1998). However, ataxic patients may present an unequivocal cerebellar hypoplasia but a normal or slightly abnormal transferrin isofocusing result (Vermeer et al., 2007). In these cases, the enzymatic activity of phosphomannomutase (PMM2) is deficient in both leukocytes and fibroblasts. Several mutations have been identified, in particular the R141H – the Danish population has a high carrier frequency of this mutation – and F119L of the PMM2 gene located on chromosome 16p13 (Matthijs et al., 1997; Kjaergaard et al., 2001). A majority of patients are compound heterozygotes. Dietary supplementation might be helpful in some cases associated with a protein-losing enteropathy (Freeze, 1998). Surgical draining of pericardial effusions or pericardiectomy should be considered when ventricular function is compromised.

Other malformations and syndromes

Lhermitte-Duclos syndrome

Children affected by this syndrome exhibit macrocephaly, seizures, and mild cerebellar deficits. Granule cells are replaced by abnormal ganglion cells, hence the name cerebellar gangliocytoma (Lhermitte & Duclos, 1920; see also Chapter 13).

Macrocerebellum

The cerebellum may appear diffusely enlarged. It may be associated with delayed white matter myelination. Children may present with developmental delay, oculomotor disorders, and hypotonia. Alexander disease is recognized as a cause of macrocerebellum (see also Chapter 20).

Aicardi syndrome

This rare neurodevelopmental disorder has a probable X-linked dominant inheritance, being identified almost exclusively in girls, with lethality in the hemizygous male (Aicardi et al., 1969; Aicardi, 2005). Some cases have been reported in 47, XXY males. The syndrome is characterized by a triad of corpus callosum agenesis, chorioretinal lacunae, and infantile spasms. Focal seizures rather than spasms are common (Aicardi, 2005). Symptoms typically appear before the age of 5 years, usually in the first year. EEG recordings show suggestive bilateral independent bursts (BIBs), which are pseudo-periodic discharges occurring asynchronously over both hemispheres (Ohtsuka et al., 1993). BIBs may evolve to hypsarrhythmia or multiple focal spikes in the middle of infancy. Brain MRI shows polymicrogyria predominating in the frontal and perisylvian regions, periventricular heterotopia, widening of the operculum, and intracranial cysts. Recent studies underline the high incidence of cerebellar abnormalities: superior foliar prominence of the vermis, inferior vermian hypoplasia, dysplasia, hypoplastic hemispheres, enlarged cisterna magna, and cerebellar cysts (Hopkins et al., 2008). The prognosis is generally unfavorable, although the course may be milder.

Smith-Lemli-Opitz syndrome

Smith-Lemli-Opitz syndrome (SLOS) is an autosomal recessive disorder caused by reduced activity of 7-dehydrocholesterol reductase. This results in an increased concentration of 7-dehydrocholesterol and 8-dehydrocholesterol in body fluids and tissues, whereas levels of cholesterol are decreased (Porter, 2008). SLOS is characterized by multiple developmental malformations, including cerebellar hypoplasia. SLOS is an example of the link between cholesterol metabolism and cerebellar development (see discussion of SHH in Chapter 1). Combined treatment of a cholesterol-enriched diet and simvastatin is recommended (Chan et al., 2009).

References

Aicardi J. Aicardi syndrome. *Brain Dev* 2005;**27**(3):164–71.

Aicardi J, Chevrie JJ, Rousselie F. Spasma-in-flexion syndrome, callosal agenesis, chorioretinal abnormalities. *Arch Fr Pediatr* 1969;**26**(10):1103–20.

Alkan O, Kizilkilic O, Yildirim T. Malformations of the midbrain and hindbrain: a retrospective study and review of the literature. *Cerebellum* 2009;**8**: 355–65.

Barkovich A. *Pediatric Neuroimaging*. New York: Raven Press, 1995.

Barkovich AJ, Kjos BO, Norman D, Edwards MS. Revised classification of posterior fossa cysts and cystlike malformations based on the results of multiplanar MR imaging. *Am J Roentgenol* 1989;**153**:1289–1300.

Barth PG. Ponto-cerebellar hypoplasias: an overview of a group of inherited neurodegenerative disorders with fetal onset. *Brain Dev* 1993;**15**:411–22.

Barth PG, Blennow G, Lenard HG, et al. The syndrome of autosomal recessive pontocerebellar hypoplasia, microcephaly, and extra-pyramidal dyskinesia (pontocerebellar hypoplasia type 2): compiled data from 10 pedigrees. *Neurology* 1995;**45**:311–17.

Chan YM, Merkens LS, Connor WE, et al. Effects of dietary cholesterol and simvastatin on cholesterol synthesis in Smith-Lemli-Opitz syndrome. *Pediatr Res* 2009;**65**(6): 681–5.

Chiari H. Ueber Veränderungen des Kleinhirns infolge von Hydrocephalie des Grosshirns. *Deutsche Medicinische Wochenschrift* 1891;**17**:1172–5.

Courchesne E, Townsend J, Akshoomoff NA, et al. Impairment in shifting attention in autistic and cerebellar patients. *Behav Neurosci* 1994;**108**(5):848–65.

Dandy W, Blackfan K. Internal hydrocephalus: an experimental, clinical and pathologic study. *Am J Dis Children* 1914;**8**:406.

Dobyns WB, Truwit CL. Lissencephaly and other malformations of cortical development: 1995 update. *Neuropediatrics* 1995;**26**:132–47.

Forzano F, Mansour S, Ierullo A, et al. Posterior fossa malformation in fetuses: a report of 56 further cases and review of the literature. *Prenat Diagn* 2007;**27**(6): 495–501.

Freeze HH. Disorders in protein glycosylation and potential therapy: tip of an iceberg? *J Pediatr* 1998;**133**:593–600.

Hirsch JF, Pierre-Kahn A, Renier D, et al. The Dandy-Walker malformation: a review of 40 cases. *J Neurosurg* 1984;**61**:515–22.

Hopkins B, Sutton VR, Lewis RA, Van Den Veyver I, Clark G. Neuroimaging aspects of Aicardi syndrome. *Am J Med Genet A* 2008;**146A**(22):2871–8.

Jaeken J, Vanderschueren-Lodeweyck M, Casaer P, et al. Familial psychomotor retardation with markedly fluctuating serum prolactin, FSH and GH levels, partial TBG-deficiency, increased serum arylsulphatase A and increased CSF protein: a new syndrome? *Pediatr Res* 1980;**14**:179.

Kaiser G, Schut L, James HE, Bruce DA. Problems of diagnosis and treatment in the Dandy-Walker syndrome. *Neurology* 1977;**22**:771–80.

Kjaergaard S, Schwartz M, Skovby F. Congenital disorder of glycosylation type Ia (CDG-Ia): phenotypic spectrum of the R141H/F119 genotype. *Arch Dis Child* 2001;**85**: 236–9.

Krasnewich D, O'Brien K, Sparks S. Clinical features in adults with congenital disorders of glycosylation type Ia (CDG-Ia). *Am J Med Genet C Semin Med Genet* 2007; **145C**(3):302–6.

Lhermitte J, Duclos P. Sur un ganglioneurome diffus du cortex du cervelet. *Bull Assoc Française Etude Cancer* 1920;9:99M12.

Madsen JR, Poussaint TY, Barnes PD. Congenital malformations of the cerebellum and posterior fossa. In *The Cerebellum and Its Disorders*, ed. M. Manto and M. Pandolfo. Cambridge, UK: Cambridge University Press, 2002, pp. 161–77.

Maria BL, Boltshauser E, Palmer SC, Tran TX. Clinical features and revised diagnostic criteria in Joubert syndrome. *J Child Neurol* 1999;**14**:583–90.

Matthijs G, Schollen E, Pardon E, et al. Mutations in PMM2, a phosphomannomutase gene on chromosome 16p13, in carbohydrate-deficient glycoprotein type 1 syndrome (Jaecken syndrome). *Nat Genet* 1997;**16**:88–92.

Messerschmidt A, Prayer D, Brugger PC, et al. Preterm birth and disruptive cerebellar development: assessment of perinatal risk factors. *Eur J Paediatr Neurol* 2008;**12**(6):455–60.

Metry DW, Dowd CF, Barkovich AJ, Frieden IJ. The many faces of PHACE syndrome. *J Pediatr* 2001;**139**:117–23.

Millen KJ, Gleeson JG. Cerebellar development and disease. *Curr Opin Neurobiol* 2008;**18**:12–19.

Naidich TP, Pudlowski RM, Naidich JB. Computed tomographic signs of Chiari II malformation. II: midbrain and cerebellum. *Radiology* 1980;**134**:391–8.

Niesen CE. Malformations of the posterior fossa: current perspectives. *Sem Pediatr Neurol* 9:320–34.

Ohtsuka Y, Oka E, Terasaki T, Ohtahara S. Aicardi syndrome: a longitudinal clinical and electroencephalographic study. *Epilepsia* 1993;**34**(4): 627–34.

Oldfield EH, Muraszko K, Shawker TH, Patronas NJ. Pathophysiology of syringomyelia associated with Chiari I malformation of the cerebellar tonsils.

Implications for diagnosis and treatment. *J Neurosurg* 1994;**80**:3–15.

Ozgen HM, Overweg-Plandsoen WC, Blees-Pelk J, Besselaar PP, Hennekam RC. Cerebellar hypoplasia-endosteal sclerosis: a long term follow-up. *Am J Med Genet A* 2005;**134A**(2):215–9.

Parisi MA, Dobyns WB. Human malformations of the midbrain and hindbrain: review and proposed classification scheme. *Mol Genet Metabol* 2003;**80**:36–53.

Patel S, Barkovich AJ. Analysis and classification of cerebellar malformations. *Am J Neuroradiol* 2002;**23**(7):1074–87.

Porter FD. Smith-Lemli-Opitz syndrome: pathogenesis, diagnosis and management. *Eur J Hum Genet* 2008;**16**(5):535–41.

Ramaekers VT, Heimann G, Reul J, Thron A, Jaeken J. Genetic disorders and cerebellar structural abnormalities in childhood. *Brain* 1997;**120**:1739–51.

Raynes HR, Shanske A, Goldberg S, et al. Joubert syndrome: monozygotic twins with discordant phenotypes. *J Child Neurol* 1999;**14**:649–54.

Ross ME, Swanson K, Dobyns WB. Lissencephaly with cerebellar hypoplasia (LCH): a heterogeneous group of cortical malformations. *Neuropediatrics* 2001;**32**:256–63.

Sarnat HB. Molecular genetic classification of central nervous system malformations. *J Child Neurol* 2000;**15**(10):675–87.

Stibler H, Holzbach U, Kristiansson B. Isoforms and levels of transferrin, antithrombin, alpha(1)-antitrypsin and thyroxine-binding globulin in 48 patients with carbohydrate-deficient glycoprotein syndrome type I. *Scand J Clin Lab Invest* 1998;**58**:55–61.

Taggart J, Walker A. Congenital atresias of the foramens of Luschka and Magendie. *Arch Neurol Psychiatry* 1942;**48**:583.

Toelle SP, Yalcinkaya C, Kocer N, et al. Rhombencephalosynapsis: clinical findings and neuroimaging in 9 children. *Neuropediatrics* 2002;**33**:209–14.

Truwit CL, Barkovich AJ, Shanahan R, Maroldo TV. MR imaging of rhombenvephalosynapsis: report of three cases and review of the literature. *Am J Neuroradiol* 1991;**12**:957–65.

Vermeer S, Kremer HP, Leijten QH, et al. Cerebellar ataxia and congenital disorder of glycosylation Ia (CDG-Ia) with normal routine CDG screening. *J Neurol* 2007;**254**(10):1356–8.

Utsunomiya H, Takano K, Ogasawara T, et al. Rhombencephalosynapsis: cerebellar embryogenesis. *Am J Neuroradiol* 1998;**19**(3):547–9.

Wan SM, Khong PL, Ip P, Ooi GC. Partial rhombencephalosynapsis and Chiari II malformation. *Hong Kong Med J* 2005;**11**(4):299–302.

Wolpert SM, Anderson M, Scott RM, et al. Chiari II malformation: MR imaging evaluation. *Am J Roentgenol* 1987;**149**:1033–42.

Zelnik N, Dobyns WB, Forem SL, Kolodny EH. Congenital pontocerebellar atrophy in three patients: clinical, radiologic, and etiologic considerations. *Neuroradiology* 1996;**38**:684–87.

Cerebellar stroke

Anatomy of cerebellar vessels

The cerebellum is supplied by the two vertebral arteries and the basilar artery located anteriorly to the brainstem (the vertebrobasilar system is illustrated in Figure 8.1, see Chapter 1 for the embryology of cerebellar vessels). Therefore, given the shared artery supply, the cerebellum and brainstem are often damaged together in cases of arterial occlusion. Vertebral arteries enter the skull via the foramen magnum. In about 60% of the population, vertebral arteries are asymmetrical.

Vascularization of the cerebellar cortex is divided into a pial network and intracortical vessels (Duvernoy et al., 1983). Three superficial vascular layers follow approximately the three subdivisions of the cerebellar cortex (see Chapter 1).

The three main cerebellar arteries are, from the origin of the vertebral artery, the posterior inferior cerebellar artery (PICA), the anterior inferior cerebellar artery (AICA), and the superior cerebellar artery (SCA). The arterial territories of the major cerebellar vessels are illustrated in the anatomical sections presented in Figure 8.2.

The PICA is the largest branch emerging from the vertebral artery. The PICA is a sinuous artery which takes its origin in most cases from the V4 segment (intradural) of the vertebral artery (Amarenco et al., 1998). In some cases, it may arise from the basilar artery on one side or, rarely, from the ascending pharyngeal artery. It is estimated that the PICA is missing in 7% to 9% of the patients. Hypoplasia occurs in 5% of cases. The PICA irrigates the posterior and caudal part of the cerebellum (sections I to VII of the Figure). The artery gives off medial (mPICA) and lateral (lPICA) branches. mPICA supplies the inferior vermis and the inferior part of the inferior semilunar lobule, gracilis lobule, and tonsil. lPICA irrigates the inferior parts of the biventer lobule, the inferior semilunar and gracilis lobules, and the ventrolateral part of the tonsil.

The dorsal medullary area (comprising the middle and inferior vestibular nuclei, the restiform body, the dorsal nucleus of the vagus, the area postrema, the gracilis, and cuneiform nuclei) is vascularized by the PICA and the posterior spinal arteries.

The AICA emerges from the first third of the basilar artery in about 75% of subjects. It takes its origin more distally on the basilar artery in the remaining cases. The point of origin is asymmetrical in most individuals. The AICA supplies a territory involving the pons and the cerebellum (sections IV to VII). The AICA supplies cranial nerve V (which may be vascularized by the basilar artery also) and is the origin of the auditory and labyrinthine arteries. Unusually, the AICA shares its origin with the internal auditory artery. The territory of the brainstem irrigated by the AICA includes the lateral region of the pons, the facial nucleus, the lateral lemniscus, the spinothalamic tract, the vestibular nuclei (superior, lateral, and medial), and the cochlear nucleus. The middle cerebellar peduncles are also vascularized by branches of the AICA. The artery divides in two branches: the lateral branch irrigates the lateral portion of the biventer lobule, and the medial branch irrigates the inferior surface of the cerebellum. Branches of the AICA and branches of the SCA make an anastomosis in the posterior superior fissure.

The SCA arises either from the top or from the rostral part of the basilar artery, before the origin of posterior cerebral arteries. The SCA is the main source of arterial supply for the superior part of the cerebellum (sections V to XII). The SCA gives off two main branches: the medial branch (mSCA) and the lateral (lSCA) division. SCA supplies the dorsolateral tegmental area of the upper pons, including the superior cerebellar peduncle, the lateral lemniscus, the spinothalamic tract, and the root of the contralateral cranial nerve IV. It irrigates the medial half of the superior cerebellar surface, the lobulus simplex, the

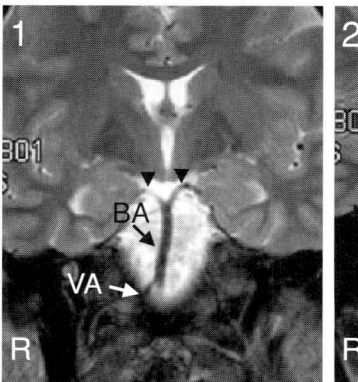 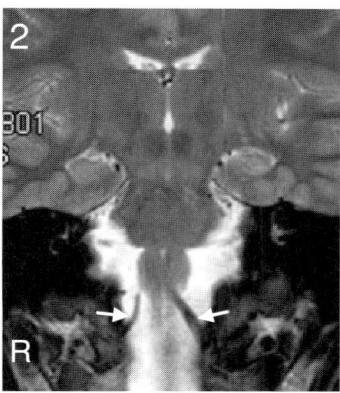 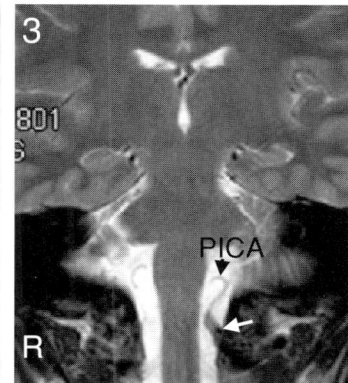

Figure 8.1 Illustration of the vertebrobasilar system on T2-weighted coronal MRI. Vertebral arteries (VA, white arrows) and basilar artery (BA) are identified. The posterior cerebral arteries originate from the top of the BA (arrowheads in panel 1). Note the asymmetry in size of the VAs (panel 2). The origin of the posterior inferior cerebellar artery (PICA) is visible in panel 3. R: right side.

superior semilunar lobule, the culmen, the central lobule, the tuber, and the lingula of the vermis. The rostral part of the cerebellar nuclei also depends on the arterial blood of the SCA.

The venous drainage of the cerebellum is characterized by relatively large zones of venous return and anatomical variations between subjects. Three main groups of veins are identified: the superior or Galenic group, the anterior or petrosal group, and the posterior or tentorial group (Figure 8.3). The superior group drains the upper brainstem and the superior portion of the cerebellum. The superior cerebellar vein reaches the great cerebral vein of Galen. The anterior group drains the anterior parts of the brainstem and cerebellum. The veins of this group empty mostly in the superior petrosal vein near the pons (Braun et al., 1996). The posterior group drains the inferior parts of the cerebellar vermis and medial parts of the cerebellar hemispheres. Veins from this group will empty in the straight sinus and the transverse sinus.

Cerebellar infarctions

Cerebellar infarctions account for about 3% to 4% of strokes. A majority of cerebellar strokes are ischemic (80%). Given the arterial distribution, the simultaneous involvement of the cerebellum and the brainstem is frequent (Macdonnel et al., 1987).

PICA infarctions

PICA infarcts account for 40% to 50% of patients with cerebellar infarctions (Amarenco, 1993; Kase et al., 1993). Partial infarcts are the most common, with the whole territory of the PICA being involved in only

7% to 8% in autopsy series. Other cerebellar infarctions in the territory of the AICA or SCA may be associated.

Symptoms are given in Table 8.1. Six patterns of PICA infarctions may occur (Table 8.2). Ataxia in dorsal lateral medullary syndrome (Wallenberg syndrome; Figure 8.4) is mainly due to a lesion of the dorsal spinocerebellar tract (DSCT), which runs in the inferior cerebellar peduncle. The intact ventral spinocerebellar tract cannot fully compensate for the loss of key information due to DSCT damage (see Chapter 1).

AICA infarctions

AICA infarctions are relatively rare. These infarcts are typically small and usually affect the middle cerebellar peduncle, the caudal pons, and the flocculus. In individuals with hypoplastic PICA, the AICA supplies the territory normally irrigated by the posterior inferior artery. Therefore, the infarction can include signs usually observed in PICA infarcts. Four main clinical presentations may occur (Table 8.3).

SCA infarctions

SCA infarctions are the most common after PICA infarcts. In three of five patients, signs of brainstem infarction are present, usually at the level of the mesencephalon. Autopsy series reveal concomitant infarctions in the occipital/temporal lobes and thalamic-subthalamic areas in 70% of patients (Amarenco & Hauw, 1990). Six clinical presentations are described (Table 8.4).

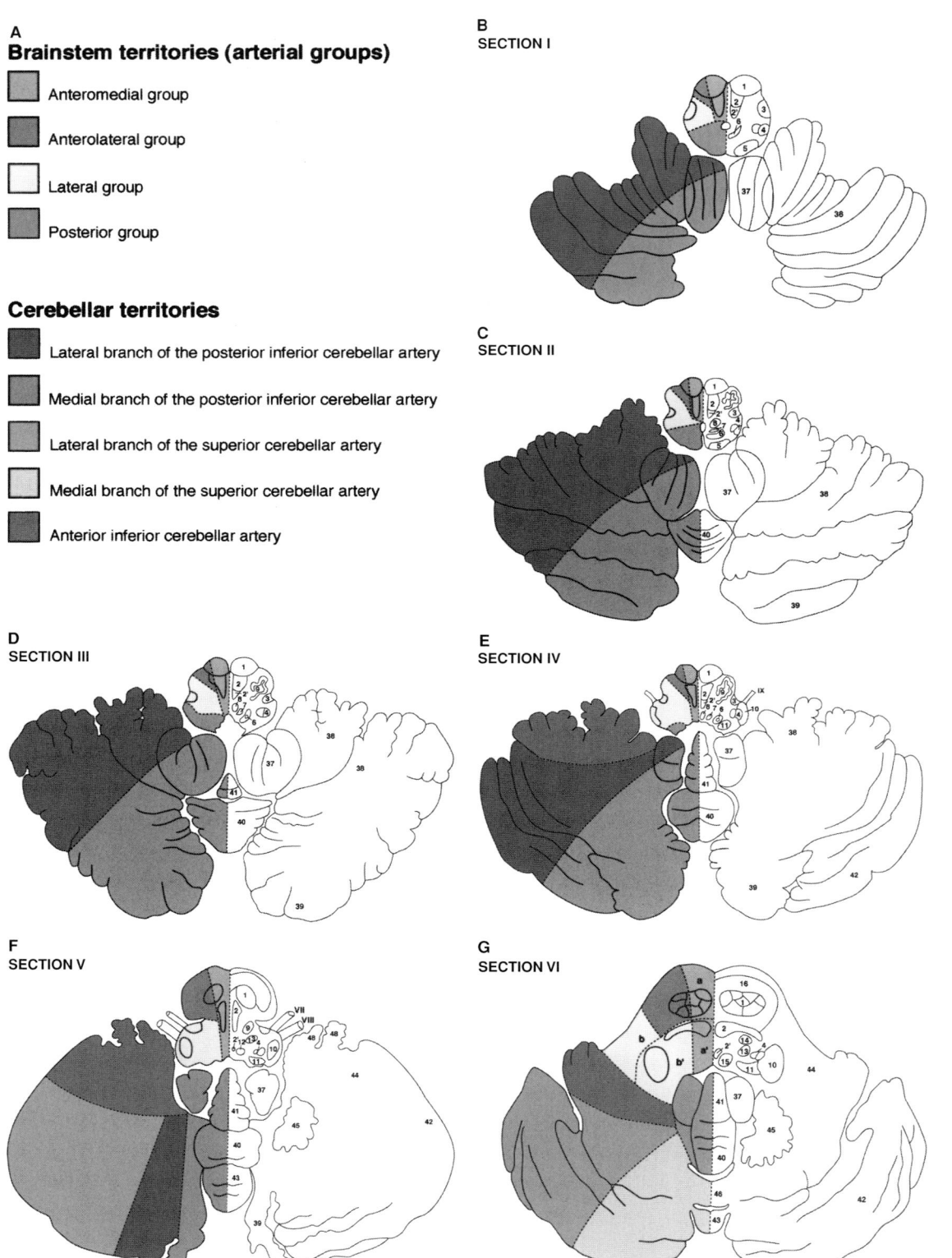

Figure 8.2 Arterial groups and cerebellar territories supplied by the main cerebellar arteries. Illustration of serial sections (4-mm thick) based on a bicommissural plane passing through the anterior and posterior commissures. From: Tatu et al., 1996. With permission. (See color section.)

Anatomic structures of sections I to XII

1 Corticospinal tract; 2 Medial lemniscus; 2′ Medial longitudinal fasciculus; 3 Spinothalamic tract; 4 Spinal trigeminal tract/nuclei; 5 Gracile and cuneate nuclei; 6 Nucleus of solitary tract; 7 Dorsal motor vagal nucleus; 8 Hypoglossal nucleus; 9 Inferior olivary nucleus; 10 Inferior

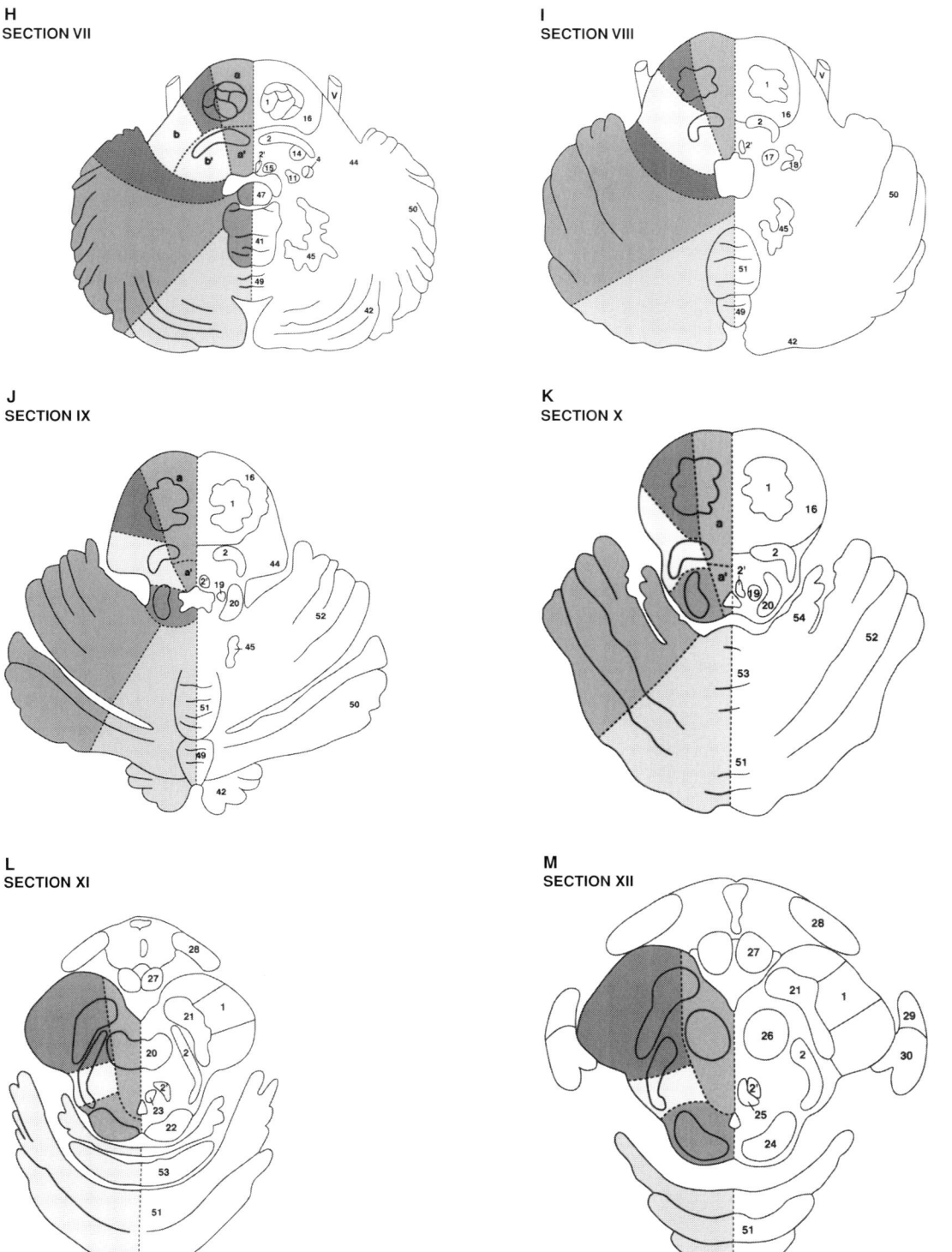

Figure 8.2 (*cont.*) cerebellar peduncle; 11 Vestibular nucleus; 12 Nucleus prepositus; 13 Facial nucleus; 14 Superior olivary nucleus; 15 Abducens nucleus; 16 Pontine nuclei; 17 Motor trigeminal nucleus; 18 Principal sensory trigeminal nucleus; 19 Nucleus ceruleus; 20 Superior cerebellar peduncle; 21 Substantia nigra; 22 Inferior colliculus; 23 Trochlear nucleus; 24 Superior colliculus; 25 Oculomotor nucleus; 26 Red nucleus; 27 Mammillary body; 28 Optic tract; 29 Lateral geniculate nucleus; 30 Medial geniculate body; 31 Pulvinar; 32 Mamillothalamic tract; 33 Column of fornix; 34 Caudate nucleus; 35 Putamen; 36 Anterior commissure; 37 Tonsil; 38 Biventer lobule; 39 Inferior semilunar lobule; 40 Pyramid of vermis; 41 Uvula; 42 Superior semilunar lobule; 43 Tuber of vermis; 44 Middle cerebellar peduncle; 45 Dentate nucleus; 46 Folium of vermis; 47 Nodulus; 48 Flocculus; 49 Declive; 50 Simple lobule; 51 Culmen; 52 Quadrangular lobule; 53 Central lobule; 54 Ala of the central lobule, V Trigeminal nerve, VII Facial nerve, VIII Vestibulocochlear nerve, X Glossopharyngeal nerve.

Table 8.1 Symptoms in territorial cerebellar infarctions

Symptoms	SCA	AICA	PICA
Deafness	Absent	Frequent	Absent
Dizziness	Frequent	Absent	Frequent
Drowsiness	Frequent	Frequent	Uncommon
Tinnitus	Uncommon	Frequent	Absent
Vertigo	Frequent	Frequent	Very common
Nausea/vomiting	Frequent	Very common	Frequent
Hallucinations	Uncommon	Uncommon	Absent
Headache/facial pain	Uncommon	Absent	Uncommon
Pain in limbs/trunk	Absent	frequent	Absent
Sleep disturbances	Uncommon	Absent	Absent

Abbreviations: AICA: anterior inferior cerebellar artery; PICA: posterior inferior cerebellar artery; SCA: superior cerebellar artery.

Figure 8.5 illustrates an example of a stroke in the territory of the lateral branch of the superior cerebellar artery.

Border zone infarctions (watershed)

Border zone infarctions are more frequent than presumed (Amarenco et al., 1993). MRI is the technique of choice to identify the lesions, which have an area usually less than 2 cm in diameter (Rodda, 1971). Brain imaging shows small infarctions mainly found at the boundaries between the SCA and PICA territories, either on the surface of the cortex or around cerebellar nuclei (Amarenco, 1995). They are classified in three categories:

- Cortical border zone infarcts are perpendicular to the cerebellar cortex. They are located at the boundary zones between the SCA and PICA territories, or between the PICA and AICA territories.
- Cortical dorsal infarcts are parallel to the cortex, distributed between the SCA and PICA territories.
- Small deep infarcts are located either in the border zone of the AICA and lateral branches of PICA territories, or between the vermal branches of the two SCA arteries.

Clinically, symptoms are similar to those described in SCA, PICA, or AICA infarctions. Symptoms tend to be transient and may be recurrent. Position-related symptoms are common (vertigo, disequilibrium, etc.). They are probably due to states of low blood flow in the posterior circulation.

Lacunar infarctions

Lacunar infarctions probably do not exist in the cerebellum, due to the fact that cerebellar arteries show a progressive reduction in diameter in their course, without penetrating branches arising from middle-size arteries (Fisher, 1977).

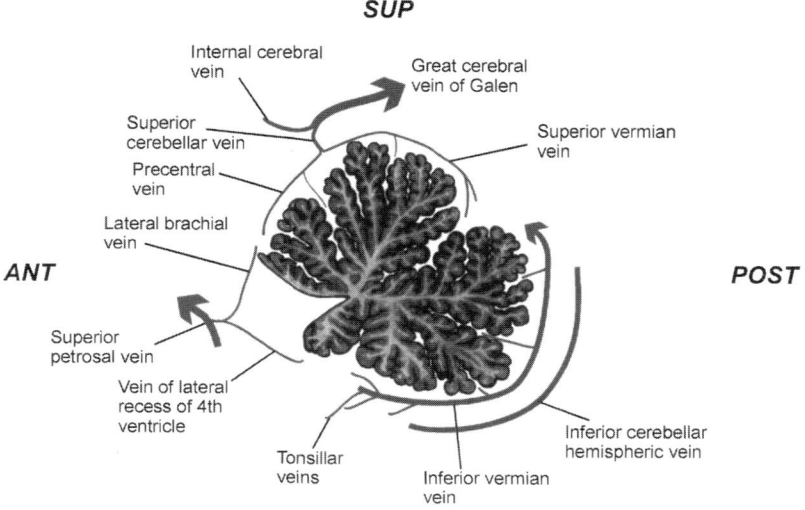

Figure 8.3 Cerebellar venous anatomy. The Galenic group, the petrosal group, and the posterior group empty into the vein of Galen, the superior/inferior petrosal sinuses, and the straight sinus, respectively. Abbreviations: ANT: anterior; SUP: superior; POST: posterior; INF: inferior. With permission from: Blecic and Bogousslavsky, 2002.

Table 8.2 Patterns of posterior inferior cerebellar artery infarctions

Type	Incidence	Presentation
Dorsal lateral medullary syndrome (Wallenberg syndrome)	25–30%	Vertigo Nystagmus Ipsilateral Horner sign Appendicular ataxia Cranial nerve palsies (V, IX, X) Contralateral loss of pain/temperature Lateropulsion
PICA infarct sparing brainstem	15–20%	Vertigo Limb and gait ataxia Nystagmus Lateropulsion Headache Risk of brainstem compression
Isolated acute vertigo	5%	Mimics a peripheral labyrinthitis
mPICA	10%	Vertigo Lateropulsion Dysmetria Possible associated Wallenberg syndrome
lPICA	10%	Vertigo Dysmetria
Multiple infarcts	25–30%	Multiple infarcts in PICA, AICA, SCA Possible pseudotumoral presentation Impaired consciousness, coma

Abbreviations: AICA: anterior inferior cerebellar artery; PICA: posterior inferior cerebellar artery; SCA: superior cerebellar artery.

LATERAL MEDULLARY INFARCTION (Wallenberg syndrome)

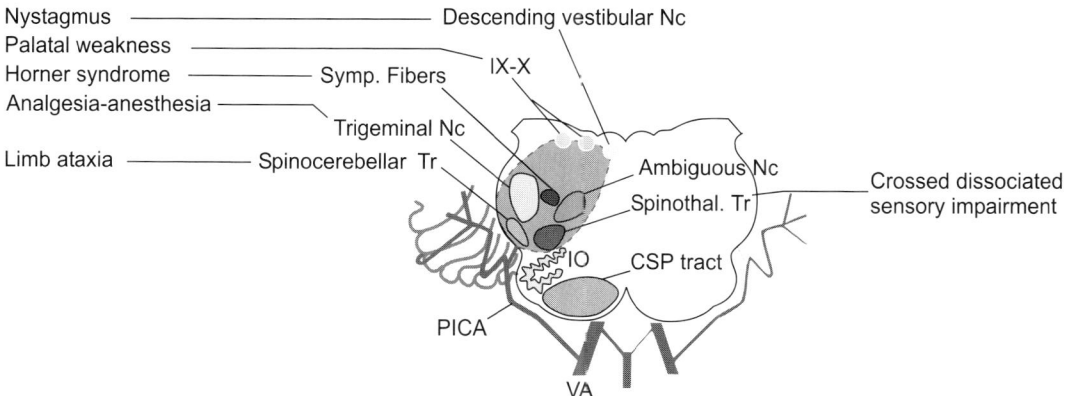

Figure 8.4 Anatomical basis of the symptoms in lateral medullary infarction. The lateral region of the medulla (gray zone) is supplied by small perforating branches. Abbreviations: Ambiguous Nc: ambiguous nucleus; Spinothal. Tr: spinothalamic tract; CSP tract: corticospinal tract; VA: vertebral artery; PICA: posterior inferior cerebellar artery; Trigeminal Nc: trigeminal nucleus; Symp. Fibers: sympathetic fibers; IX–X: cranial nerves IX–X. (See color section.)

Table 8.3 Patterns of anterior inferior cerebellar artery infarctions

Type	Incidence	Presentation
Classic syndrome	30–50%	Vertigo Vomiting Tinnitus Dysarthria Ipsilateral facial palsy Facial sensory loss Horner syndrome Dysmetria Contralateral loss of sensation Hearing loss Gaze palsy Dysphagia Ipsilateral motor weakness
Isolated vertigo	10–15%	Mimics a labyrinthitis
Massive infarction	10%	Coma Tetraplegia Ophthalmoplegia
Isolated cerebellar signs	5%	

Table 8.4 Patterns of superior cerebellar artery (SCA) infarctions

Type	Incidence	Presentation
Classical infarct	3–5%	Ipsilateral limb dysmetria Ipsilateral Horner syndrome Contralateral loss of pain/temperature Sleep disorders Ipsilateral slow involuntary movements Hearing loss (uncommon) Contralateral nerve palsy (IV; rare) Palatal myoclonus/jaw myoclonus
Rostral basilar artery syndrome	20–25%	Diplopia Dizziness Paresthesias Drowsiness Balint syndrome Thalamic-mesencephalic signs Hemiballism Benedikt syndrome Claude syndrome Weber syndrome
Concomitant infarction in the anterior circulation		Signs of SCA occlusion Aphasia Brachiofacial weakness
Vestibular form of SCA		Headache Unsteadiness Dizziness Vomiting Dysarthria Dysmetria Kinetic tremor Nystagmus
Lateral SCA syndrome		Ipsilateral limb dysmetria Axial lateropulsion Dysarthria Nystagmus Contrapulsion of ocular saccades
Medial SCA syndrome		Gait ataxia Ataxia of limbs Increased tone in extensor muscles Isolated dysarthria
Multiple infarctions		Drowsiness, coma Tetraparesis/tetraplegia Ophthalmoplegia

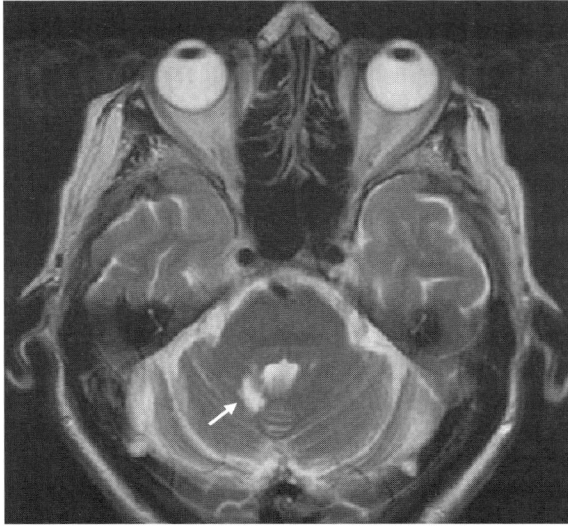

Figure 8.5 Hyperintense lesion (arrow) in the territory of the lateral branch of the superior cerebellar artery. This patient had a history of abrupt-onset unilateral cerebellar dysmetria with kinetic tremor.

Extra-cerebellar lesions causing hemiataxia

Homolateral ataxia may be accompanied by signs of corticospinal tract involvement in the so-called ataxic hemiparesis (Hiraga et al., 2007). This lacunar syndrome is associated with lesions in the pons, internal capsule, corona radiate, and precentral gyrus. Lacunae involve the fibers of the frontopontocerebellar system. A resulting cerebellar diaschisis can be observed. Pontine lesions involve the anteromedial pontine arteries. Pontocerebellar fibers disperse among numerous divergent fascicles before converging to enter into the contralateral middle cerebellar peduncle (Schmahmann et al., 2004). Contralateral hemiataxia and motor paresis may arise from lesions affecting corticopontine and corticospinal fibers descending close to each other to the midpontine level (Marx et al., 2008).

Lesions at the rostral pontomesencephalic level affect the decussation of the dentate-rubrothalamic pathways as they leave the cerebellum via the upper cerebellar peduncle and cause a bilateral ataxia due to outflow tract impairment (Marx et al., 2008).

Posterior and lateral thalamic stroke can mimic a cerebellar lesion (thalamic ataxia). Patients often show sensory deficits and various degrees of pain according to the location of the stroke. Patients with a thalamic infarct in the territory of the posterior choroidal artery involving the posterior thalamic nuclei may develop delayed complex hyperkinetic motor syndromes, combining ataxia, tremor, dystonia, myoclonus, and chorea ("jerky dystonic unsteady hand") (Ghika et al., 1994). These patients have sensory dysfunction. Brain MRI shows infarcts in the territory of the posterior cerebral artery involving the posterior choroidal territory, with an abnormal signal in the posterior area of the thalamus. The other thalamic, subthalamic, and midbrain structures are spared. Dystonia, athetosis, and chorea are associated with position sensory loss, whereas the tremor and myoclonic movements are related to the presence of ataxia (Kim, 2001).

Pure or predominant brainstem sensory stroke is most often caused by small infarcts or hemorrhages in the paramedian dorsal pontine area and may be distinguished from thalamic pure sensory stroke by the following features: frequent association of dizziness and gait ataxia, predominant lemniscal sensory symptoms, occasional leg dominance or cheiro-oral pattern, and frequent bilateral perioral involvement (Kim & Bae, 1997).

Outcome of cerebellar infarctions

The pseudotumoral complication with brainstem compression and herniation is a major life-threatening consequence of cerebellar infarctions. Patients develop hydrocephalus, impaired consciousness, and coma. The compression may develop from a few hours after the stroke up to 8 days after the stroke, although the first 4 days involve greater risk. Full PICA infarctions lead to brainstem compression and tonsillar herniation in 25% of cases (Kase et al., 1993). Isolated

Table 8.5 Mechanisms of cerebellar infarctions

Atherosclerosis

Dissection

Embolism

Hypoperfusion

Small artery disease

Aneurysm

Infection

Migraine

AICA infarctions have a more benign course. However, the prognosis of proximal occlusion of the AICA may be worse, since AICA infarcts may herald a massive occlusion of the basilar artery. Full SCA infarctions have a pseudotumoral presentation in 20% of cases. Nevertheless, partial SCA infarcts usually have a benign course. This is typically the case in lateral SCA infarction (Barth et al., 1993).

Pathogenesis of cerebellar infarcts

The main mechanisms of ischemic stroke in the vertebrobasilar system are listed in Table 8.5. Atherosclerosis is the leading cause. Plaques can be observed in the vertebrobasilar system. They may be calcified or ulcerated, especially in vertebral arteries. In the vertebrobasilar system, plaques evolve in a local clot in most cases. The thrombus may extend to the basilar artery when the occlusion occurs into the intra-cranial part of the vertebral artery (Castaigne et al., 1973). The proximal portion of the basilar artery is more regularly involved than the distal part. Atherosclerosis progresses by involving the orifice of the AICA and SCA arteries. The top of the basilar artery is also damaged by atherosclerosis. While PICA infarctions are due to atherosclerosis in about 60% of cases, cardio-embolism is the leading cause of SCA infarction (Amarenco et al., 1994). AICA infarction is due to atherosclerosis in the large majority of patients, especially those who present with diabetes.

Stroke following a dissection may be due to arterial occlusion, especially in young patients (Barinagarrementeria et al., 1997). The extra-cranial vertebral artery is the most vulnerable site of dissection, especially at the level of the C2 vertebra (Frumkin & Baloh, 1990). Trauma, neck manipulation, vasculitis, and several congenital pathologies (Marfan disease, Ehlers-Danlos disease, Grönblad-Strandberg syndrome, fibromuscular dysplasia) are risk factors.

The recurrence rate is about 1% in the general population. Dissection of the basilar artery is rare. Patients usually develop a coma very rapidly.

Embolism generates a clinical deficit which is usually abrupt and culminating at onset. Main sources are the heart (about 45% of cases), the aortic arch, and the vertebral artery. Embolism is either focal or multiple. Cardio-embolism is the cause of border zone infarcts in about half of cases (Mounier-Vehier et al., 1995). The heart disorders which cause embolism are atrial fibrillation, valvular diseases, myocardial infarct, congestive heart failure, and patent foramen ovale.

Another cause of border zone infarction is hypoperfusion, leading to low flow ischemia. However, this is uncommon, due to the numerous anastomoses in the cerebellum.

Lipohyalinosis affects the small penetrating branches in the brainstem, occluding the lumen of the vessel as a result of subintimal proliferation. Involvement of the cerebellar parenchyma is not demonstrated.

Saccular aneurysms of the vertebral artery or the basilar artery can lead to cerebellar infarction, probably following a clot in the aneurysmal sac. This is the case in particular for the distal part of the basilar artery and the vertebral/PICA junction.

Aspergillosis can involve the posterior circulation vessels, occluding the distal branches of the cerebellar arteries and leading to either infarction or hemorrhage (Walsh et al., 1985). Rare causes of cerebellar stroke also include migraine and vasculitis (systemic lupus erythematosus, granulomatous angiitis, polyarteritis nodosa, giant cell arteritis, Takayasu arteritis, syphilis, isolated angiitis of the central nervous system) (Caplan, 1991; Mclean et al., 1993; Klos et al., 2003). Cocaine can cause a cerebellar stroke by several mechanisms (vasculitis, vasospasm, peak of hypertension, cardiac arrhythmia) (Daras et al., 1991).

Fabry disease is an X-linked lysosomal disorder resulting from alpha-galactosidase deficiency. The disorder affects hemizygous males, as well as both heterozygous and homozygous females. Symptoms are usually more severe in males (probably due to X-inactivation patterns during embryonic development). The deficiency causes accumulation of glycosphingolipids, causing neuropathic pain, with predominant involvement of small nerve fibers, progressive renal dysfunction, cardiomyopathy, and stroke (Morel & Clarke, 2009). Stroke usually presents around the age of 40 years. The vertebrobasilar circulation is symptomatic in about two-thirds of patients, with numerous silent lesions, increasing with age, affecting mainly small perforant arteries (periventricular white matter, brainstem, cerebellum, basal ganglia). Mechanisms are multiple: progressive stenosis of small vessels, arterial remodeling, endothelial dysfunction, cerebral hypoperfusion consecutive to dysautonomy, and cardiac embolism (Clavelou et al., 2006). Patients often show suggestive skin lesions (angiokeratoma) which should prompt the diagnosis. A peculiar corneal opacity (cornea verticillata) may be observed. Proteinuria is often the first sign of kidney involvement.

Cerebellar hemorrhage

The clinical presentation in adults is usually very similar to cerebellar infarcts. Nevertheless, the sudden onset of occipital headache, dizziness, vomiting, and stance/gait ataxia is very suggestive of bleeding (Gilman et al., 1981). Stupor and coma may be the initial presentation. Patients may deteriorate in a few hours or days, suggesting a pseudo-tumoral course.

The hemorrhage is located around the lateral nuclei in most cases. This region is particularly sensitive to peaks of arterial hypertension. Hemorrhage can extend to the middle cerebellar peduncle, the brainstem, and the fourth ventricle.

The hemorrhage results from hypertension in most cases, but some patients may be carriers of a silent aneurysm (about 10–15% of aneurysms are located in the posterior fossa). Aneurysms are located in the following zones: bifurcation of the basilar artery in the posterior cerebral arteries, along the basilar artery, the junction of the vertebral artery with PICA, and along the cerebellar arteries (Hudgins et al., 1983). Patients may develop classical signs of subarachnoid hemorrhage, followed by vasospam in some cases. Grading varies from I to IV in the Hunt and Hess scale (Redekop et al., 1997). Intraventricular hemorrhage and hydrocephalus are common in ruptured aneurysms of cerebellar arteries. The clinical presentation of a giant aneurysm of the basilar artery can mimic a tumor of the posterior fossa. Other sources of hemorrhage in the cerebellum are anticoagulation therapy, angiomas and hemangioblastomas, arteriovenous malformations, brain metastases, trauma, and disorders of coagulation. In addition, cerebellar hemorrhage may be the consequence of a primary infarction, usually an embolism from the heart or the vertebral arteries. In this case, the hemorrhage is commonly

A POST-RESECTION OF SPHENOIDAL MENINGIOMA

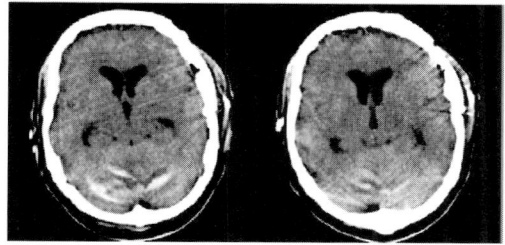

B POST-LUMBAR SURGERY

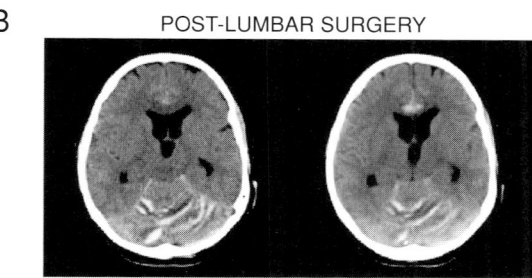

C POST-THORACIC SURGERY

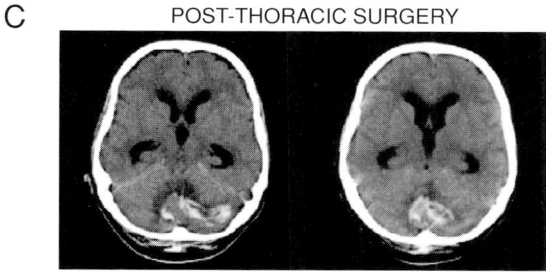

Figure 8.6 Remote cerebellar hemorrhage. (A) Axial CT scan obtained 2 hours after resection of a large left-sided sphenoidal meningioma. The zebra coat–like pattern of remote cerebellar hemorrhage with a typical streaky, curvilinear bleeding pattern is located in the upper cerebellar sulci. (B) CT scan of a comatose patient obtained 4 hours after lumbar surgery. More than 500 mL of serous fluid, which retrospectively was considered to be CSF, had been drained within this time. Curvilinear bleeding pattern with blood in the cerebellar sulci facing the tentorium is seen. Note likewise the small hemorrhage in the interhemispheric fissure (interpreted as being related to acute loss of CSF). (C) CT scan of a patient who underwent resection of a Pancoast tumor with subsequent insertion of a thoracic suction drain. From: Brockman, 2006. With permission.

detected on serial scans performed in the days following stroke onset (Chaves et al., 1996).

Isolated venous angiomas of the posterior fossa are common and are very often asymptomatic. They are managed conservatively.

Remote cerebellar hemorrhage is a rare complication of supra-tentorial, thoracic, or lumbar spinal surgery (Brockmann & Groden, 2006). Brain imaging shows a typical bleeding pattern (Figure 8.6). Remote cerebellar hemorrhage should not be mistaken for a hemorrhagic infarction. Outcome is good in more than half of cases, with only mild remaining neurological symptoms or complete recovery. However, death occurs in approximately 10% to 15% (Brockmann & Groden, 2006). Close monitoring of patients undergoing surgery that involves the risk of draining large volumes of cerebrospinal fluid is mandatory. Patients with post-operative drainage of large amounts of fluid are at risk.

Extremely low birth weight infants (≤ 1000 g) are at high risk for cerebellar hemorrhage (Maddalena & Gibbins, 2008). Associated risk factors include immaturity, fetal distress, and cardiorespiratory instability.

Cerebellar vein thrombosis

Cerebellar venous infarction is a rare cause of cerebellar stroke (<5 %). The initial occlusion involves either the surface veins (draining in the transverse sinus) or the superior cerebellar vein (draining in the great vein of Galen). Thrombosis of the vein of Galen or the straight sinus is a life-threatening condition. The cerebellum is affected bilaterally, in association with the rostral brainstem and supratentorial structures.

Cerebellar vein occlusion can be either hemorrhagic or ischemic. Surrounding edema is very common. Patients may develop cerebellar herniation (tonsillar or upward) and brainstem compression. This pseudo-tumoral presentation results from compression of posterior fossa structures (Rousseaux et al., 1988). Signs of intra-cranial pressure in the posterior fossa may evolve abruptly or develop progressively over several weeks.

Predisposing factors are given in Table 8.6 (Bousser & Russel, 1997). In patients with pterional craniotomy, symptoms of brainstem compression and obstructive hydrocephalus develop within 24 hours following surgery (Papanastassiou et al., 1996). Diagnosis is made with MRI/MRA demonstrating the vein occlusion. Increased venous blood flow velocity is used as an indirect indicator of venous thrombosis (Stolz et al., 1999).

Diagnosis of cerebellar stroke

The techniques and ancillary tests used for the diagnosis of cerebellar stroke are given in Table 8.7.

Conventional MRI is the recommended test to evaluate stroke in the posterior fossa. It has a marked superiority as compared with other techniques. MRI

97

Table 8.6 Predisposing factors to cerebellar vein thrombosis

Pregnancy
Oral contraceptives
Hyperosmolar states
Coagulation disorders (antithrombin III deficiency, R-APC)
Infection (mastoiditis, facial pyodermitis, sinusitis)
Pterional craniotomy

Abbreviation: R-APC: resistance to activated protein C.

Table 8.7 Techniques and ancillary tests used for the diagnosis of cerebellar stroke

MRI
MRA
CT scan
Conventional angiography in selected cases
Ultrasound imaging
Single-photon emission CT
Blood studies
Cardiac investigations
Lumbar puncture in selected cases

Table 8.8 Management of cerebellar stroke

Identification/management of risk factors (hypertension, diabetes mellitus, hyperlipemia, cigarette smoking, exposure to vasoconstrictive agents)
Control of vital functions
Intensive follow-up (stroke unit)

Ischemia
  Thrombolysis
  Anticoagulants
  Antiplatelet agents
  Neurosurgery
  Endovascular prosthesis in selected cases

Hemorrhage   Neurosurgery

Vein thrombosis
  Anticoagulants
  Monitoring of intra-cranial pressure
  Surgical removal of the lesion if required
  Endovascular thrombolysis in selected cases
  Antibiotics in case of infection

allows one to determine the precise location of the lesion(s) and therefore to make a presumption about the cause of the stroke (Tohgi et al., 1993). MRA is a useful complement to MRI. It allows the investigation of the vertebrobasilar system. The technique is non-invasive. Brain CT is useful for the diagnosis and follow-up of acute hemorrhage.

Conventional angiography is performed if an aneurysm or a vascular malformation is suspected. It may prove to be superior to MRA when a dissection is suspected. The technique carries a risk.

Due to anatomical reasons, ultrasound of the posterior circulation is less informative as compared with that of the carotid arteries. Nevertheless, continuous-wave Doppler and duplex systems are non-invasive techniques which can detect stenosis and even dissection (Trattnig et al., 1990). Transcranial Doppler (TCD) is used to evaluate hemodynamics. It detects microbubbles during the Valsalva maneuver in patients presenting with a patent foramen ovale in whom microbubbles are injected in the veins of the upper limbs, confirming a right-left shunt (paradoxical embolism). However, transcranial Doppler of the vertebrobasilar system requires technical skills and also depends on the anatomical variability between subjects.

Single-photon emission computed tomography with technetium-99 hexamethylpropyleneamine oxime may reveal a reduction in blood flow in the territory of a cerebellar infarct. A contralateral diaschisis, clinically silent or not, may be detected (Rousseaux & Steinling, 1999).

Blood tests should include cell counts, hematocrit, lipid levels, glucose level, and coagulation studies. Coagulation studies should be detailed in patients with unexplained strokes or a positive family history of stroke.

Electrocardiographic studies may demonstrate an arrhythmia or signs of congestive heart failure. Transesophageal echocardiography – which is superior to transthoracic echocardiography for detecting cardiac sources of embolism – with contrast administration is recommended when a cardiac source of embolism is suspected, as well as 24-hour Holter monitoring.

Lumbar puncture should be performed in patients complaining of severe headache, without known cause. Mass effect in the posterior fossa should first be ruled out by a CT scan.

Treatment of cerebellar stroke

Management of cerebellar stroke is discussed in Table 8.8. General management in the acute phase includes cardiac and respiratory care, metabolic maintenance, blood pressure control, and prevention of bed sores and phlebitis.

Enzyme replacement therapy (agalsidase alfa/beta) in Fabry disease improves pain and stabilizes renal function and might prevent stroke and adverse cardiac events.

Vasculitis is usually treated with steroids or immunosuppressants (cyclophosphamide therapy to induce remission, commonly followed by maintenance treatment with a less toxic immunosuppressant, such as azathioprine or methotrexate).

Thrombolysis within a few hours should be considered in patients with recent thrombotic occlusions (Hacke et al., 1988). The role of heparin in the acute treatment of ischemic stroke is not established. However, patients with transient ischemic episodes might have some benefit (Amarenco et al., 1998). Long-term oral anticoagulation is recommended in patients presenting with cardio-embolism (atrial fibrillation, myocardial infarction, intra-cardiac thrombus, valvular disease). Prothrombin time should be maintained between 1.2 and 2.5. Patent foramen ovale can be managed with percutaneous closure. Antiplatelet agents (aspirin, ticlopidine, clopidogrel, dipyridamole) are active in the secondary prevention of ischemic stroke in the vertebrobasilar circulation (Sivenius et al., 1991).

Decompressive surgery with monitoring of intra-cranial pressure needs to be performed as soon as possible in patients presenting with a pseudo-tumoral ischemic stroke. Most authors recommend external ventricular drainage (intra-cranial pressure >35 mm H_2O as detected by monitoring of intra-cranial pressure requires ventricular drainage in most cases) and/or suboccipital craniectomy when acute hydrocephalus develops. Third ventriculocisternostomy is a treatment option which may obviate the placement of an external ventricular drainage (Roux et al., 2002). The absence of a hypodense lesion on CT scan in the cerebellum in the first hours after stroke onset should be kept in mind. Early surgery in both cerebellar hemorrhage and infarction (external drainage or evacuation of the lesion) may have a good outcome (Mathew et al., 1995). About three-quarters of patients with hematoma will require a neurosurgical procedure. Brain MRI should be performed immediately in patients presenting with severe weakness, hemiplegia, or tetraplegia. Indeed, a massive pontine infarction might be detected. In these patients, the neurosurgical procedure is not advised.

Aneurysms are managed with neurosurgery (clipping) or endovascular treatments. A decision-making algorithm has been suggested for dissecting aneurysms of the vertebral artery (Iihara et al., 2002). Embolization of arteriovenous malformations may facilitate the resection of the lesion. Multimodality therapy (combinations of radiosurgery, surgery, and endovascular techniques) of arteriovenous malformations of the posterior fossa is associated with a better clinical outcome (Kelly et al., 2008). Vasospasm is treated with "triple H" therapy (hemodilution, hypertension, hypervolemia), calcium channel blockers, recombinant tissue plasminogen activator, and percutaneous transluminal angioplasty (Chiappetta et al., 1998).

References

Amarenco P. Cerebellar stroke syndrome. In *Stroke Syndrome*, ed. J. Bogousslavsky and L. Caplan. Cambridge, UK: Cambridge University Press, 1995, pp. 344–57.

Amarenco P. Les infarctus du cervelet et leurs mécanismes. *Rev Neurol* (Paris) 1993;**149**:728–48.

Amarenco P, Caplan LR, Pessin MS. Vertebrobasilar occlusive disease. In *Stroke*, ed. H.J.M. Barnett, J.P. Mohr, B.M. Stein, and F.M. Yatsu. New York: Churchill Livingstone, 1998, pp. 513–98.

Amarenco P, Hauw JJ. Cerebellar infarction in the territory of the superior cerebellar artery: a clinicopathologic study of 33 cases. *Neurology* 1990;**40**:1383–90.

Amarenco P, Kase CS, Rosengart A, et al. Very small (border zone) cerebellar infarcts. Causes, mechanisms, distribution and clinical features. *Brain* 1993;**116**:161–86.

Amarenco P, Levy C, Cohen A, et al. Causes and mechanisms of territorial and non territorial cerebellar infarcts in 115 consecutive cases. *Stroke* 1994;**25**:105–12.

Barinagarrementeria F, Amaya LE, Cantu C. Causes and mechanisms of cerebellar infarction in young patients. *Stroke* 1997;**28**:2400–4.

Barth A, Bogousslavsky J, Regli F. The clinical and topographic spectrum of cerebellar infarcts: a clinical-magnetic resonance imaging correlation study. *Ann Neurol* 1993;**33**:451–6.

Blecic S, Bogousslavsky J. Cerebellar stroke. In *The Cerebellum and Its Disorders*, ed. M. Manto and M. Pandolfo. Cambridge, UK: Cambridge University Press, 2002, pp. 202–27.

Bousser MG, Russel RR. Cerebellar vein thrombosis. In *Major Problems in Neurology*, ed. M.G. Bousser and R.R. Russel. London: Saunders Ltd, 1997, pp. 40–2.

Braun M, Bracard S, Huot JC, et al. Pontine veins. MRI cross-sectional anatomy. *Surg Radiol Anat* 1996;**18**:315–21.

Brockmann MA, Groden C. Remote cerebellar hemorrhage: a review. *Cerebellum* 2006;**5**(1):64–8.

Caplan LR. Migraine and vertebrobasilar ischemia. *Neurology* 1991;**41**:55–61.

Castaigne P, Lhermitte F, Gauthier JC, et al. Arterial occlusions in the vertebro-basilar system. A study of 44 patients with post-mortem data. *Brain* 1973;**96**: 133–54.

Chaves CJ, Caplan LR, Chung CS, et al. Cerebellar infarcts in the New England Medical Center Posterior Circulation Stroke Registry. *Neurology* 1994;**44**:1385–90.

Chiappetta F, Brunori A, Bruni P. Management of intracranial aneurysms: 'state of the art'. *J Neurosurg Sci* 1998;**42**(suppl 1):5–13.

Clavelou P, Besson G, Elziere C, et al. Neurological aspects of Fabry's disease. *Rev Neurol (Paris)* 2006;**162**(5):569–80.

Daras M, Tuchman AJ, Marks S. Central nervous system infarction related to cocaine abuse. *Stroke* 1991;**22**:1320–5.

Duvernoy H, Delon S, Vannson JL. The vascularization of the human cerebellar cortex. *Brain Res Bull* 1983;**11**:419–80.

Fisher CM. Bilateral occlusion of basilar artery branches. *J Neurol Neurosurg Psychiatry* 1977;**40**:566–7.

Frumkin L, Baloh RW. Wallenberg's syndrome following neck manipulation. *Neurology* 1990;**40**:611–5.

Ghika J, Bogousslavsky J, Henderson J, Maeder P, Regli F. The "jerky dystonic unsteady hand": a delayed motor syndrome in posterior thalamic infarctions. *J Neurol* 1994;**241**(9):537–42.

Gilman S, Bloedel JR, Lechtenberg R. *Disorders of the Cerebellum*: Contemporary Neurology Series. Philadelphia: FA Davis, 1981.

Hacke W, Zeumer H, Ferbert A, et al. Intra-arterial thrombolytic therapy improves outcome in patients with acute vertebrobasilar occlusive disease. *Stroke* 1988;**19**:1216–22.

Hiraga A, Uzawa A, Kamitsukasa I. Diffusion weighted imaging in ataxic hemiparesis. *J Neurol Neurosurg Psychiatry* 2007;**78**(11):1260–2.

Hudgins RJ, Day AL, Quisling RG, et al. Aneurysms of the posterior inferior cerebellar artery. A clinical and anatomical analysis. *J Neurosurg* 1983;**58**:381–7.

Iihara K, Sakai N, Murao K, et al. Dissecting aneurysms of the vertebral artery: a management strategy. *J Neurosurg* 2002;**97**:259–67.

Kase CS, Norrving B, Levine SR, et al. Cerebellar infarction: clinical and anatomic observations in 66 cases. *Stroke* 1993;**24**:76–83.

Kelly ME, Guzman R, Sinclair J, et al. Multimodality treatment of posterior fossa arteriovenous malformations. *J Neurosurg* 2008;**108**(6):1152–61.

Kim JS. Delayed onset mixed involuntary movements after thalamic stroke: clinical, radiological and pathophysiological findings. *Brain* 2001;**124** (Pt 2):299–309.

Kim JS, Bae YH. Pure or predominant sensory stroke due to brain stem lesion. *Stroke* 1997;**28**(9):1761–4.

Klos K, Flemming KD, Petty GW, Luthra HS. Takayasu's arteritis with arteriographic evidence of intracranial vessel involvement. *Neurology* 2003;**60**(9):1550–1.

Macdonnel RA, Kalnins RN, Donnan GA. Cerebellar infarction: natural history, prognosis and pathology. *Stroke* 1987;**19**:847–55.

Maddalena P, Gibbins S. Cerebellar hemorrhage in extremely low birth weight infants: incidence, risk factors, and impact on long-term outcomes. *Neonatal Netw* 2008;**27**(6):387–96.

Marx JJ, Iannetti GD, Thömke F, et al. Topodiagnostic implications of hemiataxia: an MRI-based brainstem mapping analysis. *Neuroimage* 2008;**39**(4):1625–32.

Mathew P, Teasdale G, Bannan A, Oluoch-Olunya D. Neurosurgical management of cerebellar haematoma and infarct. *J Neurol Neurosurg Psychiatry* 1995;**59**:287–92.

Mclean CA, Gonzales MF, Dowling JP. Systemic giant cell arteritis and cerebellar infarction. *Stroke* 1993;**24**(6):899–902.

Morel CF, Clarke JT. The use of agalsidase alfa enzyme replacement therapy in the treatment of Fabry disease. *Expert Opin Biol Ther* 2009;**9**(5):631–9.

Mounier-Vehier F, Degaey I, Leclerc X, Leys D. Cerebellar border zone infarcts are often associated with presumed cardiac sources of ischemic stroke. *J Neurol Neurosurg Psychiatry* 1995;**59**:87–89.

Papanastassiou V, Kerr R, Adamc C. Contralateral cerebellar hemorrhagic infarction after pterional craniotomy: report of five cases and review of the literature. *Neurosurgery* 1996;**39**:841–51.

Redekop GJ, Durity FA, Woodhurst WB. Management-related morbidity in unselected aneurysms of the upper basilar artery. *J Neurosurg* 1997; **87**: 836–42.

Rodda R. The vascular lesions associated with cerebellar infarcts. *Proc Aust Assoc Neurol* 1971;**8**:101–10.

Rousseaux M, Lesoin F, Barbaste P, Jomin M. Pseudotumoral cerebellar infarction of venous origin. *Rev Neurol (Paris)* 1988;**144**:209–11.

Rousseaux M, Steinling M. Remote regional cerebral blood flow consequences of focused infarcts of the medulla, pons and cerebellum. *J Nucl Med* 1999; **40**:721–9.

Roux FE, Boetto S, Tremoulet M. Third ventriculocisternostomy in cerebellar haematomas. *Acta Neurochir (Wien)* 2002;**144**:337–42.

Schmahmann JD, Rosene DL, Pandya DN. Ataxia after pontine stroke: insights from pontocerebellar fibers in monkey. *Ann Neurol* 2004;**55**(4):585–9.

Sivenius J, Riekkinen J, Smets P, et al. The European Stroke Prevention Study (ESPS): results by arterial distribution. *Ann Neurol* 1991;**29**:596–600.

Stolz E, Kaps M, Dorndorf W. Assessment of intracranial venous hemodynamics in normal individuals and patients with cerebral venous thrombosis. *Stroke* 1999;**30**:70–75.

Tatu L, Moulin T, Bogousslavsky J, Duvernoy H. Arterial territories of human brain: brainstem and cerebellum. *Neurology* 1996;**47**(5):1125–35.

Tohgi H, Takahashi S, Chibra K, Hirata Y. Cerebellar infarction. Clinical and neuroimaging analysis in 293 patients. *Stroke* 1993;**24**:1697–1701.

Trattnig S, Hubsch P, Shuster H, Polzleitner D. Color-coded Doppler imaging of normal vertebral arteries. *Stroke* 1990;**21**:1222–5.

Walsh TJ, Hier DB, Caplan LR. Aspergillosis of the central nervous system: clinicopathologic analysis of 17 patients. *Ann Neurol* 1985;**18**:574–82.

Immune diseases

Multiple sclerosis

Multiple sclerosis (MS) is a chronic inflammatory-demyelinating disease of the central nervous system which typically presents as an acute clinically isolated syndrome attributable to a monofocal or multifocal demyelinating lesions. MS is a common chronic neurological disorder in young and middle-aged adults, with a prevalence up to 100 to 200 cases per 100 000. The disorder affects mainly Caucasians. African American individuals have a more severe disease course, an older age at onset, and clinical manifestations usually restricted to the optic nerves and spinal cord (opticospinal MS) as compared with White persons (Cree et al., 2009). Demyelination usually affects the optic nerve, brain, and spinal cord. The relapsing-remitting and secondary progressive forms of MS are the most common presentations (70% of cases). A majority of patients with late-onset MS (diagnosed after 50 years of age) have a primary progressive disease course, whereas a majority of younger patients with age at diagnosis of less than 40 years have a relapsing-remitting course (Kis et al., 2008). Other presentations include the primary progressive (15–20% of cases), the progressive relapsing, and the benign course, which continues for years after onset (benign MS).

Clinical manifestations

Clinical manifestations are multiple. Fatigue is a common and disabling symptom, impairing quality of life. Prevalence of depression is high, and a systematic screening for depression is now recommended. Roughly two-thirds of individuals with MS experience significant cognitive dysfunction, especially in the domains of learning/memory, processing speed, and working memory. Sensory manifestations are present in nearly all the patients, reflecting spinal and/or supra-spinal plaques. Lhermitte sign is suggestive of MS, although it is not entirely specific. Optic neuritis is common and usually unilateral. Uhthoff sign (temporary decrease in vision during exercise or while taking a hot bath) and heat intolerance reflect impaired conductivity in demyelinated axons. Eye movement disorders, such as nystagmus and internuclear ophthalmoplegia, are related to brainstem and cerebellar lesions. Many patients have action tremor, either postural or kinetic (Alusi et al., 2001). Tremor severity ranges from minimal to severe. Tremor severity correlates with the degree of dysarthria, dysmetria, and dysdiadochokinesia. The association of nystagmus, scanning speech, and kinetic tremor is called the Charcot triad of cerebellar signs. These latter are a major factor of incapacity. Dysarthria can be paroxysmal (Blanco et al., 2008). Paresis is usual in lower limbs and may be associated with spasticity, tendon hyperreflexia, and extensor plantar reflexes, reflecting lesions along the pyramidal tracts. Bladder symptoms (failure to store urine) are common. Patients often complain of constipation and anal incontinence due to anorectal dysfunction, which occurs more commonly in progressive forms (Munteis et al., 2008). Patients with anorectal dysfunction are older and have greater disability, longer disease duration, and a greater association with urinary dysfunction (Munteis et al., 2006). Sexual dysfunction is a significant and often underestimated symptom of multiple sclerosis, affecting 50% to 90% of men and 40% to 80% of women (Kessler et al., 2009).

Diagnostic criteria

Diagnostic criteria are based on the objective demonstration of dissemination of lesions in time and space (Table 9.1). New criteria allow the occurrence of lesions of MRI to fulfill the requirements for dissemination (McDonald et al., 2001). Attacks must have a duration of at least 24 hours, and two successive attacks must be separated by at least 30 days between the onset of events. In patients with abnormalities in

Table 9.1 Diagnostic criteria for multiple sclerosis

Presentation	Additional studies required
2 or more attacks 2 or more objective clinical lesions	None (desirable, must be consistent with MS)
2 or more attacks 1 objective clinical lesion	Demonstration of a dissemination in space by MRI, or positive CSF and at least 2 MRI lesions, or a new attack in another site
1 attack 2 or more clinical lesions	Dissemination in time demonstrated by MRI or a second clinical attack
1 attack 1 objective clinical lesion	Dissemination in space demonstrated by MRI or positive CSF with at least 2 MRI lesions Dissemination in time demonstrated by MRI or a second clinical attack
Neurological progression suggestive of MS	Positive CSF Dissemination in space demonstrated by brain MRI (9 lesions or more), or at least 2 spinal cord lesions, or 4–8 brain lesions and 1 spinal cord lesion, or positive visual evoked potential (VEP) with 4 to 8 MRI lesions, or positive VEP with fewer than 4 brain lesions with 1 spinal cord lesion Dissemination in time demonstrated by MRI or continued progression for 1 year

cerebrospinal fluid (CSF) (see below), the presence of two or more lesions is sufficient to disclose dissemination in space. New T2- or gadolinium-enhancing lesions appearing at least 3 months after the onset of the clinical event satisfy the MRI criteria for dissemination in time. Failure to perform follow-up MRI in patients with clinically isolated syndromes may become a practical difficulty for compliance with the criteria (McHugh et al., 2008).

Differential diagnosis

Several disorders can mimic MS:

- Neuromyelitis optica (NMO) is characterized by optic neuritis and myelitis. Revised diagnostic criteria for definite NMO also require at least two of three supportive criteria: MRI evidence of a contiguous spinal cord lesion (three or more segments in length), onset brain MRI nondiagnostic for multiple sclerosis, or NMO immunoglobulin (Ig) G seropositivity (NMO-IgG, an autoantibody targeting aquaporin-4, is a biomarker for NMO) (Wingerchuk et al., 2006).
- Other causes of optic neuritis
- Transverse myelitis
- The group of vasculitis disorders affecting the central nervous system
- Fabry disease (Saip et al., 2007): patients present with unexplained stroke-like episodes, angiokeratomas, and proteinuria (see Chapter 8)
- Fulminant or acute inflammatory-demyelinating diseases, such as the Marburg variant of MS, Baló concentric sclerosis, Schilder disease, and acute disseminated encephalomyelitis (see Chapter 11)
- Erdheim-Chester disease (see Chapter 13)
- Congenital adrenal hyperplasia is an inherited recessive disorder of adrenal steroidogenesis caused by a total or partial deficiency in 21-hydroxylase due to a deletion of or mutations in the CYP21 gene (Bergamaschi et al., 2004). Impaired cortisol biosynthesis results in corticotropin hypersecretion. Patients may present with cerebellar signs. Repeated brain MRI shows focal white matter lesions in periventricular areas, the corpus callosum, the cerebellum, and the brainstem.

Neurophysiology

Multimodality evoked potentials (visual evoked potentials, somatosensory evoked potentials, auditory evoked potentials, and motor evoked potentials) document spatial dissemination of lesions. These lesions may be clinically silent. Evoked potentials are particularly useful when symptoms are atypical without any objective impairment and when symptoms have already recovered at the time of clinical examination (Fischer et al., 2001). Transcranial magnetic stimulation measures have a high sensitivity in detecting lesions in MS, and abnormalities in central motor conduction time may correlate with motor impairment and disability (Chen et al., 2008). Cerebellar stimulation may detect lesions in the cerebellum or the cerebellar output pathways.

About half of the patients have impaired sympathetic skin responses. Sudomotor regulation failure might be correlated with the total lesion volume in the whole brain and focal lesion volumes in the temporal lobe, in the pons, and in the cerebellum (Saari et al., 2008).

Neuroimaging

MRI has a unique sensitivity to demonstrate the spatial and temporal dissemination of demyelinating plaques in the brain and spinal cord (Rovira & León, 2008). Conventional MRI techniques, such as T2-weighted and gadolinium-enhanced T1-weighted sequences, are sensitive in detecting MS plaques and provide a quantitative assessment of inflammatory activity and lesion load. However, there is often a discrepancy between clinical efficacy and MRI-based estimation of the effects of treatments.

T2-weighted images of the optic nerve usually show a hyperintense lesion in optic neuritis, and gadolinium enhancement is seen in the acute attack (Kolappan et al., 2009). Quantifying atrophy of the optic nerve using MRI gives an indication of the degree of axonal loss. Magnetization transfer ratio (MTR) of the optic nerve provides an indication of myelination, and diffusion tensor imaging of the optic nerve/optic radiation gives information about the involvement of the visual white matter tracts. Infratentorial T1-weighted hypointense lesions are often found on brain MRI in patients with MS and chronic cerebellar ataxia. The Expanded Disability Status Scale score correlates with both the number and the volume of these lesions. Lesions may predominate in the cerebellar peduncles in some patients. Overall, cerebellar lesions are less frequent in late-onset MS as compared with young-onset MS (Kis et al., 2008).

Cortical and subcortical atrophy in MS relates to clinical outcomes. Voxel-based automated studies for brain reconstruction show that cerebellum white matter volumes are significantly lower in MS from the earliest clinical stages (Ramasamy et al., 2009). MS patients have lower volumes of thalamus as well as cortical thinning, which increases as the disease progresses.

Diffusion tensor MRI scans might become a useful tool for detecting abnormalities which are not apparent in T2-weighted sequences. In primary progressive MS patients, mean diffusivity changes involve several cortical-subcortical structures in all cerebral lobes and the cerebellum (Ceccarelli et al., 2009). An overlap between decreased white matter fractional anisotropy and increased white matter mean diffusivity is found in the middle cerebellar peduncles.

CSF studies

More than 95% of patients have positive oligoclonal bands or raised IgG index in the CSF.

Neuropathology

Plaques are found in both gray and white matter. The most likely sites are periventricular and peri-aqueductal areas. Acute plaques typically spread out from the post-capillary venules. Early plaques are usually hypercellular, with diffuse demyelination, swollen astrocytes, and attack of the myelin by macrophages. Inflammation and edema will slowly decrease thereafter. The cerebellar cortex is a predilection site for demyelination, in particular in patients with primary and secondary progressive MS (Kutzelnigg et al., 2007). In these patients, about 40% of the cerebellar cortical area is affected. Cerebellar cortical demyelination occurs mainly in a band-like manner. There is no correlation between demyelination in the cortex and the white matter.

Pathogenesis

MS is characterized by immune attack(s) against myelin and myelin-forming cells in the central nervous system. Multiple causes have been suggested. In particular, damage to oligodendrocytes might follow a viral or a bacterial infection, myelin repair by oligodendroglia might be defective, and MS might develop following complex genetic–environmental interactions. Increased family risks range from 300-fold for monozygotic twins to 20- to 40-fold for biological first-degree relatives (Ebers et al., 1995). MRI shows abnormalities consistent with demyelination in some monozygotic and dizygotic co-twins who are clinically unaffected (Mumford et al., 1994). Episodes of demyelination and axonal damage are mediated primarily by CD4-positive T-helper cells with a pro-inflammatory Th1 phenotype, macrophages, and soluble mediators of inflammation. Experimental allergic encephalomyelitis is a commonly used model of MS in animals.

Treatment

Therapies are summarized in Table 9.2. It is now possible to diagnose patients with MS earlier than

Table 9.2 Treatment of multiple sclerosis

Corticosteroids

Beta-interferons

Glatiramer acetate

Plasma exchange

Immunosuppressants

Monoclonal antibodies

Cladribine

Treatment of tremor (deep brain stimulation, thalamotomy)

previously due to the integration of MRI parameters into the diagnostic criteria. This provides a window of opportunity to treat patients before clinically manifest tissue destruction (Tintoré, 2009).

Corticosteroids remain a mainstay of treatment for acute relapses in MS and optic neuritis (Tumani, 2008). High-dose short-term intravenous steroid therapy (methylprednisolone 500–1000 mg/day for 3–5 days) provides symptomatic relief, improves motor function, and accelerates the recovery, but there is no evidence that long-term corticosteroid treatment delays progression of long-term disability. Young-onset MS patients usually respond to steroids to a significantly greater degree as compared with late-onset MS patients (Kis et al., 2008). Oral applications of steroids may be proposed for the treatment of exacerbations if intravenous administration poses practical problems (Tumani, 2008). Acute monitoring in patients with diabetes mellitus, patients receiving anticoagulation, or those having a history of glaucoma is recommended. Behavioral disturbances and gastritis are potential side effects. Supplements of vitamin D and calcium (1 g/day) may be added in patients with osteoporosis. Some authors suggest bisphosphonates or calcitonin.

Patients suffering from severe steroid-resistant relapses may benefit from plasma exchange. This therapy has become an integral part of escalating relapse therapy in relapsing-remitting MS (Linker & Gold, 2008). Best effects can be expected when plasma exchange is administered within 4 to 6 weeks after onset of symptoms and require usually at least three sessions. Possible complications are related to the use of central venous access (infections, thrombosis, pneumothorax), anticoagulation, and hypocalcemia due to citrate infusion.

Beta-interferons and glatiramer acetate, a complex heterogenous mixture of polypeptides with immunomodulatory activity, can decrease the frequency and severity of relapses. Patients with relapsing multiple sclerosis randomized to interferon-beta 1b or glatiramer acetate show similar MRI and clinical activity (Cadavid et al., 2009). Patients treated with an interferon-beta should be monitored systematically for the appearance of neutralizing antibodies. Interferon-beta treatment should be discontinued in case of persistent neutralizing antibodies.

Monoclonal antibodies such as natalizumab might reduce relapses and progression in relapsing-remitting and secondary progressive MS. The risk of progressive multifocal leukoencephalopathy (see also Chapter 11) is increased with this agent (Langer-Gould et al., 2005). The interleukin-2 receptor antagonist daclizumab leads to both clinical improvement and a reduction in MRI activity (Rose et al., 2007).

Brief immunosuppression with mitoxantrone followed by maintenance therapy with glatiramer acetate might provide a synergistic effect on control of disease activity (Boggild, 2009).

Cladribine is a novel immunosuppressant currently under investigation. Cladribine triggers anti-inflammatory effects on MRI evaluation, but may not influence the neurodegenerative process (Filippi et al., 2000).

Fatigue may improve with modafinil and glatiramer acetate (Lange et al., 2009; Ziemssen, 2009).

Sildenafil (50–100 mg) is effective in the treatment of sexual dysfunction in some patients.

Paroxysmal dysarthria responds to carbamazepine (Blanco et al., 2008).

Improvement of tremor with medical treatment (clonazepam, gabapentin, topiramate, primidone Mysoline@) is often modest. Stereotactic surgery targeting the vim nucleus of the thalamus is successful in alleviating MS tremor. Tremor with a poor response to vim deep brain stimulation monotherapy may respond favorably to vim plus ventralis oralis anterior/ventralis oralis posterior (Foote et al., 2006). Stimulation of the zona incerta nucleus may have the advantage of improving proximal components of tremor (Plaha et al., 2008). Gamma knife radiosurgical thalamotomy is an effective alternative to stereotactic surgery (Mathieu et al., 2007). Patients experience improvement in tremor after a median latency period of 2.5 months. More improvement was noted in tremor amplitude than in writing and drawings. Transient contralateral hemiparesis is a potential complication which may respond to steroids.

Recent studies suggest that vagus nerve stimulation might improve postural cerebellar tremor associated with MS, probably by acting at multiple levels in the brainstem (Marrosu et al., 2007).

Repetitive transcranial magnetic stimulation over the motor cortex in MS subjects with cerebellar symptoms improves hand dexterity, but the therapeutical implications remain to be determined.

Ataxia with anti-GAD antibodies

Glutamic acid decarboxylase (GAD) is the enzyme converting glutamate to GABA (see also Chapter 1). Antibodies against GAD (GAD-Ab) may be associated with neurological disorders such as cerebellar ataxia or stiff-man syndrome (Saiz et al., 1997). Patients may suffer from insulin-dependent diabetes or autoimmune polyendocrine syndrome (APS; see section Other immune disorders affecting the cerebellum).

Clinical presentation

Neurological examination shows various degrees of severity of cerebellar ataxia, ranging from mild to severe. Nystagmus (gaze-evoked, periodic alternating, downbeat) may be the predominant finding. Patients are at risk for aspiration pneumonia in advanced cases.

Neuroimaging

Brain MRI reveals various degrees of cerebellar atrophy after several years of evolution.

Neuropathology

Autopsy shows depletion of Purkinje cells and diffuse proliferation of the Bergmann glia (Ishida et al., 2007). This is reminiscent of pathological changes that are observed in paraneoplastic cerebellar degeneration (see Chapter 13). Basket cells appear relatively preserved (Ishida et al., 2007). Lymphocytic infiltration in the pancreas and selective decrease in the pancreatic islets are suggestive of an antibody-mediated diabetes mellitus (Nakanishi et al., 1993).

Blood studies

GAD-Ab are considered as a serological diagnostic marker of the disease. There is a significant link between GAD-Ab and cerebellar symptoms (Honnorat et al., 2001). Purkinje cells, particularly enriched in GAD, are probably very sensitive to GAD-Ab (Manto

et al., 2007). Purkinje cells might have the ability to uptake immunoglobulins from the CSF, so that GAD-Ab would reach their target. GAD-Ab suppress cerebellar GABAergic transmission and impair NMDA-mediated synaptic regulation of neurotransmitters (Ishida et al., 1999; Manto et al., 2007). Muscle spasms are presumably due to dysfunction of inhibitory circuits in the spinal cord.

Treatment

Ataxia may respond to intravenous immunoglobulins (Abele et al., 1999). Plasma exchanges and immunosuppressive therapy might improve slightly cerebellar ataxia (Ishida et al., 2007). Baclofen tends to reduce oculomotor deficits. Spasms and rigidity may improve with diazepam and baclofen administration. Oculomotor deficits may respond to gabapentin (900–3000 mg/day).

Celiac disease and gluten ataxia

Gluten ataxia is an immune-mediated disorder which is triggered by ingestion of gluten in susceptible individuals (Hadjivassiliou et al., 2008). It is one of the extraintestinal manifestations of gluten sensitivity, which is a systemic illness. Gluten ataxia can be defined as a sporadic cerebellar ataxia associated with circulating antigliadin antibodies in absence of an alternative etiology for ataxia (Hadjivassiliou et al., 2008).

There is a high prevalence of antigliadin antibodies in sporadic ataxias as compared with healthy individuals. The prevalence of antigliadin antibodies in a control population is about 5% to 12%, depending on the technique used and the local prevalence of celiac disease (Hadjivassiliou et al., 2008). Some authors argue that this high prevalence in controls decreases the value of antigliadin antibodies as a marker of disease. Nevertheless, these antibodies remain the most sensitive marker for gluten ataxia, until the discovery of more specific ones. The prevalence of occult gluten sensitivity in subjects with positive antigliadin antibodies and no enteropathy is unknown.

Clinical presentation

Mean age of gluten ataxia is 53 years, with a male-to-female ratio of 1:1. The onset of ataxia is usually insidious. Gait is always abnormal, with limb ataxia being present in most cases. Severe gait ataxia occurs usually after a long disease duration. Subacute course mimicking a paraneoplastic cerebellar degeneration may occur. Patients presenting with gluten ataxia may exhibit other neurological features. In particular, gluten ataxia is often accompanied by peripheral neuropathy involving large fibers or small fibers (more than 50% of patients with gluten ataxia present with evidence of sensorimotor axonal neuropathy; Hadjivassiliou et al., 2003), autonomic insufficiency, and can be associated, although uncommonly, with cognitive impairment, pyramidal signs, myoclonus, palatal tremor, opsoclonus-myoclonus, parkinsonism or chorea, and myopathy (Cooke & Thomas-Smith, 1966; Luostarinen et al., 1999; Hadjivassiliou et al., 2002; Pereira et al., 2004). The clinical picture may be suggestive of multiple system atrophy (see Chapter 23).

Blood studies

By definition, all patients have positive IgG and/or IgA antigliadin antibodies (Hadjivassiliou et al., 2008). Anti-endomysium antibodies are detected in 1 in 5 patients. However, these antibodies have a high specificity for the presence of enteropathy. It should be noted that the specificity of IgG antigliadin antibodies is lower than that of IgA antigliadin antibodies in the diagnosis of celiac disease (Farrell & Kelly, 2002). Tissue transglutaminase antibodies are positive in up to 56% of patients with gluten ataxia. Concomitant auto-immune disease is not exceptional (especially Hashimoto thyroiditis, type 1 diabetes mellitus, and pernicious anemia) (Hadjivassiliou et al., 2008).

Neuroimaging

Brain MRI shows various degrees of cerebellar atrophy. White matter lesions also can be found. They tend to be confluent. Single-photon emission CT images may demonstrate decreased cerebellar blood flow (Ihara et al., 2006). Proton MR spectroscopy reveals abnormal ratios of N-acetylaspartate to creatine in the cerebellum (Wilkinson et al., 2005). Oligoclonal bands are found in the CSF in 50% of cases.

Small bowel biopsy

Small bowel biopsy shows evidence of enteropathy in about 35% of patients with gluten ataxia. Duodenal biopsy demonstrates infiltration of plasma cells and lymphocytes in the lamina propria, crypt hyperplasia, and villous blunting. It should be kept in mind

that extra-intestinal manifestations of gluten sensitivity can exist in the absence of an enteropathy disclosed by biopsy specimen.

Pathogenesis

Gluten sensitivity is probably genetically determined. Many patients presenting with gluten ataxia express HLA-DQ2, found in 70% of cases and in about 90% of patients with celiac disease (Hadjivassiliou et al., 2003; Hadjivassiliou et al., 2008). The other patients are HLA-DQ8 and HLA-DQ1 positive. There is growing evidence for impaired immunoregulation in gluten ataxia. Post-mortem studies have provided evidence of neuroinflammation in the cerebellum and posterior columns (Hadjivassiliou et al., 2002). Patchy losses of Purkinje cells are found in the cerebellar cortex, and the cerebellar white matter is characterized by astrocytic gliosis, vacuolation, and diffuse infiltrate with a majority of T-lymphocytes, which are also identified in perivascular cuffing. Experimental studies indicate an antibody cross-reactivity between antigenic epitopes on Purkinje cells and gluten peptides (Hadjivassiliou et al., 2002). Some authors have hypothesized that positivity for antigliadin antibodies might be a consequence rather than the origin of the cerebellar degeneration, raising some controversy about the entity of gluten ataxia (Bushara et al., 2004). Malabsorption of vitamins (such as vitamin E) and nutrients could contribute to cerebellar deficits (Harding et al., 1982).

Treatment

A gluten-free diet should be initiated immediately. This can lead to symptomatic relief in ataxic patients (Ihara et al., 2006). In others, diet will stop the progression of ataxia. The best marker of strict adherence to a gluten-free diet is serological demonstration of the elimination of circulating antigliadin antibodies (Hadjivassiliou et al., 2008). Intravenous immunoglobulins can be considered also. They may improve gluten ataxia without enteropathy (Burk et al., 2001). Main additional immunosuppressive treatments used are cyclosporin and cyclophosphamide. They are used in refractory cases and require a close follow-up.

Other immune disorders affecting the cerebellum

Cogan syndrome is a disorder which is probably overlooked. It affects young adults and is characterized by episodes of acute interstitial keratitis with vestibu-loauditory dysfunction (Cogan, 1945). From 2% to 50% of patients present with neurological deficits, mainly meningoencephalitis, seizures, organic mental syndrome, and peripheral neuropathy. Patients may present with thrombosis of the PICA artery or multiple acute cerebellar lesions mimicking cerebellar infarctions (Norton & Cogan, 1959; Fair & Levi, 1960; Manto & Jacquy, 1996). The diagnosis should be considered in any patients presenting with a combination of eye and ear symptoms with cerebellar signs. The pathogenesis consists of a vasculitis. Cerebellar ataxia may improve with steroids (Manto & Jacquy, 1996).

Behçet disease usually starts between 16 and 55 years of age, with a predominance in males. The disorder is a vasculitis characterized by a triad of oral and genital aphthous ulcers, meningoencephalitis, and relapsing uveitis. The disease has a wide systemic spectrum, involving joints, nervous system, gastrointestinal tract, and vessels. About 10% to 25% of patients exhibit neurological deficits (Nakasu et al., 2001; Wolf et al, 1965; Hadfield et al., 1997). Usually, patients have fever during or preceding CNS manifestations (O'Duffy & Goldstein, 1976). The most common symptoms of neuro-Behçet disease are headache, paresthesia, unsteadiness, diplopia, and weakness (Ashjazadeh et al., 2003). Neurological examination shows various combinations of gait deficits, sensory abnormalities, ophthalmoplegia, cerebellar ataxia, pseudobulbar syndrome, and hemiplegia. The most common presentation is a "brainstem-plus" type. Intracranial hypertension is not rare. Subacute onset or a relapsing-remitting course may first suggest a multiple sclerosis (MS). Patients are particularly at risk for venous sinus thrombosis, arterial occlusion, or thrombophlebitis. Most intra-cranial aneurysms which have been described are located supra-tentorially. The superior cerebellar artery is a potential site (Ho & Deruytter, 2005). The most common neuropathologic findings are focal necrotic lesions in the brain. Perivascular inflammation is particularly marked (Arai et al, 2006). Although some aneurysms disappear after steroid therapy, others require surgery, keeping in mind that aneurysms may be the site of an inflammatory process and therefore are friable (Nakasu et al., 2001; Chun et al., 2001). Regarding CSF, neuro-Behçet disease is characterized by pleocytosis with predominant lymphocytosis, as well as elevated protein levels (O'Duffy & Goldstein, 1976). MRI is the investigation of choice, revealing iso-/hypointense lesions in T1-weighted images and hyperintense lesions in T2-weighted images, mainly in the mesodiencephalic junction, cerebellar peduncles, or other brainstem areas (Haghighi et al., 2005). Steroids are usually effective to reduce or stop the progression of the neurological deficits. Immunosuppressive agents used are cyclophosphamide, azathioprine, and chlorambucil (Benamour et al., 2006). Anticoagulation and anti-epileptic agents may be required for dural sinus thrombosis. The prognosis is usually worse in cases of parenchymal CNS involvement.

Systemic lupus erythematosus may affect cerebellar structures in an acute or subacute mode. Patients are at risk for acute vasculopathy in the territory of cerebellar arteries or may develop a subacute pancerebellar syndrome (Manto et al., 1996; Chan et al., 2006; Parikh et al., 2007). Multiple infarctions in the vertebrobasilar territory may be the initial manifestation (Kwon et al., 1999). Sjögren syndrome and Hashimoto encephalopathy might share some pathophysiological mechanisms with lupus. Antibodies directed against Purkinje cells have been reported in patients with lupus ataxia (Shimomura et al., 1993). Treatments include prednisone, cyclophosphamide, and anticoagulation. Ataxia may respond promptly to steroids in some cases.

Polyarteritis nodosa is characterized by a necrotizing arteritis of small and medium arteries. The disorder manifests from childhood to midlife and affects mainly the skin, joints, kidneys, gastrointestinal tract, and peripheral nerves in a context of fever and weight loss (Conn, 1990). Hypertension is common. CNS involvement includes diffuse encephalopathy, focal deficits, and seizures. Infarctions are found in the cortical and subcortical regions of cerebral hemispheres, in basal ganglia, internal capsule, brainstem, and cerebellum (Provenzale & Allen, 1996). Cerebral angiography shows alternating sites of narrowing and dilatation in middle-size and small arteries, consistent with arteritis. Diagnosis can be confirmed by nerve, muscle, or kidney biopsy. Neurological symptoms usually respond to steroid and cytotoxic agents.

Auto-immune polyglandular syndromes (APS) comprise a wide spectrum of auto-immune disorders and are divided into a rare juvenile (PAS type I) and a more common adult type with (PAS II) or without adrenal failure (PAS III) (Kahaly, 2009). Autosomal recessive PAS I is caused by mutations in the

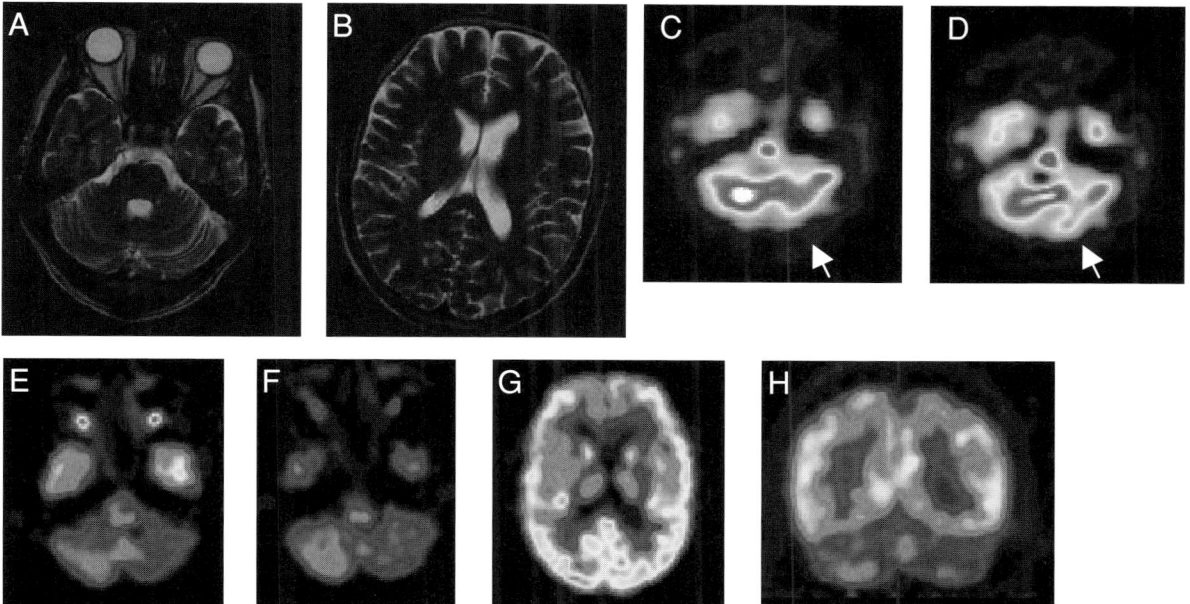

Figure 9.1 Auto-immune polyglandular syndrome (APS) type 2 in a young man presenting with a disabling cerebellar syndrome. (A,B) T2-weighted brain MRI. Cerebellar sulci are widened (A). There is a moderate cerebral diffuse cortical atrophy (B). (C,D) Single-photon emission CT imaging showing an asymmetry of cerebellar blood flow, with hypoperfusion of right cerebellar hemisphere (arrows). (E–H) ^{18}F-Fluorodeoxyglucose positron emission tomography study shows an asymmetry of cerebellar metabolism and a diffuse cerebral cortical hypometabolism.

auto-immune regulatory (AIRE) gene on chromosome 21. Mutations in the AIRE gene result in defective proteins which cause auto-immune destruction of target organs. Neurologic deficit may result from the associated endocrinopathies (hypoparathyroidism, hypothyroidism, diabetes mellitus), vitamin deficiencies (vitamins B12 and E), and celiac sprue (Berger et al., 2008). Cerebellar syndrome may be prominent in APS type I or type II. Brain MRI can demonstrate a cerebellar atrophy, and positron emission tomography studies can reveal a cerebellar hypometabolism (Figure 9.1). Diagnosis of PAS involves serological measurement of organ-specific autoantibodies and subsequent functional testing.

Vogt-Koyanagi-Harada disease is an inflammatory disorder characterized by posterior uveitis, iridocyclitis, and papillitis. Hair loss and vitiligo are commonly observed. Patients may present with diplopia, dysarthria, and cerebellar ataxia as a result of a brainstem encephalitis extending into the middle cerebellar peduncle (Hashimoto et al., 2009). Wallenberg syndrome due to stroke is a complication. Ataxia may respond to administration of steroids.

Kikuchi-Fujimoto disease (histiocytic necrotizing lymphadenitis) is a benign and self-limiting disease of unknown etiology affecting mainly young women. It presents with localized lymphadenopathy, usually cervical, accompanied by various systemic manifestations including fever, weight loss, night sweats, leukopenia, and high erythrocyte sedimentation rate. Patients may present with acute aseptic meningitis. Kinetic tremor and gait ataxia may precede cervical lymphadenopathy (Moon et al., 2009). Diagnosis is based upon the biopsy of cervical lymph nodes, showing areas of necrosis with abundant debris and reactive histiocytes. Acute cerebellar symptoms resolve spontaneously. Kikuchi-Fujimoto disease has been described in association with other auto-immune disorders, mainly systemic lupus erythematosus.

Graft-versus-host disease after a bone-marrow transplant is a cause of cerebral vasculitis (Campbell & Morris, 2005). Lesions may predominate in the cerebellum. Cerebral angiography shows dilated and narrowed segments of the posterior circulation. Steady improvement with immunosuppressant therapy is reported.

References

Abele M, Weller W, Merscheriakov S, et al. Cerebellar ataxia with glutamic acid decarboxylase antibodies. *Neurology* 1999;**52**:857–9.

Alusi SH, Worthington J, Glickman S, Bain PG. A study of tremor in multiple sclerosis. *Brain* 2001;**124**(Pt 4):720–30.

Arai Y, Kohno S, Takahashi Y, Miyajima Y, Tsutsui Y. Autopsy case of neuro-Behçet's disease with multifocal neutrophilic perivascular inflammation. *Neuropathology* 2006;**26**:579–85.

Ashjazadeh N, Borhani Haghighi A, Samangooie Sh, Moosavi H. Neuro-Behçet's disease: a masquarader of multiple sclerosis. A prospective study of neurologic manifestations of Behçet's disease in 96 Iranian patients. *Exp Mol Pathol* 2003;**74**:17–22.

Benamour S, Naju T, Alaoui FZ, El-Kabli H, El-Aidouni S. Neurological involvement in Behçet's disease. 154 cases from a cohort of 925 patients and review of the literature. *Rev Neurol* (Paris) 2006;**162**:1084–90.

Bergamaschi R, Livieri C, Candeloro E, et al. Congenital adrenal hyperplasia and multiple sclerosis: is there an increased risk of multiple sclerosis in individuals with congenital adrenal hyperplasia? *Arch Neurol* 2004;**61**(12):1953–5.

Berger JR, Weaver A, Greenlee J. Neurologic consequences of autoimmune polyglandular syndrome type 1. *Neurology* 2008;**70**(23):2248–51.

Blanco Y, Compta Y, Graus F, Saiz A. Midbrain lesions and paroxysmal dysarthria in multiple sclerosis. *Mult Scler* 2008;**14**(5):694–7.

Boggild M. Immunosuppression followed by immunomodulation. *J Neurol Sci* 2009;**277** (suppl 1):S50–4.

Burk K, Melms A, Schulz JB, Dichgans J. Effectiveness of intravenous immunoglobulin therapy in cerebellar ataxia associated with gluten sensitivity. *Ann Neurol* 2001;**50**:827–8.

Bushara KO, Nance M, Gomez CM. Antigliadin antibodies in Huntington's disease. *Neurology* 2004;**62**:132–3.

Cadavid D, Wolansky LJ, Skurnick J, et al. Efficacy of treatment of MS with IFN beta-1b or glatiramer acetate by monthly brain MRI in the BECOME study. *Neurology* 2009;**72**(23):1976–83.

Campbell JN, Morris PP. Cerebral vasculitis in graft-versus-host disease: a case report. *AJNR Am J Neuroradiol* 2005;**26**(3):654–6.

Ceccarelli A, Rocca MA, Valsasina P, et al. A multiparametric evaluation of regional brain damage in patients with primary progressive multiple sclerosis. *Hum Brain Mapp* 2009 Jan 26 [Epub ahead of print].

Chan AY, Li EK, Wong GL, Liu DT. Cerebellum vasculopathy and normal tension glaucoma in systemic lupus erythematosus: report of a case and review of the literature. *Rheumatol Int* 2006;**27**:101–2.

Chen R, Cros D, Curra A, et al. The clinical diagnostic utility of transcranial magnetic stimulation: report of an IFCN committee. *Clin Neurophysiol* 2008;**119**(3):504–32.

Chun JY, Smith W, Halbach VV. Current multimodality management of infectious intracranial aneurysms. *Neurosurgery* 2001;**48**:1203–13.

Cogan DG. Syndrome of nonsyphilitic interstitial keratitis and vestibuloauditory symptoms. *Arch Ophtalmol* 1945;**33**:144–9.

Conn DL. Polyarteritis. *Rheum Dis Clin North Am.* 1990;**16**(2):341–62

Cooke WT, Thomas-Smith W. Neurological disorders associated with adult celiac disease. *Brain* 1966;**89**:683–22.

Cree BA, Reich DE, Khan O, et al. Modification of multiple sclerosis phenotypes by African ancestry at HLA. *Arch Neurol* 2009;**66**(2):226–33.

Ebers GC, Sadovnick AD, Risch NJ. A genetic basis for familial aggregation in multiple sclerosis. Canadian Collaborative Study Group. *Nature* 1995;**377**(6545):150–1.

Fair JR, Levi GA. Keratitis and deafness. *Am J Ophtalmol* 1960;**49**:1017–21.

Farrell RJ, Kelly CP. Celiac sprue. *N Engl J Med* 2002;**346**:180–8.

Filippi M, Rovaris M, Iannucci G, et al. Whole brain volume changes in patients with progressive MS treated with cladribine. *Neurology* 2000;**55**(11):1714–8.

Fischer C, André-Obadia N, Mauguière F. Diagnostic criteria of multiple sclerosis: electrophysiological criteria. *Rev Neurol* (Paris) 2001;**157**(8–9 Pt 2): 974–80.

Foote KD, Seignourel P, Fernandez HH, et al. Dual electrode thalamic deep brain stimulation for the treatment of posttraumatic and multiple sclerosis tremor. *Neurosurgery* 2006;**58**(4 suppl 2):ONS-280–5.

Hadfield MG, Aydin F, Lippman HR, et al. Neuro-Behçet's disease. *Clin Neuropathol* **16**;55–60.

Hadjivassiliou M, Grunewald R, Sharrack B, et al. Gluten ataxia in perspective: epidemiology, genetic susceptibility and clinical characteristics. *Brain* 2003;**26**:685–91.

Hadjivassiliou M, Grunewald RA, Davies-Jones GA. Gluten sensitivity as a neurological illness. *J Neurol Neurosurg Psychiatry* 2002;**72**:560–3.

Hadjivassiliou M, Sanders DS, Woorroofe N, Williamson C. Gluten ataxia. *Cerebellum* 2008;**7**(3):494–8.

Haghighi AB, Pourmand R, Nikseresht AR. Neuro-Behçet disease: a review. *Neurologist* 2005;**11**:80–9.

Harding AE, Muller DP, Thomas PK, Willison HJ. Spinocerebellar degeneration secondary to chronic intestinal malabsorption: a vitamin E deficiency syndrome. *Ann Neurol* 1982;**12**:419–24.

Hashimoto T, Takizawa H, Yukimura K, Ohta K. Vogt-Koyanagi-Harada disease associated with brainstem encephalitis. *J Clin Neurosci* 2009;**16**(4): 593–5.

Ho CL, Deruytter MJ. Manifestations of Neuro-Behçet's disease. Report of two cases and review of the literature. *Clin Neurol Neurosurg* 2005;**107**:310–4.

Honnorat J, Saiz A, Giometto B, et al. Cerebellar ataxia with anti-glutamic acid decarboxylase antibodies: study of 14 patients. *Arch Neurol* 2001;**58**:225–30.

Ihara M, Makino F, Sawada H, et al. Gluten sensitivity in Japanese patients with adult-onset cerebellar ataxia. *Intern Med* 2006;**45**(3):135–40.

Ishida K, Mitoma H, Song SY, et al. Selective suppression of cerebellar GABAergic transmission by an autoantibody to glutamic acid decarboxylase. *Ann Neurol* 1999;**46**:263–7.

Ishida K, Mitoma H, Wada Y, et al. Selective loss of Purkinje cells in a patient with anti-glutamic acid decarboxylase antibody-associated cerebellar ataxia. *J Neurol Neurosurg Psychiatry* 2007;**78**(2):190–2.

Kahaly G. Polyglandular Autoimmune Syndromes. *Eur J Endocrinol* 2009;**161**(1):11–20.

Kessler TM, Fowler CJ, Panicker JN. Sexual dysfunction in multiple sclerosis. *Expert Rev Neurother* 2009;**9**(3):341–50.

Kis B, Rumberg B, Berlit P. Clinical characteristics of patients with late-onset multiple sclerosis. *J Neurol* 2008;**255**(5):697–702.

Kolappan M, Henderson AP, Jenkins TM, et al. Assessing structure and function of the afferent visual pathway in multiple sclerosis and associated optic neuritis. *J Neurol* 2009;**256**(2):305–19.

Kutzelnigg A, Faber-Rod JC, Bauer J, et al. Widespread demyelination in the cerebellar cortex in multiple sclerosis. *Brain Pathol* 2007;**17**(1):38–44

Kwon SU, Koh JY, Kim JS. Vertebrobasilar artery territory infarction as an initial manifestation of systemic lupus erythematosus. *Clin Neurol Neurosurg* 1999;**101**(1):62–7.

Lange R, Volkmer M, Heesen C, Liepert J. Modafinil effects in multiple sclerosis patients with fatigue. *J Neurol* 2009;**256**(4):645–50.

Langer-Gould A, Atlas SW, Green AJ, et al. Progressive multifocal leukoencephalopathy in a patient treated with natalizumab. *N Engl J Med* 2005;**353**(4):375–81.

Linker RA, Gold R. Use of intravenous immunoglobulin and plasma exchange in neurological disease. *Curr Opin Neurol* 2008;**21**(3):358–65.

Luostarinen L, Pirtilla T, Collin P. Coeliac disease presenting with neurological disorders. *Eur Neurol* 1999;**42**:132–5.

Manto M, Jacquy J. Cerebellar ataxia in Cogan syndrome. *J Neurol Sci* 1996;**136**:189–91.

Manto MU, Laute MA, Aguera M, et al. Effects of anti-glutamic acid decarboxylase antibodies associated with neurological diseases. *Ann Neurol* 2007;**61**(6):544–51.

Manto MU, Rondeaux P, Jacquy J, Hildebrand J. Subacute pancerebellar syndrome associated with systemic lupus erythematosus. *Clin Neurol Neurosurg* 1996;**98**: 157–60.

Marrosu F, Maleci A, Cocco E, et al. Vagal nerve stimulation improves cerebellar tremor and dysphagia in multiple sclerosis. *Mult Scler* 2007;**13**(9):1200–2.

Mathieu D, Kondziolka D, Niranjan A, Flickinger J, Lunsford LD. Gamma knife thalamotomy for multiple sclerosis tremor. *Surg Neurol* 2007;**68**(4):394–9.

McDonald WI, Compston A, Edan G, et al. Recommended diagnostic criteria for multiple sclerosis: guidelines from the International Panel on the diagnosis of multiple sclerosis. *Ann Neurol* 2001;**50**(1):121–7.

McHugh JC, Galvin PL, Murphy RP. Retrospective comparison of the original and revised McDonald criteria in a general neurology practice in Ireland. *Mult Scler* 2008;**14**(1):81–5.

Moon JS, II Kim G, Koo YH, et al. Kinetic tremor and cerebellar ataxia as initial manifestations of Kikuchi-Fujimoto's disease. *J Neurol Sci* 2009;**277**(1–2):181–3.

Mumford CJ, Wood NW, Kellar-Wood H, et al. The British Isles survey of multiple sclerosis in twins. *Neurology* 1994;**44**(1):11–5.

Munteis E, Andreu M, Martinez-Rodriguez J, et al. Manometric correlations of anorectal dysfunction and biofeedback outcome in patients with multiple sclerosis. *Mult Scler* 2008;**14**(2):237–42.

Munteis E, Andreu M, Téllez MJ, et al. Anorectal dysfunction in multiple sclerosis. *Mult Scler* 2006;**12**(2):215–8.

Nakanishi K, Kobayashi T, Miyashita H, et al. Relationships among residual beta cells, exocrine pancreas, and islet cell antibodies in insulin-dependent diabetes mellitus. *Metabolism* 1993;**42**:196–203.

Nakasu S, Kaneko M, Matsuda M. Cerebral aneurysms associated with Behçet's disease: a case report. *J Neurol Neurosurg Psychiatry* 2001;**70**:682–4.

Norton HWD, Cogan DG. Syndrome of nonsyphilitic interstitial keratitis and vestibuloauditory symptoms: long-term follow-up. *Arch Ophtalmol* 1959;**61**: 695–7.

O'Duffy JD, Goldstein NP. Neurologic involvement in seven patients with Behçet's disease. *Am J Med* 1976;**61**:170–8.

Parikh T, Shifteh K, Lipton ML, Bello JA, Brook AL. Deep brain reversible encephalopathy: association with secondary antiphospholipid antibody syndrome. *Am J Neuroradiol* 2007;**28**:76–8.

Pereira AC, Edwards MJ, Buttery PC, et al. Choreic syndrome and coeliac disease: a hitherto unrecognised association. *Mov Disord* 2004;**19**:478–82.

Plaha P, Khan S, Gill SS. Bilateral stimulation of the caudal zona incerta nucleus for tremor control. *J Neurol Neurosurg Psychiatry* 2008;**79**(5):504–13.

Provenzale JM, Allen NB. Neuroradiologic findings in polyarteritis nodosa. *AJNR Am J Neuroradiol* 1996;**17**(6):1119–26.

Ramasamy DP, Benedict R, Cox JL, et al. Extent of cerebellum, subcortical and cortical atrophy in patients with MS A case-control study. *J Neurol Sci* 2009;**282**(1–2):47–54.

Rose JW, Burns JB, Bjorklund J, et al. Daclizumab phase II trial in relapsing and remitting multiple sclerosis: MRI and clinical results. *Neurology* 2007;**69**(8):785–9.

Rovira A, León A. MR in the diagnosis and monitoring of multiple sclerosis: an overview. *Eur J Radiol* 2008;**67**(3):409–14.

Saari A, Tolonen U, Pääkkö E, et al. Sympathetic skin responses in multiple sclerosis. *Acta Neurol Scand* 2008;**118**(4):226–31.

Saip S, Uluduz D, Erkol G. Fabry disease mimicking multiple sclerosis. *Clin Neurol Neurosurg* 2007;**109**(4):361–3.

Saiz A, Arpa J, Sagasta A, et al. Autoantibodies to glutamic acid decarboxylase in three patients with cerebellar ataxia, late-onset insulin-dependent diabetes mellitus and polyendocrine autoimmunity. *Neurology* 1997;**49**:1026–30.

Shimomura T, Kuno M, Takenaka T, Maeda M, Takahashi K. Purkinje cell antibody in lupus ataxia. *Lancet* 1993; **342**:375–376.

Tintoré M. New options for early treatment of multiple sclerosis. *J Neurol Sci* 2009;**277**(suppl 1):S9–11.

Tumani H. Corticosteroids and plasma exchange in multiple sclerosis. *J Neurol* 2008;**255**(Suppl 6):36–42.

Wilkinson ID, Hadjivassiliou M, Dickson JM, et al. Cerebellar abnormalities on proton MR spectroscopy in gluten ataxia. *J Neurol Neurosurg Psychiatry* 2005;**76**:1011–13.

Wingerchuk DM, Lennon VA, Pittock SJ, Lucchinetti CF, Weinshenker BG. Revised diagnostic criteria for neuromyelitis optica. *Neurology* 2006;**66**(10):1485–9.

Wolff SM, Schotland DL, Phillips LL. Involvement of nervous system in Behçet's syndrome. *Arch Neurol* 1965;**12**:315–25.

Ziemssen T. Multiple sclerosis beyond EDSS: depression and fatigue. *J Neurol Sci* 2009;**277**(suppl 1):S37–41.

Endocrine disorders

Thyroid disorders

The main cause of cerebellar ataxia of endocrine origin is a dysfunction of the thyroid gland. Thyroid hormones exert a trophic action during growth of the cerebellum and throughout the lifespan. They are involved in proliferation, migration, and maturation of cerebellar neurons and promote myelination as well as gliogenesis. They also interact with growth factors.

Both hypothyroidism and hyperthyroidism are associated with cerebellar ataxia. The stage of development of the cerebellum and the severity of the endocrine dysfunction are main factors for influencing cerebellar function. Ataxia predominates for trunk and limb movements. Patients may exhibit kinetic tremor, dysmetria, and dysdiadochokinesia. Oculomotor disturbances are usually subtle. The main deficit is saccadic pursuit. Speech is usually normal. Concomitant vestibular signs may render the clinical examination equivocal.

In all ataxic patients, thyrotropin hormone (TSH) and free T4 levels should be determined.

Hypothyroidism

The general signs and the neurological deficits associated with hypothyroidism are summarized in Table 10.1. Cerebellar ataxia is associated with extra-cerebellar signs in most cases. Cerebellar ataxia may be the first manifestation of hypothyroidism (Gilman et al., 1981). When present, the cerebellar signs commonly develop gradually over a period of several months. Patients report unsteadiness and gait difficulties (Harayama et al., 1983; Pinelli et al., 1990). This is due to the fact that the superior vermis is the cerebellar region that is most affected (Barnard et al., 1971). The slowness of muscle contractions as well as the involvement of peripheral nerves also contributes.

Levothyroxine is the principal treatment of hypothyroidism. The initial dose is usually about 50 μg/day. Doses are increased by steps of 25 μg/day according to basal levels of TSH. The goal is to reach both clinical and biological euthyroid status.

Cerebellar ataxia resulting from a congenital hypothyroidism carries a poor prognosis if the therapy is not initiated immediately after birth, leading to permanent sequelae. In adult-onset hypothyroidism, ataxia usually resolves with levothyroxine therapy. Regression of ataxia may be complete in a few weeks or months, although ataxia may not improve in some patients (Bonuccelli et al., 1991).

Hyperthyroidism

In hyperthyroidism, patients show combinations of general symptoms such as sweating and heat intolerance, restlessness, palpitations, and diarrhea. The thyroid may be enlarged, and endocrine ophthalmopathy is common. Patients show an enhanced physiological tremor, myopathic signs, seizures, choreoathetosis, pyramidal deficits, and psychiatric symptoms. Ataxia predominates on posture and gait and may have a recurrent course.

Hyperthyroidism is treated with the following methods: anti-thyroid drugs (propylthiouracil, methimazole), radioactive iodine therapy, and surgical thyroid ablation. Beta-blockers such as propranolol are often used in the management of hyperthyroidism, including for the management of tremor.

Hashimoto ataxia

About 30% of patients with Hashimoto ataxia have a history of other auto-immune disorders. Hashimoto thyroiditis is associated with two principal neurological presentations: encephalopathy and vasculitis-like syndrome (Kothbauer-Margreiter et al., 1996). The encephalopathy presents with dementia, seizures,

Table 10.1 General and neurological signs associated with hypothyroidism

	General signs	Neurological deficits
Congenital hypothyroidism	Deficient growth	Mental retardation
Endemic cretinism	Delayed skeletal maturation Constipation Skin mottling	Lethargy Deaf mutism Spastic diplegia Cerebellar ataxia
Adult-onset hypothyroidism	Dry/coarse skin Cold intolerance Decreased sweating Periorbital puffiness Constipation Bradycardia	Hearing deficit Dementia Depression Coma Myoclonus Myopathy Entrapment neuropathy Polyneuropathy Cerebellar ataxia

psychotic episodes, agitation, hallucinations, or altered consciousness ranging from drowsiness to coma. Symptoms may have a fluctuating course. Ataxic jerks occur in about 10% of cases, but gait ataxia affects up to two-thirds of patients (Castillo et al., 2006). Patients are usually middle-aged women who have often been misdiagnosed as presenting with a psychiatric disorder. The clinical picture can mimic a Creutzfeldt-Jakob disease (see Chapter 11), with a combination of dementia, myoclonus, and ataxia (Seipelt et al., 1999). Status epilepticus is a rare presentation (Aydin-Ozemir et al., 2006), but it should be kept in mind that seizure is a potential presentation in young children or adolescents (Hoffmann et al., 2007). The stroke-like presentation combines focal neurological deficits, including cerebellar deficits, and confusion. Ataxic signs are acute, subacute, or even recurrent if the disorder remains untreated. Thyroid sonography shows a hypoechoic thyroid (Seipelt et al., 1999). Blood studies show high titers of autoantibodies against thyroglobulin and thyroid peroxidase. One difficulty is that these antibodies can be detected in elevated titers in the healthy general population (Mocellin et al., 2007). Autoantibodies against the amino terminal of alpha-enolase are detected in about 70% of cases and might become a useful serological diagnostic marker for Hashimoto encephalopathy (Yoneda et al., 2007). In some patients, anti-TSH receptor antibodies are identified. Patients may be euthyroid at the time of neurological presentation. Increased erythro-

cyte sedimentation rate is not rare. Cerebrospinal fluid (CSF) studies are abnormal in 80% of cases, showing an increased leukocyte count and/or raised protein levels and increased CSF/serum concentration ratio of albumin. Oligoclonal bands may be present. Protein 14–3–3 is not detected. Electroencephalogram (EEG) recordings show a slowing of the background activity in half of cases and epileptic activity in about 15% of cases, but periodic sharp wave complexes (see Chapter 11) are usually absent. Brain CT shows hypodense areas in 30% of cases. Areas of increased signal are found on brain MRI in most cases. MRI signal abnormalities may have a diffuse subcortical pattern (Bohnen et al., 1997). Atrophy of gray matter may be detected also (Takahashi et al., 1994). Single-photon emission CT/positron emission tomography studies show decreased tracer uptake with a patchy pattern or a global hypoperfusion (Forchetti et al., 1997). MRI spectroscopy shows decreased levels of N-acetylaspartate and increased levels of the choline-containing compounds. Clinical deficits respond to immunosuppressive therapy. Steroid administration is the treatment of choice (hence the terminology of steroid-responsive encephalopathy associated with auto-immune thyroiditis [SREAT]). High-dose methylprednisolone (1 g/day for 5 days) is recommended in cases of encephalopathy (Shaw et al., 1991). Levothyroxine may be added. There is usually a good clinical response to steroids, especially in the encephalopathic presentation, provided the treatment is initiated early in the course of the disease. In some patients, addition of other drugs like azathioprine or methotrexate is required. Seizures respond to anticonvulsant drugs. Clonazepam is useful to decrease myoclonus. Steroid administration is often associated with a drop of antibody titers and normalization of the CSF results, the EEG, and MRI lesions (Bohnen et al., 1997). Doses of steroids are progressively reduced after the acute episode. Plasmapheresis (four exchanges with a volume of plasma exchanged per treatment of 1.5 times to twice the total plasma volume; Boers & Colebatch, 2001) and intravenous immunoglobulins can be considered in patients refractory to steroids (Mocellin et al., 2007). Thyroidectomy can be considered in rare cases of thyrotoxic Hashimoto encephalopathy with poorly controlled relapses (Yuceyar et al., 2007). Some authors add antipsychotics in case of psychotic-like symptoms. In patients in whom therapy has been delayed for years, neurological deficits may be irreversible.

Table 10.2 Parathyroid disorders associated with cerebellar ataxia

Disorder	General features	Neurological deficits	Cerebellar deficits
Hypoparathyroidism		Increased neuromuscular excitability Seizures Choreoathetosis Parkinsonism Dystonia Hemiballism Mental retardation	Bilateral cerebellar syndrome with dysarthria, dysmetria, dysdiadochokinesia, and ataxia of gait
Pseudohypoparathyroidism Pseudopseudohypoparathyroidism	Short stature Round face Short metacarpals Obesity Hypertension	Seizures Mental deterioration Extra-pyramidal deficits	Bilateral cerebellar syndrome
Hyperparathyroidism		Cognitive deficits Psychiatric symptoms Ophthalmoplegia Pyramidal signs Fasciculations Myopathy	Minor cerebellar deficits

Drug-induced dysfunction of the thyroid gland

Amiodarone and lithium salts can generate a genuine cerebellar syndrome (see Chapter 15).

Parathyroid disorders

Parathyroid hormone plays a key role in the regulation of calcemia. The parathyroid disorders associated with cerebellar ataxia are given in Table 10.2.

Hypoparathyroidism is idiopathic or acquired (resection of glands during thyroidectomy for cancer, multinodular goiter, or Graves disease; complication of thalassemia major due to iron overload). Hypoparathyroidism may also be part of a spectrum of multiple endocrine deficits, such as auto-immune polyglandular syndrome type 1 (Berger et al., 2008). Patients usually exhibit signs of increased neuromuscular excitability due to hypocalcemia: tetany, paresthesias, cramps, and muscle spasms, with Chvostek and Trousseau signs. Patients exhibit a pancerebellar syndrome (Ertaş et al., 1997). Laboratory findings show hypocalcemia and hyperphosphatemia, with decreased levels of parathyroid hormone. In chronic hypoparathyroidism, deposits of calcium are commonly observed in the dentate nuclei, cerebellar white matter, and granular layer of the cerebellum. However, despite these deposits, cerebellar syndrome may be reversible with calcium administration. Calcium

deposits also occur in the so-called Fahr syndrome involving the cerebellum, thalami, lentiform nuclei, and white matter of cerebral lobes. Bilateral calcifications in the globus pallidus are common after the age of 55 years and may be an incidental finding. The correlation between deposits of calcium in the cerebellum and ataxia is poor. Treatment of hypoparathyroidism includes supplements of calcium and vitamin D.

Pseudohypoparathyroidism (PHP) is a genetic disorder characterized by a resistance to the parathyroid hormone. Patients have low serum calcium and high phosphate levels, but the parathyroid hormone level is high. Some of these patients have a phenotype of Albright hereditary osteodystrophy in absence of disorders of calcium metabolism (pseudopseudohypoparathyroidism [pseudo PHP]). Patients show massive, symmetrical calcifications located in the basal ganglia, dentate nuclei, and cerebral sulci (Nyland & Skre, 1977; Araki et al., 1990). The mutations in the gene (GNAS1) encoding the alpha subunit of the stimulatory G protein (this signaling protein is essential for the actions of parathormone) cause at least three different forms of the disease: PHP type 1A, PHP type 1B, and pseudo-PHP (Bastepe, 2008)

Hyperparathyroidism may be primary (adenoma), secondary to hypocalcemia (malabsorption, pancreatic failure, vitamin D deficiency), or tertiary (renal failure). Hyperparathyroidism may be associated with cerebellar hemangioblastomas (see Chapter 13)

Table 10.3 Differential diagnosis of cerebellar ataxia associated with diabetes mellitus

Friedreich ataxia (see Chapter 20)

Mitochondrial disorders (see Chapter 21)

Anti–glutamic acid decarboxylase antibodies (see Chapter 9)

Auto-immune polyendocrine syndromes (see Chapter 9)

Aceruloplasminemia (see Chapter 20)

Hemochromatosis

Cytomegalovirus infection

Von Hippel-Lindau disease (see Chapter 13)

Langerhans histiocytosis (see Chapter 13)

Wolfram disease (see Chapter 20)

Cerebellar and pancreatic agenesis (neonatal diabetes mellitus with cerebellar hypoplasia/agenesis and dysmorphism: see also Chapter 1)

Table 10.4 Disorders combining cerebellar ataxia and diabetes insipidus

Langerhans histiocytosis (see Chapter 13)

Erdheim-Chester disease (see Chapter 13)

Wolfram disease (see Chapter 20)

De Morsier syndrome (septo-optic dysplasia)

(Gaymard et al., 1989). Residual sequelae are often observed following removal of a parathyroid adenoma or hyperplastic parathyroid glands (Patten & Pages, 1984).

Cerebellar ataxia and diabetes

Cerebellar patients may present with diabetes mellitus or diabetes insipidus. The differential diagnosis of the disorders combining cerebellar ataxia and diabetes mellitus or insipidus is shown in Tables 10.3 and 10.4, respectively. In addition to primary cerebellar damage, it should be kept in mind that both hyperglycemia (a risk factor for stroke) and hypoglycemia may be associated with cerebellar deficits. Although the cerebellum is relatively protected from hypoglycemia due to differences in glucose metabolism, a cerebellar syndrome may develop following a severe hypoglycemia, such as after an overdose of insulin (Berz & Orlander, 2008). Cerebellar deficits are usually reversible. The delay for recovery ranges from a few hours to several days.

Cerebellar ataxia and hypogonadism

Holmes ataxia and Boucher-Neuhauser syndrome are discussed in Chapter 20. Septo-optic dysplasia (De Morsier syndrome) is characterized by unilateral or bilateral hypoplasia of the optic nerve (Willnow et al., 1996). Patients may exhibit diabetes insipidus centralis or hypothyroidism. Brain MRI shows a cavum septum pellucidum, aplasia of the corpus callosum, aplasia of the fornix, and cerebellar hypoplasia. An empty sella with or without an ectopic pituitary has been reported in some cases. Differential diagnosis includes Kallmann syndrome, which combines hypogonadotropic hypogonadism and anosmia. Hypogonadism is due to gonadotropin-releasing hormone deficiency. Anosmia is related to the absence or hypoplasia of the olfactory bulbs and tracts. The disorder is genetically heterogeneous and can be transmitted in an autosomal dominant form, as an autosomal recessive trait, or in an X chromosome–linked form. It has been shown recently that anosmin-1, the protein defective in the X-linked form of Kallmann syndrome, stimulates outgrowth and branching of developing Purkinje axons (Gianola et al., 2009). Hypogonadism occurs also in carbohydrate-deficient glycoprotein syndrome (see Chapter 7). The so-called 4H syndrome is characterized by progressive encephalopathy, cerebellar ataxia, central hypomyelination, hypodontia, and hypogonadotropic hypogonadism (Timmons et al., 2006). Electron microscopy and myelin protein immunohistochemistry of sural nerves show granular debris–lined clefts, expanded abaxonal space, outpocketing with vacuolar disruption, and loss of normal myelin periodicity. Decreased levels of galactocerebroside, sphingomyelin, and GM1-N-acetylglucosamine and increased levels of esterified cholesterol are found. Brain MRI shows diffuse hypomyelination, which is confirmed with diffusion and spectroscopy studies.

References

Araki Y, Furukawa T, Tsuda K, Yamamoto T, Tsukaguchi I. High field MR imaging of the brain in pseudohypoparathyroidism. *Neuroradiology* 1990;**32**(4):325–7.

Aydin-Ozemir Z, Tüzün E, Baykan B, et al. Autoimmune thyroid encephalopathy presenting with epilepsia partialis continua. *Clin EEG Neurosci* 2006;**37**(3): 204–9.

Barnard RO, Campbell MJ, McDonald WI. Pathological findings in a case of hypothyroidism with ataxia.

J Neurol Neurosurg Psychiatry 1971;**34**(6): 755–60.

Bastepe M. The GNAS locus and pseudohypoparathyroidism. *Adv Exp Med Biol* 2008;**626**:27–40.

Berger JR, Weaver A, Greenlee J. Neurologic consequences of autoimmune polyglandular syndrome type 1. *Neurology* 2008;**70**(23):2248–51.

Berz JP, Orlander JD. Prolonged cerebellar ataxia: an unusual complication of hypoglycemia. *J Gen Intern Med* 2008;**23**(1):103–5.

Boers PM, Colebatch JG. Hashimoto's encephalopathy responding to plasmapheresis. *J Neurol Neurosurg Psychiatry* 2001;**70**(1):132.

Bohnen NI, Parnell KJ, Harper CM. Reversible MRI findings in a patient with Hashimoto's encephalopathy. *Neurology* 1997;**49**(1):246–7.

Bonuccelli U, Nuti A, Monzani F, De Negri F, Muratorio A. Familial occurrence of hypothyroidism and cerebellar ataxia. *Funct Neurol* 1991;**6**(2):171–5.

Castillo P, Woodruff B, Caselli R, et al. Steroid-responsive encephalopathy associated with autoimmune thyroiditis. *Arch Neurol* 2006;**63**(2):197–202.

Ertaş NK, Hanoğlu L, Kirbaş D, Hatemi H. Cerebellar syndrome due to hypoparathyroidism. *J Neurol* 1997;**244**(5):338–9.

Forchetti CM, Katsamakis G, Garron DC. Autoimmune thyroiditis and a rapidly progressive dementia: global hypoperfusion on SPECT scanning suggests a possible mechanism. *Neurology* 1997;**49**(2):623–6.

Gaymard B, Jan M, Gouaze A, et al. Cerebellar hemangioblastoma and primary hyperparathyroidism. *Surg Neurol* 1989;**31**(5):369–75.

Gianola S, de Castro F, Rossi F. Anosmin-1 stimulates outgrowth and branching of developing Purkinje axons. *Neuroscience* 2009;**158**(2):570–84.

Gilman S, Bloedel JR, Lechtenberg R. *Disorders of the Cerebellum*: *Contemporary Neurology Series*. Philadelphia: FA Davis, 1981.

Harayama H, Ohno T, Miyatake T. Quantitative analysis of stance in ataxic myxoedema. *J Neurol Neurosurg Psychiatry* 1983;**46**(6):579–81.

Hoffmann F, Reiter K, Kluger G, et al. Seizures, psychosis and coma: severe course of Hashimoto encephalopathy in a six-year-old girl. *Neuropediatrics* 2007;**38**(4):197–9.

Kothbauer-Margreiter I, Sturzenegger M, Komor J, Baumgartner R, Hess CW. Encephalopathy associated with Hashimoto thyroiditis: diagnosis and treatment. *J Neurol* 1996;**243**(8):585–93.

Mocellin R, Walterfang M, Velakoulis D. Hashimoto's encephalopathy: epidemiology, pathogenesis and management. *CNS Drugs* 2007;**21**(10):799–811.

Nyland H, Skre H. Cerebral calcinosis with late onset encephalopathy. Unusual type of pseudo-pseudohypoparathyreoidism. *Acta Neurol Scand* 1977;**56**(4):309–25.

Patten BM, Pages M. Severe neurological disease associated with hyperparathyroidism. *Ann Neurol* 1984;**15**(5):453–6.

Pinelli P, Pisano F, Miscio G. Ataxia in myxoedema: a neurophysiological reassessment. *J Neurol* 1990;**237**(7):405–9.

Seipelt M, Zerr I, Nau R, et al. Hashimoto's encephalitis as a differential diagnosis of Creutzfeldt-Jakob disease. *J Neurol Neurosurg Psychiatry* 1999;**66**(2):172–6.

Shaw PJ, Walls TJ, Newman PK, Cleland PG, Cartlidge NE. Hashimoto's encephalopathy: a steroid-responsive disorder associated with high anti-thyroid antibody titers—report of 5 cases. *Neurology* 1991;**41**(2 Pt 1): 228–33.

Takahashi S, Mitamura R, Itoh Y, Suzuki N, Okuno A. Hashimoto encephalopathy: etiologic considerations. *Pediatr Neurol* 1994;**11**(4):328–31.

Timmons M, Tsokos M, Asab MA, et al. Peripheral and central hypomyelination with hypogonadotropic hypogonadism and hypodontia. *Neurology* 2006;**67**(11):2066–9.

Willnow S, Kiess W, Butenandt O, et al. Endocrine disorders in septo-optic dysplasia (De Morsier syndrome): evaluation and follow up of 18 patients. *Eur J Pediatr* 1996;**155**(3):179–84.

Yoneda M, Fujii A, Ito A, et al. High prevalence of serum autoantibodies against the amino terminal of alpha-enolase in Hashimoto's encephalopathy. *J Neuroimmunol* 2007;**185**(1–2):195–200.

Yuceyar N, Karadeniz M, Erdogan M, et al. Thyrotoxic autoimmune encephalopathy in a female patient: only partial response to typical immunosuppressant treatment and remission after thyroidectomy. *Clin Neurol Neurosurg* 2007;**109**(5):458–62.

Infectious diseases

Bacterial infections

Most of the abscesses in the brain occur in the supratentorial areas. Nevertheless, the cerebellum may be the site of a bacterial infection, in particular following an otogenic infection (Brydon & Hardwidge, 1994; Kurien et al., 1998). About 8% to 18% of purulent brain abscesses are located in the cerebellum (Beller et al., 1973; Gilman et al., 1981). The incidence of cerebellar abscesses is higher between the ages of 3 and 8 years, and between 18 and 40 years.

Cerebellar abscesses require a particular attention, due to the risk of brainstem compression, tonsillar herniation, and obstructive hydrocephalus. The clinical presentation is acute in most patients and depends on the location, the size, and the number of infectious lesions. Patients usually complain of headache and develop cerebellar signs very rapidly. Fundus examination may reveal papilledema due to raised intra-cranial pressure.

The causes are summarized in Table 11.1. Otogenic infection may disseminate to the cerebellum by direct extension from the temporal bone or by retrograde thrombosis from the lateral inferior petrosal or superior petrosal sinuses (Nager, 1967). Petrous apex osteitis or labyrinthitis is usually associated with medial and deep cerebellar infections (Shaw & Russell, 1975). Infection located in the sinodural angle or thrombophlebitis of the lateral sinus tends to disseminate laterally or superficially. The proportion of abscesses located in the hemispheres is higher as compared with midline infections (Carey et al., 1972; Shaw & Russell, 1975). Culture of CSF specimen is positive in up to 50% of cases. Blood studies commonly reveal a leukocytosis, usually in the range of 11 000 to 25 000 white blood cells/mL, and increased erythrocyte sedimentation rate.

Neuroimaging

The role of imaging techniques is crucial for the diagnosis and follow-up of cerebellar abscesses.

Brain CT scan is often the first technique available. The degree and pattern of contrast enhancement help to differentiate a cerebellar abscess from another pathology. At an early stage (days 1–3 of abscess formation, called early cerebritis), a low-density nonenhancing lesion is observed. Contrast enhancement changes from mild peripheral enhancement to thick, taking a ring appearance. The late cerebritis is characterized by a hypodense necrotic core, with a surrounding capsule usually taking the contrast intensely. Enhancement can diffuse from the periphery towards the central area, making the radiological lesion more homogeneous. With time, the necrotic center becomes decreased in size while the capsule becomes thicker. After 2 weeks and up to several months later, the capsule still enhances, but there is only a minimal contrast diffusion into the core, if any (Dobkin et al., 1984). Peripheral edema around the abscess is observed early in the course of abscess formation. Steroids may decrease contrast enhancement at the cerebritis stage (Enzmann et al., 1982). Differential diagnosis of a ring-like enhancing lesion on CT scan includes high-grade gliomas and metastases, infarction, resolving hematoma, granulomas, and radiation necrosis (Osborn, 1994).

MRI detects very small lesions (which may be overlooked by CT scan) and allows a detailed anatomical description. Its superiority to CT scan makes MRI the technique of choice when a cerebellar abscess is suspected. Peripheral edema appears mildly hypointense in T1-weighted images and hyperintense in T2-weighted images. The core is usually rich in proteins and appears hyperintense as compared with

Table 11.1 Causes of cerebellar abscesses

Otogenic infection

Cyanotic heart disease

Congenital dermal sinus

Tuberculosis

Traumatic injury

Post-operative complication

Septic emboli

CSF but is usually hypointense relative to white matter (T1-weighted sequences). In T2-weighted sequences, the necrotic core is usually isointense or hyperintense as compared with CSF and gray matter. The capsule may enhance with gadolinium. It is isointense or hyperintense to white matter in T1-weighted sequences and usually hypointense to gray matter in T2-weighted sequences (Sze & Zimmerman, 1988).

Magnetic resonance spectroscopy (MRS) is a good complement to MRI. MRS can detect metabolites normally not found in other disorders. Peaks of aspartate, amino acids (due to proteolysis), lactate (resulting from bacterial anaerobic activity), pyruvate, and lipids are found. Gliomas display increased peaks of choline and smaller peaks of N-acetyl-aspartate, creatine, lactate, and lipids and usually near absence of amino acids or acetate (Dev et al., 1998).

Single-photon emission CT (SPECT) and positron emission tomography studies may provide additional information. Leukocyte scintigraphy may detect inflammatory foci in the brain, but may be inaccurate in the presence of steroids (Belloti et al., 1986). False positives occur with brain tumors.

Treatment of cerebellar abscesses

Due to the small volume of posterior fossa, mass effect and obstructive hydrocephalus may develop rapidly. Therefore, surgical management may be required. Antibiotics and steroids are usually in the front line. Antibiotics should be started immediately. Whenever possible, a culture should be performed before the initiation of drug administration. Broad-spectrum antibiotics are selected initially in an empirical mode, and the drugs and doses are adapted when the micro-organism is identified. Selection of antibiotics takes into account the blood–brain barrier. Lipophilic and non–protein-bound antibiotics penetrate the brain.

Antibiotics may resolve the abscess if lesions are small, especially at an early stage of abscess prior to capsule formation. The earlier the diagnosis, the greater is the chance for antibiotics to resolve the abscess (Heineman et al., 1971). Many abscesses of a diameter <2.5 cm can be completely resolved with antibiotics (Dyste et al., 1988). Steroids are used in abscesses producing mass effect and significant perilesional edema.

If the medical treatment does not resolve the abscess or in cases of large infectious lesions (diameter >2.5 cm), surgery may be indicated. When brain imaging is not informative or in immunocompromised patients, surgical treatment should be discussed (Osenbach & Loftus, 1992). Surgery may consist of aspiration and drainage, or full resection. The risk of obstructive hydrocephalus may justify an externalized ventricular drain. Aspiration by a burr hole is less invasive, provides a rapid decompressing effect, reduces mass effect, and allows the identification of the germ(s), thus enabling one to adapt the antibiotics. This technique is recommended in patients in whom a general anesthesia is contraindicated or in those presenting with multiple lesions (Shahzadi et al., 1996). The reduction in the size of the abscess may also increase the efficacy of drugs (Black et al., 1973). Aspiration may be performed under CT guidance. Transmastoid drainage is possible (Coin et al., 1983). A stereotactic approach may be particularly useful for deep lesions. Some authors recommend the endoscopic approach, which allows a direct visualization of the cavity (Fritsch & Manwaring, 1997). The resection of the abscess has the advantage to decrease drastically the mass effect, to provide a large specimen for culture or histological study, and to remove fragments following a trauma. These fragments may be the source of an abscess after a penetrating injury (Rish et al., 1981). Fungal abscesses and multiloculated infections may require excision. Subtotal excision may be performed when the cyst capsule adheres firmly to vital structures, as observed in abscesses associated with posterior fossa dermoid cysts (Manto, 2002). The most common primary sites of infection are the gastrointestinal tract and the respiratory airways (Klockgether et al., 1993). Cerebellitis may also start after a skin rash or a vaccination. Usually, the deficits occur in children aged 1 to 6 years and in young adults. Nevertheless, cerebellitis may also develop in the elderly. Males are more affected. The male-to-female ratio varies from 2:1 to 4.3:1.

Cerebellitis

Clinical presentation

Fever may be absent at the time of neurological deficits, with body temperature being considered an unreliable clinical sign (Clearly et al., 1980). Headache is common. The clinical presentation is characterized by an acute or subacute cerebellar syndrome developing in the hours, days, or weeks (usually up to 5 weeks) following the infection. A history of orchitis or parotitis may point to mumps, myalgia and myocarditis suggest a coxsackie infection, and rash may occur in enterovirus infection. History of insect bite should prompt a search for tick-borne diseases, in particular Lyme disease and rickettsial infection. Cerebellar ataxia is either isolated or part of a diffuse inflammation of the CNS (Table 11.2). Children usually present with a combination of abrupt-onset limb clumsiness, gait difficulties, and muscle hypotonia. A majority of patients exhibit oculomotor disturbances (impaired smooth pursuit, dysmetria, impaired suppression of the VOR, nystagmus, opsoclonus). Patients with brainstem signs usually exhibit cranial nerve palsies (especially nerves VI and VII), sensory deficits (bilateral or unilateral), pyramidal signs, and increased muscle tone sometimes localized to the neck muscles (Alfaro, 1993; Yuki et al., 1997; Aylett et al., 1998). Vertigo may be particularly intense, often associated with vomiting. Rarely, mutism followed by dysarthria is observed in patients with swelling of the cerebellum (Papavasiliou et al., 2004). Opsoclonus may be an early sign of neonatal herpes simplex cerebellitis (Krolczyk et al., 2003). Cerebellar signs may be accompanied by seizures, headaches, and drowsiness in cases of generalized meningoencephalitis or acute diffuse encephalomyelitis (ADEM). Ataxia combined with ophthalmoplegia and tendon areflexia suggests a Miller Fisher syndrome. There may be an overlap between a predominant brainstem syndrome

Table 11.2 Clinical presentation of cerebellitis

Pure cerebellar syndrome bilateral or with unilateral predominance ("hemicerebellitis")

"Cerebellar plus"
- Miller Fisher syndrome
- Bickerstaff brainstem encephalitis
- Opsoclonus-myoclonus (Kinsbourne syndrome)
- Acute hydrocephalus due to edema
- Dystonia-rigidity of neck and limbs
- Spinocerebellar syndrome
- Part of diffuse encephalitis

(Bickerstaff encephalitis), cerebellitis, and Guillain-Barré syndrome. Acute hemorrhagic leukoencephalitis (Hurst disease) may involve predominantly the brainstem and the cerebellum (Hofer et al., 2005). It usually evolves following an unspecific respiratory infection. Progressive neurological deficits predominate, leading to reduced consciousness and coma. Human T-lymphotropic virus types I and II, usually associated with tropical spastic paraparesis, may cause a spinocerebellar syndrome characterized by a combination of cerebellar deficits (dysarthria, nystagmus, dysmetria, ataxic gait) and signs due to spinal cord involvement (spastic paraparesis, bladder and sphincter disturbances) (Castillo et al., 2000). Spastic paraparesis may develop several years after the onset of cerebellar symptoms.

Infectious agents

Table 11.3 lists the infectious diseases and the vaccinations associated with cerebellitis. Varicella, measles, mumps, and rubella are the most common in children. About 0.05% to 0.10% of children with varicella infection present with cerebellar ataxia. In adults, cerebellar ataxia is common in enteric fever, with an incidence of 2.3% (Wadia et al., 1985). Ataxia usually develops in the second week. Even with the use of polymerase chain reaction (PCR) or the search for antigens, the causative agent remains unknown in one-third of the cases.

Pathogenesis

Different factors contribute to cerebellar ataxia. Cerebellitis following a viral infection is related to a direct viral replication and post-infectious demyelination. Viruses penetrate the CNS via the bloodstream or via the peripheral nerves. Immuno-allergic reactions participate in the pathogenesis of demyelination (Johnson et al., 1985). The latent interval of several days to weeks is reminiscent of a delayed antigen-antibody reaction. The possibility of molecular mimicry between antigens of infectious agents and epitopes in the cerebellum is raised. Familial association; favorable response to steroids in some patients; increased levels of tumor necrosis factor alpha, interleukin (IL) 6, and IL-2 in blood and CSF; and serum antibodies to gangliosides (mainly GM1, GM2, and GT1b) argue in favor of an immunological mechanism (Woody et al., 1989; de Silva et al., 1992; Komatsu et al.,

120

Table 11.3 Infections and vaccinations associated with cerebelitis

Infections in children	Vaccinations	Infectious agents in adults
Varicella	Diphteria-tetanus-poliomyelitis	Epstein-Barr virus
Measles	Mumps-measles-rubella	Influenza
Mumps	Varicella	Parainfluenza
Rubella	Influenza	Enterovirus (poliovirus, coxsackie,
Infectious mononucleosis	Hepatitis B	echovirus)
Enterovirus (poliovirus, coxsackie, echovirus)		Herpes simplex virus
Whooping cough		Varicella zoster virus
Legionellosis		Cytomegalovirus
Parvovirus B19 infection		Adenovirus
Hepatitis A		HIV-1
Q fever		Human T-lymphotropic virus types I
Rotavirus gastroenteritis		and II
		Borrelia burgdorferi
		Rickettsia
		Mumps virus
		Mycoplasma pneumoniae
		Legionella pneumophila
		Salmonella typhi
		Plasmodium falciparum

1998). Autoantibodies to triosephosphate isomerase have been discovered recently in patients with a preceding Epstein-Barr virus (EBV) infection (Uchibori et al., 2005). Autoantibodies against glutamate receptor delta 2 (predominantly expressed in the cerebellum) have been reported also (Shimokaze et al., 2007). Cerebellitis associated with whooping cough might be triggered by an exogenous toxin. *Bordetella pertussis* liberates an exotoxin called lymphocytosis-promoting factor (LPF; a membrane-associated protein). The cerebellum might be one of the most vulnerable regions in the brain to this exotoxin (Askelöf & Bartfai, 1979). LPF increases cellular levels of $3',5'$ cyclic guanosine monophosphate, a second messenger involved in cerebellar neurotransmission. Another possible mechanism of cerebellitis is a direct toxicity of the virus to cellular populations, as suggested in cerebellar degeneration associated with HIV infection (Tagliati et al., 1998). In this case, atrophy of the cerebellum is greatest in the posterior cerebellar vermis and is not correlated with CD4+ T-cell counts or viral load (Klunder et al., 2008). Hurst disease is characterized at pathological examination by perivascular hemorrhages, vessel wall necrosis, and extensive necrotic areas. The possible role of EBV in its pathogenesis has been recently underlined (Hofer et al., 2005).

Lymphocytic choriomeningitis virus (LCMV) is a prevalent human pathogen causing substantial neurological disorders (Peters, 2006). Mechanisms of neurological deficits are directly related to infection and due to a consecutive cascade of neuro-

teratogenic events. Rodents are the reservoir, especially the common house mouse. Children and adults acquire LCMV infection by contact with contaminated fomites, by inhalation, or via transplantation (Fischer et al., 2006). Classic signs of post-natal infection are those of an aseptic meningitis, with full recovery within 4 weeks. By contrast, pre-natal infection can cause severe and permanent disease for the fetus. Children with congenital LCMV infection develop chorioretinitis and variable structural brain deficits including microencephaly, periventricular calcifications, ventriculomegaly, pachygyria, cerebellar hypoplasia, cysts, and hydrocephalus (Bonthius et al., 2007). Epilepsy and cerebral palsy are common. All these children will have permanent neurological deficits. Those with isolated cerebellar hypoplasia present with jitteriness and are ataxic at follow-up, with only mild mental deficits and relatively less affected vision.

Tick-borne diseases can induce a severe meningoencephalitis, with meningeal lymphoid infiltrates, widespread loss of Purkinje neurons, and marked Bergmann gliosis in the cerebellum (Tavakoli et al., 2009).

Investigations

Blood studies

Serology may point to the diagnosis. Miller Fisher syndrome is associated with anti-GQ1b antibodies. The anti-GQ1b immunoglobulin G (IgG) antibody titer

121

may also be increased in Guillain-Barré syndrome and Bickerstaff encephalitis, two disorders which might be closely related or part of a continuous spectrum (Lo, 2007). Anti-GQ1b antibodies have also been associated with ocular flutter, generalized myoclonus, and trunk ataxia (Zaro-Weber et al., 2008). Anti-GD1b antibodies may be associated with the ataxic variant of Guillain-Barré syndrome in the absence of ophthalmoplegia or severe loss of proprioceptive sense (Yuki et al., 2000). These antibodies bind to the cerebellar granular layer or spinocerebellar Ia fibers (Sugimoto et al., 2002). Anti-GM1b and GalNAc-GD1a have been reported in Bickerstaff encephalitis following *Campylobacter jejuni* enteritis (Matsuo et al., 2004).

CSF studies

Opening pressure is either normal or slightly increased. In the majority of cases, a pleocytosis is found. White blood cells are increased up to $250/\mu L$, with a predominance of lymphocytes from 60% to 99%. Protein levels are increased up to 300 mg/dL. The CSF IgG/albumin ratio is increased in 60% of cases. Oligoclonal bands are relatively rare in pure cerebellitis. Glucose level is normal in most cases, but may be found to be reduced. Culture of virus may be positive. PCR of virus DNA is very useful. Demonstration of a viral infection can be made very early (Dangond et al., 1993), allowing early diagnosis and treatment and preventing unnecessary investigations.

Clinical neurophysiology

Non-specific slowing in the EEG records and abnormal evoked potentials (somatosensory evoked potentials, visual evoked potentials, brainstem auditory evoked potentials) are found in patients with extracerebellar lesions.

MRI

MRI is clearly superior to brain CT scan. MRI shows inflammatory lesions in the white matter of the cerebellar hemispheres and diffuse lesions in the cerebellar cortex and may reveal round-shaped lesions in the cerebellar peduncles (Hayakawa & Katoh, 1995). Lesions may be asymmetrical and may predominate on one side. Swelling of the cerebellum occurs in 10% to 15% of cases, with possible obstructive hydrocephalus and tonsillar herniation into the foramen magnum (Sawaishi et al., 1999). Variable degrees of enhancement occur with gadolinium administration. Cerebellar involvement may appear on one side in hemicere-

bellitis, with a pseudotumoral presentation (Amador et al., 2007). A pattern of predominantly pial contrast enhancement, absence of a well-defined mass, and decline of the abnormalities in follow-up examinations help to exclude a malignancy (de Mendonca et al., 2005). Hemicerebellitis may have a recurrent course with a mirror pattern of involvement of the contralateral cerebellar hemisphere (Oguz et al., 2008). MRI lesions may either persist or disappear with time. In some patients, an irreversible cerebellar atrophy may be demonstrated in the months following the acute episode.

MRS

In the acute phase, low N-acetylaspartate-to-creatine and N-acetylaspartate-to-choline ratios can be detected (Guerrini et al, 2002). These changes can be reversible.

SPECT

Technetium-99m (^{99m}Tc) hexamethylpropyleneamine oxime shows a decreased regional perfusion in the cerebellum. Iodine-123 N-isopropyl-p-iodoamphetamine SPECT may be superior to MRI (Figure 11.1; Nagamitsu et al., 1999).

Ultrasound

Cranial ultrasound in the neonatal period may reveal a small cerebellum in children with congenital cytomegalovirus infection (de Vries et al., 2004). Other concomitant findings are periventricular calcifications, lenticulostriate vasculopathy, ventricular dilatation, cysts, polymicrogyria, and foci of dysplasia.

Differential diagnosis

ADEM is a differential diagnosis of demyelinating diseases of the CNS, especially MS. ADEM is characterized by a monophasic course. Although lesions have similar features, MS is a progressive disease with a relapsing-remitting or progressive course.

Table 11.4 shows the disorders mimicking cerebellitis, and Table 11.5 lists the causes of opsoclonus-myoclonus (Kinsbourne syndrome). Metabolic encephalopathies and paraneoplastic disorders are the main differential diagnoses of para-infectious opsoclonus-myoclonus. In patients with AIDS, prevalent brainstem and cerebellar signs may be found in cytomegalovirus encephalitis, which should be distinguished from *Listeria monocytogenes*

Figure 11.1 Post-infectious cerebellitis. (A,B) T1- and T2-weighted images show no abnormality. (C) By contrast, ^{123}I-SPECT demonstrates a decreased regional cerebral blood flow (rCBF) in the cerebellum. (D) SPECT in a control subject. From: Nagamitsu et al., 1999. With permission. (See color section.)

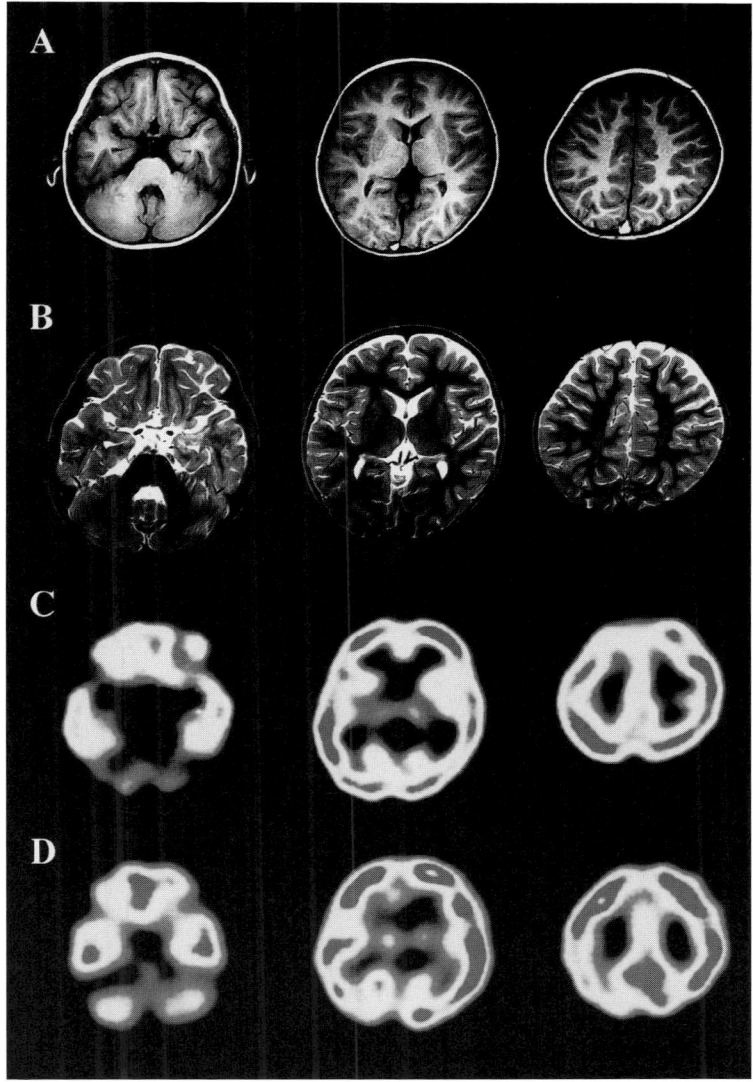

rhombencephalitis (Pierelli et al., 1997), a potentially serious illness, especially in pregnant women, neonates, the elderly, and immunocompromised patients. A vacuolar cerebellar leukoencephalopathy as a complication of AIDS has been reported (Aboulafia & Taylor, 2002).

Cerebellitis can mimic a tumor on brain imaging (pseudo-tumoral presentation). The lesion may be unilateral (Amador et al., 2007). Predominant pial contrast enhancement, absence of a well-defined mass, and regression of the lesion in follow-up argue for cerebellitis (de Mendonca et al., 2005).

Progressive multifocal leukoencephalopathy (PML) is a demyelinating infectious disease due to a neurotrophic papovavirus (John Cunningham [JC] virus). PML affects patients with impaired cell-mediated immune status (Brooks & Walker, 1984). Its incidence has markedly increased with AIDS pandemia. The JC virus has a particular tropism for oligodendroglia, the myelin-producing cells. Cerebellar signs occur in about 13% of patients (Morriss et al., 1997). CSF studies show pleocytosis in up to 20% of cases and increased protein levels in up to 30% of patients (Tornatore et al., 1994). Detection

Table 11.4 Differential diagnosis of cerebellitis

Labyrinthitis

Migraine

Post-infectious or inflammatory acute sensory neuropathy

Accidental exposure to toxins/drugs

Opsoclonus-myoclonus

Tumor

Heat stroke

Table 11.5 Causes of opsoclonus-myoclonus

Post-infectious	Epstein-Barr virus, enterovirus, herpes zoster, herpes simplex type 2, lymphocytic choriomeningitis, mumps, rubella
Metabolic encephalopathies	
Paraneoplastic	Neuroblastoma, leukemia, Hodgkin disease, lung cancer, breast or gynecologic cancer, renal cancer
Cranial trauma	
Hydrocephalus	
Thalamic hemorrhage	
Brainstem lesion	
Toxins	Herbal medicine, cocaine, chlordecone
Progressive encephalopathy with rigidity	
Sarcoidosis	
Idiopathic	

of viral DNA confirms the diagnosis in up to 70% of cases (Gibson et al., 1993). Brain CT may disclose a low-density lesion in the white matter, in the absence of a mass effect. Middle cerebellar peduncles and the adjacent white matter are particularly involved. MRI shows asymmetrical or symmetrical white matter lesions appearing hypointense in T1-weighted sequence and hypersignal in T2-weighted images. Lesions are usually not enhanced by gadolinium – unlike in lymphoma and abscess – although enhancement occurs in atypical cases (Rosas et al., 1999). MRS demonstrates low levels of N-acetylaspartate and increased levels of choline, lipids, and lactate (Chang et al., 1997). Another syndrome, called JC virus granule cell neuronopathy, has been described recently in association with the JC virus (Koralnik et al., 2005). The infection is restricted to the granule cells, with preservation of Purkinje neurons and absence of white matter lesions suggestive of PML. Several drugs aiming to inhibit virus replication have been suggested for the treatment, with variable responses (Brink & Miller, 1996; Brambilla et al., 1999).

Cerebellar ataxia is also encountered in Whipple disease. This infectious disease is due to an intracellular Gram-positive actinomycete called *Tropheryma whippelii* (Relman et al., 1992). Whipple disease causes four groups of symptoms: gastrointestinal, articular, cardiac, and neurologic (Verhagen et al., 1996). There is often a context of diarrhea and weight loss. Oculomasticatory myorhythmia, characterized by a convergence nystagmus associated with mandibular/tongue/neck involuntary movements taking a bruxism-like or dystonic aspect, are pathognomonic (Tison et al., 1992). Their frequency is usually between 2 and 4 Hz. Patients may develop a cerebellar syndrome that includes scanning speech and limb and truncal ataxia leading to frequent falls. Duodenal or jejunal biopsy may demonstrate periodic acid-

Schiff–positive foamy macrophages in the lamina propria. Similar macrophages may be found in the CSF, in which an increased protein level and elevated cell count are common. PCR (on intestinal tissues, CSF fluid, vitreous specimen, or brain tissue when a biopsy has been performed) discloses a portion of 16S ribosomal RNA gene sequence specific for Whipple disease (Relman et al., 1992). Its sensitivity and specificity are high. Brain MRI shows hypointense areas in T1-weighted sequence and hyperintense lesions on T2-weighted images. Lesions are usually enhanced by gadolinium. Enhancement may be restricted to ependymal zones. Penicillin G, streptomycin, and co-trimoxazole are recommended (Singer, 1998).

Progressive ataxia in patients with a history of chronic liver disease following hepatitis B infection should raise the possibility of acquired hepatocerebral degeneration (Park & Heo, 2004). Cerebellar symptoms may be prominent.

Treatment of cerebellitis

Antibiotics and steroids are the main treatments. Intravenous acyclovir 10 mg/kg three times/day for 10 to 15 days reduces the duration and severity of the varicella infection if administered very early. However, it becomes ineffective if initiation starts after a few days. Ceftriaxone (4 g/day intravenously for 2 weeks) remains a treatment of choice for cerebellitis associated with Lyme disease (Manto, 1995). Minocycline (4 mg/kg per day) is recommended for *Coxiella brunetti* infection (Sawaishi et al., 1999).

The usual doses of steroids are the following: oral prednisolone 1 to 5 mg/kg per day during 10 to 15 days, followed by a progressive tapering of doses. In case of ADEM, doses up to 1 g/day of methylprednisolone for 5 days are usually administered. Due to the self-limited character of cerebellitis in a substantial number of cases, the effects of steroids on the clinical course are not established. Steroids should be used cautiously in cerebellitis associated with enterovirus infection, due to the risk of worsening (Tabarki et al., 1998). Adrenocorticotrophic hormone reduces symptoms in up to 85% of children with Kinsbourne syndrome and is more effective than prednisone.

Nausea, vomiting, and vertigo require an immediate treatment. Nausea can be managed with metoclopramide, domperidone, or ondansetron. Neuroleptics may improve vertigo. Transtentorial or transforaminal herniations are life-threatening conditions treated with posterior fossa decompression and external ventricular drainage in most cases, although herniated tonsils compressed by a swollen vermis may respond to glycerol and dexamethasone (Asenbauer et al., 1997; de Ribaupierre et al, 2005). Plasmapheresis might be effective in some patients presenting with Miller Fisher syndrome and Bickerstaff encephalitis (Yuki, 1995), as well as in cerebellitis associated with EBV (Schmahmann, 2004). High-dose immunoglobulins (0.4 g/kg daily for 5 days) may stop the progression in Miller Fisher syndrome (Zifko et al., 1994).

Prognosis

Prognosis is usually good in children and adults before the age of 40 years. About 80% to 90% of patients return to normal life. Moderate residual cerebellar deficits are observed in 10% to 20% of cases. Recovery occurs between 1 week and 30 weeks. Cerebellar ataxia associated with *Plasmodium falciparum* infection carries an excellent prognosis (Senanayake & de Silva, 1994).

Despite the favorable prognosis in the majority of patients, some patients may develop permanent sequelae, especially the elderly (Klockgether et al., 1993). Yawning and hiccoughs appearing during the acute phase might carry a bad prognosis. Cerebellar atrophy may occur, especially in young patients and after

the age of 60 years. Atrophy may be localized to one cerebellar hemisphere in patients with a history of hemicerebellitis. Congenital cytomegalovirus infection can lead to severe neurological sequelae, with cerebellar atrophy (de Vries et al., 2004).

Hurst disease has a fatal outcome in most cases.

Human prion diseases

Human prion disorders, a group of neurodegenerative and infectious disorders with a fatal course, include sporadic Creutzfeldt-Jakob disease (CJD), variant CJD, fatal familial insomnia, Gerstmann-Sträussler-Scheinker disease, and kuru (Collinge, 2001). About 85% of cases are sporadic CJD, with a worldwide incidence of about 1.2 cases/million population per year. Iatrogenic causes include contamination via growth hormone from cadavers, implantation of contaminated dura mater grafts, corneal transplantation, contaminated EEG electrodes, and surgical procedures with contaminated instruments (Brown et al., 2000). Incubation periods can extend up to 30 years. Acquired prion disease resulting from a dietary origin presents as kuru, affecting patients in Eastern Highlands of Papua New Guinea (transmission due to ingestion of infected tissues from deceased relatives), and variant CJD (due to exposure of prions from cattle).

Prions appear to be composed principally or entirely of abnormal isoforms of a host-encoded glycoprotein (prion protein). Prion propagation involves recruitment of host cellular prion protein PrPc, composed primarily of alpha-helical structure, into a disease-specific isoform rich in beta-sheet structure PrPsc (Prusiner, 1982).

Clinical presentation

The main clinical presentation of sporadic CJD is a rapidly progressive dementia in people between the ages of 60 and 65 in about 70% of cases. Mean illness duration is 9 months.

Patients develop myoclonus, parkinsonism, cerebellar ataxia, seizures (partial or generalized seizures), and akinetic mutism. In any sporadic ataxic patient developing dementia and myoclonus, the diagnosis of sporadic CJD should be suspected. Only 5% of patients with sporadic CJD have an isolated cerebellar onset (Cooper et al., 2006). These patients subsequently develop myoclonus and pyramidal deficits.

The variant CJD (reported in UK, France, Ireland, Italy, and United States) occurs in younger people (average age of onset of around 27 years) and manifests with prodromal symptoms consisting of sensory disturbances and joint pains in the legs, as well as psychiatric symptoms (Collinge et al., 1996). Depression is common. Ataxia develops in all cases, and patients develop akinetic mutism. The mean duration of illness is 13 to 14 months, with a range of 9 to 35 months (Zeidler et al., 1997).

Iatrogenic CJD is characterized by a progressive cerebellar syndrome. Patients usually present with gait ataxia and psychiatric symptoms (Lowden et al., 2008).

Fatal familial insomnia manifests with prominent insomnia, generally in combination with dysautonomia, myoclonus, and eventual dementia.

The clinical presentation of kuru is stereotyped. Following a prodromal phase, three consecutive stages occur: an ambulatory phase, a sedentary phase, and a tertiary stage. Progressive cerebellar ataxia is a dominant clinical feature, while dementia is less prominent and occurs later (Wadsworth et al., 2008).

Differential diagnosis

Differential diagnosis of prion disorders includes Alzheimer disease, dementia with Lewy bodies, frontotemporal dementia, and spinocerebellar ataxias (see Chapter 23). The possibility of Hashimoto encephalopathy should not be overlooked, because this is a treatable condition which can mimic a sporadic CJD (see also Chapter 10) (Sakurai et al., 2008). Lymphomatosis cerebri (infiltrating form of primary central nervous system lymphoma) has to be considered in the differential diagnosis of rapidly progressive dementia (Vital & Sibon, 2007). The 14–3–3 protein may be positive in the CSF, and brain MRI is characterized by diffuse leukoencephalopathy without contrast enhancement (Kanai et al., 2008).

Neuroimaging

Brain MRI shows brain atrophy and high signal intensity in the caudate nucleus and putamen bilaterally on T2-weighted images. Diffusion-weighted imaging (DWI) and fluid-attenuated inversion recovery appear to be the most sensitive techniques. DWI can show cortical hyperintensities, cortical and subcortical abnormalities, or isolated subcortical anomalies. In cases of isolated cortical involvement, frontal and parietal lobes are the most affected (Meissner et al., 2008). An involvement of the thalamus can be observed. Thalamic lesions are common in variant CJD. The "pulvinar sign" (hyperintense signals in the posterior thalamus) is observed in about 70% of cases. Ataxic patients may show a predominant cerebellar atrophy on MRI. Cerebellar atrophy may not be detected on clinical reading of standard MRI images and becomes apparent on statistical group analysis, with elevated diffusion in the cerebellum (Figure 11.2).

^{18}F-Fluorodeoxyglucose positron emission tomography shows a pronounced regional decrease in glucose brain metabolism, indicative of neuronal dysfunction (Engler et al., 2003). Changes are usually most pronounced in the frontal, occipital, and parietal cortices, and in the cerebellum. In some patients, regional cerebral glucose metabolism is increased in temporal lobes and basal ganglia.

^{99m}Tc-ethyl cysteinate diethylester SPECT images demonstrate an overall decrease in the accumulation of ^{99m}Tc in the cerebrum. SPECT of the dopamine transporter shows putaminal dopaminergic presynaptic alterations in sporadic CJD (Ragno et al., 2009).

Neurophysiology

EEG is usually suggestive in sporadic CJD. Recordings show characteristic changes depending on the stage of the disease, ranging from non-specific findings such as diffuse slowing and frontal rhythmic delta activity in early stages to typical periodic sharp wave complexes (PSWC) in middle and late stages, areactive coma traces, or even alpha coma in preterminal state (Wieser et al., 2006). PSWC tend to disappear during sleep and may be attenuated by sedative medication and external stimulation. PSWC have a positive predictive value of about 95%. In iatrogenic CJD, PSWC are usually found with more regional EEG findings corresponding to the site of inoculation of the transmissible agent. PSWC are often absent in the variant CJD, and they are uncommon in familial prion disorders since they occur in about 10% of patients (Wieser et al., 2006).

Fatal familial insomnia is characterized by severe disturbances of sleep, with major disturbances in spindle formation (Cortelli et al., 2006). Sporadic CJD patients also have marked sleep EEG abnormalities, with very low sleep efficiency and virtual absence of REM sleep (Landolt et al., 2006).

Figure 11.2 Cerebellar involvement in Creutzfeldt-Jakob disease. The larger cerebellar loci of significantly elevated apparent diffusion coefficient (ADC) and CSF volume (respectively in A and B) are found bilaterally in the cerebellar nodule, shown here in three orthogonal projections. Focal atrophy cannot be detected on clinical reading of standard MRI sequences but is highly significant on statistical group analysis. Degenerative changes are reflected in elevated diffusion in the cerebellum, presumably due to tissue destruction and replacement by CSF. From: Cohen et al., 2009. With permission. (See color section.)

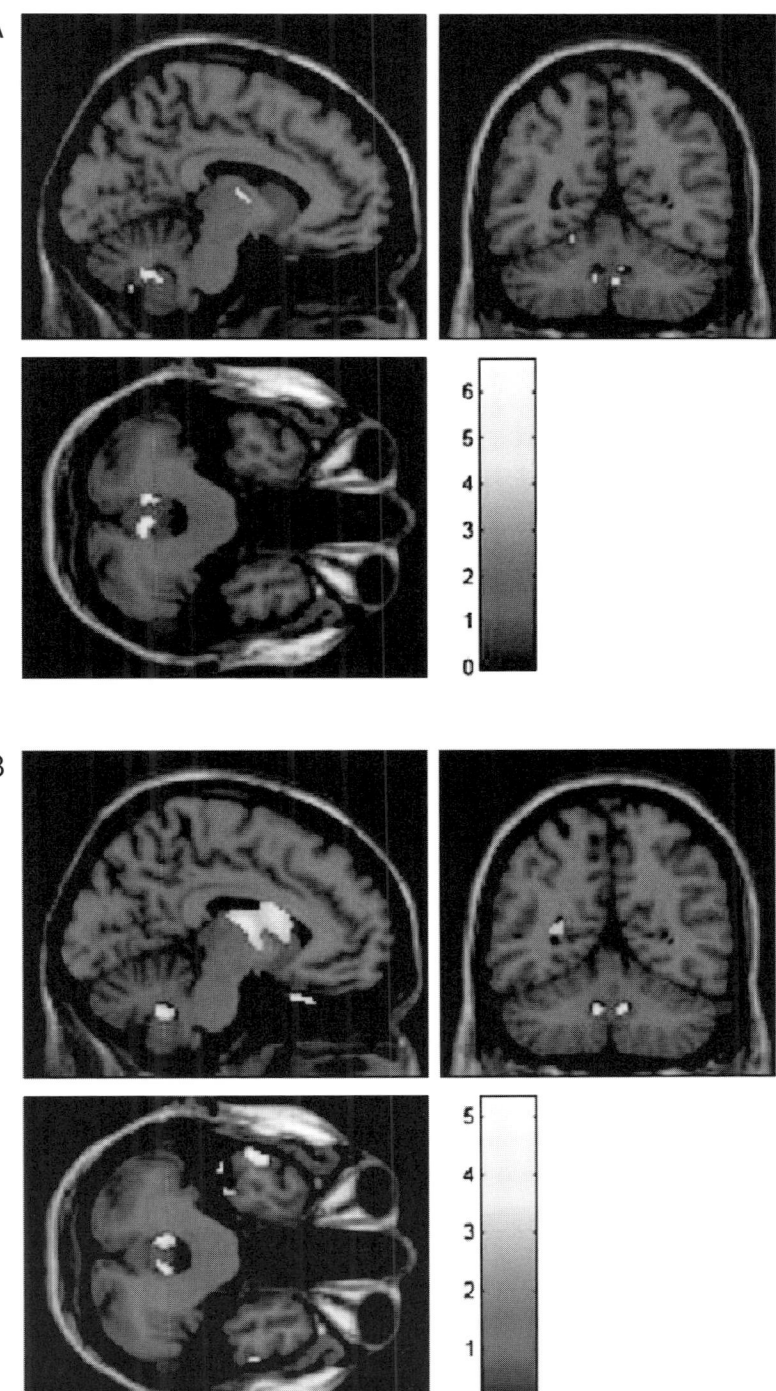

CSF studies

Classically, CSF shows a non-inflammatory profile in sporadic CJD, although a significant CSF pleocytosis has been reported in some cases (Bui et al., 2008).

Testing for 14–3–3 protein (a cellular protein whose release reflects extensive neuronal damage) in the CSF is useful when considered in an appropriate clinical context. However, the classical assay cannot be used for screening because of the high rate of false positives in sporadic CJD (Brechlin et al., 2008). False-positive results include stroke, meningoencephalitis, and dementia with Lewy bodies (Collins et al., 2000; Lemstra et al., 2000). Results of 14–3–3 protein testing are often negative in variant CJD. Detection of total tau protein in CSF might be more sensitive than the assessment of 14–3–3 protein (Satoh et al., 2007)

Genetic aspects

Gerstmann-Sträussler-Scheinker disease is due to mutations of the prion protein gene (PRNP) and presents as an autosomal dominant disease. More than 30 mutations have been identified. The mutation in the PRNP gene resulting in a Pro102Leu amino acid substitution is traditionally associated with Gerstmann-Sträussler-Scheinker syndrome. Fatal familial insomnia is due to a mutation at codon 178 of the PRNP gene.

The advent of variant CJD has confirmed one of the most powerful human genetic susceptibility factors, since all tested patients have an identical genotype at polymorphic codon 129 of PRNP (Mead, 2006). Homozygosity confers genetic susceptibility to both sporadic and acquired forms of CJD.

Neuropathology

Histology shows neuronal loss, spongiform changes with numerous vacuoles, and diffuse astrogliosis. Cortical involvement is detectable in most cases and is usually associated with spongiform changes in the basal ganglia, thalamus, and cerebellar cortex. Cerebellar involvement is present in most cases, although the severity and distribution of the spongiform change are variable. There is often an irregular loss of neurons in the granular and Purkinje cell layer. About 10% of CJD cases are characterized by PrP plaques, which are usually visible as rounded eosinophilic structures. These are most frequently observed in the cerebellum.

Unicentric PrP plaques are prominent and widespread in kuru (Hainfellner et al., 1997). Plaques are prominent in the striatum, thalamus, and granular layer of the cerebellar cortex. The occurrence of kuru-type plaques is noticeable in iatrogenic CJD (Liberski & Budka, 2004). The predominant pathologic changes of fatal familial insomnia lie within the thalami. There is little or no spongiosis and usually no PrPsc deposition.

Differential diagnosis of spongiosis includes Pick disease, Alzheimer disease, cortical ischemia, and viral encephalitis. Metabolic encephalopathies and neuronal storage disorders can mimic spongiosis in gray matter.

Treatment

There is no cure for prion disorders.

The antimalarial drug quinacrine is known to prevent the conversion of PrPc to PrPsc in vitro. In a recent trial, quinacrine at a dose of 300 mg/day did not significantly affect the clinical course of sporadic CJD, iatrogenic CJD, variant CJD, or inherited prion disease (Collinge et al., 2009).

References

Aboulafia DM, Taylor L. Vacuolar myelopathy and vacuolar cerebellar leukoencephalopathy: a late complication of AIDS after highly active antiretroviral therapy-induced immune reconstitution. *AIDS Patient Care STDS* 2002;**16**:579–84.

Alfaro A. Cerebellar encephalitis in adults. *J Neurol* 1993;**240**:505–6.

Amador N, Scheithauer BW, Giannini C, Raffel C. Acute cerebellitis presenting as tumor. Report of two cases. *J Neurosurg* 2007;**107**(1 suppl):57–61.

Asenbauer B, McConachie NS, Allcutt D, et al. Acute near-fatal parainfectious cerebellar swelling with favourable outcome. *Neuropediatrics* 1997;**28**: 122–5.

Askelöf P, Bartfai T. Effect of whopping-cough vaccine on cyclic-GMP levels in the brain. *FEMS Microbiol Lett* 1979;**6**:223–5.

Aylett SE, O'Neill KS, De Sousa C, Britton J. Cerebellitis presenting as acute hydrocephalus. *Childs Nerv Syst* 1998;**14**:139–41.

Beller AJ, Sahar A, Praiss I. Brain abscess. Review of 89 cases over a period of 30 years. *J Neurol Neurosurg Psychiatry* 1973;**36**:757–68.

Belloti C, Aragno M, Medina M, et al. Differential diagnosis of CT-hypodense cranial lesions with indium-111-oxine-labeled leukocytes. *J Neurosurg* 1986;**64**: 750–3.

Billette de Villemeur T, Gelot A, et al. Iatrogenic Creutzfeldt-Jakob disease in three growth hormone recipients: a neuropathological study. *Neuropathol Appl Neurobiol* 1994;**20**(2):111–7.

Black P, Graybill JR, Charache P. Penetration of brain abscess by systemically administered antibiotics. *J Neurosurg* 1973;**38**:705–9.

Bonthius DJ, Wright R, Tseng B, et al. Congenital lymphocytic choriomeningitis virus infection: spectrum of disease. *Ann Neurol* 2007;**62**(4):347–55.

Brambilla AM, Castagna A, Novati R, et al. Remission of AIDS-associated progressive multifocal leukoencephalopathy after cidofovir therapy. *J Neurol* 1999;**246**:723–5.

Brechlin P, Jahn O, Steinacker P, et al. Cerebrospinal fluid-optimized two-dimensional difference gel electrophoresis (2-D DIGE) facilitates the differential diagnosis of Creutzfeldt-Jakob disease. *Proteomics* 2008;**8**(20):4357–66.

Brink NS, Miller RF. Clinical presentation, diagnosis and therapy of progressive multifocal leukoencephalopathy. *J Infect* 1996;**32**:97–102.

Brooks BR, Walker DL. Progressive multifocal leukoencephalopathy in AIDS. *Neurol Clin* 1984;**2**:299–313.

Brown P, Preece M, Brandel JP, et al. Iatrogenic Creutzfeldt-Jakob disease at the millennium. *Neurology* 2000;**55**(8):1075–81.

Brydon HL, Hardwidge C. The management of cerebellar abscess since the introduction of CT scanning. *Br J Neurosurg* 1994;**8**:447–455.

Bui E, Ehrensperger E, Sahlas DJ, et al. Inflammatory cerebrospinal fluid in sporadic Creutzfeldt-Jakob disease. *Can J Neurol Sci* 2008;**35**(5):625–9.

Carey M, Shou S, French L. Experience with brain abscesses. *J Neurosurg* 1972;**34**:652–6.

Castillo LC, Gracia F, Román GC, et al. Spinocerebellar syndrome in patients infected with human T-lymphotropic virus types I and II (HTLV-I/HTLV-II): report of 3 cases from Panama. *Acta Neurol Scand* 2000;**101**(6):405–12.

Chang L, Ernst T, Tornatore C, et al. Metabolite abnormalities in progressive multifocal leukoencephalopathy by proton magnetic resonance spectroscopy. *Neurology* 1997;**48**:836–45.

Clearly TG, Henle W, Pickering LK. Acute cerebellar ataxia associated with Epstein-Barr virus infection. *J Am Med Assoc* 1980;**243**:148–9.

Cohen OS, Hoffmann C, Lee H, et al. MRI Detection of the cerebellar syndrome in Creutzfeldt-Jakob disease. *Cerebellum* 2009;**8**(3):373–81.

Coin CG, Hucks-Folliss AG, Mehegan CC. Computed-tomographically guided percutaneous transmastoid drainage of a cerebellar abscess. *Surg Neurol* 1983;**20**:387–90.

Collinge J. Prion diseases of humans and animals: their causes and molecular basis. *Annu Rev Neurosci* 2001;**24**:519–50.

Collinge J, Gorham M, Hudson F, et al. Safety and efficacy of quinacrine in human prion disease (PRION-1 study): a patient-preference trial. *Lancet Neurol* 2009;**8**(4): 334–44.

Collinge J, Sidle KC, Meads J, Ironside J, Hill AF. Molecular analysis of prion strain variation and the aetiology of 'new variant' CJD. *Nature* 1996;**383**(6602):685–90.

Collins S, Boyd A, Fletcher A, et al. Creutzfeldt-Jakob disease: diagnostic utility of 14–3–3 protein immunodetection in cerebrospinal fluid. *J Clin Neurosci* 2000;**7**:203–8.

Cooper SA, Murray KL, Heath CA, Will RG, Knight RS. Sporadic Creutzfeldt-Jakob disease with cerebellar ataxia at onset in the UK. *J Neurol Neurosurg Psychiatry* 2006;**77**(11):1273–5.

Cortelli P, Perani D, Montagna P, et al. Pre-symptomatic diagnosis in fatal familial insomnia: serial neurophysiological and 18FDG-PET studies. *Brain* 2006;**129**(Pt 3):668–75.

Dangond F, Engle E, Yessayan L, Sawyer MH. Pre-eruptive varicella cerebellitis confirmed by PCR. *Pediatr Neurol* 1993;**9**:491–493.

de Mendonca JL, Barbosa H, Viana SL, et al. Pseudotumoural hemicerebellitis: imaging findings in two cases. *Br J Radiol* 2005;**78**(935):1042–6.

de Ribaupierre S, Meagher-Villemure K, Villemure JG, et al. The role of posterior fossa decompression in acute cerebellitis. *Childs Nerv Syst* 2005;**21**:970–4.

de Silva HJ, Hoang P, Dalton H, et al. Immune activation during cerebellar dysfunction following Plasmodium falciparum malaria. *Trans R Soc Trop Med Hyg* 1992;**86**:129–131.

De Vries LS, Gunardi H, Barth PG, et al. The spectrum of cranial ultrasound and magnetic resonance imaging abnormalities in congenital cytomegalovirus infection. *Neuropediatrics* 2004;**35**:113–9.

Dev R, Gupta R, Poptani H, et al. Role of in vivo proton magnetic resonance spectroscopy in the diagnosis and management of brain abscesses. *Neurosurgery* 1998;**42**: 37–43.

Dobkin J, Healton E, Dickinson P, Brust JC. Nonspecificity of ring-enhancement in 'medically cured' brain abscesses. *Neurology* 1984;**34**:139–44.

Dyste GN, Hitchon PW, Menezes AH, et al. Stereotaxic surgery in the treatment of multiple brain abscesses. *J Neurosurg* 1988; **69**:188–94.

Engler H, Lundberg PO, Ekbom K, et al. Multitracer study with positron emission tomography in Creutzfeldt-Jakob disease. *Eur J Nucl Med Mol Imaging* 2003;**30**(1):85–95.

Enzmann DR, Britt R, Placone RJ, et al. The effect of short-term corticosteroid treatment on the CT appearance of experimental brain abscesses. *Radiology* 1982;**45**:79–84.

Fischer SA, Graham MB, Kuehnert MJ, et al. Transmission of lymphocytic choriomeningitis virus by organ transplantation. *N Engl J Med* 2006;**354**(21):2235–49.

Fritsch M, Manwaring KH. Endoscopic treatment of brain abscess in children. *Minim Invasive Neurosurg* 1997;**40**:103–6.

Gibson PE, Knowles WA, Hand JF, Brown DWG. Detection of JC virus DNA in the cerebrospinal fluid from patients with progressive multifocal leukoencephalopathy. *J Med Virol* 1993;**39**:278–81.

Gilman S, Bloedel JR, Lechtenberg R. Disorders of the cerebellum. Contemporary Neurology series. Philadelphia: FA. Davis, 1981.

Guerrini L, Belli G, Cellerini M, et al. Proton MR spectroscopy of cerebellitis. *Magn Reson Imaging* 2002;**20**:619–22.

Hainfellner JA, Liberski PP, Guiroy DC, et al. Pathology and immunocytochemistry of a kuru brain. *Brain Pathol* 1997;7(1):547–53.

Hayakawa H, Katoh T. Severe cerebellar atrophy following acute cerebellitis. *Pediatr Neurol* 1995;**12**:159–61.

Heineman HS, Braude AI, Osterholm JL. Intracranial suppurative disease. Early presumptive diagnosis and successful treatment without surgery. *J Am Med Assoc* 1971;**218**:1542–7.

Hofer M, Weber A, Haffner K, et al. Acute hemorrhagic leukoencephalitis (Hurst's disease) linked to Epstein-Barr virus infection. *Acta Neuropathol* 2005;**109**:226–30.

Johnson RT, Griffin DE, Gendelman HE. Postinfectious encephalomyelitis. *Semin Neurol* 1985;**5**:180–90.

Kanai R, Shibuya M, Hata T, et al. A case of 'lymphomatosis cerebri' diagnosed in an early phase and treated by

whole brain radiation: case report and literature review. *J Neurooncol* 2008;**86**(1):83–8.

Karagoz Guzey F, Bas NS, Sencer A, et al. Posterior fossa dermoid cysts causing cerebellar abscesses. *Pediatr Neurosurg* 2007;**43**:323–26.

Klockgether T, Döller G, Wüllner U, et al. Cerebellar encephalitis in adults. *J Neurol* 1993;**240**(1):17–20.

Klunder AD, Chiang MC, Dutton RA, et al. Mapping cerebellar degeneration in HIV/AIDS. *Neuroreport* 2008;**19**(17):1655–9.

Komatsu H, Kuroki S, Shimizu Y, et al. Mycoplasma pneumoniae meningoencephalitis and cerebellitis with antiganglioside antibodies. *Pediatr Neurol* 1998;**18**: 160–4.

Koralnik IJ, Wüthrich C, Dang X, et al. JC virus granule cell neuronopathy: a novel clinical syndrome distinct from progressive multifocal encephalopathy. *Ann Neurol* 2005;**57**:576–80.

Krolczyk S, Pacheco E, Valencia P, et al. Opsoclonus: an early sign of neonatal herpes encephalitis. *J Child Neurol* 2003;**18**:356–8.

Kurien M, Job A, Mathew J, Chandy M. Otogenic intracranial abscess: concurrent craniotomy and mastoidectomy – changing trends in a developing country. *Arch Otolaryngol Head Neck Surg* 1998;**124**:1353–1356.

Landolt HP, Glatzel M, Blättler T, et al. Sleep-wake disturbances in sporadic Creutzfeldt-Jakob disease. *Neurology* 2006;**66**(9):1418–24.

Lemstra AW, van Meegen MT, Vreyling JP, et al. 14–3–3 testing in diagnosing Creutzfeldt-Jakob disease: a prospective study in 112 patients. *Neurology* 2000;**55**(4):514–6.

Liberski PP, Budka H. Gerstmann-Sträussler-Scheinker disease. I. Human diseases. *Folia Neuropathol* 2004;**42**(Suppl B):120–40.

Lo YL. Clinical and immunological spectrum of the Miller Fisher syndrome. *Muscle Nerve* 2007;**36**(5):615–27.

Lowden MR, Scott K, Kothari MJ. Familial Creutzfeldt-Jakob disease presenting as epilepsia partialis continua. *Epileptic Disord* 2008;**10**(4):271–5.

Manto M. Cerebellitis associated with Lyme disease. *Lancet* 1995;**345**:1060.

Matsuo M, Odaka M, Koga M, et al. Bickerstaff's brainstem encephalitis associated with IgM antibodies to GM1b and GalNAc-GD1a. *J Neurol Sci* 2004;**217**(2):225–8.

Mead S. Prion disease genetics. *Eur J Hum Genet* 2006;**14**(3):273–81.

Meissner B, Kallenberg K, Sanchez-Juan P, et al. Isolated cortical signal increase on MR imaging as a frequent lesion pattern in sporadic Creutzfeldt-Jakob disease. *AJNR Am J Neuroradiol* 2008;**29**(8):1519–24.

Meissner B, Kallenberg K, Sanchez-Juan P, et al. MRI and clinical syndrome in dura materrelated Creutzfeldt-Jakob disease. *J Neurol* 2009;**256**(3):355–63.

Morriss MC, Rutstein RM, Rudy B, et al. Progressive multifocal leukoencephalopathy in an HIV-infected child. *Neuroradiology* 1997;**39**:142–4.

Nagamitsu S, Matsuishi T, Ishibashi M, et al. Decreased cerebellar blood flow in postinfectious acute cerebellar ataxia. *J Neurol Neurosurg Psychiatry* 1999;**67**:109–12.

Nager G. Mastoid and paranasal sinus infections and their relation to the central nervous system. *Clin Neurosurg* 1967;**14**:288–313.

Oguz KK, Haliloglu G, Alehan D, Topcu M. Recurrent pseudotumoral hemicerebellitis: neuroimaging findings. *Pediatr Radiol* 2008;**38**(4):462–6.

Osborn A. *Diagnostic Neuroradiology*. St Louis: Mosby-Year Book, 1994.

Osenbach RK, Loftus CM. Diagnosis and management of brain abscess. *Neurosurg Clin N Am* 1992;**3**:403–20.

Papavasiliou AS, Kotsalis C, Trakadas S. Transient cerebellar mutism in the course of acute cerebellitis. *Pediatr Neurol* 2004;**30**:71–4.

Park SA, Heo K. Prominent cerebellar symptoms with unusual magnetic resonance imaging findings in acquired hepatocerebral degeneration. *Arch Neurol* 2004;**61**:1458–60.

Peters CJ. Lymphocytic choriomeningitis virus–an old enemy up to new tricks. *N Engl J Med* 2006;**354**(21):2208–11.

Pierelli F, Tilia G, Damiani A, et al. Brainstem CMV encephalitis in AIDS: clinical case and MRI features. *Neurology* 1997;**48**:529–30.

Prusiner SB. Novel proteinaceous infectious particles cause scrapie. *Science* 1982;**216**(4542):136–44.

Ragno M, Scarcella MG, Cacchiò G, et al. Striatal [123I] FP-CIT SPECT demonstrates dopaminergic deficit in a sporadic case of Creutzfeldt-Jakob disease. *Acta Neurol Scand* 2009;**119**(2):131–4.

Relman DA, Schmidt TM, MacDermott RP, Falkow S. Identification of the uncultured bacillus of Whipple's disease. *N Engl J Med* 1992;**327**:293–301.

Rish B, Caveness W, Dillon J, et al. Analysis of brain abscess after penetrating cranio-cerebral injuries in Vietnam. *Neurosurgery* 1981;**9**:535–41.

Rosas MJ, Simoes-Ribeiro F, An SF, Sousa N. Progressive multifocal leukoencephalopathy: unusual MRI findings and prolonged survival in a pregnant woman. *Neurology* 1999;**52**:657–9.

Sakurai T, Tanaka Y, Koumura A, et al. Case report of a patient with Hashimoto's encephalopathy associated with Basedow's disease mimicking Creutzfeldt-Jakob disease. *Brain Nerve* 2008;**60**(5):559–65.

Satoh K, Shirabe S, Tsujino A, et al. Total tau protein in cerebrospinal fluid and diffusion-weighted MRI as an early diagnostic marker for Creutzfeldt-Jakob disease. *Dement Geriatr Cogn Disord* 2007;**24**(3):207–12.

Sawaishi Y, Takahashi I, Hirayama Y, et al. Acute cerebellitis caused by Coxiella burnetii. *Ann Neurol* 1999;**45**:124–7.

Schmahmann JD. Plasmapheresis improves outcome in postinfectious cerebellitis induced by Epstein-Barr virus. *Neurology* 2004;**62**:1443.

Senanayake N, de Silva HJ. Delayed cerebellar ataxia complicating falciparum malaria: a clinical study of 74 patients. *J Neurol* 1994;**241**:456–9.

Shahzadi S, Lozano AM, Bernstein M, et al. Stereotactic management of bacterial brain abscesses. *Can J Neurol Sci* 1996;**23**:34–9.

Shaw MD, Russell JA. Cerebellar abscess. A review of 47 cases. *J Neurol Neurosurg Psychiatry* 1975;**38**:429–35.

Shimokaze T, Kato M, Yoshimura Y, et al. A case of acute cerebellitis accompanied by autoantibodies against glutamate receptor delta 2. *Brain Dev* 2007;**29**:224–6.

Singer R. Diagnosis and treatment of Whipple's disease. *Drugs* 1998;**55**:699–704.

Sugimoto H, Wakata N, Kishi M, et al. A case of Guillain-Barré syndrome associated with cerebellar ataxia and positive serum anti-GD1b IgG antibody. *J Neurol* 2002;**249**(3):346–7.

Sze G, Zimmerman RD. The magnetic resonance imaging of infections and inflammatory diseases. *Radiol Clin N Am* 1988;**26**:839–59.

Tabarki B, Palmer P, Lebon P, Sebire G. Spontaneous recovery of opsoclonus-myoclonus syndrome caused by enterovirus infection. *J Neurol Neurosurg Psychiatry* 1998;**64**:406–7.

Tagliati M, Simpson D, Morgello S, et al. Cerebellar degeneration associated with human immunodeficiency virus infection. *Neurology* 1998;**50**:244–51.

Tavakoli NP, Wang H, Dupuis M, et al. Fatal case of deer tick virus encephalitis. *N Engl J Med* 2009;**360**(20):2099–107.

Tison F, Louvet-Giendaj C, Henry P, et al. Permanent bruxism as a manifestation of the oculofacial syndrome related to systemic Whipple's disease. *Mov Disord* 1992;**7**:82–5.

Tornatore C, Amemiya K, Atwood W, et al. JC virus: current concepts and controversy in the molecular virology and pathogenesis of progressive multifocal leukoencephalopathy. *Rev Med Virol* 1994;**4**: 197–219.

Uchibori A, Sakuta M, Kusunoki S, Chiba A. Autoantibodies in postinfectious acute cerebellar ataxia. *Neurology* 2005; **65**:1114–16.

van Dellen JR, Bullock R, Postma MH. Cerebellar abscess: the impact of computed tomographic scanning. *Neurosurgery* 1987;**21**:547–50.

Verhagen WI, Huygen PL, Dalman JE, Schuurmans MM. Whipple's disease and the central nervous system. A case report and review of the literature. *Clin Neurol Neurosurg* 1996;**98**:299–304.

Vital A, Sibon I. A 64-year-old woman with progressive dementia and leukoencephalopathy. *Brain Pathol* 2007;**17**(1):117–8, 121.

Wadia RS, Ichaporia NR, Kiwalkar RS, et al. Cerebellar ataxia in enteric fever. *J Neurol Neurosurg Psychiatry* 1985;**48**:695–7.

Wadsworth JD, Joiner S, Linehan JM, et al. The origin of the prion agent of kuru: molecular and biological strain typing. *Philos Trans R Soc Lond B Biol Sci* 2008;**363** (1510):3747–53.

Wieser HG, Schindler K, Zumsteg D. EEG in Creutzfeldt-Jakob disease. *Clin Neurophysiol* 2006;**117**(5):935–51.

Woody RC, Street RW, Charlton RK, Smith S. Histocompatibility determinants in childhood postinfectious encephalomyelitis. *J Child Neurol* 1989;**4**:204–7.

Yuki N. Successful plasmapheresis in Bickerstaff's brain stem encephalitis associated with anti-GQ1b antibody. *J Neurol Sci* 1995;**131**:108–10.

Yuki N, Susuki K, Hirata K. Ataxic form of Guillain-Barré syndrome associated with anti-GD1b IgG antibody. *J Neurol Neurosurg Psychiatry* 2000;**69**(1):136–7.

Yuki N, Wakabayashi K, Yamada M, Seki K. Overlap of Guillain-Barré syndrome and Bickerstaff's brainstem encephalitis. *J Neurol Sci* 1997;**145**:119–121.

Zaro-Weber O, Galldiks N, Dohmen C, Fink GR, Nowak DA. Ocular flutter, generalized myoclonus, and trunk ataxia associated with anti-GQ1b antibodies. *Arch Neurol* 2008;**65**(5):659–61.

Zeidler M, Stewart GE, Barraclough CR, et al. New variant Creutzfeldt-Jakob disease: neurological features and diagnostic tests. *Lancet* 1997;**350**(9082):903–7.

Zifko U, Drlicek M, Senautka G, Grisold W. High dose immunoglobulin therapy is effective in the Miller Fisher syndrome. *J Neurol* 1994;**241**:178–9.

Corticobasal degeneration

Clinical features

Corticobasal ganglionic degeneration (CBD) is a sporadic neurodegenerative disorder usually appearing after the age of 50 years. Most patients die within 10 years of onset. CBD is characterized by asymmetrical parkinsonism, ideomotor apraxia, stimulus-sensitive myoclonus, dystonia, cortical sensory loss (agraphesthesia, extinction, astereognosis), and the alien hand syndrome, which is an inability to recognize one's own limb in absence of vision (Doody & Jankovic, 1992). A substantial number of patients report complaints related to a jerky, stiff, or clumsy upper limb (Rinne et al., 1994). The arm is akinetic, rigid, and apraxic and may be held in a suggestive fixed dystonic posture. Difficulties in walking are related to clumsiness and loss of fine motor control of one leg due to apraxia or disequilibrium. Symptoms progressively spread to four limbs. Neuropsychiatric features include depression, apathy, irritability, and agitation (Litvan et al., 1998). Minor features are blepharospasm, choreoathetosis, cerebellar ataxia, cognitive deficits, and supranuclear gaze deficits. A genuine cerebellar syndrome may develop in CBD, but ataxia is often masked by the extrapyramidal deficits and the concomitant parietal ataxia.

Brain imaging

Brain MRI shows asymmetrical atrophy of the frontoparietal cortex and may demonstrate a cerebellar atrophy, which tends to be symmetrical. Volumetric studies reveal atrophy of the corpus callosum also (Gröschel et al., 2004).

Single-photon emission CT and positron emission tomography studies show an asymmetrical involvement of the cortical structures around the perirolandic cortex and thalamus (Eidelberg et al., 1991).

Neurophysiology

Electroencephalographic recordings show a slowing, which is often asymmetrical. Action myoclonus is not preceded by a cortical discharge, and the amplitude of sensory evoked potentials is normal. The jerks consist of hypersynchronous short-duration bursts of electromyographic activity coincident in agonist and antagonist muscles (Thompson et al., 1994). Reflex myoclonus to stimulation of the median nerve at the wrist has a latency of approximately 40 msec in the hand, suggesting that myoclonus is mediated by direct sensory input to motor cortical areas that activates corticospinal tract output. Magnetic, but not electrical, brain stimulation elicits repetitive bursts of myoclonus due to enhanced cortical excitability.

Upper limb tremor is rapid (5–8 Hz) and irregular, and combines jerky components and myoclonic-like movements. In some patients, fast movements are hypermetric, and the overshoot is enhanced by the addition of mass.

Neuropathology

Neuropathological studies show an asymmetry of the cortical atrophy at the level of frontoparietal areas. The temporal and occipital cortices are usually spared. At a cellular level, neuronal loss, "ballooned" neurons, and gliosis are commonly observed in the cortical and subcortical areas. Degeneration of the substantia nigra is classical. Variable degrees of cell loss occur in the thalamic nuclei, red nuclei, dentate nuclei, and inferior olivary complex. In some patients, a marked degeneration of the dentatorubrothalamic pathway is found (Litvan et al., 1996). CBD is classified in tauopathies with parkinsonism, a group of disorders sharing the pathologic accumulation of hyperphosphorylated tau protein fragments within the CNS (Ludolph et al., 2009). Tau deposition is found in both gray and white matter of the cortical regions and basal ganglia and to a lesser extent in cerebellar white matter. Purkinje cell somata show diffuse granular accumulation of cytoplasmic tau in about half of cases (Piao et al., 2002). Neuropathological criteria have been proposed: the minimal pathologic features for CBD are cortical and striatal tau-positive neuronal and glial lesions, especially astrocytic plaques and thread-like lesions in both white matter and gray matter, along with neuronal loss in focal cortical regions and in the substantia nigra (Dickson et al., 2002).

Differential diagnosis

Signs of cortical involvement and lack of response to anti-parkinsonian drugs are two important clues to differentiate CBD from Parkinson disease, which also presents as an asymmetrical disease. Progressive supranuclear palsy is characterized by early falls, vertical supranuclear ophthalmoplegia, and axial rigidity. Clinical symptoms of frontotemporal dementia included personality and behavioral changes. Dementia with Lewy bodies manifests with parkinsonism, fluctuating cognition, parasomnia, and hallucinations. Other neurodegenerative disorders which can mimic CBD with ataxia are multiple system atrophy, Wilson disease, neuronal ceroid lipofuscinosis, and Creutzfeldt-Jakob disease. Alien hand sign may occur in multiple infarcts.

Treatment

Treatment of CBD is primarily supportive. Extrapyramidal deficits may respond to levodopa and dopamine agonists. Myoclonus usually responds to clonazepam. Dystonia in upper limbs is improved with botulinum toxin injections. Physiotherapy, occupational therapy, and speech rehabilitation are recommended. Assisting devices such as a rolling walker reduce falls (Reich & Grill, 2009). Gastrostomy is often required at an advanced stage.

References

Dickson DW, Bergeron C, Chin SS, et al. Office of Rare Diseases of the National Institutes of Health. Office of Rare Diseases neuropathologic criteria for corticobasal degeneration. *J Neuropathol Exp Neurol* 2002;**61**(11):935–46.

Doody RS, Jankovic J. The alien hand and related signs. *J Neurol Neurosurg Psychiatry* 1992;**55**(9):806–10.

Eidelberg D, Dhawan V, Moeller JR, et al. The metabolic landscape of cortico-basal ganglionic degeneration: regional asymmetries studied with positron emission tomography. *J Neurol Neurosurg Psychiatry* 1991;**54**(10):856–62.

Gröschel K, Hauser TK, Luft A, et al. Magnetic resonance imaging-based volumetry differentiates progressive supranuclear palsy from corticobasal degeneration. *Neuroimage* 2004;**21**(2):714–24.

Litvan I, Cummings JL, Mega M. Neuropsychiatric features of corticobasal degeneration. *J Neurol Neurosurg Psychiatry* 1998;**65**(5):717–21.

Litvan I, Hauw JJ, Bartko JJ, et al. Validity and reliability of the preliminary NINDS neuropathologic criteria for progressive supranuclear palsy and related disorders. *J Neuropathol Exp Neurol* 1996;**55**(1):97–105.

Ludolph AC, Kassubek J, Landwehrmeyer BG, et al. Reisensburg Working Group for Tauopathies With Parkinsonism. Tauopathies with parkinsonism: clinical spectrum, neuropathologic basis, biological markers, and treatment options. *Eur J Neurol* 2009;**16**(3):297–309.

Piao YS, Hayashi S, Wakabayashi K, et al. Cerebellar cortical tau pathology in progressive supranuclear palsy and corticobasal degeneration. *Acta Neuropathol* 2002;**103**(5):469–74.

Reich SG, Grill SE. Corticobasal degeneration. *Curr Treat Options Neurol* 2009;**11**(3):179–85.

Rinne JO, Lee MS, Thompson PD, Marsden CD. Corticobasal degeneration. A clinical study of 36 cases. *Brain* 1994;**117**(Pt 5):1183–96.

Thompson PD, Day BL, Rothwell JC, et al. The myoclonus in corticobasal degeneration. Evidence for two forms of cortical reflex myoclonus. *Brain* 1994;**117**(Pt 5):1197–207.

Tumors and paraneoplastic disorders

Six main causes of cerebellar lesions occur in cancer patients: primary tumors, metastases, complications of treatments, vascular lesions, infectious disorders, and paraneoplastic phenomena (Table 13.1). Medulloblastomas, astrocytomas, ependymomas, and brainstem gliomas principally affect children. The most common malignancies in adults are metastases, meningiomas, and schwannomas (neurinomas). Both schwannomas and meningiomas occur in type 1 (von Recklinghausen disease) – diagnosed usually in the first decade – or in type 2 neurofibromatosis – diagnosed usually between 18 and 40 years. In children, primary tumors of the cerebellum are more common than in adults, in whom metastases have a higher incidence.

Lesions exerting a mass effect generate a displacement of posterior fossa structures with a risk of herniation, obstructive hydrocephalus, and signs of intracranial hypertension (triad of headache, vomiting, and papilledema and palsy of nerve VI). Headache tends to be located in the occipital region and is enhanced by coughing or Valsalva maneuver. Vomiting may be abrupt. In children, enlarged head, tense fontanels, and separation of cranial sutures point towards intracranial hypertension. Upwards transtentorial herniation presents clinically with impaired upwards gaze, impaired consciousness, and coma. Obstructive hydrocephalus is common. Tonsillar herniation presents with neck stiffness, head tilt, ataxia, and nystagmus. Breathing may become irregular, and patients may exhibit apnea or impaired heart rhythm/blood pressure regulation. An unsuitable lumbar puncture may provoke tonsillar herniation.

Brain MRI represents the technique of choice for diagnosis and follow-up, being superior to CT scan. Brain magnetic resonance spectroscopy and positron emission tomography (PET) provide additional useful information. Fusion of CT (or MRI) and PET images (^{18}F-fluorodeoxyglucose [FDG], methionine [MET]) is now performed on a routine basis in many centers. As a general rule, lesions producing mass effect and

enhanced by gadolinium are suggestive of a tumor (see also Chapter 11). The decision to make a cerebellar biopsy is often made case-by-case. Stereotactic biopsies are usually suggested when the primary tumor is undetermined (the advent of combination of whole-body CT scan combined with PET might change this attitude), when intra-tumoral bleeding is suspected, or when antibiotics do not cure a mass initially suspected to be an abscess.

Medulloblastomas

These primitive neuroectodermal tumors affect children, with a peak incidence between 5 and 11 years. They are usually located in the vermis, with a predominance in the lower part. In adults, their origin is usually more lateral. Medulloblastomas may develop in Gorlin syndrome or ataxia-telangiectasia. The tumor has a propensity to invade the fourth ventricle and the leptomeninges, or to generate spinal seedings. Patients usually present with headache, signs of raised intracranial pressure, and ataxia of posture/gait. MRI shows a hypointense mass in T1-weighted sequences and a heterogeneous tumor in T2-weighted images, around the fourth ventricle (Figure 13.1). There is a marked enhancement, usually heterogeneous, with gadolinium. Neuropathology shows high cell density, hyperchromatic nuclei, and numerous mitosis. Treatment consists of surgery, radiotherapy, and chemotherapy. Total tumor resection is generally recommended (Tait et al., 1990). Radiation therapy plays a critical role. Standard doses for the posterior fossa are 5000 to 5500 cGy given in 30 fractions. Adjuvant chemotherapy consists of an association of vincristine, lomustine (CCNU), and cisplatin (Goldwein et al., 1993; Cohen & Packer, 1996). Chemotherapy may be used to delay radiation therapy in very young children (younger than 3 years) to minimize the effects of irradiation on cognitive functions or growth. Indeed, in very young children, craniospinal irradiation has a greater

Table 13.1 Cerebellar lesions in cancer

Primary tumors	Intrinsic: Medulloblastomas Astrocytomas Extrinsic: Brainstem gliomas Hemangioblastomas Ependymomas Meningiomas Schwannomas (neurinomas) Epidermoids and dermoid tumors Primary lymphomas of the CNS Lhermitte-Duclos disease (gangliocytoma)
Metastases	
Following treatment	Chemotherapy: 5-Fluorouracil Cytosine arabinoside Surgery Radiation-induced Phenytoin Lithium salts Superficial siderosis
Vascular	Stroke
Infections	Mainly abscesses
Paraneoplastic	Anti-Yo, Anti-Hu, Anti-Ri, Anti-CV2, Anti-Tr, Anti-Ma1, Anti-Zic4
Langerhans histiocytosis	

Adapted from: Hildebrand and Balériaux (2002). With permission.

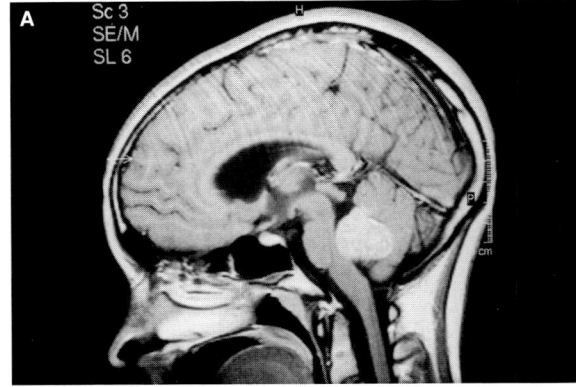

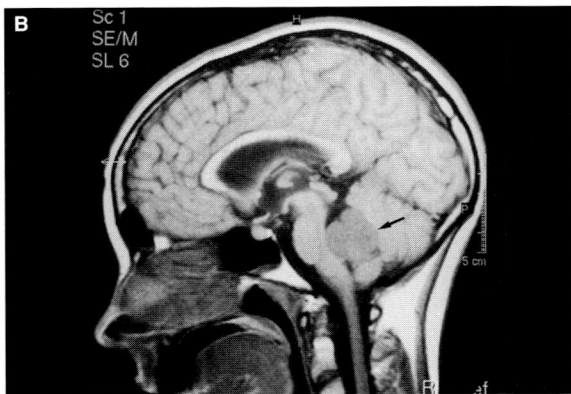

Figure 13.1 Medulloblastoma. Sagittal T1-weighted image showing a hypointense mass in the fourth ventricle (A), enhancing following contrast injection (B). With permission from: Hildebrand and Balériaux, 2002.

detrimental effect (Clarke et al., 2007). Prognostic factors appear similar in children and in adults (Padovani et al., 2007). Brainstem involvement, fourth ventricle invasion, and radiation dose to the posterior fossa and the spine are prognostic factors. The 10-year overall survival rate is 50% to 55%. Medulloblastoma is associated with a deregulation of the sonic hedgehog pathway (see Chapter 1) (Wetmore, 2003; Ferretti et al., 2008).

Cerebellar astrocytomas

The peak incidence of cerebellar astrocytomas is seen in the first decade of life. This group of tumors includes benign juvenile pilocytic astrocytoma (80% of cerebellar astrocytomas), grade II infiltrating fibrillary astrocytoma, and grade IV glioblastoma. Juvenile pilocytic astrocytoma arises mainly from cerebellar hemispheres, and therefore patients initially may exhibit unilateral signs. MRI shows a usually cystic lesion, with a solid component markedly enhanced with contrast media (Figure 13.2). Juvenile pilocytic astrocytomas are made of bipolar elongated cells, with presence of small vessels without endothelial proliferation (microvascular proliferation). Intracellular inclusions

known as Rosenthal fibers are suggestive. Mitoses are rare. Total resection is recommended. However, infiltrating grade II astrocytoma and grade IV glioblastoma render total resection difficult. Adjuvant radiotherapy is commonly applied in high-grade tumors, but the use of adjuvant chemotherapy is still questionable, although it is used in many centers by analogy with chemotherapy used in supratentorial glioblastomas.

Brainstem gliomas

A majority of brainstem gliomas occur before the age of 25 years. They can also develop with preference in adults aged 35 to 50 years. The three main localizations are the tectal region, the pons, and the cervicomedullary junction. The pons is infiltrated in two-thirds of brainstem gliomas. Cranial nerve palsies are common. MRI shows a widening of the pons (Figure 13.3). In T1-weighted images, the lesion is

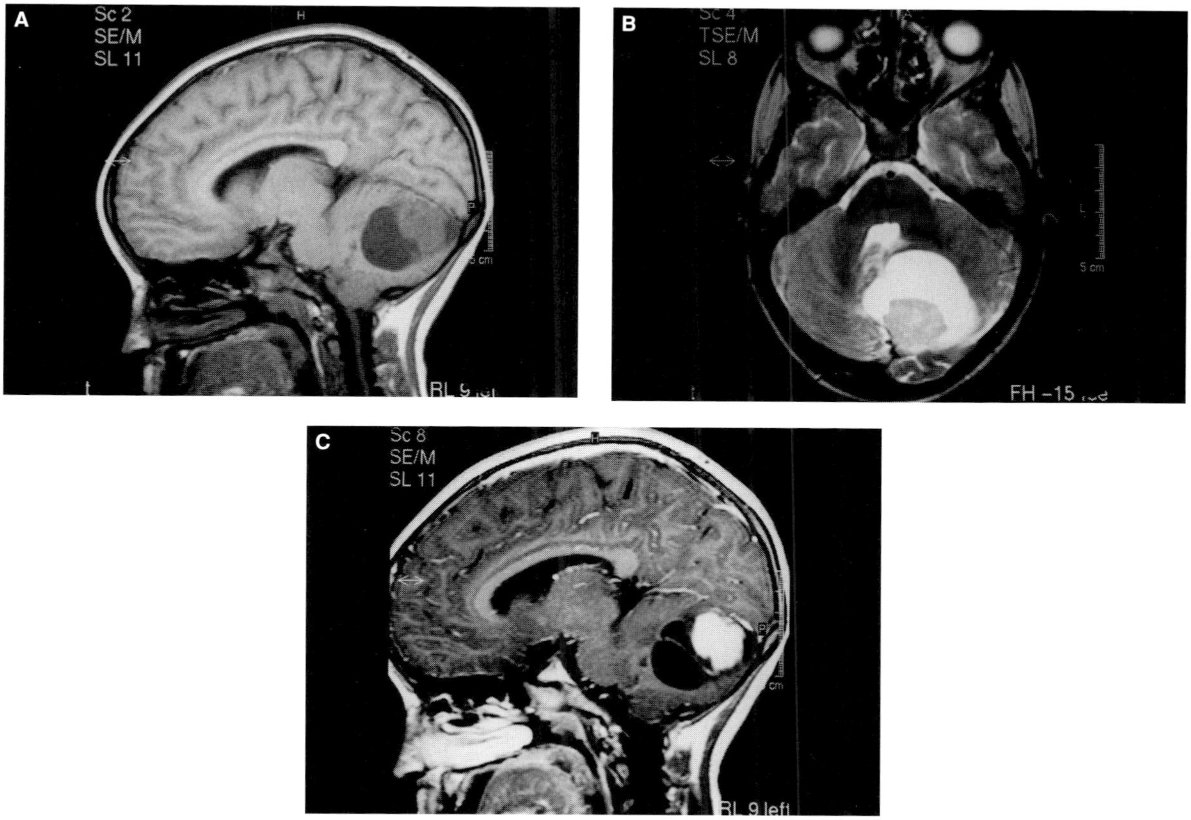

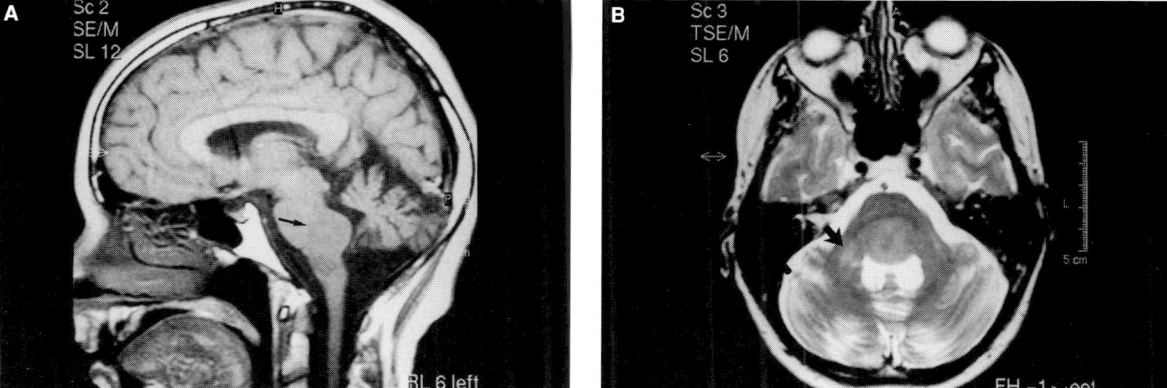

Figure 13.2 Left cerebellar cystic grade II astrocytoma. On T1-weighted sequence (A), the tumor appears as a partially cystic mass causing tonsillar herniation. The solid component is moderately hypointense. The cyst appears uniformly hyperintense on T2 sequence (B). Post-contrast T1-weighted image shows enhancement of the solid component, also observed in the cyst wall (C). With permission from: Hildebrand and Balériaux, 2002.

Figure 13.3 MRI of brainstem glioma. (A) Sagittal T1-weighted image shows a widening of the pons and medulla by a slightly hypointense tumor (arrow). (B) The tumor is moderately hyperintense on T2-weighted sequence, extending into the middle cerebellar peduncle (arrow). With permission from: Hildebrand and Balériaux, 2002.

Table 13.2 Lesions in von Hippel-Lindau disease

Hemangioblastoma (retina, cerebellum, spinal cord, brainstem)

Kidney tumors (cyst, carcinoma)

Pheochromocytoma

Pancreatic tumors (adenoma, cyst)

Epididymal cyst

Liver tumors

Cyst of the spleen

Cyst of the lung

Sympathetic paraganglioma

usually slightly hypointense. In T2-weighted images, the glioma appears moderately hyperintense. Contrast enhancement is mild. Combination and integration of PET data (FDG, MET) with MRI could improve target selection for stereotactic biopsies. The suboccipital transcerebellar approach is associated with low morbidity and has a high diagnostic yield (Roujeau et al., 2007). Radiation therapy (up to 5500 cGy in up to 200-cGy daily fractions) is the principal treatment (Littman et al., 1980). Recurrent tumors are treated with chemotherapy (etoposide [VP-16], cisplatin, cyclophosphamide, vincristine, lomustine). Efficacy of adjuvant chemotherapy is not proven. Mean overall survival at 5 years for high-grade tumors ranges from 15% (infants) to 36% (children) (Bertolone et al., 2003).

Hemangioblastomas

Hemangioblastomas occur mainly in patients with the dominantly transmitted von Hippel-Lindau disease (gene on chromosome 3p). The incidence of this disease is 1 per 39 000, with a high penetrance. Patients are usually diagnosed between the second and the fifth decade. The mean age at presentation is 33 years. Hemangioblastoma may occur in association with multiple endocrine neoplasia in Von Hippel-Lindau disease (Table 13.2). Indeed, these patients are at risk to develop neoplasias in various organs (Richard et al., 1998). Hemangioblastomas may also develop sporadically. Sporadic tumors are nearly always solitary. Neurological symptoms and signs include headache, gait ataxia, dysmetria, and symptoms of hydrocephalus. Brain MRI shows a large cystic lesion with a small solid nodule in the cerebellum (80% in hemispheres, 15% in vermis, 5% in the floor of the fourth ventricle). Lesions are usually posterior and medial. They are isointense or hypointense on T1-weighted images (Figure 13.4).

On T2-weighted images, the nodule is hypointense within a hyperintense cystic cavity. The nodule is enhanced by contrast media, unlike the wall of the cyst. Hemangioblastoma may be solely solid. Patients usually die from nervous system hemangioblastomas, followed by kidney tumors. Polycythemia is found in up to 30% of patients and is due to production of erythropoietin-like substances by hemangioblastomas. Treatment is surgical removal of the tumor. The midline suboccipital approach is often used to resect the tumor (Jagannathan et al., 2008). Hydrocephalus may require a ventriculoperitoneal shunt. Most patients benefit immediately from surgical removal of the hemangioblastoma. Recurrence rates vary from 20% to 33% (Conway et al., 2001). Radiation therapy has been used as an adjunct to resection. Small hemangioblastomas not associated with cysts might be candidates for radiosurgery, but its efficacy remains to be determined. Genetic counseling is recommended.

Ependymomas

Ependymomas occur usually within the first two decades of life. Signs of raised intra-cranial pressure are the common clinical presentation. The tumor is commonly located in the floor of the fourth ventricle, filling and molding this area. This is often very suggestive on brain MRI (Figure 13.5). The main differential diagnosis is medulloblastoma. Total resection is recommended (Healey et al., 1991). Radiation therapy (5000–5500 cGy in up to 200-cGy daily fractions) is used in patients with partial resection. Because craniospinal dissemination is possible, some authors recommend prophylactic spinal irradiation. However, this is a matter of debate. In order to delay irradiation, chemotherapy (mainly platinum derivatives) can be administered in very young children. Chemotherapy can also be used for recurrence. The 5-year overall survival rate varies from 60% to 84% according to series (Metellus et al., 2007; Shu et al., 2007). Favorable prognosis is associated with age older than 3 years, absence of spinal cord extension, complete resection, low histological grade, and dose greater than 54 Gy (Metellus et al., 2007; Shu et al., 2007). Histological grade is a main prognostic factor in adults (Metellus et al., 2007).

Meningiomas

Meningiomas usually grow from the tentorium of the cerebellum, the cerebellar convexity, or the ponto-cerebellar angle. Patients exhibit various combinations

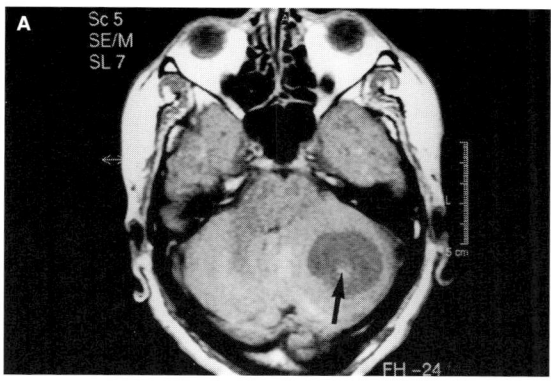
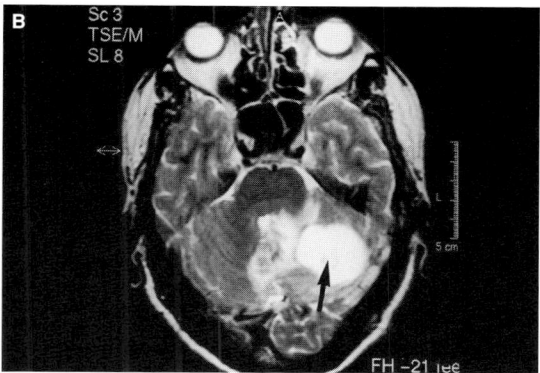
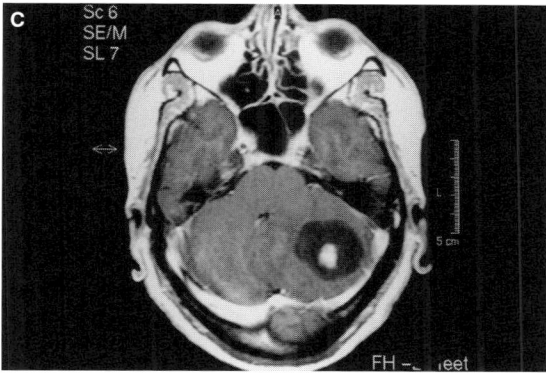

Figure 13.4 Cerebellar hemangioblastoma. (A) Axial T1-weighted sequence shows a cystic lesion with a small isointense nodule (arrow). (B) The nodule appears hypointense on T2-weighted images. (C) Post-contrast T1-weighted images show enhancement of the solid nodule. There is no enhancement within the wall of the cyst. With permission from: Hildebrand and Balériaux, 2002.

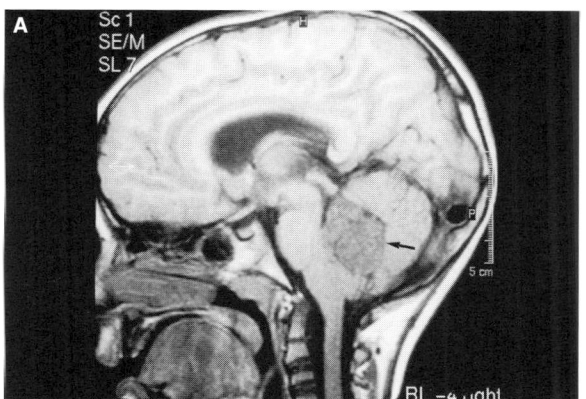
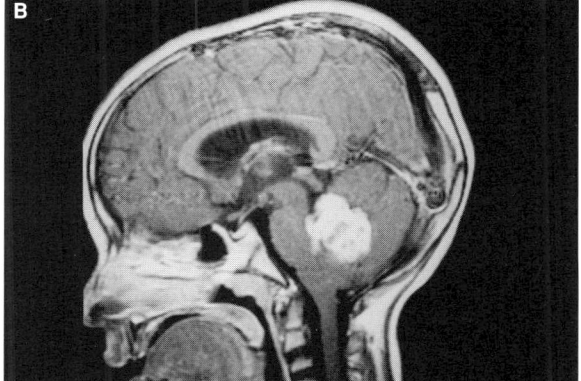

Figure 13.5 Ependymoma of the fourth ventricle. MRI shows a molding of the ventricle by the tumor. (A) T1-weighted image shows a lobulated mass which appears inhomogeneously hypointense (arrow). (B) Post-contrast T1-weighted image reveals a strong and heterogeneous enhancement. With permission from: Hildebrand and Balériaux, 2002.

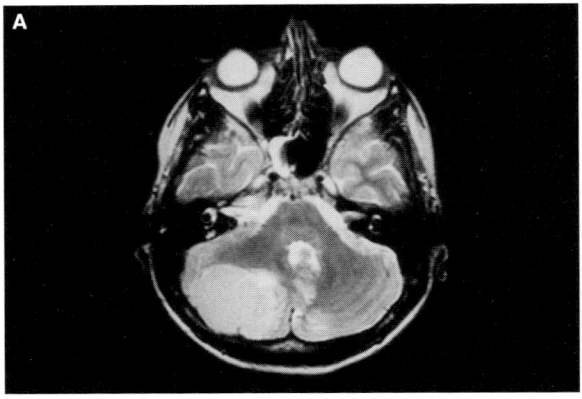
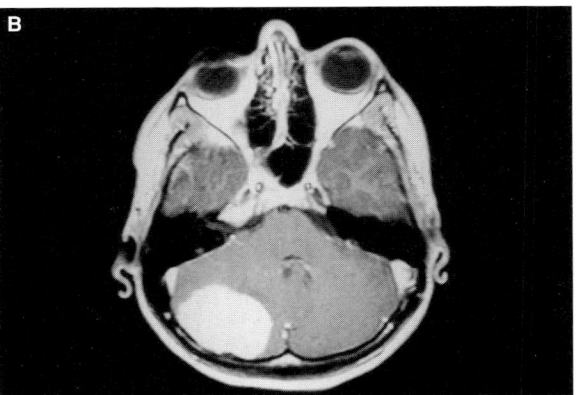
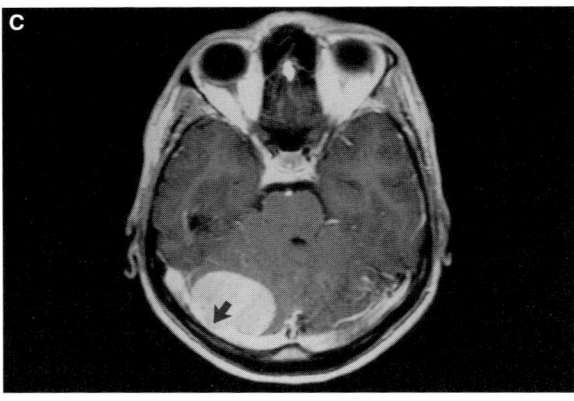

Figure 13.6 Posterior fossa meningioma. (A) Axial T2-weighted image shows a slightly hyperintense mass. (B, C) Post-contrast T1-weighted image reveals a homogeneous enhancement, with invasion of the transverse sinus (arrow). With permission from: Hildebrand and Balériaux, 2002.

of cerebellar deficits, cranial nerve palsy, and intracranial hypertension. They are sometimes referred to otolaryngologists due to predominant vertigo (Fujino et al., 2007). In T1-weighted sequence, the lesion is nearly isointense, whereas it is slightly hyperintense and homogeneous on T2-weighted images (Figure 13.6). Contrast enhancement is intense. Invasion of venous sinuses may occur. Total resection is recommended. Adjuvant radiation therapy is used in cases of partial resection (Barbaro et al., 1987). Hydroxyurea has been suggested for recurrent tumors (Schrell et al., 1997). Extensive meningiomas of the skull base should not be misinterpreted as idiopathic hypertrophic pachymeningitis (IHPM) (Rudnik et al., 2007). Indeed, IHPM affecting the posterior fossa may manifest with headache, cranial nerve palsies, and cerebellar ataxia. MRI shows thickening of the cranial base pachymeninx compressing the lower brainstem, with presence of contrast enhancement. Dura mater biopsy shows inflamma-

tion with abundant lymphocytic infiltrations, without neoplastic infiltration. IHPM responds to corticosteroids and/or azathioprine or other immunosuppressant drugs. Suboccipital decompression may be required.

Schwannomas (neurinomas)

Most schwannomas are tumors growing from the vestibular nerve. Patients present with symptoms related to the invasion of the cerebellopontine angle, affecting especially nerves V and VIII (acousticofacial complex). With time, cerebellar signs develop. Treatment consists of microsurgery or radiosurgery for lesions less than 3 cm (Pollock et al., 1995). Low-dose treatments using a marginal tumor dose of about 12 Gy achieve tumor growth control in 91% to 96% of patients along with low trigeminal and facial nerve dysfunction (Iwai et al., 2007). Transient swelling may occur in up to 60% of cases

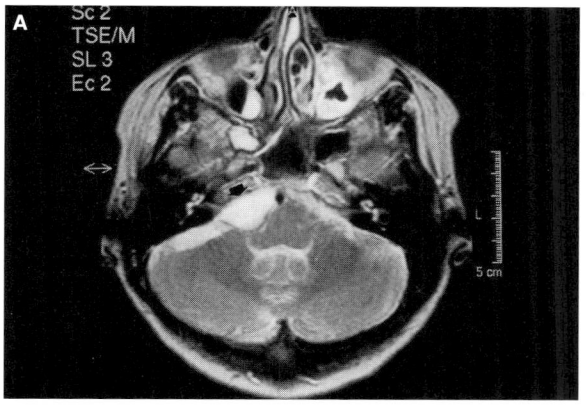
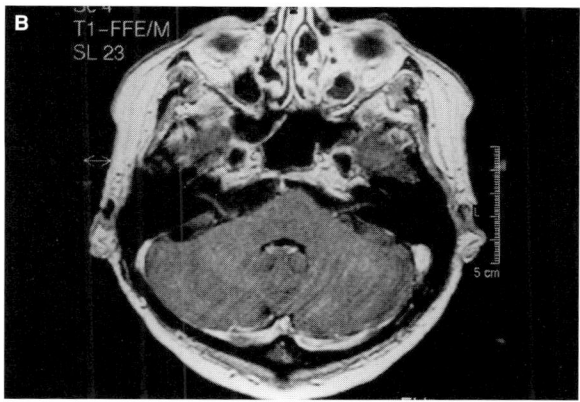

Figure 13.7 Epidermoid tumor of the pontocerebellar angle cistern. (A) T2-weighted image shows a hyperintense lesion (arrow) which mimics the aspect of cerebrospinal fluid. (B) The lesion is not enhanced by contrast administration (T1-weighted image). With permission from: Hildebrand and Balériaux, 2002.

treated with gamma knife radiosurgery, and large tumors are usually those associated with neurological deterioration (Yu et al., 2000). Swelling usually peaks about 6 months after radiosurgery, but it may persist for up to 2 years and it may not respond to steroids. Nevertheless, because radiosurgery is less invasive than surgical resection and provides good functional preservation along with long-term tumor growth control, it is becoming the preferred therapy for small to medium acoustic neuromas. However, about 5% of patients require surgical resection after radiosurgery, in the presence of increased intra-cranial pressure or cerebellar ataxia (Iwai et al., 2007). These surgeries are complicated by fibrosis and adhesions between the tumor and the surrounding tissues (Lee et al., 2003). When surgery is performed during the transient swelling period, surgical results are poor in terms of cranial nerve function preservation, especially facial nerve function (Iwai et al., 2007). Subtotal removal/resection of the tumor is more successful in preserving cranial nerve dysfunction. In patients with tumor enlargement several years after radiosurgery, the possibility of chronic intratumoral bleeding due to delayed radiation injury should be considered (Iwai et al., 2007). Close follow-up in very old patients with slowly growing tumors and mild deficits may be an alternative.

Epidermoid and dermoid tumors

The cerebellopontine angle is the principal site of posterior fossa epidermoid tumors. The tumor is usually discovered between the ages of 30 and 55 years, unlike dermoid tumors, which are usually diagnosed in the first 3 decades of life. Patients may develop symptoms and signs related to the involvement of the acoustico-facial complex or signs of intracranial hypertension or may present with an acute aseptic meningitis due to rupture of the cyst. Due to a signal behavior similar to the CSF and the usual lack of contrast enhancement (Figure 13.7), the tumor may be difficult to diagnose.

Primary lymphomas of the CNS

The majority of primary CNS lymphomas (PCNSL) are non-Hodgkin lymphoma of the B type. They may develop in immunocompetent patients (usually aged between 50 and 70 years) or in immunocompromised patients (mainly in the following cases: Wiskott-Aldrich syndrome, transplantation, HIV infection, myelopathy associated with human T-lymphotropic virus type I infection, chemotherapy). These latter patients are usually younger. Basal ganglia and the regions around the lateral ventricles are the most common sites. About 20% of patients develop a tumor starting in the posterior fossa (brainstem, cerebellum). Involvement of the eyes occurs in up to 10% of cases. On T1-weighted images, the lesions appear hypointense or isointense. On T2-weighted images, lesions are usually isointense or moderately hyperintense. Gadolinium enhancement is homogeneous. Treatment includes chemotherapy (methotrexate) and radiotherapy. Irradiation carries the risk of cognitive deficits. Steroids exert a rapid cytolytic effect and should be used very cautiously if the neuropathological diagnosis has not been established yet.

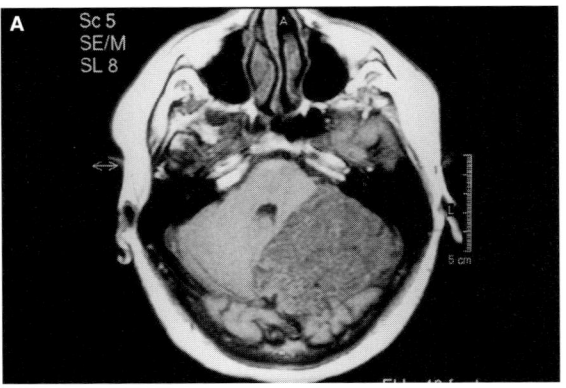
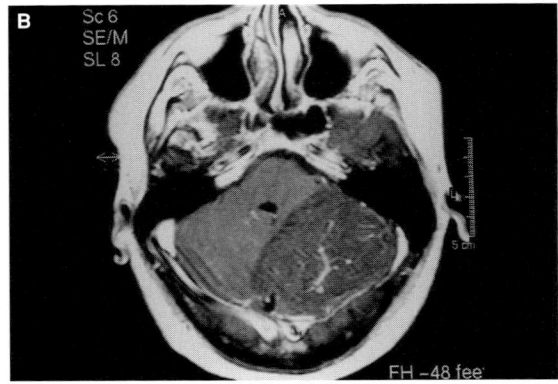
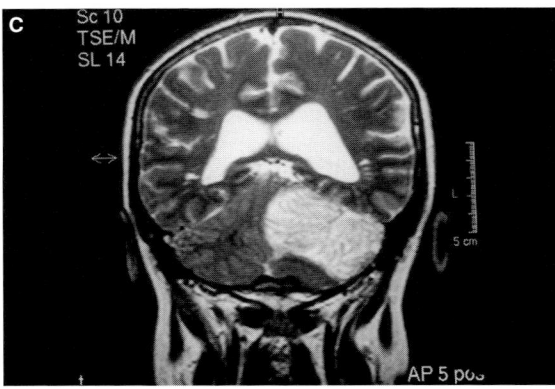

Figure 13.8 Lhermitte-Duclos disease. (A) T1-weighted image showing a heterogeneous mass displacing the fourth ventricle. (B) A suggestive linear enhancement (dilated veins) is visible following contrast administration. (C) Tigroid pattern on coronal T2-weighted image. With permission from: Hildebrand and Balériaux, 2002.

Lhermitte-Duclos disease

This disease may present as an expanding cerebellar lesion, occasionally associated with Cowden disease (multiple hamartoma-neoplasia syndrome). Some authors still consider that Lhermitte-Duclos disease is a malformation rather than a tumor (see Chapter 7). The lesion has a peculiar aspect on brain MRI (Figure 13.8). Typical linear enhancement is observed after contrast injection. T2-weighted images show a folial, "tigroid" aspect. The disease is characterized by high carbon-11 methionine uptake on PET imaging (Van Calenbergh et al., 2006). Surgical removal is recommended. However, recurrence is possible.

Cerebellar metastases

About 10% to 12% of brain metastases are located in posterior fossa. Metastases in the cerebellum have a poorer prognosis than those in the supratentorial compartment. The 1-year survival rate is around 30%. Primary tumors have the following sites: pelvis (prostate, uterus, ovary), digestive tract, lungs, and skin (Pompili et al., 2008). Patients exhibit various combinations of headache (located chiefly in the occipital region), nausea, vomiting, and ataxia of gait/limbs. With time, signs of increased intra-cranial pressure predominate. Metastases in the cerebellum may result in brainstem compression, tonsillar or upwards herniation of the cerebellar tissue. Gadolinium-enhanced MRI is more sensitive than contrast-enhanced CT for detection of metastases. In addition, MRI is superior in differentiating between solitary and multiple lesions. Steroids provide a rapid and effective attenuation of symptoms within 48 hours. Dexamethasone is preferred due to its low mineralocorticoid activity and high CNS penetration (4 mg every 6 hours, preceded by a loading dose if clinically required). Surgery is indicated when there is a need to establish the diagnosis, especially in patients who have no known primary lesion, or in cases of obstructive hydrocephalus to relieve cerebral edema and neurological deficits. Techniques of whole body PET, CT, or MRI allow an earlier detection of occult cancer. Open microneurosurgery with resection should be considered when the lesions appear removable and there is an expected survival of 6 months or more (Hildebrand & Balériaux, 2002). This supposes that the primary cancer is under control. The high postoperative complication rate is rather typical for posterior cranial fossa metastatic disease, especially because a small hematoma in the posterior fossa leads to neurological deterioration that requires a reintervention (Pompili et al., 2008). A large size (>3 cm) is a risk factor. Radiation therapy (usually 30 Gy in 10 fractions) is recommended, both in patients undergoing surgery and those in whom the metastases are not removed. Lesions with a diameter less than 3 cm may benefit from external stereotactic irradiation. Stereotactic radiosurgery (gamma knife, linear accelerator) is gaining attention in brain metastases. Indeed, small metastases are good targets for stereotaxy. They are often well defined with distinct margins on contrast enhancement, and they have a displacing rather than infiltrative effect, unlike gliomas. These characteristics help to achieve highly conformal dose distributions, with minimal damage to surrounding tissues (Wadasadawala et al., 2007). Chemotherapy may control brain seedings in chemosensitive tumors. It should be kept in mind that death is due to systemic cancer lesions in half of patients.

Complications of chemotherapy, phenytoin, lithium salts

The reader is referred to Chapter 15.

Superficial siderosis

Superficial siderosis is a late complication characterized clinically by slowly progressive bilateral hearing loss associated with a cerebellar syndrome, appearing usually in the 5 to 25 years after surgery for a primary cerebellar tumor (Anderson et al., 1999). Other causes include brain trauma and vascular malformations. Patients may also exhibit cognitive deficits and pyramidal signs. The origin of bleeding requires a detailed search, although it may remain undetermined. Fluid-filled collections may be discovered in patients with or without a history of injury or surgical procedure. Occult bleeding in the spinal cord may also cause superficial siderosis; therefore, the workup should also include a detailed search of causes of

bleeding at this level. A dynamic CT myelography may localize the defect, such as a transdural leak. The disease is characterized by deposits of hemosiderin on the leptomeninges. Brain MRI is very suggestive, showing a hypointense rim in T2-weighted images around the cerebellum, brainstem, and cranial nerves (Bracchi et al., 1993; Figure 13.9). A cerebellar cortical atrophy may evolve. CSF analysis shows red blood cells and xanthochromia. Iron-chelating drugs may be tried. Response is limited, but some patients may present with stabilization of symptoms. A favorable response to steroids has been reported (Angstwurm et al., 2002; Le Rhun et al., 2008).

Stroke

Incidence of stroke is higher in cancer patients. Hemorrhagic stroke may be related to intra-tumoral bleeding (especially metastases from germ cell tumors, melanomas, and lung cancer), a coagulation disorder (mainly in leukemia), and hypertension. Ischemic stroke may be due to disseminated intravascular coagulation and embolism from heart disease. Hematomas exerting a mass effect require surgical removal when possible (see also Chapter 8). Control of bleeding related to metastases is favored by radiochemotherapy. Infections and coagulation disorders require specific treatments.

Infections

Opportunistic infections occur mainly in immunocompromised patients or in cases of neutropenia. Patients with leukemia and lymphoma are at risk. The following agents are encountered: *Nocardia asteroides*, *Aspergillus*, *Cryptococcus neoformans*, and *Toxoplasma gondii*. Infections due to *Staphylococcus aureus* or *epidermidis* are found in patients with a previous neurosurgical intervention or carrying a shunt. Treatment of cerebellar abscess is discussed in Chapter 11. Patients who do not respond to antibiotics and those presenting with a mass effect require neurosurgical intervention.

Paraneoplastic cerebellar degeneration

About 50% of the patients who develop paraneoplastic cerebellar degeneration (PCD) have detectable antibodies in serum and/or CSF acting on autoantigens (Table 13.3). Some of these antibodies are

143

Table 13.3 Antibodies found in paraneoplastic cerebellar syndrome

Antibody	Other paraneoplastic syndromes	Primary cancer
Anti-Yo		Gynecologic cancer (ovarian, breast)
Anti-Hu (ANNA-1)	Sensory neuronopathy Encephalomyelitis Limbic encephalitis Autonomic dysfunction	Small-cell lung carcinoma (++) Non–small-cell lung carcinoma Neuroblastoma Prostate carcinoma Sarcoma
Anti-CV2	Limbic encephalitis Encephalomyelitis Polyneuropathy	Small-cell lung carcinoma (++) Uterine sarcoma Malignant thymoma Germ cell tumors of testis
Anti-Tr		Hodgkin disease
Anti-Ri (ANNA-2)	Opsoclonus-myoclonus (++) Encephalomyelitis	Breast carcinoma Small-cell lung carcinoma
Anti-MA1	Brainstem dysfunction Myoclonus	Parotid carcinoma Breast carcinoma Colon carcinoma
Anti-Zic4[a]		Small-cell lung carcinoma Merkel cell tumor
Anti-mGluR1		Hodgkin disease

[a]Possible association with other onconeuronal antibodies (Hu, CV2, Ri).

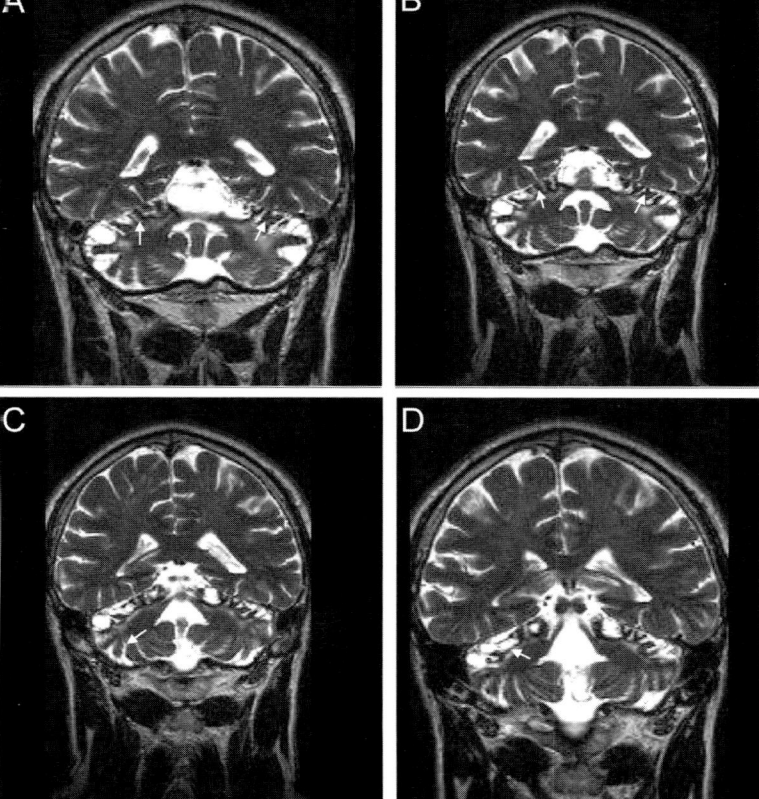

Figure 13.9 Superficial siderosis. Coronal brain MRI images showing hypointense rim around the cerebellum in T2-weighted sequence (arrows in A, B). Widened cerebellar sulci are visible (arrows in C, D). Note the moderate atrophy of cerebral sulci.

specific for a given cancer. The development of PCD prior to the diagnosis of PCD is a common finding (Hildebrand & Balériaux, 2002). The cerebellar syndrome often has a subacute course, evolving over a period of several weeks, although some patients are admitted for a pseudo-acute cerebellar ataxia mimicking cerebellitis or a systemic immune disease with neurological complications (see Chapter 9 and Chapter 11). Other possibilities to consider are the use of toxic agents (such as 5-fluorouracil [5-FU]) or alcohol abuse. Investigations are listed in Table 13.4. CSF shows typically inflammatory changes, and oligoclonal bands may be found. FDG-PET scan and single-photon emission CT may reveal cerebellar hypermetabolism and increased regional perfusion at the acute stage of the disease due to the inflammatory reaction (Choi et al., 2006). Follow-up of brain imaging may demonstrate cerebellar atrophy, despite a stability or even a slight improvement of the neurological status (Figures 13.10 and 13.11). Immunostaining (serum, CSF) is an important step for the diagnosis of PCD. False-positive high titers of antibodies are very rare.

The leading hypothesis regarding the pathogenesis of PCD is an immune reaction triggered or mediated by antibodies. Several immunomodulatory treatments have been proposed (plasmapheresis, intravenous immunoglobulins, immunoabsorption). Steroids are used by some authors, but the scientific basis is often unclear. A proportion of patients may improve clin-

Table 13.4 Recommended investigations in patients presenting with paraneoplastic cerebellar degeneration

Thorough physical examination and clinical follow-up

Blood studies (including tumor markers)

Serum and CSF antibody testing

Whole-body PET, CT, or MRI

Mammography

Bronchoscopy

ically if the treatment is administered at an early phase (Stark et al., 1995). Rapid treatment of the primary cancer (tumor resection, radiation, and/or chemotherapy, according to the cancer) might stop the progression of PCD in some cases. Functional outcome depends on the type of antibody and the primary cancer. Anti-Ri syndrome may recover spontaneously and might carry the best prognosis in PCD. However, surviving patients may exhibit a severe residual pancerebellar syndrome, becoming wheelchair-bound. Close follow-up for several years should be performed in all patients developing a subacute cerebellar syndrome with positive antibodies and in whom a primary tumor has not been found. The majority of these patients will develop a detectable malignancy.

Langerhans histiocytosis

Langerhans histiocytosis (histiocytosis X) is a rare disease characterized by proliferation of Langerhans cells,

Figure 13.10 A 66-year-old man with paraneoplastic cerebellar degeneration. Anti-Tr antibodies were found to be associated with Hodgkin lymphoma. (A, B) Sagittal T1-weighted images at 4 years of interval show progressive atrophy of the vermis with enlargement of the pericerebellar spaces, despite a favorable response of Hodgkin lymphoma to treatment. The pons is spared. (C, D) Coronal T2-weighted images show the development of atrophy of the cerebellar hemisphere, with enlargement of the fourth ventricle.

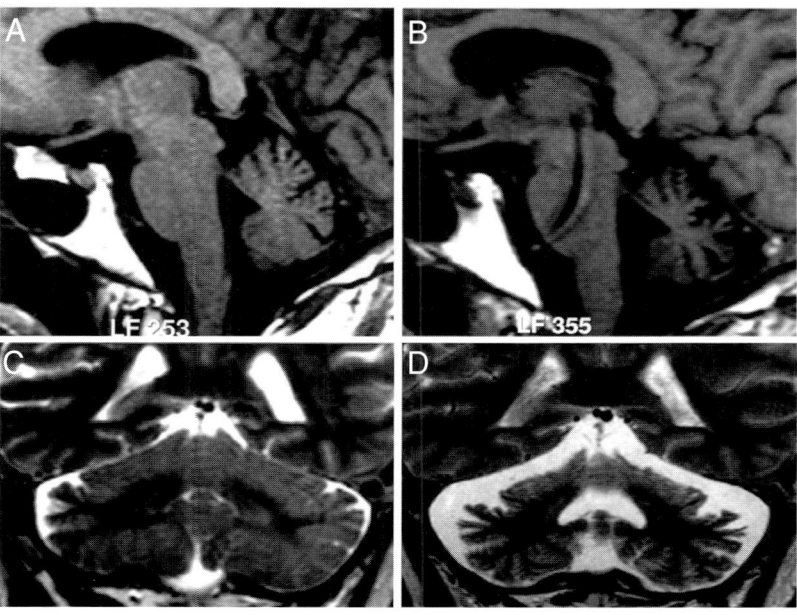

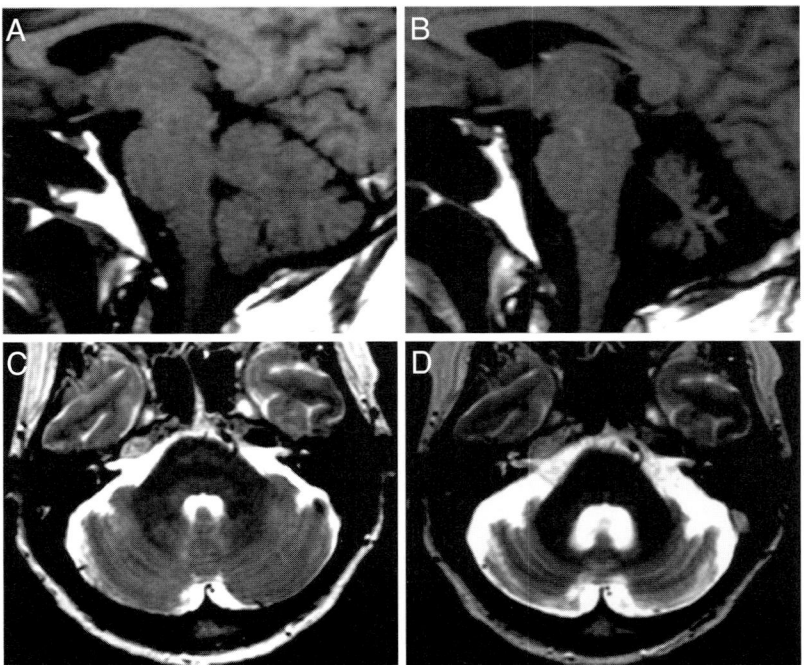

Figure 13.11 A 57-year-old man with paraneoplastic cerebellar degeneration (anti-CV2 antibodies associated with a thymic carcinoma). (A, B) Sagittal T1-weighted images at 4 years of interval show progressive atrophy of the vermis with enlargement of the cerebellar sulci. Cerebellar peduncles are spared. (C, D) Axial T2-weighted images show progressive atrophy of the cerebellar hemispheres.

usually affecting children and young adults. Definitive diagnosis relies upon the demonstration of characteristic Birbeck granules in cells and CD1a antigen on the cell surface. The clinical presentation is variable. All organs can be affected. CNS complications, classified as "tumor-like" or "neurodegenerative-like," occur in about 5% of cases (Donadieu et al., 2004). Intra-cranial granulomatous infiltration generates raised intra-cranial pressure and focal deficits. Diabetes insipidus is due to a direct hypothalamic or pituitary invasion. Cerebellar ataxia associated with brainstem deficits and cognitive decline is a known complication. Cerebellar white matter lesions are found on MRI, appearing as symmetrical non-enhancing T2 hyperintense and variable T1 hypointense areas. An evocative butterfly aspect of the dentate nuclei may be observed on coronal images (Martin-Duverneuil et al., 2006). Cerebellar atrophy has been reported. Its severity might be correlated to the gravity of cerebellar symptoms. Acute ataxia in children is an exceptional presentation (Polizzi et al., 2002). Differential diagnosis includes in particular leukodystrophies, mitochondrial encephalopathies, and toxic lesions. A remote effect of the disease on cerebellar tissue (paraneoplastic presentation, see previous section Paraneoplastic cerebellar degeneration) has been advocated by some authors when the cerebellar deficits are not associated with a direct infiltration (Goldberg-Stern et al., 1995). Treatment of Langerhans histiocytosis manifesting with cerebellar ataxia with a combination of intravenous immunoglobulin (given monthly or twice monthly at the dosage of 250–400 mg/kg/dose) and chemotherapy (steroids ± vinblastine ± 6-mercaptopurine ± methotrexate) has been associated with a stabilization of neurological deficits during a 30-month follow-up period (Imashuku et al., 2008). Further studies are needed to confirm these observations.

Erdheim-Chester disease

Erdheim-Chester disease is a non-Langerhans form of histiocytosis characterized by xanthomatous tissue infiltration with foamy histiocytes. The disease typically infiltrates the medullary portion of the diaphysis and metaphysis of long bones, with a characteristic radiological pattern dominated by bone sclerosis. Intra-cranial manifestations are rare. The usual localizations are the retro-orbital space, causing exophthalmos or diplopia, and the hypothalamic area, explaining the neurogenic diabetes insipidus. Patients may present with a progressive cerebellar syndrome associated with pyramidal deficits (Pautas et al., 1998). Cerebral MRI shows bilateral increased signal intensity in peridentatal regions on T2-weighted sequences. In other cases, ataxia is associated with histiocytic infiltration of the pons and middle cerebellar peduncles (Evidente et al., 1998). Lesions can mimic demyelinating plaques in the periventricular white matter (Bohlega et al., 1997). Bone radiography shows suggestive lesions with patchy sclerosis and osteolysis in the distal parts of the long bones. Skeletal scintigraphy shows symmetrically increased uptake of the tracer. A "hairy kidney" appearance on abdominal CT scan is evocative. The other organs which can be affected by the disorder are the lungs and heart. Treatment with pulsed corticosteroids, cyclophosphamide, or interferon-alpha is recommended (Haroche et al., 2006). Bisphosphonates might be helpful. Some authors suggest radiation therapy for bone involvement (Matsui et al., 2007). However, prognosis is poor in aggressive cases.

References

Anderson NE, Sheffield S, Hope JK. Superficial siderosis of the central nervous system: a late complication of cerebellar tumors. *Neurology* 1999;**52**:163–9.

Angstwurm K, Schielke E, Zimmer C, Kivelitz D, Weber JR. Superficial siderosis of the central nervous system: response to steroid therapy. *J Neurol* 2002;**249**(9):1223–5.

Barbaro NM, Gutin PH, Wilson CB, et al. Radiation therapy in the treatment of partially resected meningiomas. *Neurosurgery* 1987;**20**:525–8.

Bertolone SJ, Yates AJ, Boyett JM, et al. Combined modality therapy for poorly differentiated gliomas of the posterior fossa in children: a Children's Cancer Group report. *J Neurooncol* 2003;**63**:49–54.

Bohlega S, Alwatban J, Tulbah A, Bakheet SM, Powe J. Cerebral manifestation of Erdheim-Chester disease: clinical and radiologic findings. *Neurology* 1997;**49**(6):1702–5.

Bracchi M, Savoiardo M, Triulzi F, et al. Superficial siderosis of the CNS: MR diagnosis and clinical finding. *Am J Neuroradiol* 1993;**14**:227–36.

Choi KD, Kim JS, Park SH, et al. Cerebellar hypermetabolism in paraneoplastic cerebellar degeneration. *J Neurol Neurosurg Psychiatry* 2006;**77**:525–8.

Clarke JW, Hadziahmetovic M, Tzou K, et al. What is the best adjuvant treatment for very young patients with medulloblastoma? *Expert Rev Neurother* 2007;**7**:373–81.

Cohen BH, Packer RJ. Chemotherapy for medulloblastoma and primitive neuroectodermal tumors. *J Neurooncol* 1996;**29**:55–68.

Conway JE, Chou D, Clatterbuck RE, et al. Hemangioblastomas of the central nervous system in von Hippel-Lindau syndrome and sporadic disease. *Neurosurgery* 2001;**48**(1):55–62.

Donadieu J, Rolon MA, Thomas C, et al. Endocrine involvement in pediatric-onset Langerhans' cell histiocytosis: a population-based study. *J Pediatr* 2004;**144**:344–50.

Evidente VG, Adler CH, Giannini C, et al. Erdheim-Chester disease with extensive intraaxial brain stem lesions presenting as a progressive cerebellar syndrome. *Mov Disord* 1998;**13**(3):576–81.

Ferretti E, De Smaele E, Miele E, et al. Concerted microRNA control of Hedgehog signalling in cerebellar neuronal progenitor and tumour cells. *EMBO J* 2008;**27**(19):2616–27.

Fujino K, Naito Y, Tsuji J, et al. Vertigo as the sole presenting symptom of cerebellopontine angle meningioma. *Acta Otolaryngol Suppl* 2007;**557**: 12–14.

Goldberg-Stern H, Weitz R, Zaivov R, et al. Progressive spinocerebellar degeneration "plus" associated with Langerhans cell histiocytosis: a new paraneoplastic syndrome? *J Neurol Neurosurg Psychiatry* 1995;**58**:180–3.

Goldwein JW, Radcliffe J, Packer RJ, et al. Results of a pilot study of low-dose craniospinal radiation therapy plus chemotherapy for children younger than 5 years with primitive neuroectodermal tumors. *Cancer* 1993;**71**:2647–52.

Haroche J, Amoura Z, Trad SG, et al. Variability in the efficacy of interferon-alpha in Erdheim-Chester disease by patient and site of involvement: results in eight patients. *Arthritis Rheum* 2006;**54**(10):3330–6.

Healey EA, Barnes PD, Kupsky WJ, et al. The prognostic significance of postoperative residual tumor in ependymoma. *Neurosurgery* 1991;**28**:666–72.

Hildebrand J, Balériaux D. In The *Cerebellum and Its Disorders*, ed. M. Manto and M. Pandolfo. Cambridge, UK: Cambridge University Press, 2002, pp. 265–87.

Imashuku S, Okazaki NA, Nakayama M, et al; Japan LCH Study Group. Treatment of neurodegenerative CNS disease in Langerhans cell histiocytosis with a combination of intravenous immunoglobulin and chemotherapy. *Pediatr Blood Cancer* 2008;**50**(2):308–11.

147

Iwai Y, Yamanaka K, Yamagata K, Yasui T. Surgery after radiosurgery for acoustic neuromas: surgical strategy and histological findings. *Neurosurgery* 2007;**60**(2 suppl 1):ONS75–82.

Jagannathan J, Lonser RR, Smith R, DeVroom HL, Oldfield EH. Surgical management of cerebellar hemangioblastomas in patients with von Hippel-Lindau disease. *J Neurosurg* 2008;**108**(2):210–22.

Lee DJ, Westra WH, Staecker H, et al. Clinical and histopathologic features of recurrent vestibular schwannoma (acoustic neuroma) after stereotactic radiosurgery. *Otol Neurotol* 2003;**24**(4):650–60.

Le Rhun E, Soto Ares G, Pécheux N, Destée A, Defebvre L. Superficial hemosiderosis of the central nervous system improved by corticosteroids. *Rev Neurol (Paris)* 2008;**164**(3):264–70.

Littman P, Jarret P, Bilaniuk LT, et al. Pediatric brainstem gliomas. *Cancer* 1980;**45**:2787–92.

Martin-Duverneuil N, Idbaih A, Hoang-Xuan K, et al. MRI features of neurodegenerative Langerhans cell histiocytosis. *Eur Radiol* 2006;**16**:2074–82.

Matsui K, Nagata Y, Hiraoka M. Radiotherapy for Erdheim-Chester disease. *Int J Clin Oncol* 2007;**12**(3):238–41.

Metellus P, Barrie M, Figarella-Branger D, et al. Multicentric French study on adult intracranial ependymomas: prognostic factors analysis and therapeutic considerations from a cohort of 152 patients. *Brain* 2007;**130**:1338–49.

Padovani L, Sunyach MP, Perol D, et al. Common strategy for adult and pediatric medulloblastoma: a multi-center series of 253 adults. *Int J Radiat Oncol Biol Phys* 2007;**68**:433–40.

Pautas E, Chérin P, Pelletier S, Vidailhet M, Herson S. Cerebral Erdheim-Chester disease: report of two cases with progressive cerebellar syndrome with dentate abnormalities on magnetic resonance imaging. *J Neurol Neurosurg Psychiatry* 1998;**65**(4):597–9.

Polizzi A, Coghill S, McShane MA, Squier W. Acute ataxia complicating Langerhans histiocytosis. *Arch Dis Child* 2002;**86**:130–1.

Pollock BE, Lundsford LD, Kondziolka D, et al. Outcome analysis of acoustic neuroma management: a comparison of microsurgery and stereotactic radiosurgery. *Neurosurgery* 1995;**36**:215–25.

Pompili A, Carapella CM, Cattani F, et al. Metastases to the cerebellum. Results and prognostic factors in a consecutive series of 44 operated patients. *J Neurooncol* 2008;**88**(3):331–7.

Richard S, Giraud S, Beroud C, et al. Von Hippel-Lindau disease: recent genetic progress and patient management. Francophone Study Group of von Hippel-Lindau Disease (GEFVH). *Ann Endocrinol (Paris)* 1998;**59**(6):452–8.

Roujeau T, Machado G, Garnett MR, et al. Stereotactic biopsy of diffuse pontine lesions in children. *J Neurosurg* 2007;**107**(1 suppl):1–4.

Rudnik A, Larysz D, Gamrot J, et al. Idiopathic hypertrophic pachymeningitis: case report and literature review. *Folia Neuropathol* 2007;**45**(1):36–42.

Schrell UM, Rittig MG, Anders M, et al. Hydroxyurea for treatment of unresectable and recurrent meningiomas. Decrease in the size of meningiomas in patients treated by hydroxyurea. *J Neurosurg* 1997;**86**:840–5.

Shu HK, Sall WF, Maity A, et al. Childhood intracranial ependymoma: twenty-year experience from a single institution. *Cancer* 2007;**110**:432–41.

Stark E, Wurster U, Patzold U, et al. Immunological and clinical response to immunosuppressive treatment in paraneoplastic cerebellar degeneration. *Arch Neurol* 1995;**52**:814–8.

Tait DM, Thornton-Jones H, Bloom HJ, et al. Adjuvant chemotherapy for medulloblastoma: the first multicentre control trial of the International Society of Paediatric Oncology (SIOP I). *Eur J Cancer* 1990;**26**:464–9.

Van Calenbergh F, Vantomme N, Flamen P, et al. Lhermitte-Duclos disease: 11C-methionine positron emission tomography data in 4 patients. *Surg Neurol* 2006;**65**:293–6.

Wadasadawala T, Gupta S, Bagul V, Patil N. Brain metastases from breast cancer: management approach. *J Cancer Res Ther* 2007;**3**(3):157–65.

Wetmore C. Sonic hedgehog in normal and neoplastic proliferation: insight gained from human tumors and animal models. *Curr Opin Genet Dev* 2003;**13**(1):34–42.

Yu CP, Cheung JY, Leung S, Ho R. Sequential volume mapping for confirmation of negative growth in vestibular schwannomas treated by gamma knife radiosurgery. *J Neurosurg* 2000;**93**(suppl 3):82–9.

Trauma of the posterior fossa

The cerebellum and brainstem are often damaged simultaneously following traumatic injuries, due to their proximity and anatomical links. Penetrating injuries or fractures usually cause liquorrhea in open head injuries (Maschke et al., 2002). The vertebrobasilar system may be involved, with dissection of the vessels and secondary infarction (see also Chapter 8). The primary trauma carries the risk of secondary complications triggered by edema, increased intra-cranial pressure, or infection (Keidel & Miller, 1996), contributing to morbidity and mortality. Trauma of the posterior fossa is indeed a potential cause of death, especially in children, young adults, and the elderly. Car and motorcycle accidents, falls, ethanol consumption, and abuse in children are the most common causes.

Clinical presentation

When consciousness is impaired (up to coma on admission), cerebellar deficits cannot be assessed, so that the cerebellar syndrome is overlooked. Patients awake or with mild impairment of consciousness complain of mild to severe headache and vertigo. Nausea and vomiting should immediately raise the possibility of increased intra-cranial pressure. Cerebellar deficits associated with acute injuries of the cerebellum have been extensively described by Holmes, extending from mild unilateral deficits to a pancerebellar syndrome (Holmes, 1917). Partial or full Wallenberg syndrome in patients with a history of cervical trauma suggests a vessel dissection (see below). Cerebellar mutism has been described in children with cerebellar trauma (Bramanti et al., 1994).

Types of trauma

Categories of lesions are given in Table 14.1.

Concussion is associated with transient dysfunction of neural function. Patients may exhibit impaired consciousness. Amnesia of the trauma is common.

Some such patients are at risk for developing a post-traumatic concussion disorder characterized by headache, anxiety, disequilibrium, and fatigue, even following a "minor" head injury (Levin et al., 1987). *Contusion* of the posterior fossa, occurring in most cases after a severe injury, is due to the peak forces evolving at the site of the impact ("coup") or may result from a "contrecoup" phenomenon (Figure 14.1). Microhemorrhages around small vessels generate local hematoma, with dimensions varying according to the intensity and location of the trauma. Microbleedings occasionally merge in a larger hematoma several hours after the impact (Gudeman et al., 1979).

Contusion is often associated with *diffuse axonal injury* resulting from shearing forces (Adams et al., 1982). The following brain areas are the usual sites: mesencephalon, diencephalon, corpus callosum, periventricular zones, and gray matter–white matter junctions. Repeated head injuries (e.g. as in boxing) generate a traumatic encephalopathy made of frontal signs, memory deficits, parkinsonian signs, and cerebellar deficits, including dysarthria, kinetic tremor, and imbalance.

Uncal and tonsillar herniation are life-threatening complications. When penetrating brainstem vessels are elongated, a secondary brainstem hemorrhage occurs by a mechanism of ischemia-reperfusion (also called "Duret hemorrhage") (Figure 14.2).

Subarachnoid hemorrhage is classical in severe trauma. One of the complications is vasospasm generating ischemic insults.

Table 14.1 Types of posterior fossa trauma

Intra-axial lesions	Extra-axial lesions
Concussion	Epidural hematoma
Contusion	Subdural hematoma
Diffuse axonal injury	Subarachnoid hemorrhage
Secondary lesions (herniation, ischemia, bleeding)	Traumatic vascular lesion

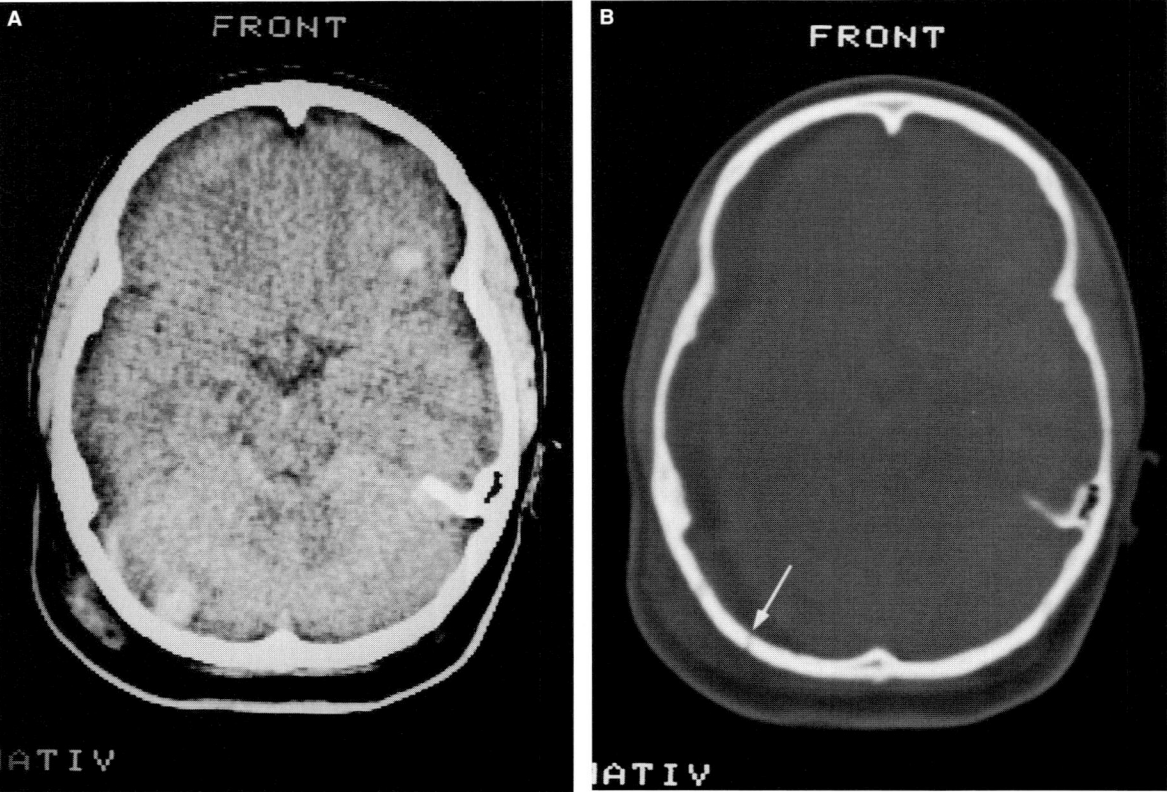

Figure 14.1 Cerebellar contusion of the cerebellum. (A) A hyperdense hematoma is visible on the right cerebellar hemisphere, with a concomitant frontobasal hematoma (contrecoup contusion). (B) Bone window showing an occipital fracture with overlying soft tissue swelling. With permission from: Maschke et al., 2002.

Subdural hematoma of the posterior fossa with collection of blood between the arachnoid and the meningeal layer of the dura is relatively rare in traumatic lesions of the brain. Brain MRI is very suggestive, showing a "hematocrit effect" in T1-weighted images (Figure 14.3).

Epidural hematoma – due to bleeding of meningeal vessels, diploic veins, or sinuses – appears more frequently in children than in adults. A majority of patients have a skull fracture. A lucid interval between the trauma and the clinical deficits usually lasts a few hours and happens in up to half of patients. The hematoma appears biconvex (Figure 14.4).

Dissection of the vessel wall is another potential complication of head trauma. This latter is sometimes minor in intensity and may even be overlooked. Occlusion of the lumen of the vessel, arterioarterial embolism, may result, with possible cerebellar stroke (Figure 14.5). Sudden cervico-occipital pain combined with brainstem deficits or lateral medullary syndrome is suggestive of a dissection of the vertebral artery. Exceptionally, traumatic aneurysm of cerebellar arteries develops. Traumatic dissection of the vertebral arteries has a higher incidence than dissection of carotid arteries (Reid & Weigelt, 1988).

Investigations

The evaluation of posterior fossa trauma is given in Table 14.2. Imaging plays a key role. CT scan is a sensitive technique which has the capacity to confirm hemorrhage or mass effect. Nevertheless, MRI is superior for detecting small lesions in the posterior fossa. Results of neuroimaging investigations are summarized in Table 14.3. Single-photon emission CT and positron emission tomography studies may detect subtle abnormalities in various regions of the brain and may show a crossed cerebellar diaschisis, characterized by a decreased perfusion or metabolism in a cerebellar

Table 14.2 Evaluation of posterior fossa trauma

Detailed repeated physical/neurological examination

Glasgow Coma Scale

Ultrasonography of neck vessels (Doppler)

Brain imaging: CT, MRI, MRA, single-photon emission CT, positron emission tomography

Conventional angiography (in case of suspicion of a dissection not detected by Doppler/MR)

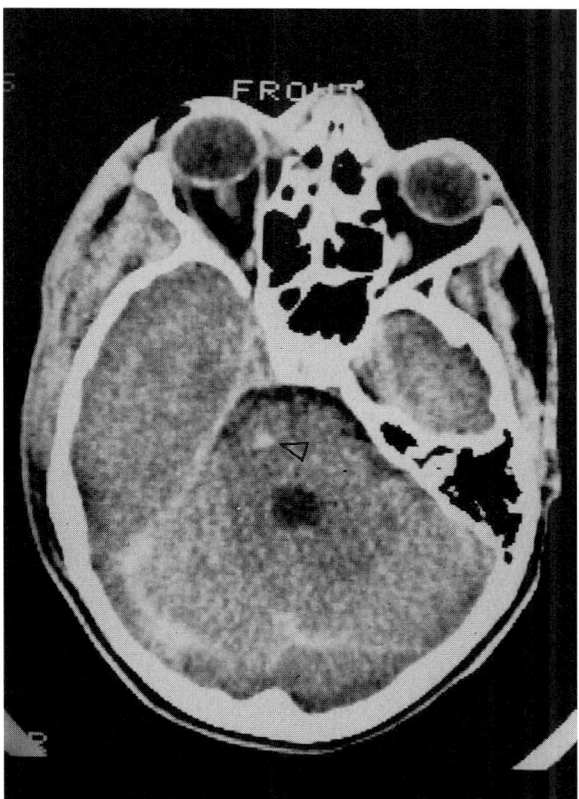

Figure 14.2 Duret hemorrhage. Brain CT scan in a patient with delayed hemorrhage in the pons (open triangle) following head injury with brain swelling and subarachnoid hemorrhage. With permission from: Maschke et al., 2002.

hemisphere contralaterally to a cerebral hemispheric trauma (Alavi et al., 1997). A hypermetabolic cerebellar vermis is a common finding (Lupi et al., 2007; Figure 14.6).

Management

The first line in the management of posterior fossa trauma aims to control vital functions and to treat increased intra-cranial pressure (see Table 14.4) (Miller, 1997). Steroids are not recommended (Miller, 1997). Patients should be transferred to a rehabilitation unit after the acute phase. Intense physical therapy with a focus on postural training and speech rehabilitation might improve functional capacities.

Late complications

Patients may develop late complications. *Delayed onset cerebellar syndrome* refers to the appearance of cerebellar deficits between 3 weeks and 2 years after trauma (Louis et al., 1996). The syndrome may take a progressive course, with a worsening over a few months. The pathogenesis might be a hypersensitivity of post-synaptic sites within the cerebellar outflow tracts (see Chapter 1). A proportion of patients exhibit a so-called "delayed-onset intention tremor." In others, tremor is present at rest, during postural tasks, and during movement (midbrain tremor). Children with a history of moderate to severe traumatic brain injury (Glasgow Coma Scale raging from 3 to 11) due to a vehicle, bicycle, or pedestrian–vehicle crash develop cerebellar atrophy of the white matter as demonstrated by quantitative MRI performed at a mean post-injury interval of 3.1 ± 2.4 years (Spanos et al., 2007). Loss of cerebellar gray matter has been documented (Gale et al., 2005). Autopsy studies confirm a loss of Purkinje neurons and activation of microglia (Matschke et al., 2007). Inflammation, axonal lesions, and excitotoxic mechanisms might contribute to delayed neuronal loss. Deep brain stimulation of the Vim nucleus can improve post-traumatic cerebellar tremor in adults. However, kinetic tremor is more difficult to treat than rest or postural tremor, and proximal tremor tends to be refractory, although there are exceptions (Deuschl & Bain, 2002).

Olivary hypertrophy may be associated with palatal myoclonus (see also Chapter 3), as a consequence of a lesion of the Guillain-Mollaret triangle. Other involuntary movements may be associated, such as myoclonias of the neck or the shoulder. Cerebellar symptoms are contralateral to the site of hypertrophy when this latter develops unilaterally. Olivary hypertrophy develops several months to several years after the trauma. Brain MRI shows abnormal signals in the inferior olive (Birbamer et al., 1994). Figure 14.7 illustrates an example. Lesions need to be distinguished from vascular, infectious, inflammatory, or neoplastic causes.

Table 14.3 Results of imaging studies in posterior fossa trauma

Lesion	CT scan	MRI
Cerebellar contusion	Ill-defined hypodense area (edema) Punctuate hyperdense areas (bleeding) Note: possible bone fracture and often swelling of soft tissues	T1-weighted images: from hypointense (early stage) to hyperintense area (later stage) T2-weighted images: hyperintense area (edema)
Cerebellar hematoma	Hyperdense area, possible mass effect with hydrocephalus Possible ring enhancement surrounding the hematoma	
Subarachnoid hemorrhage	Hyperdense fluid in the cisterns, in the sulci, around the falx of cerebellum, in ventricles	
Diffuse axonal injury	Diffuse hypodensity (swelling) Possible mass effect	Multiple areas of increased signal intensity on T2-weighted images
Epidural hematoma	Hyperdense lesion, with a biconvex shape Mass effect is common	T1-weighted images: isointense mass T2-weighted images: hypointense mass
Subdural hematoma	Hyperdense lesion, with a concavo/convex shape Often unilateral in adults and bilateral in children	T1-weighted images: hypo/isointense on the top and hyperintense on the bottom ("hematocrit-like effect") T2-weighted images: hyperintense/isointense on the top and hypointense on the bottom
Dissection of vessels	Hypodense area (infarction)	Intramural hematoma, vessel occlusion, pseudoaneurysm[a]

[a]May be demonstrated by MRA.

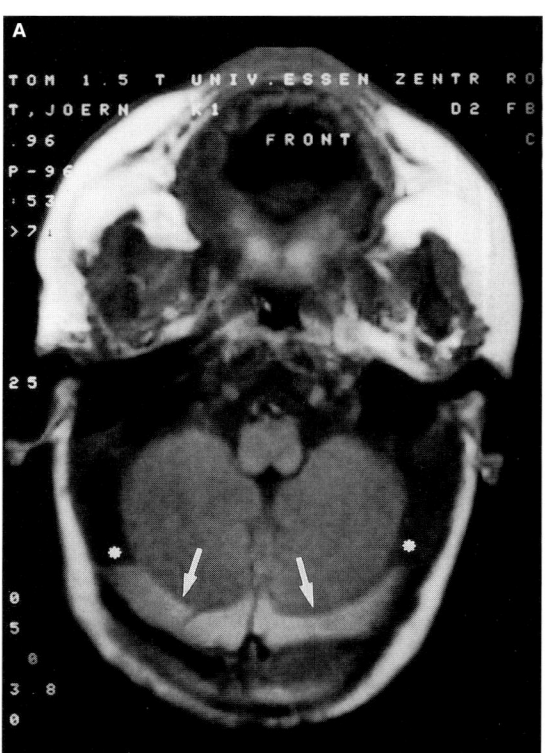 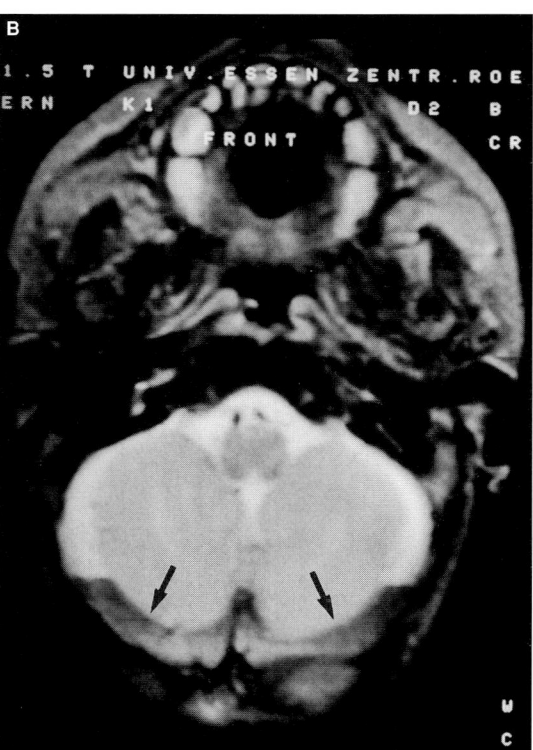

Figure 14.3 Bilateral subdural hematoma of the posterior fossa. (A) T1-weighted axial MRI shows fluid levels ("hematocrit effect") due to sedimentation of erythrocytes (arrows). Asterisks corresponds to serum. (B) T2-weighted image showing a dark aspect of the hematoma (arrows). With permission from: Maschke et al., 2002.

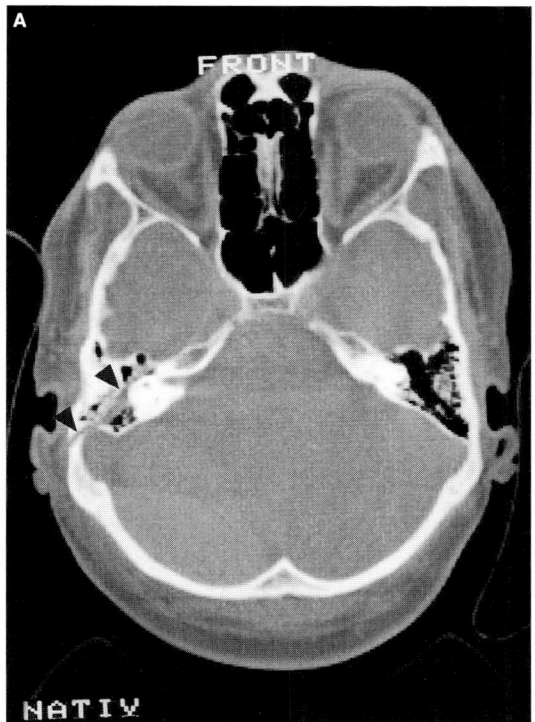

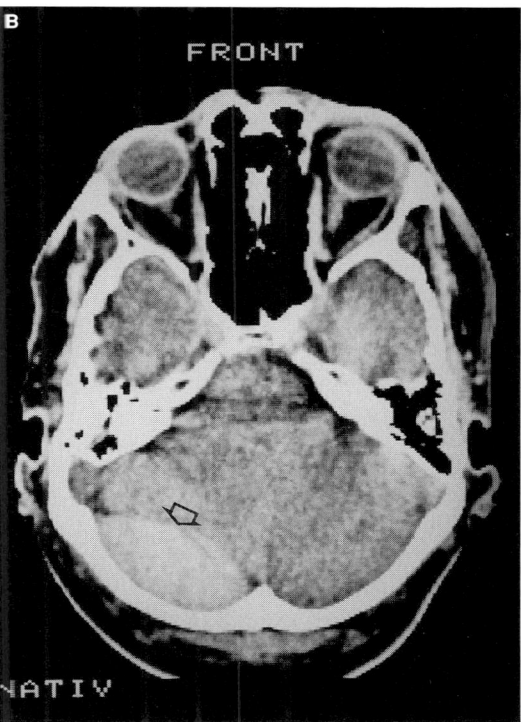

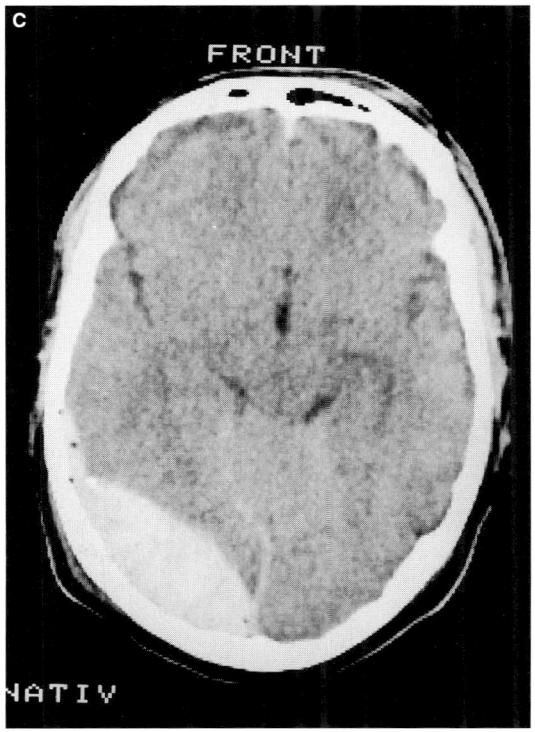

Figure 14.4 Epidural hematoma of the posterior fossa. (A) (bone w ndow) Triangles indicate a fracture of the right temporal bone extending to the sulcus of the sigmoid sinus. (B, C) Biconvex hematoma extending above the tentorium cerebella. With permission from: Maschke et al., 2002.

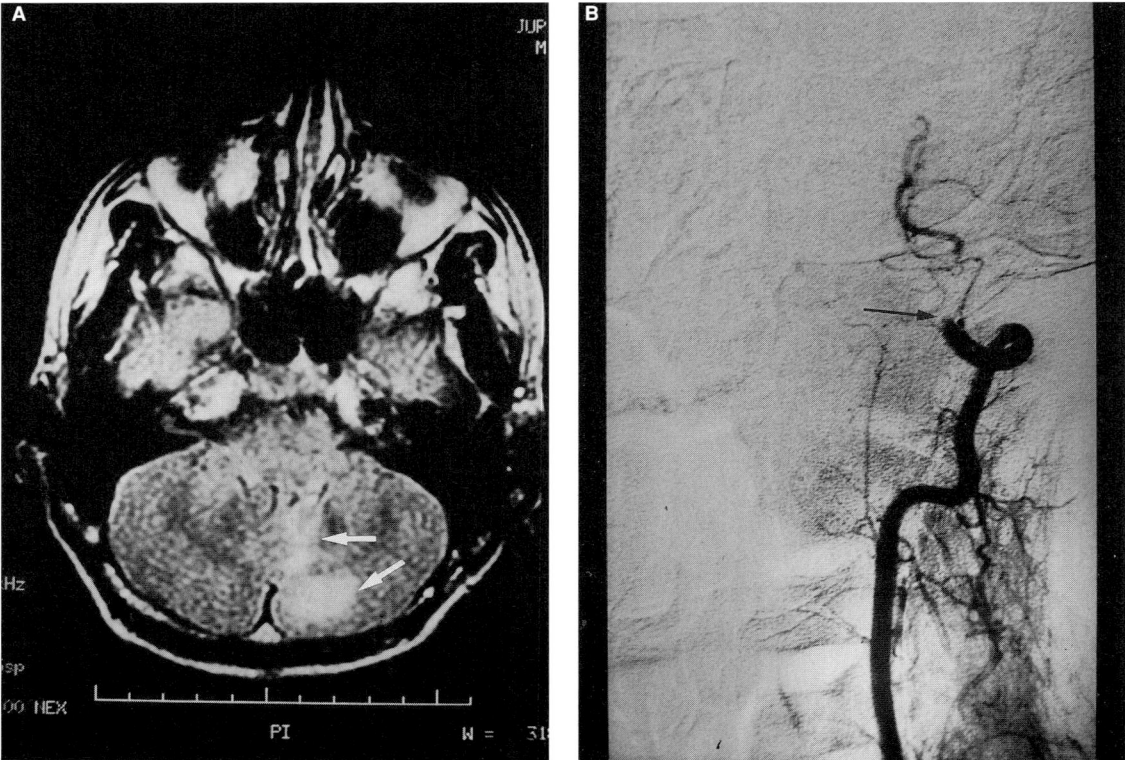

Figure 14.5 Dissection of the vertebral artery. (A) Infarction in the territory of the PICA (arrows) on axial MRI. (B) Angiography shows an arterial occlusion of the vertebral artery (arrow). From: Maschke et al., 2002. With permission.

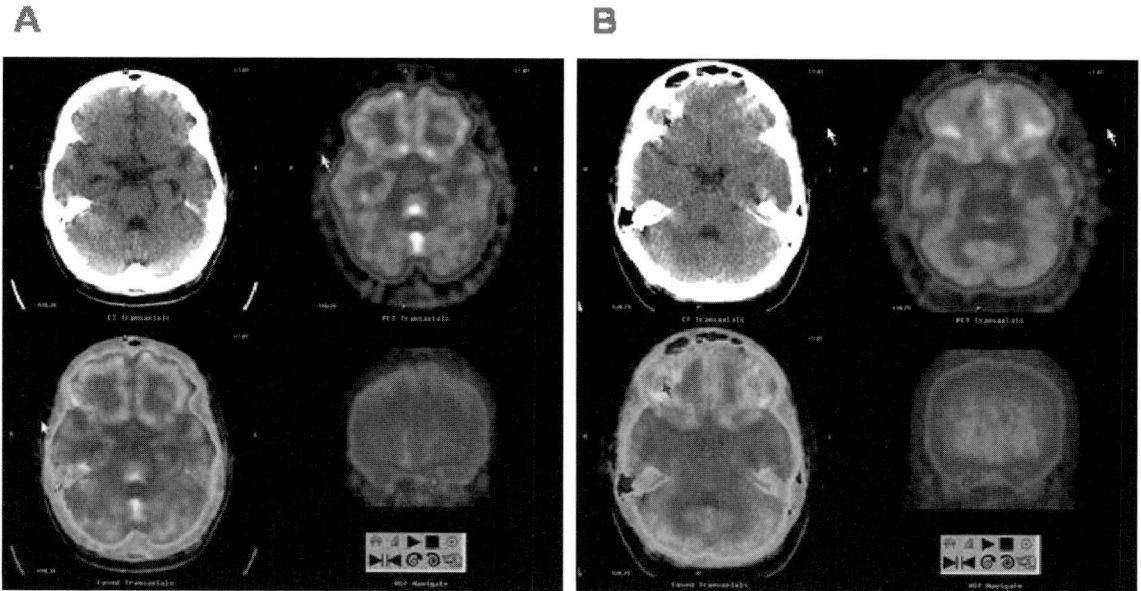

Figure 14.6 (A) Relative hypermetabolism of the cerebellar vermis and pons in a patient with post-anoxic coma. (B) Control case. From: Lupi et al., 2007. With permission. (See color section.)

Table 14.4. Management of posterior fossa trauma

Acute phase
  Cautious mobilization of patients
  Monitoring and management of vital functions (stabilization
    of vital parameters)
  Immediate brain imaging (CT or MRI)
  Monitoring of intra-cranial pressure in severe head injury
  Increased intra-cranial pressure

  Hyperventilation
    Administration of osmotic agents (mannitol), diuretics,
      barbiturates
    Drainage in case of obstructive hydrocephalus
    Surgical decompression in case of severe edema

  Management of space-occupying lesions
    Surgical evacuation of hematoma (epidural, subdural)
  Dissection
    Anticoagulation (intravenous heparin, followed by
      warfarin)

Chronic phase
  Management of tremor (drugs, Vim stimulation, Botulinum
    toxin)
  Rehabilitation
    Speech rehabilitation
    Physical therapy
    Assistive devices

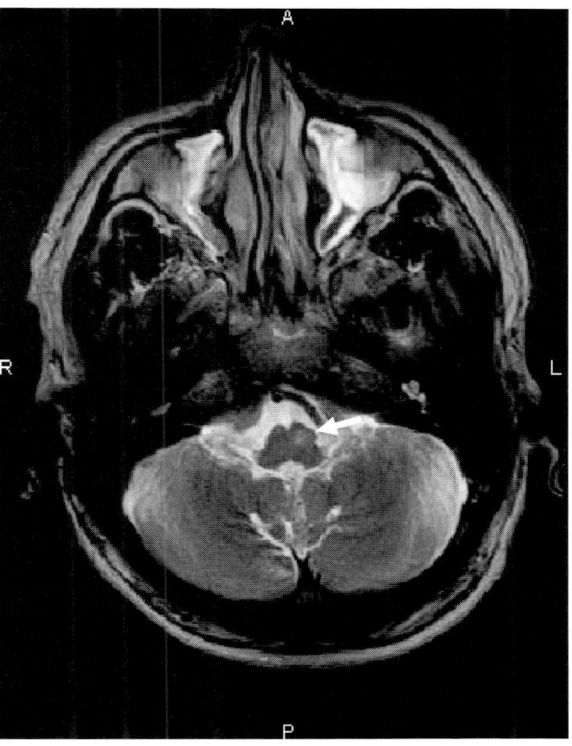

Figure 14.7 Hypertrophy of the left inferior olive (arrow) in a patient with a history of severe brain trauma (axial T2-weighted brain MRI).

Crossed atrophy of the cerebellum develops several months or years after a traumatic cerebral lesion, either by anterograde degeneration of the corticopontocerebellar tract or by retrograde trans-synaptic degeneration of the cerebello-rubrothalamic tract (Tien & Ashdown, 1992). *Superficial siderosis* in discussed in Chapter 13.

Mood disorders and neuropsychological deficits developing several months to a year after trauma of the posterior fossa may occur. There is an association between cerebellar lesions and deficits in visual recognition memory, dyscalculia, and IQ in children after severe traumatic brain injury (Braga et al., 2007).

References

Adams JH, Graham DI, Murray LS, Scott G. Diffuse axonal injury due to non-missile head injury in humans: an analysis of 45 cases. *Ann Neurol* 1982;**12**:557–63.

Alavi A, Mirot A, Newberg A, et al. Fluorine-18-FDG evaluation of crossed cerebellar diaschisis in head injury. *J Nucl Med* 1997;**38**:1717–20.

Birbamer G, Gerstenbrand F, Aichner F, et al. MR imaging of post-traumatic olivary hypertrophy. *Funct Neurol* 1994;**9**:183–7.

Braga LW, Souza LN, Najjar YJ, Dellatolas G. Magnetic resonance imaging (MRI) findings and neuropsychological sequelae in children after severe traumatic brain injury: the role of cerebellar lesion. *J Child Neurol* 2007;**22**(9):1084–9.

Bramanti P, Sessa E, Saltuari L. Post-traumatic mutism. *J Neurosurg Sci* 1994;**38**(2):117–22.

Deuschl G, Bain P. Deep brain stimulation for tremor: patient selection and evaluation. *Mov Disord* 2002; **3**(suppl):S102–11.

Gale SD, Baxter L, Roundy N, Johnson SC. Traumatic brain injury and grey matter concentration: a preliminary voxel based morphometry study. *J Neurol Neurosurg Psychiatry* 2005;**76**(7):984–8.

Gudeman SK, Kishore PR, Miller JD, et al. The genesis and significance of delayed traumatic intracerebral hematoma. *Neurosurgery* 1979;**5**:309–13.

Holmes G. The symptoms of acute cerebellar injuries due to gunshot injuries. *Brain* 1917;**40**:461–535.

Keidel M, Miller JD. Head trauma. In *Neurological Disorders*, ed. T. Brandt, L.R. Caplan, J. Dichgans,

H.C. Diener, and C. Kennard C. San Diego, CA: Academic Press, 1996, pp. 531–44.

Levin HS, Mattis S, Ruff RM, et al. Neurobehavioral outcome following minor head injury. *J Neurosurg* 1987;**66**:234–43.

Louis ED, Lynch T, Ford B, et al. Delayed-onset cerebellar syndrome. *Arch Neurol.* 1996;**53**:450–4.

Lupi A, Bertagnoni G, Salgarello M, et al. Cerebellar vermis relative hypermetabolism: an almost constant PET finding in an injured brain. *Clin Nucl Med* 2007;**32**(6):445–51.

Maschke M, Dietrich U, Timmann-Braun D. Posterior fossa trauma. In *The Cerebellum and Its Disorders*, ed. M. Manto and M. Pandolfo. Cambridge, UK: Cambridge University Press, 2002, pp. 288–304.

Matschke J, Laas R, Schulz F. Cerebellar atrophy following mild head injury in a 4-year-old girl. *Pediatr Neurosurg* 2007;**43**(4):330–3.

Miller JD. Head injury. In *Neurological Emergencies*, ed. R.A.C. Hughes. London: British Medical Group, 1997, pp. 29–49.

Reid JD, Weigelt JA. Forty-three cases of vertebral artery trauma. *J Trauma* 1988;**28**:1007–12.

Spanos GK, Wilde EA, Bigler ED, et al. Cerebellar atrophy after moderate-to-severe pediatric traumatic brain injury. *AJNR Am J Neuroradiol* 2007;**28**(3): 537–42.

Tien RD, Ashdown BC. Crossed cerebellar diaschisis and crossed cerebellar atrophy: correlation of MR findings, clinical symptoms, and supratentorial diseases in 26 patients. *Am J Roentgenol* 1992;**158**:1155–9.

Chapter 15

Toxic agents

Cerebellar toxicity of alcohol

Epidemiological studies have estimated the prevalence of alcohol dependence at about 0.5% to 3% of the population in Europe and in the United States. Chronic ingestion of ethanol can impair both the peripheral nervous system and the CNS. The cerebellum is probably one of the most vulnerable targets to ethanol ingestion in the CNS.

Clinical findings

Cerebellar signs are observed following both acute and chronic ingestion (Gilman et al., 1981). The chief symptom in patients presenting with a cerebellar dysfunction related to alcohol ingestion is difficulty in standing and walking. Most patients report a loss of coordination in lower limbs (Gilman et al., 1990). A suggestive postural lower limb tremor may be observed. Neurological signs observed in adult alcoholic patients are listed in Table 15.1.

Acute intoxication is characterized clinically by slurred speech, gaze-evoked nystagmus, impaired Romberg test, and broad-based ataxic gait. The cerebellar signs tend to become chronic features with chronic alcohol abuse (Gilman et al., 1981). Gait may worsen progressively or may rapidly turn to severe irreversible deficits in cases of malnutrition. Unpredictable exacerbations are uncommon. Typically, legs appear stiff during gait, contrasting with an absence of stiffness in the lying position (Victor et al., 1959).

Patients exhibiting Wernicke encephalopathy present with a combination of mental confusion, oculomotor deficits, and ataxic gait (Zubaran et al., 1997). Typically, a nystagmus is associated with a paralysis of the external rectus muscles causing diplopia. Onset is usual abrupt. Cerebellar ataxia associated with memory deficits and confabulation suggest Korsakoff syndrome. The terminology of Wernicke-Korsakoff is often used. Table 15.2 lists the conditions associated with Wernicke-Korsakoff syndrome.

Patients with chronic alcoholism are at risk for pontine and extra-pontine myelinolysis. Extra-pontine lesions are generally found in the cerebellum, midbrain, thalamus, basal ganglia, and periventricular white matter (Gocht & Colmant, 1987). Myelinolysis can extend in particular to middle cerebellar peduncles (cerebellar peduncular myelinolysis, also reported in patients undergoing hemodialysis for renal failure [Kim et al., 2007]). Hyponatremia, a well-known key factor in the pathogenesis of myelinolysis, is often found (Garzon et al., 2002).

Cerebellar atrophy

Between 27% and 42% of patients presenting with alcoholism have a cerebellar degeneration (Worner, 1993). Although about 25% of these patients have severe liver disease, more than one-fifth of patients with hepatic cirrhosis have no cerebellar signs. It is considered that a daily consumption of 150 g of alcohol during 10 years is associated with significant cerebellar atrophy as demonstrated by brain CT in one-third of patients (Haubek & Lee, 1979).

Concomitant widening of the cerebral sulci is common. A non-enhancing hypodense area around the aqueduct during the acute phase of Wernicke encephalopathy is found in 10% to 20% of cases, often in association with superior vermian atrophy (Gallucci et al., 1990). The discovery of severe cerebellar atrophy on brain CT/MRI in young alcoholic patients in whom neurological examination either is normal or shows only subtle deficits is not rare. Most of them will develop cerebellar deficits several months later. MRI may show various combinations of cerebellar atrophy predominating in the anterior lobe, widening of cerebral sulci, dilatation of ventricles and aqueduct, symmetrical lesions in the periventricular areas and dorsal thalamus, atrophy of mamillary bodies, or enhancement with gadolinium injection. Figure 15.1 illustrates an example of cerebral cortical and cerebellar atrophy.

157

Table 15.1 Neurological features in alcoholic patients

Cerebellar signs

    Gaze-evoked nystagmus, ocular dysmetria

    Slurred speech

    Kinetic tremor

    3-Hz postural leg tremor

    Ataxic gait

    Titubation

    Hypotonia

Decreased tendon reflexes

Amyotrophy

Wernicke encephalopathy

Korsakoff psychosis, dementia

Alcohol withdrawal syndrome

Asterixis

Myoclonus

Seizures

Extensor plantar reflexes

Table 15.2 Conditions associated with Wernicke-Korsakoff syndrome

Alcoholism

Hyperemesis gravidarum

Dialysis

Gastroplasty, intestinal surgery

Prolonged parenteral nutrition without vitamin supplementation

Psychogenic food refusal, beriberi

Patients in critical care units

Therapy-induced: AIDS, chemotherapy, immunosuppressants

Thyrotoxicosis

Pre-natal exposure (fetal alcohol syndrome) may be associated with atrophy of the anterior region of the vermis (lobules I to V), sparing lobules VI to X (Sowell et al., 1996).

Posture and gait studies

Posture and gait analysis may demonstrate an anterior-posterior tremor with a suggestive 3-Hz frequency (Figure 15.2).

Blood studies

There is no correlation between the development of cerebellar signs and laboratory findings. Blood stud-ies often show moderate to marked macrocytic anemia, platelet reduction, impaired liver function tests, sideropenia, and reduced levels of blood transketolase.

Neuropathology

Microscopic changes in the mamillary bodies are the most common findings in autopsied cases (Harper, 1983). Other common sites of damage are the diencephalon/mesencephalon, temporal lobes, frontal lobes, and cerebellum (Fadda & Rossetti, 1998). Autopsies have demonstrated widening of sulci in the cerebellar anterior lobe, with cellular loss in all layers. Purkinje cells are particularly vulnerable. Punctate hemorrhages affecting the gray matter around the third and fourth ventricles are observed in patients with a history of Wernicke encephalopathy. Patchy losses of myelin and diffuse degeneration of neurons occur in association with hepatic disease.

Pathogenesis

Ethanol interferes with neurotransmission and brain metabolism. Glutamatergic pathways, GABAergic pathways, serotoninergic and noradrenergic systems, as well as regulation of nitric oxide production, are affected (Fadda & Rossetti, 1998; Manto et al., 2005). Chronic alcoholism damages neurons containing GABA-A/benzodiazepine receptors in the superior cerebellar vermis in patients showing clinical deficits of alcoholic cerebellar degeneration (Gilman et al., 1996). Ethanol impairs cerebellar glucose metabolic rates. Hypometabolism in the superior cerebellar vermis is associated with decreased cellular and synaptic activity because of neuronal loss (Gilman et al., 1990).

Nutritional deficiencies contribute to cerebellar degeneration. Thiamine deficit is probably a determinant factor. Indeed, thiamine-deficient membranes are particularly susceptible to osmotic stress. A personal vulnerability to ethanol is known. Personal neurological sensitivity could be related to differences in thiamine enzyme systems (Greenwood et al., 1984). Advanced liver disease contributes likely to the neuronal degeneration in the cerebellum, probably because of impaired thiamine metabolism and imbalance in amino acid metabolism (Zubaran et al., 1997).

Experimental studies have revealed ethanol-induced morphometric changes in granule cells and Purkinje neurons (Pentney, 2002). Granule cells display changes in microtubular density in axons. Ethanol

Figure 15.1 Cerebral atrophy in a patient with a history of chronic alcohol abuse. (A, B) Axial T2-weighted images show widening of cerebellar sulci of the anterior lobe. (C, D) Coronal images show atrophy of the cerebellar cortex in different lobules, as well as cerebral cortical atrophy (arrows). (See color section.)

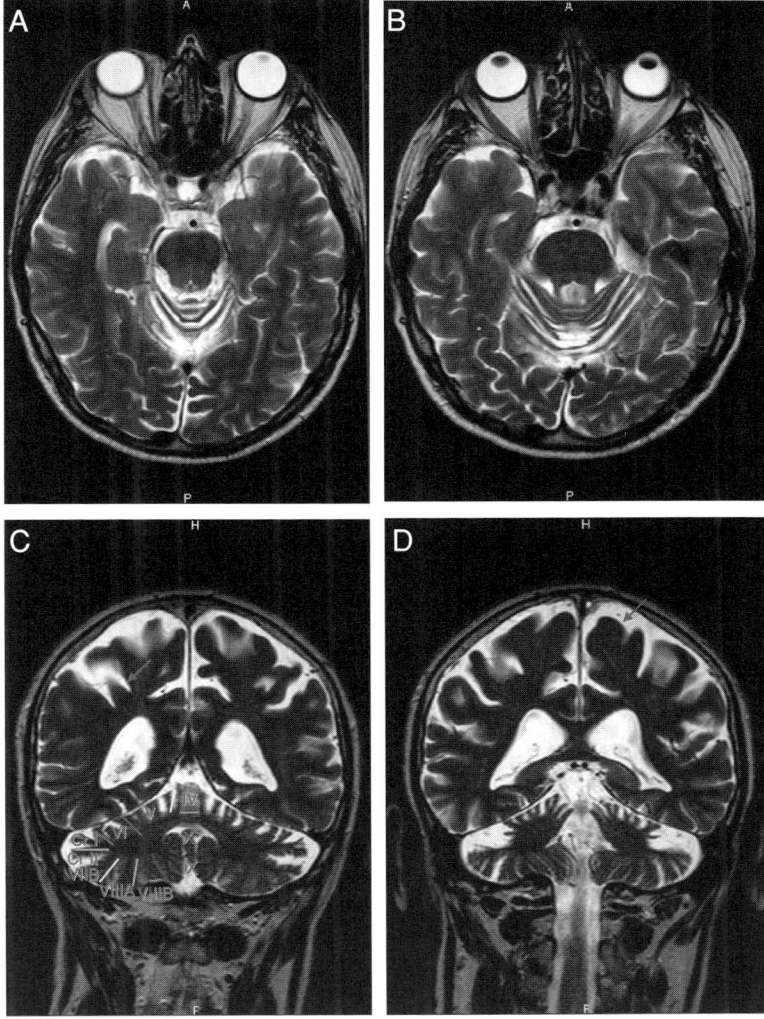

interferes with N-methyl-D-aspartic acid (NMDA) receptors of granule cells, inhibiting the expression of brain-derived neurotrophic factor (Bhave et al., 1999). Ethanol inhibits also insulin-like growth factor 1 signaling and impairs adenosine neurotransmission in granule cells, which are equipped with numerous adenosine A1 receptors. Damage in Purkinje cells results in loss of branches in the dendritic trees and finally in cell death. Increased volume in smooth endoplasmic reticulum is commonly observed

Treatment

Thiamine should be administered without delay to patients presenting a Wernicke-Korsakoff encepha-

lopathy, preferentially by the intravenous route (starting with 50–100 mg, followed by oral supplementation). Electrolyte disorders should be corrected. Balanced diet is recommended. Clonidine/fluvoxamine and benzodiazepines have shown benefits. Disulfiram, acamprosate, and naltrexone can be considered. A clinical-psychological follow-up is mandatory.

Prognosis

Ataxia of stance and gait may improve with abstinence (Diener et al., 1984). Patients who continue to drink exhibit a worsening of gait ataxia, which can lead to total inability to walk alone. The recovery of ataxia is

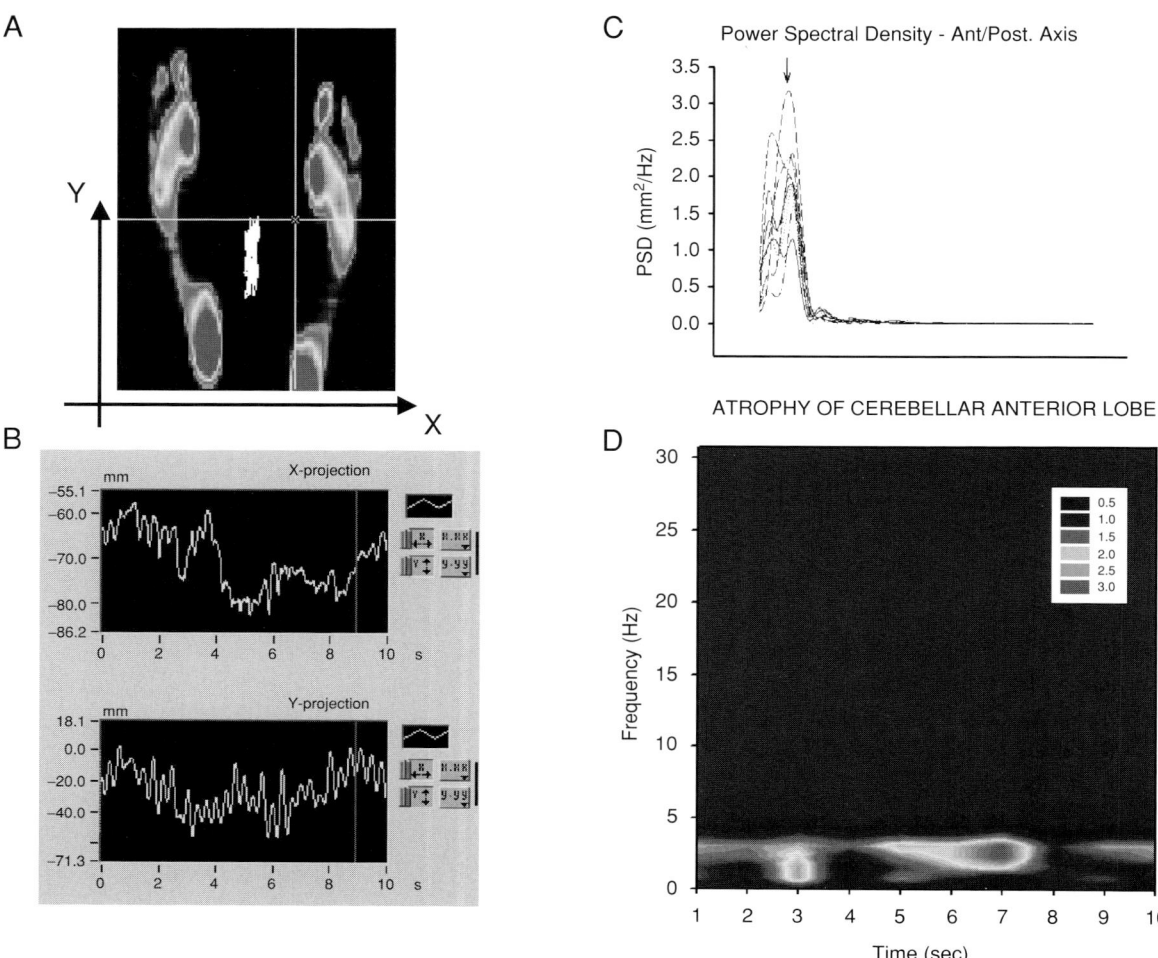

Figure 15.2 A 3-Hz body sway in chronic alcoholic cerebellar degeneration. (A) Representation of the center of pressure during a Romberg test using a pressure platform. (B) Displacements of the center of pressure in orthogonal axis X–Y. (C) Superimposition of power spectral density curves in the anterior-posterior axis. A 3-Hz tremor is found (arrow). (D) Time-frequency representation of the oscillations. (See color section.)

often incomplete in patients with Wernicke-Korsakoff syndrome, even with abstinence and thiamine replacement. About two-thirds of the patients exhibit an irreversible nystagmus with gait ataxia.

Drugs

Anticonvulsants

Phenytoin

Patients treated with phenytoin may develop ataxic signs either during a chronic treatment or following an acute intoxication. Severity of cerebellar signs ranges from subtle, such as an association of nystagmus and

mild ataxic gait, to severe (Selhorst et al., 1972). Cerebellar signs may develop several years after initiation of a chronic treatment. Dose-related nystagmus is very common for serum concentrations greater than 20 µg/mL. Patients may recover completely from cerebellar deficits, but irreversible lesions may evolve. Usually, patients who develop irreversible cerebellar deficits have been exposed to higher doses during a longer period of time. Rarely, patients present a slight cognitive deficit or a peripheral neuropathy. Some patients may be susceptible to phenytoin toxicity, for instance, in cases of a silent cerebellar disease or in myoclonic epilepsy. This rule is valid for many cerebellotoxic agents. Intra-uterine exposure to phenytoin has been associated with pontocerebellar hypoplasia (Squier et al., 1990).

Patients taking drugs increasing the half-life of phenytoin, such as ticlopidine (acting upon cytochrome P450), require a monitoring of blood levels of phenytoin, especially when ticlopidine is initiated or when the doses are increased.

Brain CT and brain MRI show cerebellar atrophy at various degrees in patients developing irreversible cerebellar signs following a chronic treatment. Cerebellar atrophy has also been described following a suicidal attempt or an acute overdose (Masur et al., 1989; Kuruvilla & Bharucha, 1997). In some cases, cerebellar atrophy is discovered in absence of cerebellar deficits. The correlation between cerebellar atrophy and the duration of epilepsy remains a matter of debate. Neuropathological studies show diffuse loss of Purkinje cells and a decreased number of granule cells and Bergmann gliosis, with a relative sparing of basket cell axons (Chatak et al., 1976; Gilman et al., 1981).

Patients presenting with acute intoxication should be monitored in an intensive care unit. Patients at risk for developing cerebellar deficits should not receive phenytoin (Eldridge et al., 1983).

Carbamazepine

Carbamazepine induces dose-dependent ataxic effects. Typically, patients complain of dizziness and exhibit a gaze-evoked nystagmus, action tremor, and ataxia of stance/gait (Masland, 1982). Impaired conscious state may mask the cerebellar deficits. Half of the patients with overdose develop cerebellar signs (Bridge et al., 1994). These signs may be related to involvement of afferent or efferent fibers to the cerebellum. Elderly patients appear more susceptible to carbamazepine than young patients (Specht et al., 1997), and patients presenting with a pre-existing cerebellar atrophy, even moderate, are at risk for developing cerebellar signs at lower serum levels. Structural lesions need to be looked for when cerebellar signs appear during treatment with carbamazepine (Hori et al., 1987).

Carbamazepine is used not only to treat focal epilepsy, but also for pain management and to treat manic-depressive disorders. In this latter case, the association of lithium salts and carbamazepine requires close clinical follow-up and biological monitoring (Rittmansberger & Lebhuler, 1992). Patients may develop a toxic syndrome made of confusion, drowsiness, nystagmus, dysarthria, hyperreflexia, coarse tremor, and ataxia of limbs and trunk. The sole addition of carbamazepine to a chronic treatment with lithium salts may trigger cerebellar signs, even when blood levels of both drugs are within the therapeutic range. Other drugs interacting with carbamazepine are sodium valproate, erythromycin/clarithromycin, verapamil, and viloxazine (Rothner et al., 1987; Zitelli et al., 1987).

Patients presenting with intoxication to carbamazepine should be monitored preferentially in an intensive care unit, due to the possibility of drowsiness or coma. Electrolyte imbalance should be corrected. Activated charcoal is still used in many centers. It should be kept in mind that total levels may be "therapeutic," whereas free levels are increased (Rothner et al., 1987).

Other anticonvulsants

Phenobarbital may induce transient ataxic signs. The most common deficits are gaze-evoked nystagmus, kinetic tremor, and ataxia of stance and gait. Most patients exhibit drowsiness. It is estimated that about 5% of epileptic patients treated with barbiturates show cerebellar deficits. Nevertheless, evidence of cellular toxicity and neuronal loss in adults is lacking. Experimental studies underline the vulnerability of the cerebellum during growth, but clinical implications are unclear.

Vigabatrin is an inhibitor of GABA transaminase that can induce mild ataxic posture in about 5% to 10% of adults with poorly controlled epilepsy. Gait ataxia is dose-related.

Gabapentin enhances GABAergic inhibition. About 7.7% of epileptic patients receiving gabapentin in add-on therapy exhibit ataxia (Baulac et al., 1998). The ataxia is reversible following discontinuation of the drug. Despite this side effect, gabapentin can also be used in patients exhibiting an isolated cerebellar atrophy. This is a paradox. We have seen several patients improving with administration of gabapentin at high doses. The initiation of the treatment may exacerbate ataxia temporarily, but this initial period is followed by an improvement of gait.

Lamotrigine added to chronic treatment with carbamazepine may induce ataxic signs, as a result of a pharmacodynamic interaction. Nevertheless, a genuine cerebellar toxicity is unlikely.

A case of cerebellar cognitive-affective syndrome induced by topiramate has been reported (Baillieux et al., 2008; see also Chapter 3). The patient exhibited impaired visuospatial memory, concentration deficits, executive dysfunctions, marked mood swings, and several disinhibited symptoms. After a gradual discontinuation of the drug, a complete remission of the cognitive and affective symptoms was observed within 6 weeks.

Antineoplastics

5-Fluorouracil

High doses of 5-fluorouracil (5-FU) may cause a disabling pancerebellar syndrome (Moertel et al., 1964). Cerebellar signs may be isolated or combined with signs of encephalopathy, raising the possibility of a Wernicke-Korsakoff syndrome. Capecitabine is an oral prodrug of 5-FU which can cause cerebellar ataxia.

Cytosine arabinoside

Doses greater than 3 g/m^2 may induce cerebellar syndrome. Signs of intoxication usually develop with cumulative doses greater than 24 g. Manifestations range from an isolated nystagmus to irreversible cerebellar deficits (Herzig et al., 1987). Patients initially develop somnolence and encephalopathy in most cases. An associated neuronopathy is common. Age is a predisposing factor.

Methotrexate

Cerebellar structures are vulnerable to methotrexate, especially when the drug is delivered by the intrathecal route (Wizniter et al., 1987; Lesnik et al., 1998).

Cisplatin, oxaliplatin, paclitaxel

These drugs may generate a polyneuropathy with predominant sensory ataxia. Oxaliplatin may induce cold-induced sensory symptoms (dysesthesia, paresthesia) early after drug infusion or a peripheral neuropathy with sensory ataxia – which can mimic cerebellar ataxia – during prolonged treatment (Gamelin et al., 2002).

Other drugs

Lithium salts

Lithium salts are used mainly for acute mania and prophylaxis of recurrent bipolar and unipolar affective disorders. Similarly to phenytoin, toxicity may occur either during maintenance therapy or following acute intoxication. The most common side effect of chronic treatment is an enhanced physiological tremor affecting mainly the hands. Lithium salts may cause hypothyroidism, a possible source of decompensation of ataxia (see also section Amiodarone). Acute intoxication may affect the cardiovascular, renal, and/or nervous system (Simard et al., 1989). The spectrum of neurological deficits is broad: coma, seizures, coarse tremor, hypokinesia, rigidity, and hyperreflexia. High fever is common during intoxication. Therefore, a neuroleptic malignant syndrome is often suspected, since neuroleptics and lithium salts are often administered in combination. Although neurological signs are usually reversible after acute intoxication, patients may exhibit a severe cerebellar syndrome in which scanning speech, tremor, and ataxic gait predominate (Manto et al., 1996). Intensive care monitoring is recommended to prevent irreversible sequelae, including a disabling cerebellar syndrome associated with marked cerebellar atrophy. Hemodialysis is the treatment of choice in the acute phase, rapidly decreasing serum levels. However, signs of intoxication may persist after normalization of blood levels due to intra-cellular accumulation of lithium.

Amiodarone

Amiodarone is a commonly used anti-arrhythmic medication, with a thyroxin-like structure. Amiodarone has an exceptionally long half-life of elimination. Daily doses of 400 mg/day bring about 8 mg of iodine/day, which is 100 times the normal daily intake. The main neurological side effects are postural tremor, peripheral neuropathy, and cerebellar deficits. Risk factors are advanced age, renal failure, diabetes mellitus, and alcoholism (Arnaud et al., 1992). About 5% to 7% of patients develop cerebellar toxicity (Garretto et al., 1994). Extra-cerebellar signs may occur also, including encephalopathy, rest tremor, dyskinesia, myoclonus, and proximal myopathy. Cerebellar ataxia may disappear very slowly following drug discontinuation or may persist several years, due to the very long half-life of elimination of the drug. Patients should be screened for a thyroid dysfunction, which is a common side effect of amiodarone and which can decompensate cerebellar signs.

Procainamide

High-dose procainamide used in cardiac arrhythmia may cause acute cerebellar ataxia resolving after discontinuation of the drug (Schwartz et al., 1984).

Cyclosporin and other calcineurin inhibitors

Calcineurin inhibitors are used in organ transplantation and in immunological diseases. The most common neurological side effect of cyclosporin is a fine tremor. Other neurological signs may develop: behavioral disorders, aphasia or mutism, seizures, cerebellar ataxia, vestibular deficits, motor spinal cord syndrome, and paresthesia (Palmer & Toto, 1991). Cerebellar toxicity of cyclosporin is probably not related to the plasma levels of the drug. Silent cerebellar lesions, such as a silent infarction, may be unraveled by the medication. Cerebellar deficits may appear several months following the initiation of treatment. Hypomagnesemia may trigger subacute episodes of ataxia (Thompson et al., 1984). A leukoencephalopathy may occur following transplantation (Belli et al., 1993). The so-called "reversible posterior leukoencephalopathy syndrome" is characterized by extensive white matter lesions predominating in the posterior regions of cerebral hemispheres. Orthotopic liver transplants might be particularly at risk for severe presentations (Bechstein, 2000). Patients previously exposed to cytotoxic agents (such as cisplatin) might be more susceptible (Rangi et al., 2005). The main differential diagnosis is progressive multifocal leukoencephalopathy (see Chapter 11). Cerebellar lesions may be reminiscent of watershed zones (Bartynski et al., 1997). Acute cerebellar edema occurs exceptionally and requires brainstem decompression (Nussbaum et al., 1995). Tacrolimus-induced mutism has been reported following liver transplant (Sokol et al., 2003). Although clinical deficits may be potentially reversible after drug withdrawal, cerebellar atrophy may develop over time after cessation of tacrolimus (Kaleyias et al., 2006). Differential diagnosis of cerebellar deficits in cases of renal failure includes stroke and action myoclonus–renal failure syndrome when there is a history of familial disease (Badhwar et al., 2004).

Metronidazole

Metronidazole exerts a peculiar toxicity on cerebellar nuclei. MRI shows edema with increased diffusion coefficients (Heaney et al., 2003). Patients may recover clinically and radiologically. This toxicity might be a property of other azole agents also.

Brimonidine tartrate

This selective alpha-2 adrenergic agonist agent is used as eye drops for the treatment of ocular hypertension (Lai Becker et al., 2009). Ingestion is the most common route of exposure for children. In addition, they may inadvertently receive a higher than intended dose. Ataxia occurs in about 4% to 5% of patients. Children younger than 5 years of age should be medically evaluated and monitored.

Drug abuse

Cocaine

Intoxication signs include seizures and impaired conscious state ranging from mild drowsiness to severe lethargy, delirium, and cerebellar ataxia. Patients may present with a clinical picture suggesting a neuroleptic malignant syndrome (Daras et al., 1995). Patients are at risk to develop mild or severe cerebellar infarctions (Aggarwal & Byrne, 1991). Other toxic agents may be added to crack cocaine and participate in neurological deficits (Katz et al., 1993). Neonates exposed to cocaine during pregnancy have been found to present with brain lesions unsuspected clinically (Dixon & Bejar, 1989).

Heroin

Heroin ingestion may induce a toxic spongiform leukoencephalopathy (Weber et al., 1998). Cerebellar signs usually start several days after the last consumption. Lesions are hypodense on brain CT and hyperintense on brain MRI (T2-weighted sequence) and are typically symmetrical, predominating in the white matter. Intoxication may be fatal (Ryan et al., 2005).

Methadone

Ingestion of methadone may cause a diffuse symmetrical swelling and edema of the cerebellum, resulting in compression of the fourth ventricle and hydrocephalus (Mills et al., 2008). Watershed injuries may be observed on brain MRI.

Phencyclidine

Phencyclidine is a non-competitive NMDA receptor antagonist with a property of neurostimulation (Deutsch et al., 1998). Complications include disorders of behavior, hallucinations, lethargy, catatonia, seizures, constricted pupils, athetosis, and dystonia. Children are at risk of presenting cerebellar signs, mainly ataxia of stance/gait and nystagmus (Schwartz & Einhorn, 1986). Intensive care therapy may be required, especially in patients with increased blood pressure, fever, and bronchospasm. The possibility of urinary retention or rhabdomyolysis should be kept in mind.

Herbs

Ceremonial herbs used for social events may induce cerebellar ataxia. Kava, used mainly in South Pacific, is an extract from a plant causing postural ataxia and limb tremor, probably via a disruption of GABAergic pathways (Singh & Singh, 2002).

Environmental causes of cerebellar ataxia

Heavy metals

Mercury

Humans are still exposed to methylmercury and mercury vapor, especially in the Amazon area, where gold mining remains an industrial activity (Clarkson, 1997; Lodenius & Malm, 1998). The intoxication in Minamata Bay resulted in an epidemic due to seafood contamination. Patients exhibit an association of constricted visual fields, sensory deficits in the extremities due to peripheral neuropathy, and cerebellar deficits (Ninomiya et al., 1995; Korogi et al., 1998). The inferior and middle parts of the vermis and cerebellar hemispheres are particularly susceptible (Korogi et al., 1994). Chelators (BAL [dimercaprol, or British anti-Lewisite] and/or penicillamine) are used to treat mercury poisoning.

Lead

The main causes of lead intoxication are ingestion of paints, sniffing of leaded gasoline, flour contamination, exposure to lead stearate, and contamination from automobile batteries. Toxicity seems greater in children (Finkelstein et al., 1998). Abdominal pain is common. Blood studies show various degrees of anemia. Lead is neurotoxic for the central (especially frontal cortex, hippocampus, and cerebellum) and the peripheral nervous system (peripheral motor neuropathy). Cerebellar ataxia may be prominent in adults (Mani et al., 1998). Cerebellar intoxication may present as a pseudo-tumor with obstructive hydrocephalus due to edema (Pappas et al., 1986; Johnson et al., 1993). Cerebral calcifications and hyperintense lesions on brain MRI are commonly found. Blood studies are mandatory when an intoxication is

suspected (Manto et al., 2002). Chelation therapy is required when intoxication is confirmed.

Toluene/benzene derivatives

Solvents can cause peripheral and CNS disturbances. Toluene exposure (glue-sniffing, occupational exposure) causes an acute encephalopathy in children characterized by coma, seizures, cerebellar ataxia, and behavior abnormalities (King, 1982). Adults present with headache, hyperactivity, memory deficits, insomnia, and cerebellar deficits (Saito & Wada, 1993). Cerebellar deficits may be irreversible. Brain MRI shows a cerebellar atrophy after a chronic exposure of several years, in addition to cerebral atrophy. Hyperintense lesions in T2-weighted or Flair sequence are common.

Cerebellar ataxia and decreased visual acuity are complications of chronic thinner intoxication (Uchino et al., 2002).

Paradichlorobenzene (PDB) is a household deodorant found in room deodorizers and toilet bowl fresheners. Addiction to PDB has been associated with gait ataxia, tremor, dysarthria, limb weakness, and bradyphrenia, in various combinations (Cheong et al., 2006). Withdrawal can trigger neurological symptoms.

Hyperthermia

Episodes of hyperthermia (usually above 40.5 °C) can induce cerebellar syndrome, either transient or permanent. Heat stroke and neuroleptic malignant syndrome are the most common causes worldwide.

Neurological examination shows deficits ranging from an isolated cerebellar dysarthria or an isolated gait ataxia to a pancerebellar syndrome (Manto & Topka, 1996). Symptoms may resolve within 3 to 10 days. Cerebellar deficits may also be part of a diffuse encephalopathy presenting clinically with seizures and confusion (Lawden et al., 1994; Bazille et al., 2005). Follow-up studies with brain CT or MRI have demonstrated that cerebellar atrophy may appear in the months following the episode of hyperpyrexia (Mohapatro et al., 1990). Cerebellar atrophy may contrast with a satisfactory clinical improvement.

Purkinje cells are particularly vulnerable to heat-induced injury. Neuropathological studies have revealed a severe diffuse loss of Purkinje cells associated with heat shock protein 70 expression by Bergmann glia (Bazille et al., 2005). Degeneration of Purkinje cell axons results in myelin pallor of the white matter of the folia and of the hilum of the dentate nuclei. DNA internucleosomal breakages are identified by in situ end labeling in the dentate nuclei and centromedian nuclei of the thalamus and are associated with degeneration of the cerebellar efferent pathways (superior cerebellar peduncles, decussation of the superior cerebellar peduncles and dentatothalamic tract). Ammon horn and other areas susceptible to hypoxia are uninjured (Bazille et al., 2005).

High fever may become an emergency. Cooling of the body and monitoring of vital functions are recommended. Prevention of heat stroke should not be underestimated in populations at risk, especially the elderly. Preventive factors include the following: limiting sun exposure, regular use of sunscreens, fluid and ion replacement, and acclimatization (Yaqub & Al Deeb, 1998).

Carbon monoxide

Carbon monoxide is a gas responsible for hypoxia leading to cardiopulmonary arrest in cases of severe intoxication. This gas is characterized by a high affinity for hemoglobin oxygen-binding sites. Carbon monoxide still accounts for a large number of deaths and notable morbidity. About 2% to 26% of patients die from acute intoxication (Pahwa, 1997). Symptoms may be initially overlooked, occasionally restricted to a mild headache.

Carbon monoxide induces immediate or delayed neurological alterations, including memory loss, cognitive impairment, neuropsychiatric manifestations, deficits linked to basal ganglia, or cerebellar dysfunction (Savoldi et al., 1973; Kulakowska et al., 2000). A free interval of several weeks between the intoxication and the presentation of neurological deficits is not rare.

Imaging studies show lesions, especially in basal ganglia (globus pallidus), thalamus, and white matter. These lesions correspond to areas of severe edema (Prockop & Naidu, 1999; O'Donnell et al., 2000). MRI may disclose extensive cerebellar white matter lesions or cerebellar atrophy (Mascalchi et al., 1996). Single-photon emission CT studies may show a reduction of cerebellar blood flow. Necropsy, histological examination, and DNA ladder assay argue for the presence of apoptosis as well as necrosis in human cases of carbon monoxide intoxication.

Experimental studies have shown that carbon monoxide induces impairment of the differentiation of cerebellar GABA-synthesizing neurons (Benagiano et al., 2005). Chronic exposure induces a delayed

impairment of soluble guanylate cyclase activation by nitric oxide (Hernández-Viadel et al., 2004). The suppression of cerebellar long-term depression (see Chapter 2) may be due to this effect (Shibuki et al., 2001).

Patients suffering from carbon monoxide intoxication should be transferred immediately to hyperbaric units.

Cyanide

Cyanide intoxication results from accidental acute exposure, suicide attempt (ingestion), or asphyxiation due to hydrocyanic fumes (Pahwa, 1997). Patients complain of headache and often exhibit coma and seizures. The mortality rate is high. Survivors may develop irreversible neurological sequelae, mainly parkinsonian signs, postural tremor, dystonia, and dementia (Carella et al., 1988). A combination of extrapyramidal and cerebellar signs has been observed (Rosenow et al., 1995). Cerebellar hemorrhage and cerebellar atrophy have been reported. Cyanide interferes with oxidative enzymes, GABAergic metabolism, and cyclic guanosine monophosphate homeostasis. Treatment includes rest, oxygen delivery, amyl nitrite, sodium thiosulfate, and hydroxocobalamin (Beasley & Glass, 1998).

Chemical weapons

Prominent brainstem-cerebellar symptoms have been reported in Japan in patients exposed to diphenylarsinic acid poisoning, derived from agents developed for use as chemical weapons (Ishii et al., 2004).

Insecticides/herbicides

Table 15.3 lists the conditions associated with intoxication to insecticides or herbicides. The cerebellum may be a privileged target of exposure.

Polychlorinated biphenyls

Polychlorinated biphenyls (PCBs) are a family of synthetic hydrocarbon compounds which have been used for a large range of industrial purposes. Although banned in the 1970s, they continue to be ubiquitous in landfills, sediments, and wildlife (Jacobson & Jacobson, 2002). They are found in significant quantities in the food chain. PCBs cross the placenta and are transferred to neonates via breast milk (Nguon et al., 2005). Consumption of PCB-contaminated salmon has been associated with cognitive deficits

Table 15.3 Cerebellotoxic insecticides and herbicides

Substance	Exposure	Clinical symptoms	Pathological studies
Chlordecone	Workers exposed to insecticides	Pleural pain Arthralgias Tremor Gait instability Opsoclonus Pseudotumor cerebri Peripheral neuropathy	
Phosphine	Toxic fumigant	Headache Nausea and vomiting Cough Paresthesias Diplopia Kinetic tremor Gait difficulties	
Carbon disulfide	Production of cellophane Industries of solvents Production of tetrachloride Pesticides	Encephalopathy Movement disorders Peripheral neuropathy	Diffuse neuronal degeneration in cerebral cortex and basal ganglia Loss of Purkinje cells

in children (Jacobson & Jacobson, 1996; Jacobson & Jacobson, 2002). Experimental studies demonstrate that perinatal PCB exposure is associated with impaired cerebellar development and abnormal motor behavior (Nguon et al., 2005). Cerebellar expression of glial fibrillary acid protein, which is involved in granule cell migration, is increased, whereas the expression of neural cell adhesion molecule L1, which is implicated in neuronal interactions, is decreased.

Eucalytpus oil

Widespread topical application of eucalyptus oil has been associated with slurred speech, ataxia, and muscle weakness progressing to unconsciousness in a child (Darben et al., 1998). The syndrome is reversible.

Saxitoxin (shellfish poisoning)

Saxitoxin is a potent neurotoxin contaminating a mollusk (*Mytilus*). It binds to voltage-sensitive sodium channels, found at high densities in the cerebellar cortex. Patients present with gastrointestinal and neurological signs. Cerebellar deficits may be predominant, hence the terminology of ataxic shellfish poisoning (Rhodes et al., 1975). Patients often complain of paresthesias.

Consumption of edible morels

Morchella esculenta and *Morchella conica*, two edible morels, can cause a self-limited cerebellar syndrome characterized by dizziness, ataxic gait, and visual disturbances. Ataxia starts after a latency of 6 to 12 hours, lasts up to 1 day, and vanishes without sequelae (Pfab et al., 2008). The mechanism of toxicity is unknown.

Animal-related cerebellar toxicity

Scorpions

Victims of scorpion envenomation exhibit local and systemic symptoms. Local manifestations include paresthesia, pain, and edema (Pardal et al., 2003). Neurological deficits may be prominent. A majority of patients present with the classical symptom of "electric shock," affecting nearly 90% of victims (Pardal et al., 2003). Myoclonus and cerebellar ataxia are the main deficits in some series. Ataxia may predominantly involve the upper limbs, with a typical dysmetria. Complications following scorpion sting can be serious and even fatal (Gadwalkar et al., 2006). In particular, cerebellar stroke is a potential complication which should be recognized immediately. Cerebellar infarctions may be bilateral and extensive (Gadwalkar et al., 2006). Stroke results from various mechanisms such as acute hypertension, myocarditis, disseminated intravascular coagulation, and toxin-induced vasculitis. Management consists of supportive care and anti-venom serum administration.

References

Aggarwal S, Byrne BD. Massive ischemic cerebellar infarction due to cocaine use. *Neuroradiology* 1991;**33**:449–50.

Arnaud A, Neau JP, Rivasseau-Jonveaux T, Marechaud R, Gil R. Neurological toxicity of amiodarone. 5 case reports. *Rev Med Interne* 1992;**13**:419–22.

Badhwar A, Berkovic SF, Dowling JP, et al. Action myoclonus-renal failure syndrome: characterization of a unique cerebro-renal disorder. *Brain* 2004;**127**:2173–82.

Baillieux H, Verslegers W, Paquier P, De Deyn PP, Mariën P. Cerebellar cognitive affective syndrome associated with topiramate. *Clin Neurol Neurosurg* 2008;**110**(5)496–9.

Bartynski WS, Grabb BC, Zeigler Z, Lin L, Andrews DF. Watershed imaging features and clinical vascular injury in cyclosporin A neurotoxicity. *J Comput Assist Tomogr* 1997; **21**:872–80.

Baulac M, Cavalcanti D, Semah F, Arzimanoglou A, Portal JJ. Gabapentin add-on therapy with adaptable dosages in 610 patients with partial epilepsy: an open, observational study. The French Gabapentin Collaborative Group. *Seizure* 1998;**7**:55–62.

Bazille C, Megarbane B, Bensimhon D, et al. Brain damage after heat stroke. *J Neuropathol Exp Neurol* 2005; **64**(11)970–5.

Beasley DM, Glass WI. Cyanide poisoning: pathophysiology and treatment recommendations. *Occup Med (Lond)* 1998;**48**(7)427–31.

Bechstein WO. Neurotoxicity of calcineurin inhibitors: impact and clinical management. *Transpl Int* 2000;**13**:313–26.

Belli LS, De Carlis L, Romani F, et al. Dysarthria and cerebellar ataxia: late occurrence of severe neurotoxicity in a liver transplant patient. *Transpl Int* 1993;**6**:176–8.

Benagiano V, Lorusso L, Coluccia A, et al. Glutamic acid decarboxylase and GABA immunoreactivities in the cerebellar cortex of adult rat after prenatal exposure to a low concentration of carbon monoxide. *Neuroscience* 2005;**135**(3):897–905.

Bhave SV, Ghoda L, Hoffman PL. Brain-derived neurotrophic factor mediates the anti-apoptotic effect of NMDA in cerebellar granule neurons: signal transduction cascades and sites of ethanol action. *J Neurosci* 1999;**19**:3277–86.

Bridge TA, Norton RL, Robertson WO. Pediatric carbamazepine overdoses. *Pediatr Emerg Care* 1994;**10**:260–3.

Carella F, Grassi MP, Savoiardo M, et al. Dystonic-Parkinsonian syndrome after cyanide poisoning: clinical and MRI findings. *J Neurol Neurosurg Psychiatry* 1988;**51**(10)1345–8.

Chatak NR, Santoso RA, McKinney WN. Cerebellar degeneration following long-term phenytoin therapy. *Neurology* 1976;**26**:818–20.

Cheong R, Wilson RK, Cortese IC, Newman-Toker DE. Mothball withdrawal encephalopathy: case report and review of paradichlorobenzene neurotoxicity. *Subst Abus* 2006;**27**(4)63–7.

Clarkson TW. The toxicology of mercury. *Crit Rev Clin Lab Sci* 1997;**34**:369–403.

Daras M, Kakkouras L, Tuchman AJ, Koppel BS. Rhabdomyolysis and hyperthermia after cocaine abuse: a variant of the neuroleptic malignant syndrome? *Acta Neurol Scand* 1995;**92**:161–5.

Darben T, Cominos B, Lee CT. Topical eucalyptus oil poisoning. *Australas J Dermatol* 1998;**39**(4)265–7.

Deutsch SI, Mastropaolo J, Rosse RB. Neurodevelopmental consequences of early exposure to phencyclidine and related drugs. *Clin Neuropharmacol* 1998;**21**:320–32.

Diener HC, Dichgans J, Bacher M, Guschlbauer B. Improvement of ataxia in alcoholic cerebellar atrophy through alcohol abstinence. *J Neurol* 1984;**231**:258–62.

Dixon SD, Bejar R. Echoencephalographic findings in neonates associated with maternal cocaine and methamphetamine use: incidence and clinical correlates. *J Pediatr* 1989;**115**:770–8.

Eldridge R, Iivanainen M, Stern R, Koerber T, Wilder BJ. 'Baltic' myoclonus epilepsy: hereditary disorder of childhood made worse by phenytoin. *Lancet* 1983;**ii**:838–42.

Fadda F, Rossetti ZL. Chronic ethanol consumption: from neuroadaptation to neurodegeneration. *Prog Neurobiol* 1998;**56**;385–431.

Finkelstein Y, Markowitz ME, Rosen JF. Low-level lead-induced neurotoxicity in children: an update on central nervous system effects *Brain Res Brain Res Rev* 1998;**27**:168–76.

Gadwalkar SR, Bushan S, Pramod K, Gouda C, Kumar PM. Bilateral cerebellar infarction: a rare complication of scorpion sting. *J Assoc Physicians India* 2006;**54**:581–3.

Gallucci M, Bozzao A, Splendiani A, Masciocchi C, Passariello R. Wernicke encephalopathy: MR findings in 5 patients. *Am J Neuroradiol* 1990;**11**:887–92.

Gamelin E, Gamelin L, Bossi L, Quasthoff S. Clinical aspects and molecular basis of oxaliplatin neurotoxicity: current management and development of preventive measures. *Semin Oncol* 2002;**29**:21–33.

Garretto NS, Rey RD, Kohler G, et al. Cerebellar syndrome caused by amiodarone. *Arq Neuropsiquiatr* 1994; **52**:575–7.

Garzon T, Mellibovsky L, Roquer J, Perich X, Diez-Perez A. Ataxic form of central pontine myelinolysis. *Lancet Neurol* 2002;**1**(8)517–8.

Gilman S, Adams K, Koeppe RA, et al. Cerebellar and frontal hypometabolism in alcoholic cerebellar degeneration studied with positron emission tomography. *Ann Neurol* 1990;**28**:775–85.

Gilman S, Bloedel JR, Lechtenberg R. *Disorders of the Cerebellum. Contemporary Neurology Series.* Philadelphia: FA Davis, 1981.

Gilman S, Koeppe RA, Adams K, et al. Positron emission tomographic studies of cerebral benzodiazepine-receptor binding in chronic alcoholics. *Ann Neurol* 1996;**40**:163–71.

Gocht A, Colmant HJ. Central pontine and extrapontine myelinolysis: a report of 58 cases. *Clin Neuropathol* 1987;**6**(6)262–70.

Greenwood J, Jeyasingham M, Pratt OE, et al. Heterogeneity of human erythrocyte transketolase: a preliminary report. *Alcohol Alcohol* 1984;**19**: 123–9.

Harper CG. The incidence of Wernicke's encephalopathy in Australia: a neuropathological study of 131 cases. *J Neurol Neurosurg Psychiatry* 1983;**46**:593–8.

Haubek A, Lee K. Computed tomography in alcoholic cerebellar atrophy. *Neuroradiology* 1979;**18**:77–9.

Heaney CJ, Campeau NG, Lindell EP. MR imaging and diffusion-weighted imaging changes in metronidazole (Flagyl)-induced cerebellar toxicity. *Am J Neuroradiol* 2003;**24**:1615–7.

Hernández-Viadel M, Castoldi AF, Coccini T, et al. In vivo exposure to carbon monoxide causes delayed impairment of activation of soluble guanylate cyclase by nitric oxide in rat brain cortex and cerebellum. *J Neurochem* 2004;**89**(5):1157–65.

Herzig RH, Hines JD, Herzig GP, et al. Cerebellar toxicity with high-dose cytosine arabinoside. *J Clin Oncol* 1987;**5**:927–32.

Hori A, Kazakuwa S, Fujii T, Kurachi M. Lennox-Gastaut syndrome with and without Dandy-Walker malformation. *Epilepsy Res* 1987;**1**:258–61.

Ishii K, Tamaoka A, Otsuka F, et al. Diphenylarsinic acid poisoning from chemical weapons in Kamisu, Japan. *Ann Neurol* 2004;**56**:741–5.

Jacobson JL, Jacobson SW. Association of prenatal exposure to an environmental contaminant with intellectual function in childhood. *J Toxicol Clin Toxicol* 2002;**40**(4)467–75.

Jacobson JL, Jacobson SW. Intellectual impairment in children exposed to polychlorinated biphenyls in utero. *N Engl J Med* 1996;**335**(11)783–9.

Johnson LM, Hubble JP, Koller WC. Effect of medications and toxins on cerebellar function. In Handbook of Cerebellar Diseases, ed. R. Lechtenberg. New York: Marcel Dekker, 1993.

Kaleyias J, Faerber E, Kothare SV. Tacrolimus induced subacute cerebellar ataxia. *Eur J Paediatr Neurol* 2006;**10**:86–9.

Katz AA, Hoffman RS, Silverman RA. Phenytoin toxicity from smoking crack cocaine adulterated with phenytoin. *Ann Emerg Med* 1993;**22**:1485–7.

Kim J, Song T, Park S, Choi IS. Cerebellar peduncular myelinolysis in a patient receiving hemodialysis. *J Neurol Sci* 2007;**253**(1–2):66–8.

King MD. Neurological sequelae of toluene abuse. *Hum Toxicol* 1982;**1**(3)281–7.

Korogi Y, Takahashi M, Okajima T, Eto K. MR findings in Minamata disease. *J Magn Reson Imaging* 1998;**8**: 308–16.

Korogi Y, Takahashi M, Sumi M, et al. MR imaging of Minamata disease: qualitative and quantitative analysis. *Radiat Med* 1994;**12**:249–53.

Kulakowska A, Drozdowski W, Halicka D, Kochanowicz J. Neurologic and psychiatric sequelae of carbon monoxide poisoning. *Neurol Neurochir Pol* 2000;**34**(3):587–95.

Kuruvilla T, Bharucha NE. Cerebellar atrophy after acute phenytoin intoxication. *Epilepsia* 1997;**38**:500–2.

Lai Becker M, Huntington N, Woolf AD. Brimonidine tartrate poisoning in children: frequency, trends, and use of naloxone as an antidote. *Pediatrics* 2009;**123**(2)e305–11.

Lawden MC, Blunt S, Matthews T, Peatfield R, Kennard C. Recurrent confusion and ataxia triggered by pyrexia in a case of occult multiple sclerosis. *J Neurol Neurosurg Psychiatry* 1994;**57**(11)1436.

Lesnik PG, Ciesielski KT, Hart BL, et al. Evidence for cerebellar-frontal subsystem changes in children treated with intrathecal chemotherapy foe leukemia: enhanced data analysis using an effect size model. *Arch Neurol* 1998;**55**:1561–8.

Lodenius M, Malm O. Mercury in the Amazon. *Rev Environ Contam Toxicol* 1998;**157**:25–52.

Mani J, Chaudhary N, Kanjalkar M, Shah PU. Cerebellar ataxia due to lead encephalopathy in an adult. *J Neurol Neurosurg Psychiatry* 1998;**65**:797.

Manto M, Godaux E, Jacquy J, Hildebrand J. Analysis of cerebellar dysmetria associated with lithium intoxication. *Neurol Res* 1996;**18**:416–24.

Manto M, Laute MA, Pandolfo M. Depression of extra-cellular GABA and increase of NMDA-induced nitric oxide following acute intra-nuclear administration of alcohol in the cerebellar nuclei of the rat. *Cerebellum* 2005;**4**(4)230–8.

Manto MU, Jacquy J. Other cerebellotoxic agents. In The *Cerebellum and Its Disorders*, ed. M. Manto and M. Pandolfo. Cambridge, UK: Cambridge University Press, 2002, pp. 342–66.

Manto MU, Topka H. Reversible cerebellar gait ataxia with postural tremor during episodes of high pyrexia. *Clin Neurol Neurosurg* 1996;**98**(3)227–30.

Mascalchi M, Petruzzi P, Zampa V. MRI of cerebellar white matter damage due to carbon monoxide poisoning: case report. *Neuroradiology* 1996;**38**(suppl 1):S73–4.

Masland RL. Carbamazepine neurotoxicity. In *Antiepileptic Drugs*, 2nd edn, ed. D.M. Woodbury, J.K. Penry, and C.E. Pippenger. New York: Raven Press, 1982, pp. 521–31.

Masur H, Elger CE, Ludolph AC, Galanski M. Cerebellar atrophy following acute intoxication with phenytoin. *Neurology* 1989;**39**:432–3.

Mills F, MacLennan SC, Devile CJ, Saunders DE. Severe cerebellitis following methadone poisoning. *Pediatr Radiol* 2008;**38**(2)227–9.

Moertel CG, Reitemeier RJ, Bolton CE, Shorter RG. Cerebellar ataxia associated with fluorinated pyrimidine therapy. *Cancer Chemother Rep* 1964;**41**:15–8.

Mohapatro AK, Thomas M, Jain S, et al. Pancerebellar syndrome in hyperpyrexia. *Australas Radiol* 1990;**34**(4)320–2.

Nguon K, Baxter MG, Sajdel-Sulkowska EM. Perinatal exposure to polychlorinated biphenyls differentially affects cerebellar development and motor functions in male and female rat neonates. *Cerebellum* 2005;**4**(2)112–22.

Ninomiya T, Ohmori H, Hashimoto K, Tsuruta K, Ekino S. Expansion of methylmercury poisoning outside of Minamata: an epidemiological study on chronic methylmercury poisoning outside of Minamata. *Environ Res* 1995;**70**:47–50.

Nussbaum ES, Maxwell RE, Bitterman PB, et al. Cyclosporine A toxicity presenting with acute cerebellar edema and brainstem compression. Case report. *J Neurosurg* 1995;**82**:1068–70.

O'Donnell P, Buxton PJ, Pitkin A, Jarvis LJ. The magnetic resonance imaging appearances of the brain in acute carbon monoxide poisoning. *Clin Radiol* 2000;**55**(4):273–80.

Pahwa R. Toxin-induced parkinsonian syndromes. In *Movement Disorders*, ed. R.L. Watts and W.C. Koller. New York: McGraw-Hill, 1997, pp. 315–23.

Palmer BF, Toto RD. Severe neurologic toxicity induced by cyclosporine A in three renal transplant patients. *Am J Kidney Dis* 1991;**1**:116–21.

Pappas CL, Quisling RG, Ballinger WE, Love LC. Lead encephalopathy: symptoms of a cerebellar mass lesion and obstructive hydrocephalus. *Surg Neurol* 1986;**26**:391–4.

Pardal PP, Castro LC, Jennings E, Pardal JS, Monteiro MR. Epidemiological and clinical aspects of scorpion envenomation in the region of Santarém, Pará, Brazil. *Rev Soc Bras Med Trop* 2003;**36**(3)349–53.

Pfab R, Haberl B, Kleber J, Zilker T. Cerebellar effects after consumption of edible morels (Morchella conica, Morchella esculenta). *Clin Toxicol (Phila)* 2008;**46**(3)259–60.

Pentney R. Alcohol toxicity in the cerebellum: fundamental aspects. In *The Cerebellum and Its Disorders*, ed. M. Manto and M. Pandolfo. Cambridge, UK: Cambridge University Press, 2002, pp. 327–35.

Prockop LD, Naidu KA. Brain CT and MRI findings after carbon monoxide toxicity. *J Neuroimaging* 1999;**9**(3):175–81.

Rangi PS, Partridge WJ, Newlands ES, Waldman AD. Posterior reversible encephalopathy syndrome: a possible late interaction between cytotoxic agents and general anaesthesia. *Neuroradiology* 2005;**47**: 586–90.

Rhodes FA, Mills CG, Popei K. Paralytic shellfish poisoning in Papua New Guinea. *P N G Med J* 1975;**8**:197–202.

Rittmannsberger H, Lebhuler F. Asterixis induced by carbamazepine. *Biol Psychiatry* 1992;**32**:364–8.

Rosenow F, Herholz K, Lanfermann H, et al. Neurological sequelae of cyanide intoxication: the patterns of clinical, magnetic resonance imaging, and positron emission tomography findings. *Ann Neurol* 1995;**38**(5) 825–8.

Rothner AD, Pippenger C, Cruse RP, et al. Carbamazepine toxicity with therapeutic total levels and elevated free levels. *Ann Neurol* 1987;**22**;413–4.

Ryan A, Molloy FM, Farrell MA, Hutchinson M. Fatal toxic leukoencephalopathy: clinical, radiological, and necropsy findings in two patients. *J Neurol Neurosurg Psychiatry* 2005;**76**:1014–16.

Saito K, Wada H. Behavioral approaches to toluene intoxication. *Environ Res* 1993;**62**(1)53–62.

Savoldi F, Mazzella GL, Bo P, Massarini M. Cerebellar ataxia due to acute carbon monoxide poisoning. *Riv Neurobiol* 1973;**19**(3-4):197–206.

Schwartz AB, Klausner SC, Yee S, Turchyn M. Cerebellar ataxia due to procainamide toxicity. *Arch Intern Med* 1984;**144**:2260–1.

Schwartz RH, Einhorn A. PCP intoxication in seven young children. *Pediatr Emerg Care* 1986;**2**:238–41.

Selhorst JB, Kaufman B, Horwitz SJ. Diphenylhydantoin-induced cerebellar degeneration. *Arch Neurol* 1972;**27**:452–5.

Shibuki K, Kimura S, Wakatsuki H. Suppression of the induction of long-term depression by carbon monoxide in rat cerebellar slices. *Eur J Neurosci* 2001;**13**(3): 609–16.

169

Simard M, Gumbiner B, Lee A, Lewis H, Norman D. Lithium carbonate intoxication. A case report and review of the literature. *Arch Intern Med* 1989;**149**: 36–46.

Singh YN, Singh NN. Therapeutic potential of kava in the treatment of anxiety disorders. *CNS Drugs* 2002;**16**:731–43.

Sokol DK, Molleston JP, Filo RS, et al. Tacrolimus (FK506)-induced mutism after liver transplant. *Pediatr Neurol* 2003;**28**:156–8.

Sowell ER, Jernigan TL, Mattson SN, et al. Abnormal development of the cerebellar vermis in children prenatally exposed to alcohol: size reduction in lobules I-V. *Alcohol Clin Exp Res* 1996;**20**:31–34.

Specht U, May TW, Rohde M, et al. Cerebellar atrophy decreases the threshold of carbamazepine toxicity in patients with chronic focal epilepsy. *Arch Neurol* 1997;**54**:427–31.

Squier W, Hope PL, Lindenbaum RH. Neocerebellar hypoplasia in a neonate following intra-uterine exposure to anti-convulsants. *Dev Med Child Neurol* 1990;**32**:737–42.

Thompson CB, June CH, Sullivan KM, Thomas ED. Association between cyclosporin neurotoxicity and hypomagnesemia. *Lancet* 1984;ii;1116–20.

Uchino A, Kato A, Yuzuriha T, et al. Comparison between patient characteristics and cranial MR findings in chronic thinner intoxication. *Eur Radiol* 2002;**12**(6)1338–41.

Victor M, Adams RD, Mancall EL. A restricted form of cerebellar cortical degeneration occurring in alcoholic patients. *Arch Neurol* 1959;**1**:579–88.

Weber W, Henkes H, Moller P, Bade K, Kuhne D. Toxic spongiform leucoencephalopathy after inhaling heroin vapour. *Eur Radiol* 1998;**8**:749–55.

Wizniter M, Packer RJ, Rorke LB, Meadows AT. Cerebellar sclerosis in pediatric cancer patients. *J Neurooncol* 1987;**4**:353–60.

Worner TM. Effects of alcohol. In *Handbook of Cerebellar Diseases*, ed. R. Lechtenberg. New Yor.k: Marcel Dekker, 1993, pp. 547–66.

Yaqub B, Al Deeb S. Heat strokes: aetiopathogenesis, neurological characteristics, treatment and outcome. *J Neurol Sci* 1998;**156**(2)144–51.

Zitelli BJ, Howrie DL, Altman H, Maroon TJ. Erythromycin-induced drug interactions. An illustrative case and review of the literature. *Clin Pediatr* 1987;**26**;117–9.

Zubaran C, Fernandes JG, Rodnight R. Wernicke-Korsakoff syndrome. *Postgrad Med J* 1997;**73**:27–31.

Autism spectrum disorders and ataxia

Description and clinical features

Autism is a neurodevelopmental disorder with an estimated prevalence of 1 in 1000. Studies of these last two decades show that autism is not a disease, but a syndrome with a strong genetic component (Polleux & Lauder, 2004). Autism is characterized by abnormalities in social interaction, impairments in verbal and non-verbal communication, and a restricted repertoire of interests and activities. It includes a large spectrum of disorders encompassing individuals at all levels of intelligence and language ability (Hill & Frith, 2003). Asperger syndrome refers to individuals with the typical social and communication impairments of autism, but who have fluent language and good academic abilities (Frith, 2004). Autism spectrum disorders also include Rett syndrome and childhood disintegrative disorder. Rett syndrome occurs almost exclusively in females. Symptoms start between 6 and 18 months of age, comprising impaired language, seizures, grinding of teeth, loss of purposeful hand skills, and gait disturbances (Rett, 1986).

Most autistic individuals exhibit motor control deficits: disturbances of gait and balance, impaired motor preparation, and defects in manual dexterity (Ghaziuddin et al., 1994; Miyahara et al., 1997; Gowen & Miall, 2005). Impairment in motor tasks is more pronounced during tasks where accuracy depends upon incoming sensory signals, such as in pointing and balancing (Gowen & Miall, 2005). Asperger subjects are slower than matched controls during rapid tasks. They have difficulties to correct end point errors.

Brain imaging

Hypoplasia and hyperplasia of the cerebellar hemispheres and vermis have been identified with MRI (Murakami et al., 1989). Children with autism spectrum disorders have reduced total vermis volumes as compared with control children after controlling for age, sex, and overall cerebral volume or cerebellum volume (Webb et al., 2009). In particular, the vermis lobe VI to VII area is reduced.

Using diffusion tensor magnetic resonance tractography, it has been shown that individuals with Asperger syndrome have significantly lower fractional anisotropy in the short intracerebellar fibers and right superior cerebellar peduncle as compared with controls, in absence of difference in the input tracts (Catani et al., 2008). The severity of social impairment is negatively correlated with diffusion anisotropy in the fibers of the left superior cerebellar peduncle. These findings indicate a possible vulnerability of specific cerebellar neural pathways in Asperger syndrome.

Hydrogen-1 magnetic resonance spectroscopy reveals significantly lower N-acetyl-aspartate/creatine ratios bilaterally in the hippocampus-amygdala but not in the cerebellum of autism spectrum disorders (Gabis et al., 2008).

Neurophysiology

Electroencephalogram (EEG) monitoring often reveals abnormal patterns of activity. EEG can show a high amplitude spike and wave pattern. Epileptiform discharges are found in up to 60% of cases.

Neuropathology

Post-mortem studies have demonstrated hyperplasia or hypoplasia of the cerebellum, with various degrees of Purkinje cell loss in the vermis and cerebellar hemispheres (Courchesne, 1997; Kemper & Bauman, 1998). Density of basket cells and stellate cells seems preserved, suggesting a late developmental loss of Purkinje cells (Whitney et al., 2009).

Genetic studies

Autism spectrum disorders are genetically heterogeneous. Several candidate genes have been reproducibly shown to display specific mutations segregating with autism because of the complex polygenic nature of this syndrome (Polleux & Lauder, 2004). These genes control the early patterning and/or the late synaptic maturation of specific neuronal subpopulations controlling the balance between excitation and inhibition in the developing cortex and cerebellum.

Rett syndrome is associated with mutations of the gene coding for methyl-CpG binding protein 2 (MECP2; Xq28). This gene encodes a transcriptional repressor modulating the expression of active genes.

Pathogenesis of autism: role of the cerebellum?

Since poor motor skills, hypotonia, and autistic features are relatively common in cerebellar hypoplasia (Wassmer et al., 2003), it has been speculated that the cerebellum could contribute to socioemotional manifestations of autism (Singer-Harris et al., 1999).

Phenotypic overlap with other disorders

From the phenotypic point of view, autism can overlap with Angelman syndrome, a neurogenetic disorder characterized by severe mental retardation, ataxia, seizures (mainly atypical absences and myoclonic seizures) and EEG abnormalities, and bouts of inappropriate laughter (Peters et al., 2004; Lalande & Calciano, 2007). In infancy, non-specific clinical features pose diagnostic challenges to the neurologist (Williams, 2005). These include a combination of microcephaly, seizure disorder, global developmental delay, or an ataxic/hypotonic cerebral palsy–like picture. In later childhood, absent speech, excessively happy behavior, ataxia, and jerky movements are more suggestive of the disorder. Brain MRI shows nonspecific or normal findings. Occasionally the EEG pattern alone is very helpful to recognize this disorder. The genetic causes are maternal deletion of chromosome 15q11-q13, paternal chromosome 15 uniparental disomy, ubiquitin protein ligase (UBE3A) mutation, and an abnormality of the imprinting process.

References

Catani M, Jones DK, Daly E, et al. Altered cerebellar feedback projections in Asperger syndrome. *Neuroimage* 2008;**41**(4)1184–91.

Courchesne E. Brainstem, cerebellar and limbic neuroanatomical abnormalities in autism. *Curr Opin Neurobiol* 1997;**7**:269–78.

Frith U. Emanuel Miller lecture: confusions and controversies about Asperger syndrome. *J Child Psychol Psychiatry* 2004;**45**:672–86.

Gabis L, Wei Huang, Azizian A, et al. 1H-magnetic resonance spectroscopy markers of cognitive and language ability in clinical subtypes of autism spectrum disorders. *J Child Neurol* 2008;**23**(7)766–74.

Ghaziuddin M, Butler E, Tsai L, Ghaziuddin N. Is clumsiness a marker for Asperger syndrome? *J Intellect Disabil Res* 1994;**3**(Pt 5)519–27.

Gowen E, Miall RC. Behavioural aspects of cerebellar function in adults with Asperger syndrome. *Cerebellum* 2005;**4**:279–89.

Hill EL, Frith U. Understanding autism: insights from mind and brain. *Philos Trans R Soc Lond B Biol Sci* 2003;**358**:281–9.

Kemper TL, Bauman M. Neuropathology of infantile autism. *J Neuropathol Exp Neurol* 1998;**57**:645–52.

Lalande M, Calciano MA. Molecular epigenetics of Angelman syndrome. *Cell Mol Life Sci* 2007;**64**(7–8): 947–60.

Miyahara M, Tsujii M, Hori M, et al. Brief report: motor incoordination in children with Asperger syndrome and learning disabilities. *J Autism Dev Disord* 1997;**27**:595–603.

Murakami JW, Courchesne E, Press GA, Yeung-Courchesne R, Hesselink JR. Reduced cerebellar hemisphere size and its relationship to vermal hypoplasia in autism. *Arch Neurol* 1989;**46**:689–94.

Peters SU, Beaudet AL, Madduri N, Bacino CA. Autism in Angelman syndrome: implications for autism research. *Clin Genet* 2004;**66**(6)530–6.

Polleux F, Lauder JM. Toward a developmental neurobiology of autism. *Ment Retard Dev Disabil Res Rev* 2004;**10**(4)303–17.

Rett A. Rett syndrome: history and general overview. *Am J Med Genet* 1986;**1**:21–5.

Singer-Harris NS, Courchesne E, Townsend J, Carper RA, Lord C. Neuroanatomic contributions to slowed orienting of attention in children with autism. *Brain Res Cogn Brain Res* 1999;**8**:61–71.

Wassmer E, Davies P, Whitehouse WP, Green SH. Clinical spectrum associated with cerebellar hypoplasia. *Pediatr Neurol* 2003;**28**:347–51.

Webb SJ, Sparks BF, Friedman SD, et al. Cerebellar vermal volumes and behavioral correlates in children with autism spectrum disorder. *Psychiatry Res* 2009;**172**(1)61–7.

Whitney ER, Kemper TL, Rosene DL, Bauman ML, Blatt GJ. Density of cerebellar basket and stellate cells in autism: Evidence for a late developmental loss of Purkinje cells. *J Neurosci Res* 2009;**87**(10):2245–54.

Williams CA. Neurological aspects of the Angelman syndrome. *Brain Dev* 2005;**27**(2)88–94.

Progressive myoclonic epilepsies

Progressive myoclonic epilepsies (PMEs) are disorders characterized by myoclonic seizures, tonic-clonic seizures, and progressive neurological deterioration, including in particular cerebellar signs and dementia (Shahwan et al., 2005). PMEs are considered to be the most severe form of the large group of myoclonic epilepsies, a collection of syndromes in which myoclonic seizures are a prominent feature (Leppik, 2003). Diagnosis of PME on pure clinical grounds can be intricate, but advances in genetics are rendering the diagnosis more and more precise.

The age of onset, the presenting symptoms, and the relative predominance of seizures or myoclonus over cerebellar ataxia or cognitive deficits vary substantially from one PME to another (Shahwan et al., 2005). The most common causes of PME are listed in Table 17.1. Myoclonic epilepsy with ragged-red fibers (MERRF) is also discussed in Chapter 21. Dentatorubral-pallidoluysian atrophy is reviewed in Chapter 23. Clues for the differential diagnosis are given in Table 17.2.

Unverricht-Lundborg disease is an autosomal recessive disorder. It is the most common PME. Its prevalence is about 1 per 20 000 births in Finland (Norio & Koskiniemi, 1979). Other clusters occur in southern Europe and North Africa. Sporadic cases are encountered worldwide. Symptoms start insidiously between 6 and 16 years. At least 50% of patients exhibit stimulus-sensitive myoclonic jerks (Lehesjoki, 2002). In many cases, the presentation is a generalized tonic-clonic seizure. Absence seizures may occur also. Action myoclonus may be global or segmental. Patients develop cerebellar ataxia later in the course of the disease. Kinetic tremor may become disabling. The disease is not associated with a progressive cognitive deficit. The electroencephalogram (EEG) may be normal initially, showing later in the course of the disease abnormalities similar to those observed in idiopathic generalized epilepsies. Subsequently, the recording will show a diffuse slow

background activity and generalized spike and wave, or polyspike and wave paroxysms with a suggestive photosensitivity (Berkovic et al., 1991). MRI results range from normal to patterns of atrophy involving the pons, medulla, cerebellar hemispheres, and cerebral cortex (Mascalchi et al, 2002). Molecular genetics is shown in Table 17.3. The disease is linked to chromosome 21q22.3. The gene encodes a cysteine protease inhibitor (Pennachio et al., 1996). The main mutation is an unstable expansion of a dodecamer repeat in the $5'$ untranslated promoter region. It is thought that apoptosis and neurodegeneration will result from the loss of inhibition of cysteine proteases.

Thanks to progress in the management of seizures, prognosis has improved substantially. The disorder has a limited progression. Patients are handicapped mostly by myoclonus. The following drugs are used for seizure and myoclonus control: valproic acid, clonazepam as add-on therapy, piracetam at high doses, levetiracetam, and zonisamide (Iivainen & Himberg, 1982; Remy & Genton, 1991; Magaudda et al., 2004). Phenytoin is contraindicated since it may worsen myoclonus and exacerbate or even trigger cerebellar signs.

Lafora disease presents with epilepsy, myoclonus, and dementia. Intracellular inclusion bodies (periodic acid–Schiff positive), called Lafora bodies, are observed in the neurons, skeletal muscles, heart, liver, and sweat-gland duct cells (Busard et al., 1986). Physical and mental development is usually normal until the age of 11 to 16 years, when seizures start. Myoclonic jerks, occipital seizures, absences, and complex partial seizures may occur. Cognitive deficit may be subtle at the beginning, and patients may be first diagnosed with juvenile myoclonic epilepsy. Dysarthria, gait, and limb ataxia appear usually early in the course of the disease. After a few years, continuous myoclonus develops (Minassian, 2002). Death within 10 to 12 years after onset of symptoms is common.

At the beginning of symptoms, the EEG is characterized by multiple spike-and-wave discharges.

Table 17.1 Main causes of progressive myoclonic epilepsies (PME)

Unverricht-Lundborg disease (PME type 1)

Lafora disease

Myoclonic epilepsy with ragged-red fibers (MEERF)

Neuronal ceroid lipofuscinosis (NCL)

Sialidoses

Dentatorubral pallidoluysian atrophy (DRPLA)

Photosensitivity is usual. Photic stimulation induces epileptiform discharges in some cases (Kobayashi et al., 1990). The background is initially relatively well organized and will worsen with time in all cases. The spike-and-wave pattern usually shifts in frequency from about 3 Hz to frequencies up to 12 Hz as the disease progresses (Yen et al., 1991). Somatosensory evoked potentials frequently show giant responses.

Skin biopsy should be performed when the diagnosis is suspected. Genetic study is also very informative. The majority of patients carry a mutation in the EPM2A gene on chromosome 6q24 (Minassian et al., 1998). The gene encodes a tyrosine phosphatase called laforin involved in translational regulation and causing polyglucosan deposits (Ganesh et al., 2000). Another locus (NHLRC1) has been mapped to chromosome 6p22 (Chan et al., 2003). This region codes for proteins involved in axonal and dendritic transport.

An effective treatment for Lafora disease is lacking. It is hoped that gene therapy or stem-cell based treatments might replace the defective protein in the next years.

Myoclonic epilepsy with ragged-red fibers (MERRF; also called Fukuhara disease) is either sporadic or familial. MERRF is typically maternally inherited (Rosing et al., 1985). There is an intrafamilial variability in terms of age of onset and severity of deficits (Chinnery et al., 1997). Clinically, the syndrome includes myoclonus, generalized seizure, and ataxia. The presentation includes various combinations of myopathy, peripheral neuropathy, behavioral and cognitive deficits (both usually mild or moderate), hearing loss, short stature, and optic atrophy. Patients may also exhibit a cardiomyopathy, oculomotor deficits with pigmentary retinopathy, lipomas, and diabetes mellitus.

The EEG reveals an abnormal background activity which progresses slowly as the disease evolves. Generalized spike-and-wave discharges at 3 to 5 Hz are common. Focal epileptiform discharges may occur (So et al., 1989).

Ragged red fibers are found in the muscles in the large majority of patients. Decreased activities of respiratory-chain enzymes in muscle extracts are common. Pathological findings include degeneration of the dentate nuclei, globus pallidus, and red nuclei, substantia nigra, inferior olivary nuclei, and cerebellar cortex. The posterior columns, spinocerebellar tracts, and Clarke columns are degenerating in the spinal cord (Fukuhara, 2008). Brain imaging may demonstrate cerebral atrophy, calcium deposits in basal

Table 17.2 Clues for the differential diagnosis of progressive myoclonic epilepsies

	Unverricht-Lundborg disease	Lafora disease	MERRF	NCL	Sialidosis
Clinical features	Severe myoclonus	Partial seizures Dementia	Severe myoclonus Deafness Lipomas Optic atrophy Myopathy Neuropathy	Fundal changes Dementia	Severe myoclonus Fundal changes Neuropathy Dysmorphism
Neurophysiology				Activation of epileptiform discharges during non-REM sleep Photosensitivity to single flashes	Vertex spikes Activation of epileptiform discharges during non-REM sleep
Laboratory findings			Elevated lactate levels in blood and CSF	Lymphocyte vacuolation	Lymphocyte vacuolation

Abbreviations: CSF: cerebrospinal fluid; MERRF: myoclonic epilepsy with ragged-red fibers; NCL: neuronal ceroid lipofuscinosis.

Table 17.3 Genetics of progressive myoclonic epilepsies

Disorder	Inheritance	Gene (locus)	Protein
Unverricht-Lundborg disease	AR	CSTB (Ch21q22.3)	Cystatin B
Lafora disease	AR	EPM2A (Ch6q24) NHLRC1 (Ch6p22)	Laforin
Myoclonic epilepsy with ragged red fibers (MEERF)	Maternal	MTTK	tRNALys
Neuronal ceroid lipofuscinosis (NCL) Late infantile Finnish-variant late infantile Juvenile Kufs disease (adult)	AR AR AR AR/AD	TPP1 (Ch11p15) CLN5 (Ch13q21-q32) CLN3 (Ch6p)	Tripeptidyl peptidase 1
Sialidoses Type I Type II	 AR AR	 NEU1 (Ch6p21.3) NEU1 (Ch20)	 Sialidase 1 Sialidase 1
Dentatorubral pallidoluysian atrophy (DRPLA)	AD	Ch12p13.31	Atrophin 1

Abbreviations: AD: autosomal dominant; AR: autosomal recessive.

ganglia, and signal changes in the white matter on brain MRI (DiMauro et al., 2002). A genetic mutation has been found in the majority of patients (point mutation A→G of nt 8344 in mitochondrial DNA), but not in all.

A specific therapy is missing. However, many patients receive an empiric treatment combining or not coenzyme Q10, L-carnitine, or various vitamins with antioxidant properties (see also Chapter 21). Valproic acid may impair carnitine uptake and should therefore be avoided if possible.

Neuronal ceroid lipofuscinosis (NCLs) consists of diseases characterized by lysosomal accumulation of abnormal amounts of lipopigment. With the exception of the adult form, NCLs have an autosomal recessive inheritance.

The late infantile form starts between 2 and 4 years. The first manifestation is usually a seizure (myoclonic, tonic-clonic, atonic, or atypical absence). Ataxia starts several months later. Macular degeneration and visual failure, dementia, and spasticity develop thereafter. Death occurs within 5 years. EEG reveals a disorganized activity, with slowing of the background and generalized epileptiform discharges. Posterior spikes may occur following photic stimulation, and flash stimuli may generate giant visual evoked potentials. Diagnosis can be confirmed by detecting a decreased enzymatic activity of TPP1, a tripeptidyl peptidase, either in fibroblasts or in leukocytes (Gardiner, 2002). A variant has been described in Finland. Symptoms start at about 5 years, and the progression is slower. Ataxia appears usually around 7 to 10 years. The

late infantile variant ("early juvenile") usually starts at the age of 5 to 7 years and leads to death within two decades. The juvenile form (Batten disease) is typically characterized by a visual failure starting at age 4 to 11 years. Blindness is very common at the age of 20 years. Patients exhibit cognitive deficits, as well as pyramidal deficits. Seizures are not prominent. Myoclonus is usually subtle. Behavioral symptoms are frequent. In particular, patients may develop a psychotic-like behavior. Fundus examination shows optic atrophy and macular degeneration. The adult form of NCL (Kufs disease) starts usually in the third decade, although onset in adolescence has been reported. First symptoms are dementia, ataxia, and extra-pyramidal deficits. Visual failure is absent. The disease is genetically heterogeneous (Boehme et al., 1971).

Brain MRI may show atrophy, including the cerebellar structures. White matter hyperintensities in T2-weighted sequences and thinning of the cerebral cortex are not uncommon. A biopsy showing intracellular inclusions (curvilinear or fingerprint-like) by electron microscopy provides the diagnosis. Inclusions are found in eccrine secretory cells, conjunctiva, and muscles or can be detected in rectal mucosa (Rapola et al., 1984).

Although antioxidants and amino acids such as methionine are administered in NCLs, the demonstration of a benefit is lacking.

Sialidosis type I (cherry spot myoclonus syndrome) is due to a deficiency in neuraminidase. The disease has a slow progression. Patients do not exhibit cognitive

Table 17.4 Rare causes of progressive myoclonic epilepsies

Action myoclonus renal failure syndrome

Juvenile form of Huntington disease

Gaucher disease (see Chapter 20)

Neuroaxonal dystrophy

Familial encephalopathy with neuroserpin inclusion bodies

GM2 gangliosidosis (see Chapter 20)

Hallevorden-Spatz disease

Table 17.5 Drugs commonly used in progressive myoclonic epilepsies

Valproic acid (caution is required in myoclonic epilepsy with ragged-red fibers)

Benzodiazepines

Phenobarbital

Piracetam

Levetiracetam

Zonisamide

deficits. Dysmorphism, gradual visual failure, tonic-clonic seizures, ataxia, and a cherry-red spot in the fundus are suggestive (Rapin et al., 1978). The clinical symptoms may be dominated by cerebellar syndrome (Palmeri et al., 2000). Sialidosis type II is a galactosialidosis starting usually between the neonatal period and the second decade. The syndrome includes learning deficits, myoclonus, corneal clouding, dysmorphism, skeletal dysplasia, and liver enlargement. Brain MRI demonstrates atrophy (cerebral cortex, pons, cerebellum) after a few years. Diagnosis is confirmed by the detection of high concentrations of sialyl oligosaccharides in urine. Lysosomal enzyme deficiency is found in leukocytes or cultured fibroblasts (Lowden & O'Brien, 1979; see also Chapter 20). Gene therapy and enzyme replacement are considered as possible therapies in the future.

Rare causes of PME are listed in Table 17.4. A syndrome affecting children presenting with generalized tonic-clonic epilepsy, ataxia, and mental retardation in absence of myoclonus recently has been described in a large consanguineous family (Gribaa et al., 2007). The gene is localized at 16q21-q23.

Familial adult myoclonic epilepsy (FAME) has an autosomal dominant inheritance. FAME has been linked to chromosome 8q24 in Japanese families (FAME1) and 2p11.1-q12.2 in European families

(FAME2) (Plaster et al., 1999; Striano et al., 2004). FAME is characterized by myoclonus, rare seizures with mild progression, and tremor. A third form (FAME3) has a more severe presentation, with clinical and radiological evidence of cerebellar impairment (Carr et al., 2007).

The management of seizures and myoclonus is essential in PME. Unfortunately, both seizures and myoclonus tend to become resistant with time. Table 17.5 summarizes the drugs commonly used. Drugs that may exacerbate myoclonus are phenytoin, carbamazepine, gabapentin, vigabatrin, and tiagabine. Lamotrigine must be used with caution (Das et al., 2003). The role of vagus nerve stimulation remains to be established.

References

Berkovic SF, So NK, Andermann F. Progressive myoclonus epilepsies: clinical and neurophysiological diagnosis. *J Clin Neurophysiol* 1991;**8**:261–74.

Boehme DH, Cottrell JC, Leonberg SC, Zeman W. A dominant form of neuronal ceroid-lipofuscinosis. *Brain* 1971;**94**:745–60.

Busard BLSM, Renier WO, Gabreels FJM, et al. Lafora's disease. *Arch Neurol* 1986;**43**:296–9.

Carr JA, Van Der Walt PE, Nakayama J, et al. A novel form of progressive myoclonus and epilepsy. *Neurology* 2007;**68**(17):1382–9.

Chan EM, Bulman DE, Paterson AD, et al. Genetic mapping of a new Lafora progressive myoclonus epilepsy locus (EPM2B) on 6p22. *J Med Genet* 2003;**40**:671–5.

Chinnery PF, Howell N, Lightwolers RN, Turnbull DM. The relationship between mutation load and clinical phenotypes. *Brain* 1997;**120**:1713–21.

Das KB, Harris C, Smyth DP, Cross JH. Unusual side effects of lamotrigine therapy. *J Child Neurol* 2003;**18**:479–80.

DiMauro S, Hirano M, Kaufmann P, et al. Clinical features and genetics of myoclonus epilepsy with ragged-red fibres. *Adv Neurol* 2002;**89**:217–29.

Fukuhara N. Fukuhara disease. *Brain Nerve* 2008;**60**(1): 53–8.

Ganesh S, Agarwala KL, Ueda K, et al. Laforin, defective in progressive myoclonus epilepsy of Lafora type, is a dual specificity phosphatase associated with polyribosomes. *Hum Mol Genet* 2000;**9**:2251–61.

Gardiner RM. Clinical features and molecular genetic basis of the neuronal ceroid lipofuscinosis. *Adv Neurol* 2002;**89**:211–5.

Gribaa M, Salih M, Anheim M, et al. A new form of childhood onset, autosomal recessive spinocerebellar ataxia and epilepsy is localized at 16q21-q23. *Brain* 2007;**130**:1921–28.

Iivanainen M, Himberg JJ. Valproate and clonazepam in the treatment of severe progressive myoclonus epilepsy. *Arch Neurol* 1982;**39**:236–8.

Kobayashi K, Iyoda K, Ohtsuka Y, et al. Longitudinal clinicoelectrophysiologic study of a case of Lafora disease proven by skin biopsy. *Epilepsia* 1990; **31**:194–201.

Lehesjoki AE. Clinical features and genetics of Unverricht-Lundborg disease. *Adv Neurol* 2002;**89**:193–7.

Leppik IE. Classification of the myoclonic epilepsies. *Epilepsia* 2003;**44**(suppl 11):2–6.

Lowden JA, O'Brien JS. Sialidosis: a review of human neuraminidase deficiency. *Am J Hum Genet* 1979;**31**:1–18.

Magaudda A, Gelisse P, Genton P. Antimyoclonic effect of levetiracetam in 13 patients with Unverricht-Lundborg disease: clinical observations. *Epilepsia* 2004;**45**: 678–81.

Mascalchi M, Michelucci R, Cosottini M, et al. Brainstem involvement in Unverricht-Lundborg disease (EPM1): an MRI and 1H MRS study. *Neurology* 2002;**58**: 1686–9.

Minassian BA. Progressive myoclonus epilepsy with polyglucosan bodies: Lafora's disease. *Adv Neurol* 2002;**89**:199–210.

Minassian BA, Lee JR, Herbrick JA, et al. Mutations in a gene encoding a novel protein tyrosine phosphatase cause progressive myoclonus epilepsy. *Nat Genet* 1998;**20**:171–4.

Norio R, Koskiniemi M. Progressive myoclonic epilepsy: genetic and nosological aspects with special reference to 107 Finish patients. *Clin Genet* 1979;**15**:382–98.

Palmeri S, Villanova M, Malandrini A, et al. Type I sialidosis: a clinical, biochemical and neuroradiological study. *Eur Neurol* 2000;**43**(2):88–94.

Pennachio LA, Lehesjoki AE, Stone NE, et al. Mutations in the gene encoding cystatin B in myoclonic epilepsy (EPM1). *Science* 1996; **271**;1731–4.

Plaster NM, Uyama E, Uchino M, et al. Genetic localization of the familial adult myoclonic epilepsy (FAME) gene to chromosome 8q24. *Neurology* 1999;**53**:1180–3.

Rapin I, Goldfisher S, Katzman R, et al. The cherry-red spot myoclonus syndrome. *Ann Neurol* 1978;**3**:234–42.

Rapola J, Santavuori P, Savilahti E. Suction biopsy of rectal mucosa in the diagnosis of infantile and juvenile types of neuronal ceroid lipofuscinoses. *Hum Pathol* 1984;**15**:352–60.

Remy C, Genton P. Effect of high dose of oral piracetam on myoclonus in progressive myoclonus epilepsy (Mediterranean myoclonus). *Epilepsia* 1991;**32**:6.

Rosing HS, Hopkins LC, Wallace DC, et al. Maternally inherited mitochondrial myopathy and myoclonic epilepsy. *Ann Neurol* 1985; **17**:228–37.

Shahwan A, Farrell M, Delanty N. Progressive myoclonic epilepsies: a review of genetic and therapeutic aspects. *Lancet Neurol* 2005;**4**:239–48.

So N, Berkovic SF, Andermann F, et al. Myoclonus epilepsy and ragged-red fibers (MERRF). 2. Electrophysiological studies and comparison with the other progressive myoclonus epilepsies. *Brain* 1989;**112**:1261–76.

Striano P, Chifari R, Striano S, et al. A new benign adult familial myoclonic epilepsy (BAFME) pedigree suggesting linkage to chromosome 2p11.1-q12.2. *Epilepsia* 2004;**45**:190–2.

Yen C, Beydoun A, Drury I. Longitudinal EEG studies in a kindred with Lafora disease. *Epilepsia* 1991; **32**:895–9.

Multiple system atrophy

Multiple system atrophy (MSA) encompasses olivo-pontocerebellar atrophy, striatonigral degeneration, and Shy-Drager syndrome (Graham & Oppenheimer, 1969) (see Figure 18.1). MSA is sporadic in the vast majority of cases, although familial occurrence has been reported (Hara et al., 2007). MSA could be defined as a degenerative disease of the nervous system causing combinations of extra-pyramidal, pyramidal, cerebellar, and autonomic features (Berciano, 2002).

Epidemiology

Based on epidemiological studies, the prevalence rate of MSA is estimated to about 3 per 100 000 population, with a range from 0.6 in the United States to 8.4 in Japan, where the prevalence might be higher than in other countries (Harada et al., 1989; Bower et al., 1997; Schrag et al., 1999). In addition, the clinical presentation is dominated by the MSA-C type (see below) in Japan. A yearly incidence of 3 new cases per 100 000 has been estimated in a population aged 50 to 99 years (Bower et al., 1997). The disease is more common in men than women, with male-to-female ratios ranging from 1.1:1 to 1.5:1 (Wenning et al., 1994). Mean age of onset is 52.2±9.0 years, with a range from 31 to 78 years.

Diagnostic criteria

Diagnosis is based upon the consensus criteria issued in 1999, which take into account four groups of symptoms: symptoms of autonomic and urinary dysfunction, parkinsonism, symptoms of cerebellar dysfunction, and corticospinal tract features (Gilman et al., 1999). Patients can be classified as having possible MSA, probable MSA, or definite MSA. Autonomic dysfunction is a major feature of MSA. MSA-P refers to patients in whom parkinsonian features predominate. MSA-C indicates that cerebellar signs dominate. Nevertheless, clinical features of MSA appear heterogeneous, and some patients initially classified

as MSA-C may fall in the basket of MSA-P during follow-up.

Diagnosis may be difficult at onset of the disease. Some patients are initially classified as having cerebellar cortical atrophy or Parkinson disease. The most common complaint is gait difficulties. Autonomic symptoms are reported in about 20% to 25% at an initial stage (Table 18.1), but signs of dysautonomia will be found in all patients during the follow-up (Watanabe et al., 2002). Bradykinesia and rigidity are relatively common. Levodopa-induced dyskinesias have been reported in up to 53% of cases, having an orofacial predominance (Hughes et al., 1992). Parkinsonism is clear in up to 80% of the patients, whereas cerebellar signs are clearly noted in 47% of cases. Pyramidal signs are reported in 6 in 10 patients. Cognitive deterioration is not rare, but marked dementia is considered to be a red flag (Table 18.2). Frontal lobe-like symptoms and dysexecutive syndrome are detected by neuropsychological evaluation (Robbins et al., 1992; Pillon et al., 1995). Supranuclear ophthalmoparesis primarily involves vertical gaze in progressive supranuclear palsy, whereas the horizontal gaze can be affected in MSA. Other manifestations include myoclonus, sleep disturbances, acroerythrocyanosis, and dystonia. Severity of clinical deficits can be estimated using the Unified Multiple System Atrophy Rating Scale (UMSARS) specifically designed for MSA (see Chapter 4). MSA-P patients usually have a more rapid functional deterioration than MSA-C patients, but survival is similar in both groups.

Neuroimaging

Brain imaging provides useful information to reach diagnosis, although diagnostic criteria do not include imaging results. Atrophy of the cerebellum and brainstem is observed in most patients (Figure 18.2). MRI can also reveal a hyperintense rim (T2-weighted sequence) at the outer margin of the putamen, and

Table 18.1 Autonomic symptoms commonly reported in multiple system atrophy

Urinary urgency

Incontinence

Retention

Postural hypotension (light-headedness, syncope)

Impotence

Constipation

Dyshidrosis

Table 18.2 Signs not suggestive of multiple system atrophy

Marked dementia

Classical "pill rolling" tremor

Good and long-standing levodopa response

Gaze palsy

Slowing of saccades

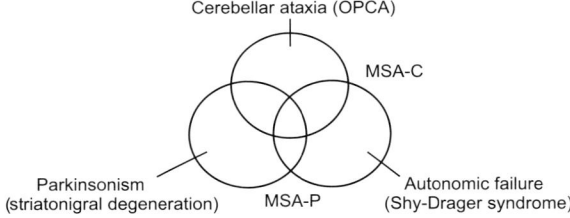

Figure 18.1 Multiple system atrophy (MSA) was originally described as olivopontocerebellar atrophy (OPCA), striatonigral degeneration, and Shy-Drager syndrome. These disorders have a noticeable overlap. MSA-C: MSA with predominance of cerebellar signs; MSA-P: MSA with predominant parkinsonian manifestations.

a "cross" sign in the pons. Positron emission tomography studies (^{18}F-fluorodeoxyglucose) show glucose hypometabolism in the cerebellum, brainstem, striatum, frontal, and motor areas in MSA (Gilman, 2005). Brain acetylcholinesterase activities are significantly decreased in the thalamus and the posterior lobe of the cerebellar cortex in MSA-C (Hirano et al., 2008). Magnetic resonance spectroscopy shows reductions in N-acetyl-aspartate/creatine ratios, reflecting neuronal loss.

Assessment of autonomic nervous system

Urodynamic studies show that 48% of patients have detrusor hyperreflexia and 29% have detrusor ato-nia (Beck et al., 1994). Denervation of the external sphincter of the urethra results from degeneration of somatic Onuf nucleus and can be assessed by sphincter electromyography (Mannen et al., 1982). Although postural hypotension (drop by 20 mm Hg systolic or 10 mm Hg diastolic) can be assessed at bedside, the use of a tilt table is recommended. Iodine-123 meta-iodobenzylguanidine (MIBG; an analogue of noradrenaline which evaluates postganglionic cardiac sympathetic neurons) cardiac scintigraphy is effective in distinguishing MSA from Parkinson disease (Druschky et al., 2000). This is based on the predominating postganglionic involvement of the autonomic nervous system in Parkinson disease, whereas the preganglionic structures are mainly affected in MSA. As a result, MIBG uptake is lower in patients with Parkinson disease as compared with MSA patients. There is no correlation between the involvement of the autonomic nervous system and the subclinical peripheral neuropathy which can be detected occasionally (Golbe, 1998).

Differential diagnosis

Differential diagnosis of MSA includes in particular sporadic cerebellar cortical atrophy, spinocerebellar ataxias presenting as pseudo-sporadic cerebellar atrophy, fragile X–associated tremor/ataxia syndrome, Parkinson disease with autonomic failure, Lewy body dementia with autonomic failure, and progressive supranuclear palsy. Other forms of sporadic ataxias need to be considered when neurological examination shows mainly cerebellar deficits, such as paraneoplastic cerebellar degeneration, ataxia with anti–glutamic acid decarboxylase antibodies, and gluten-sensitive enteropathy. Measurement of the midbrain area determined on brain MRI could differentiate MSA from progressive supranuclear palsy (Oba et al., 2005). Myocardial scintigraphy with MIBG shows an uptake significantly lower not only in Parkinson disease but also in Lewy body disease, as compared with MSA (Orimo et al., 2001). Another procedure which appears useful to distinguish Parkinson disease from MSA is the study of the growth hormone (GH) response to arginine (Pellecchia et al., 2006). A reduced GH response to arginine predicts MSA-P with an accuracy of 95%. Decreased response is due to an impairment of cholinergic central systems modulating GH release in MSA. Pure autonomy failure should be distinguished from MSA.

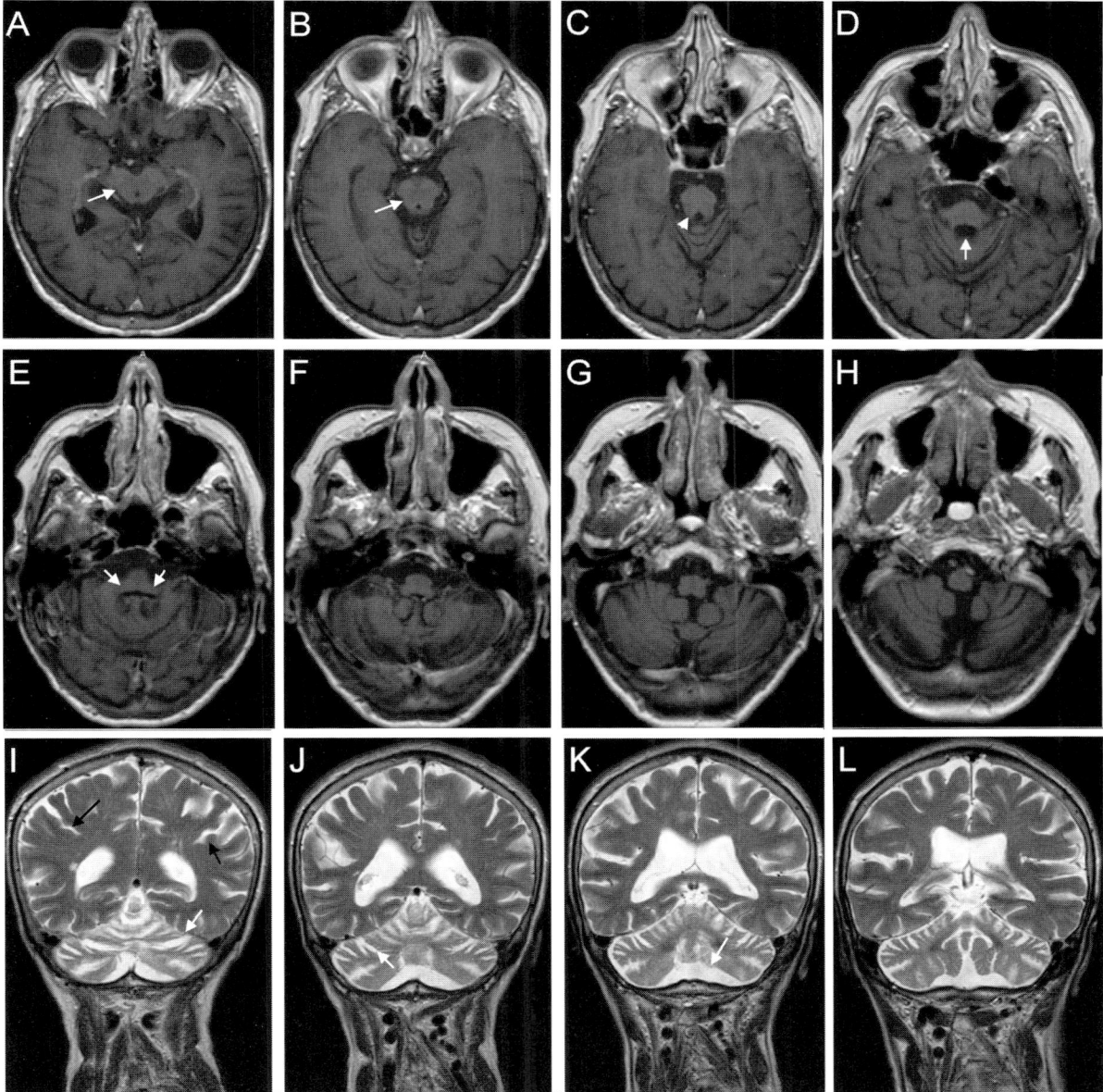

Figure 18.2 (A–H) T1-weighted axial brain MRI showing brainstem and cerebellar atrophy in a patient with the cerebellar form of MSA (MSA-C). (A, B) The mesencephalon (white arrows) is slightly atrophic. (C) Superior cerebellar peduncle (arrowhead). (D) Fourth ventricle (white arrow) is enlarged. Cerebellar sulci are widened and the pons is atrophic. (E) The middle cerebellar peduncles are shrunken (white arrows). (F–H) Atrophy of the medulla and the cerebellum. (I–L) Coronal T2-weighted images showing enlarged cerebral sulci (black arrows) and widened cerebellar sulci (white arrows in I–J). (K) Enlarged pericerebellar spaces (white arrow).

Neuropathology

Neuropathological studies show neuronal loss and glial or neuronal cytoplasmic inclusions, considered to be a pathological hallmark, in various locations of the CNS. The more severe lesions are found in the fol-lowing structures: substantia nigra, putamen, caudate, globus pallidus, inferior olivary nuclei, pons, cerebellar cortex, dentate nuclei, intermediolateral columns, anterior horns, and pyramidal tracts (Wenning et al.,

Table 18.3 Symptomatic treatment in multiple system atrophy

Extra-pyramidal signs	Carbidopa/levodopa Dopamine agonists Amantadine
Autonomic failure	Management of orthostatic hypotension Management of urinary disturbances Constipation: dietary fiber, liquid ingestion, laxatives
Respiratory difficulties	Clonazepam
Dysphagia	Modified diet Percutaneous gastrostomy
Decreased motility and speech deficits	Psychosocial support, occupational therapy, speech therapy

Adapted from: Berciano, 2002.

1997). Glial cytoplasmic inclusions are characterized by a marked alpha-synuclein immunoreactivity (Gai et al., 1998).

There is a correlation between nigrostriatal cell loss and disease severity at the time of death. Similarly, ataxia correlates with the degree of olivopontocerebellar lesions.

Treatment

Treatment is symptomatic (Table 18.3). Although levodopa (dose up to 1000 mg/day if tolerated) may improve patients exhibiting extra-pyramidal deficits at an early stage of the disease (up to 30% of MSA patients respond initially), most patients will become poor responders (Wenning et al., 1994). In a number of cases, the beneficial effect becomes evident when apparently unresponsive patients deteriorate after levodopa withdrawal (Hughes et al., 1992). Deterioration may become apparent after a delay of 3 to 6 days. Usually, dopamine agonists do not provide additional benefits. Some patients show improvements with amantadine (up to 400 mg/day). Orthostatic hypotension can be treated with elastic support stockings, head-up tilt of the bed at night, increased salt intake, fludrocortisone to expand extravascular body fluid volume (0.1–0.4 mg/day), and midodrine to cause vasoconstriction (7.5–30 mg/day). Oral L-threo-3,4-dihydroxyphenylserine (L-DOPS) also may be used (100–600 mg/day). L-DOPS is converted in norepinephrine outside the brain. Caffeine, octreotide,

and desmopressin may also provide some benefits. Some authors recommend the use of indomethacin (50–150 mg/day) to inhibit prostaglandin synthesis (resulting in vasodilatation). Drugs causing orthostatic hypotension should be avoided when possible (in particular antihypertensive agents and vasodilators). Desmopressin may provide benefits for nocturnal polyuria. Oxybutynin (5–10 mg/day) or propantheline (15–30 mg/day) is used for detrusor hyperreflexia. Clean intermittent self-catheterization of the bladder is recommended for large post-void residuals. If self-catheterization becomes difficult, a suprapubical catheter should be considered. Constipation should be treated with laxatives or clysters. Erectile dysfunction may benefit from sildenafil or penis implant. Sleep disturbances may respond to clonazepam (0.5–1 mg at bedtime). Continuous positive airway pressure therapy has been proposed for sleep apnea. Physical, occupational, and speech therapies may help the patient to remain independent for a longer period of time.

The course of the disease is characterized by worsening of symptoms. Progression tends to be faster as compared with hereditary ataxias (Klockgether et al., 1990). Patients become wheelchair-bound after a period of about 5 years (median; Watanabe et al., 2002). Death usually occurs after a median interval of 9 to 10 years. Frequent falling and dysphagia leading to aspiration pneumonia are frequent. Sudden death due to apnea and vocal fold palsy is common in MSA (Saito et al., 1994).

References

Beck RO, Betts CD, Fowler CJ. Genitourinary dysfunction in multiple system atrophy: clinical features and treatment of 62 cases. *J Urol* 1994;**151**:1336–41.

Berciano J. Multiple system atrophy and isiopathic late-onset cerebellar ataxia. In The *Cerebellum and Its Disorders*, ed. M. Manto and M. Pandolfo. Cambridge, UK: Cambridge University Press, 2002, pp. 178–97.

Bower JH, Maraganore DM, McDonnell SK, Rocca WA. Incidence of, progressive supranuclear palsy and multiple system atrophy in Olmsted County, Minnesota, 1976 to 1990. *Neurology* 1997;**49**:1284–8.

Druschky A, Hilz MJ, Platsch G, et al. Differentiation of Parkinson's disease and multiple system atrophy in early disease stages by means of I-123-MIBG-SPECT. *J Neurol Sci* 2000;**175**(1):3–12.

Gai WP, Power JHT, Blumbergs PC, Blessing WW. Multiple system atrophy: a new alpha-synuclein disease? *Lancet* 1998;**352**:547–8.

Gilman S. Functional imaging with positron emission tomography in multiple system atrophy. *J Neural Transm* 2005;**112**:1647–55.

Gilman S, Low PA, Quinn N, et al. Consensus statement on the diagnosis of multiple system atrophy. *J Neurol Sci* 1999;**163**:94–8.

Golbe LI. Multiple system atrophy. In *Neurobase*, ed. S. Gilman, G.W. Goldstein, and S.G. Waxman. San Diego, CA: Arbor Publishing, 1998.

Graham JG, Oppenheimer DR. Orthostatic hypotension and nicotine sensitivity in a case of multiple system atrophy. *J Neurol Neurosurg Psychiatry* 1969;**32**:28–34.

Hara K, Momose Y, Tokiguchi S, et al. Multiplex families with multiple system atrophy. *Arch Neurol* 2007;**64**:545–51.

Harada H, Takahashi K. Epidemiology of spinocerebellar degeneration in Tottori prefecture. *Rinsho Shinkeigaku* 1989;**29**:164–6.

Hirano S, Shinotoh H, Arai K, et al. PET study of brain acetylcholinesterase in cerebellar degenerative disorders. *Mov Disord* 2008;**23**(8):1154–60.

Hughes AJ, Colosimo C, Kleeforfer B, Daniel SE, Lees AJ. The dopaminergic response in multiple system atrophy. *J Neurol Neurosurg Psychiatry* 1992;**55**:1009–13.

Klockgether T, Schroth G, Diener HC, Dichgans J. Idiopathic cerebellar ataxia of last onset: natural history and MRI morphology. *J Neurol Neurosurg Psychiatry* 1990;**53**:297–305.

Mannen T, Iwata M, Toyokura Y, Nagashima K. The Onuf's nucleus and the external sphincter muscles in amyotrophic lateral sclerosis and Shy-Drager syndrome. *Acta Neuropathol* 1982; **58**:225–60.

Oba H, Yagishita A, Terada H, et al. New and reliable MRI diagnosis for progressive supranuclear palsy. *Neurology* 2005;**64**:2050–5.

Orimo S, Ozawa E, Oka T, et al. Different histopathology accounting for a decrease in myocardial MIBG uptake in PD and MSA. *Neurology* 2001;**57**:1140–1.

Pellecchia MT, Longo K, Pivonello R, et al. Multiple system atrophy is distinguished from idiopathic Parkinson's disease by the arginine growth hormone stimulation test. *Ann Neurol* 2006;**60**(5):611–5.

Pillon B, Gonider-Khouja N, Deweer B, et al. Neuropsychological pattern of striatonigral degeneration: comparison with Parkinson's disease and supranuclear palsy. *J Neurol Neurosurg Psychiatry* 1995;**58**:174–9.

Robbins TW, James M, Lange KW, et al. Cognitive performance in multiple system atrophy. *Brain* 1992; **115**:271–291.

Saito Y, Matsuoka Y, Takahashi A, Ohno Y. Survival of patients with multiple system atrophy. *Intern Med* 1994;**33**:321–5.

Schrag A, Ben-Shlomo Y, Quinn NP. Prevalence of progressive supranuclear palsy and multiple system atrophy: a cross-sectional study. *Lancet* 1999;**354**:1771–5.

Watanabe H, Saito Y, Terao S, et al. Progression and prognosis in multiple system atrophy: an analysis of 230 Japanese patients. *Brain* 2002;**125**:1070–83.

Wenning GK, Ben-Shlomo Y, Magalhes M, Daniel SE, Quinn NP. Clinical features and natural history of multiple system atrophy: an analysis of 100 cases. *Brain* 1994;**117**:835–45.

Wenning GK, Tison F, Ben-Shlomo Y, Daniel SE, Quinn NP. Multiple system atrophy: a review of 203 pathologically proven cases. *Mov Disord* 1997;**12**:133–47.

Essential tremor

Epidemiology

Essential tremor (ET) is the most common movement disorder in the elderly. Although the disorder usually starts after the age of 50 years in most cases, it may occur at any age. Many patients may never seek medical attention. The estimated annual incidence of essential tremor is 616 per 100 000 among individuals aged 65 years and older (Benito-Leon et al., 2005). Prevalence is higher in white than in African American populations and reaches 20% among the oldest old (age $\geq$ 95 years) (Louis et al., 2009). Relatives of patients with ET are five times more likely to develop the disease than are members of the general population (Louis et al., 2001). Patients with ET have an increased risk to develop incident Parkinson disease (Benito-Leon et al., 2009).

Clinical features

Essential tremor is now considered a progressive and clinically heterogeneous disorder with sporadic and familial forms, and motor and non-motor manifestations (Thanvi et al., 2006). In many cases, ET is familial. Dominantly inherited ET was first recognized by Dana in 1887 (Dana, 1887). One pattern of presentation is a dominant mode of inheritance with an incomplete penetrance by the age of 65 years. Age of onset is usually earlier in familial forms than in sporadic cases.

Postural/action tremor of the arms is a major feature, but the head, legs, trunk, voice, jaw, and facial muscles may also be involved. Typically, a more or less symmetrical tremor affects the extremities and progresses medially. Bilateral action arm tremor is a key diagnostic feature. Up to 70% of patients report a benefit with alcohol intake (Jankovic, 2000). Table 19.1 shows the clinical diagnostic criteria (Deuschl et al., 1998).

The Fahn-Tolosa-Marin clinical tremor rating scale is widely used to characterize the severity of ET (Fahn et al., 1987).

Neurophysiological studies

In ET, the frequency of upper limb tremor is 4 to 12 Hz. A majority of patients exhibit a tremor with a main frequency between 5 and 9 Hz (Figure 19.1). A kinetic tremor is often found in association with the postural oscillations (Brennan et al., 2002). The amplitude of the kinetic component is usually more severe. Tremor frequency decreases with time, whereas tremor amplitude tends to increase. The average annual decrease of the tremor frequency is 0.12 Hz/year (Hellwig et al., 2009).

The olivo-cerebello-thalamo-cortical pathway has been implicated in the genesis of ET. The olivocerebellar pathway is considered as the central oscillator driving the peripheral tremor. Thalamic nuclei might play a critical role since they behave as oscillators or even as resonators. Coherence analysis of electromyography signals indicates that tremor in each arm is related to independent central oscillators which may dynamically synchronize by interhemispheric coupling (Hellwig et al., 2003).

Blink reflex conditioning studies show a significantly abnormal motor learning in subjects with advanced ET (Farkas et al., 2006).

Neuroimaging studies

Recent automated volumetric methods confirm a reduction of cerebellar volume in patients with ET with respect to healthy controls after controlling for intra-cranial volume (Cerasa et al., 2009).

Proton magnetic resonance spectroscopy (MRS) studies show decreased N-acetyl-aspartate/creatine (NAA/Cr) ratios in the cerebellum of individuals with ET, suggesting a neuronal dysfunction (Louis et al., 2007).

A significant glucose hypermetabolism of the medulla and thalami has been found using positron emission tomography with ^{18}F-fluorodeoxyglucose (Hallett & Dubinsky, 1993).

Table 19.1 Diagnostic criteria of essential tremor (ET)

Definite ET
   Inclusion criteria
      Visible and persistent bilateral postural tremor with or
         without kinetic tremor, involving hands and forearms
      Duration > 5 years

   Exclusion criteria
      Other abnormal neurological signs (Except Froment sign)
      Presence of known causes of increased physiological
         tremor
      Concurrent or recent exposure to tremorogenic drugs
      Drug-withdrawal state
      Trauma within 3 months before onset of tremor
      Historical or clinical evidence of psychogenic origin
      Sudden onset or stepwise deterioration

Probable ET
   Tremor may be confined to one body part other than the
   hands
   Duration > 3 years

Possible ET
   Presence of other neurological disorders (parkinsonism)
   Presence of other isolated tremors (task-specific tremors)

Genetic studies

Essential tremor is genetically heterogeneous. Hereditary essential tremor-1 (ETM1) is associated with a polymorphism in the DRD3 gene on chromosome 3q13 (Gulcher et al., 1997). Other mapped loci include ETM2 on chromosome 2p25-p22 and ETM3 on chromosome 6p23. Pairwise concordance in monozygotic twins is approximately two times that in dizygotic twins, indicating that environmental factors may play an important role (Tanner et al., 2001).

Environmental factors

Several studies suggest that ET is triggered by environmental factors (Jiménez-Jiménez et al., 2007). High concentrations of beta-carboline alkaloids (BCAs; tremor-producing chemicals that are naturally present in the food chain) have been found in blood (Louis et al., 2002). Harmaline, a BCA, induces a temporary tremor in rodents which is reminiscent of ET. Harmaline enhances the electrical coupling in the inferior olives and also exerts dysregulation of glutamatergic pathways in cerebellar nuclei (Manto & Laute, 2008). Proton MRS studies in humans show a correlation between blood concentrations of BCAs and the NAA/Cr ratio in the cerebellar cortex (Louis et al., 2007).

Table 19.2 Drugs under investigation for the treatment of essential tremor

Zonisamide (100–200 mg/day)

Sodium oxybate (gamma-hydroxybutyrate; 1.5 g twice daily)

T2000 (DMMDPB; 600–1000 mg/day)

1-Octanol (1 mg/kg)

Lacosamide (50–400 mg/day)

Neuropathology

Neuropathological changes are observed in the cerebellum in about 75% of patients. These changes include a decreased number of Purkinje neurons, Purkinje cell heterotopias, dendrite swellings, torpedoes (Purkinje cell axonal swellings), degeneration of dentate neurons, and presence of Lewy bodies in the brainstem (Axelrad et al., 2008).

Treatment

Currently, there is still no medication developed and specifically approved for essential tremor. Most of the drugs used are approved for epilepsy. Pharmacological treatments currently available are effective in only approximately 50% of patients with ET (Lyons & Pahwa, 2008). The most commonly used medications are propranolol (40–160 mg/day) and primidone (250–750 mg/day), administered either as monotherapy or in combination. In case of insufficient reduction of tremor, other beta-adrenoceptor antagonists, such as metoprolol or atenolol, and other antiepileptic drugs, such as topiramate (50–200 mg/day) or gabapentin (600–1800 mg/day), are often tried. Beta-blockers should be used very cautiously in elderly individuals with asthma or heart disorders (conduction block). Pregabalin (50–600 mg/day) has shown some efficacy (Zesiewicz et al., 2007). Confirmation in large trials is required. Benzodiazepines can be effective in some patients, especially alprazolam and clonazepam (4 mg/day). Several drugs are under investigation (Table 19.2).

Botulinum toxin injections in the forearm muscles may provide some benefit, but carry the risk of muscle weakness. Swallowing difficulties and breathiness are complications of neck injections for head/voice tremor.

Deep brain stimulation (DBS) of the thalamic nuclei (Vim) has beneficial effects in ET. It is now an established therapy for medically intractable ET

A

UPPER LIMB OUTSTRETCHED

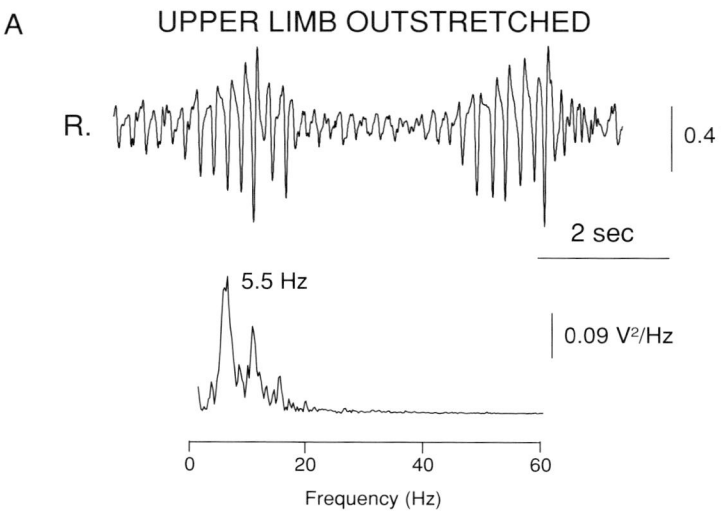

Figure 19.1 (A) Right upper limb postural tremor in a patient presenting with essential tremor. The patient is asked to maintain the upper limb outstretched in a horizontal position at the height of the shoulder. Fast Fourier Transform (FFT) shows a peak frequency of 5.5 Hz. Accelerometer fixed on the extremity of the index. Sampling rate: 512 Hz.
(B) Tremor of the index during a finger-to-finger test. The patient is asked to maintain left/right index finger near the chest, at the height of the shoulder. FFT analysis shows a peak frequency of 5 Hz on the left side and 3.9 Hz on the right side.

B

FINGER-TO-FINGER TEST

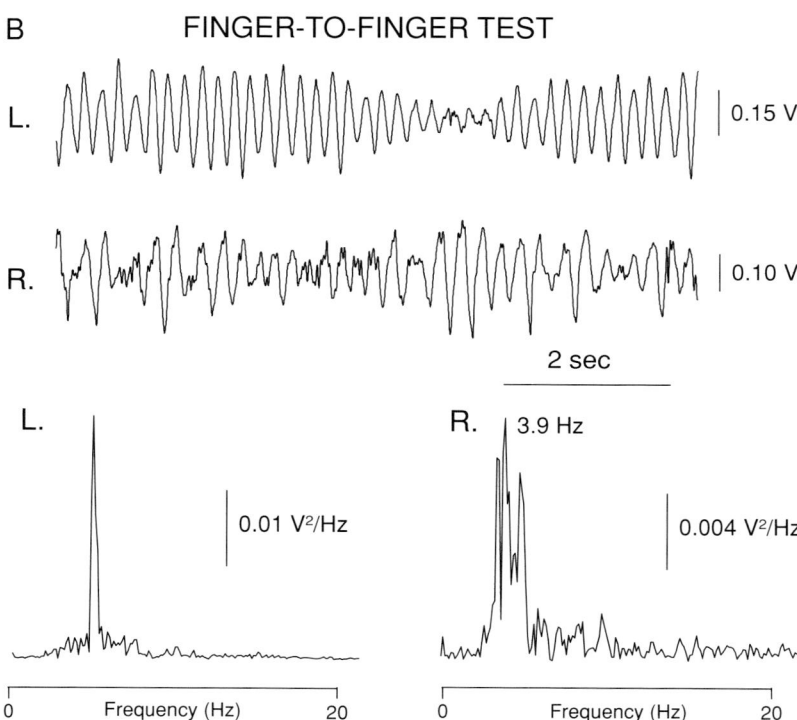

(see also Chapter 9). The benefit of stimulation of the subthalamic area might be related to a modulation of cerebellothalamic projections (Herzog et al., 2007). Risks of DBS procedures are intracranial hemorrhage (especially in patients with hypertension), seizures, and infections (Coley et al., 2009). Behavioral changes are usually transient. Although DBS has several advantages over thalamotomy, namely, the reversibility and the fact that bilateral procedures are feasible, irreversible lesion therapy is still used in some centers with good results.

Gamma-knife radiosurgery is a viable alternative in patients ineligible for DBS (Kondziolka et al., 2008). About 70% of patients show improvement in both action tremor and writing. However, patients may develop a delayed neurological deficit (hemiparesis, dysphagia, or a complex movement disorder).

Biomechanical loading has emerged as a potential tremor suppression alternative. Applying damping loads attenuates tremor in upper limbs. A wearable orthosis based on this principle has been proposed (Rocon et al., 2007). Although individuals with ET may show a dramatic reduction of tremor, the current wearable solutions require major improvements in terms of weight, aesthetics, and cosmetic aspects to be used in daily life.

Electroencephalogram-based brain–computer interfaces aiming to detect and attenuate tremor are under investigation.

Patients may benefit from a computer mouse that filters the shaking components of movements during daily use of computers.

References

Axelrad JE, Louis ED, Honig LS, et al. Reduced Purkinje cell number in essential tremor: a postmortem study. *Arch Neurol* 2008;**65**(1):101–7.

Benito-Leon J, Bermejo-Pareja F, Louis ED. Incidence of essential tremor in three elderly populations of central Spain. *Neurology* 2005;**64**:1721–5.

Benito-León J, Louis ED, Bermejo-Pareja F; Neurological Disorders in Central Spain Study Group. Risk of incident Parkinson's disease and parkinsonism in essential tremor: a population based study. *J Neurol Neurosurg Psychiatry* 2009;**80**(4):423–5.

Brennan KC, Jurewicz EC, Ford B, Pullman SL, Louis ED. Is essential tremor predominantly a kinetic or a postural tremor? A clinical and electrophysiological study. *Mov Disord* 2002;**17**(2):313–6.

Cerasa A, Messina D, Nicoletti G, et al. Cerebellar atrophy in essential tremor using an automated segmentation method. *AJNR Am J Neuroradiol* 2009;**30**(6):1240–3.

Coley E, Farhadi R, Lewis S, Whittle IR. The incidence of seizures following deep brain stimulating electrode implantation for movement disorders, pain and psychiatric conditions. *Br J Neurosurg* 2009;**23**(2):179–83.

Dana CL. Hereditary tremor, a hitherto undescribed form of motor neurosis. *Am J Med Sci* 1887;**94**:386–93.

Deuschl G, Bain P, Brin M. Consensus statement of the movement disorder society on tremor. Ad Hoc Scientific Committee. *Mov Disord* 1998;**13**(suppl 3):2–23.

Fahn S, Tolosa E, Marin C. Clinical rating scale for tremor. In *Parkinson's Disease and Movement Disorders*, ed. J. Jankovic and E. Tolosa. Baltimore, MD: Urban and Schwarzenberg, 1987, pp. 225–34.

Farkas Z, Szirmai I, Kamondi A. Impaired rhythm generation in essential tremor. *Mov Disord* 2006;**21**(8):1196–9.

Gulcher JR, Jonsson P, Kong A, et al. Mapping of a familial essential tremor gene, FET1, to chromosome 3q13. *Nat Genet* 1997;**17**:84–7.

Hallett M, Dubinsky RM. Glucose metabolism in the brain of patients with essential tremor. *J Neurol Sci* 1993;**114**(1):45–8.

Hellwig B, Mund P, Schelter B, et al. A longitudinal study of tremor frequencies in Parkinson's disease and essential tremor. *Clin Neurophysiol* 2009;**120**(2):431–5.

Hellwig B, Schelter B, Guschlbauer B, Timmer J, Lücking CH. Dynamic synchronisation of central oscillators in essential tremor. *Clin Neurophysiol* 2003;**114**(8):1462–7.

Herzog J, Hamel W, Wenzelburger R, et al. Kinematic analysis of thalamic versus subthalamic neurostimulation in postural and intention tremor. *Brain* 2007;**130**(Pt 6):1608–25.

Jankovic J. Essential tremor: clinical characteristics. *Neurology* 2000;**54**(11 suppl 4):S21–5.

Jiménez-Jiménez FJ, de Toledo-Heras M, Alonso-Navarro H, et al. Environmental risk factors for essential tremor. *Eur Neurol* 2007;**58**(2):106–13.

Kondziolka D, Ong JG, Lee JY, et al. Gamma knife thalamotomy for essential tremor. *J Neurosurg* 2008;**108**(1):111–7.

Louis ED, Ford B, Frucht S, Ottman R. Mild tremor in relatives of patients with essential tremor: what does this tell us about the penetrance of the disease? *Arch Neurol* 2001;**58**:1584–9.

Louis ED, Thawani SP, Andrews HF. Prevalence of essential tremor in a multiethnic, community-based study in northern Manhattan, New York, N.Y. *Neuroepidemiology* 2009;**32**(3):208–14.

Louis ED, Zheng W, Jurewicz EC, et al. Elevation of blood beta-carboline alkaloids in essential tremor. *Neurology* 2002;**59**(12):1940–4.

Louis ED, Zheng W, Mao X, Shungu DC. Blood harmane is correlated with cerebellar metabolism in essential tremor: a pilot study. *Neurology* 2007;**69**(6):515–20.

Lyons KE, Pahwa R. Pharmacotherapy of essential tremor: an overview of existing and upcoming agents. *CNS Drugs* 2008;**22**(12):1037–45.

Manto M, Laute MA. A possible mechanism for the beneficial effect of ethanol in essential tremor. *Eur J Neurol* 2008;**15**(7):697–705.

Rocon E, Manto M, Pons J, Camut S, Belda JM. Mechanical suppression of essential tremor. *Cerebellum* 2007;**6**(1):73–8.

Shill HA, De La Vega FJ, Samanta J, Stacy M. Motor learning in essential tremor. *Mov Disord* 2009;**24**(6):926–8.

Tanner CM, Goldman SM, Lyons KE, et al. Essential tremor in twins: an assessment of genetic vs environmental determinants of etiology. *Neurology* 2001;**57**:1389–91.

Thanvi B, Lo N, Robinson T. Essential tremor-the most common movement disorder in older people. *Age Ageing* 2006;**35**(4):344–9.

Zesiewicz TA, Ward CL, Hauser RA, et al. A pilot, double-blind, placebo-controlled trial of pregabalin (Lyrica) in the treatment of essential tremor. *Mov Disord* 2007;**22**(11):1660–3.

Chapter 20

Autosomal recessive cerebellar ataxias

Autosomal recessive cerebellar ataxias (ARCAs) are a heterogeneous group of neurological disorders involving both the central and peripheral nervous systems and, in some cases, other systems as well (Palau & Espinós, 2006). The onset is usually before the age of 20 years. The presence of multiple affected siblings in a single generation or consanguinity in parents supports the possibility of an autosomal recessive mode of inheritance. ARCAs are characterized in most cases by degeneration or abnormal development of the cerebellum and spinal cord. Due to autosomal recessive inheritance, previous familial history of affected individuals is unlikely.

Based on clinicogenetic criteria, five main types of ARCAs can be distinguished (Table 20.1): congenital ataxias (developmental disorder), ataxias associated with metabolic disorders, ataxias with a DNA repair defect, degenerative ataxias, and ataxia associated with other features.

The most commonly encountered ARCAs are as follows:

- Friedreich ataxia (the most common in Caucasian population)
- Ataxia-telangiectasia
- Wilson disease
- Lysosomal storage disorders
- Early-onset cerebellar ataxia with retained tendon reflexes
- Ataxia with vitamin E deficiency (AVED)
- Abetalipoproteinemia
- Ataxia with oculomotor apraxia (AOA1)
- Ataxia with oculomotor apraxia (AOA2)
- Ataxia associated with coenzyme Q10 deficiency
- Autosomal recessive spastic ataxia of Charlevoix-Saguenay (ARSACS)

Clinical diagnosis is confirmed by ancillary tests such as neuroimaging (MRI, scanning), electrophysiological studies, and mutation analysis when the causative gene has been identified. Correct clinical and genetic diagnosis is important for appropriate genetic counseling and prognosis and, in some instances, pharmacological treatment, especially for coenzyme Q10 deficiency and abetalipoproteinemia.

Friedreich ataxia

Clinical description

Friedreich ataxia (FRDA) affects patients from Europe, North Africa, and the Middle East. The disorder is rare among sub-Saharan Africans and does not exist in the Far East. The prevalence varies between 2 and 4.5 per 100 000. Some clusters of families have been reported in Québec and Cyprus, due to a founder effect (Barbeau, 1978; Dean et al., 1988).

The first symptoms usually start between 8 and 19 years (Friedreich, 1863a, 1863b, 1863c; Geoffroy et al., 1976; Campanella et al., 1980). However, they may start earlier or even later in the adult life, in the so-called late-onset Friedreich ataxia (LOFA; first symptoms occurring after the age of 25) or very late-onset Friedreich ataxia (VLOFA; symptoms starting after the age of 40 years) (Klockgether et al., 1993). The disease progression of LOFA and VLOFA is slower. The occurrence of skeletal deformities such as scoliosis is also lower. Variability of age onset may be observed within the same family, probably due to the characteristics of the mutation.

Diagnostic criteria have been proposed (Table 20.2).

Ataxia is typically progressive and mixed, combining cerebellar and sensory features. Truncal ataxia may be the first symptom, followed by limb dysmetria and kinetic tremor. Patients exhibit growing difficulties with walking and standing. Dysarthria is characterized by a slow and jerky speech with sudden utterances (Gentil, 1990; Cisneros & Braun, 1995). Most patients will exhibit various degrees of muscular weakness. Muscle tone is usually unaffected. When patients

Table 20.1 Autosomal recessive cerebellar ataxias

Congenital ataxias
    Joubert syndrome
    Cayman ataxia

Metabolic disorder
    Ataxia with isolated vitamin E deficiency (AVED)
    Refsum disease
    Cerebrotendinous xanthomatosis
    Abetalipoproteinemia
    Metachromatic leukodystrophy
    Niemann-Pick type C
    GM1 gangliosidosis
    GM2 gangliosidosis
    Chorea-acanthocytosis
    Wilson disease
    Aceruloplasminemia

Ataxias associated with a DNA repair defect
    Ataxia telangiectasia
    Ataxia with oculomotor apraxia 1 (AOA1)
    Ataxia with oculomotor apraxia 2 (AOA2)
    Ataxia-telangiectasia–like disorder
    Spinocerebellar ataxia with axonal neuropathy (SCAN1)

Degenerative ataxias
    Friedreich ataxia
    Coenzyme Q10 deficiency with cerebellar ataxia
    Charlevoix-Saguenay spastic ataxia
    Early-onset cerebellar ataxia with retained tendon reflexes
    Mitochondrial recessive ataxic syndrome
    Marinesco-Sjögren syndrome

Others

Table 20.2 Diagnostic criteria of Friedreich ataxia according to Harding (1981)

Onset before the age of 25

Progressive and unremitting ataxia

Hyporeflexia/areflexia in lower limbs

Babinski sign

Axonal sensory neuropathy demonstrated by neurophysiological studies

Dysarthria

become wheelchair-bound, a disuse atrophy develops. The sense of position and vibration are impaired early in the course of the disease due to peripheral nerve involvement. Although a majority of patients have an absence of tendon reflexes, some of them have increased tendon reflexes and may exhibit some degree of spasticity. This occurs in the so-called Friedreich ataxia with retained reflexes (FARR) presentation. A phenotype characterized by spastic paraparesis without obvious ataxia has been reported (Castelnovo et al., 2000). Oculomotor disturbances are common, with square wave jerks and fixation instability (Spieker et al., 1995). Nevertheless, a nystagmus is rarely

encountered. About one-third of patients exhibit optic atrophy (Livingstone et al., 1981). Patients may present with some degree of visual impairment. Sensorineural hearing loss occurs in one in five patients (El et al., 1984; Cassandro et al., 1986). Chorea has been reported in a few patients (Hanna et al., 1998).

Patients also exhibit extra-neurological features. Heart disease affects nearly all patients, although some patients remain asymptomatic. Cardiomyopathy may directly impact prognosis (Boyer et al., 1962; Maione et al., 1997). The most common symptoms are shortness of breath and palpitations. Electrocardiogram (ECG) often shows inverted T waves and signs of ventricular hypertrophy. Conduction disturbances, ectopic beats, and atrial fibrillation are less common (Alboliras et al., 1986). This latter is often considered to be a negative prognostic indicator. Decreased heart rate variability would be due to impaired parasympathetic activity (Pousset et al., 1996). Echocardiography shows a concentric hypertrophy of the ventricles or a symmetrical septal hypertrophy, with diastolic function abnormalities (Morvan et al., 1992). A transition from the hypertrophic to the hypokinetic-dilated cardiomyopathy may occur. Muscular subaortic stenosis has been described in a few cases (Elias, 1972). Another common complication is diabetes mellitus, which occurs in 10% to 12% of patients. A carbohydrate intolerance occurs in about one-fifth of the patients. Patients may develop insulin dependence. Obviously, diabetes may complicate the neurological picture. Other signs are kyphoscoliosis, pes cavus, equinovarus, and hammer toe. These orthopedic deficits may contribute to gait difficulties. Cold and cyanotic legs/feet are not uncommon in advanced cases.

Neurophysiological investigations

Reduced amplitudes or absence of sensory nerve action potentials (SNAPs) is very common, especially in the lower limbs (McLeod, 1971; Ackroyd et al., 1984). By contrast, sensorimotor nerve conduction velocities are either normal or only slightly reduced. Somatosensory evoked potentials are characterized by a dispersion with delayed responses. Central motor conduction times assessed by transcranial magnetic stimulation are increased, in parallel with disease duration (Santoro et al., 1999). Visual evoked potentials are often reduced in amplitude (Rabiah et al., 1997).

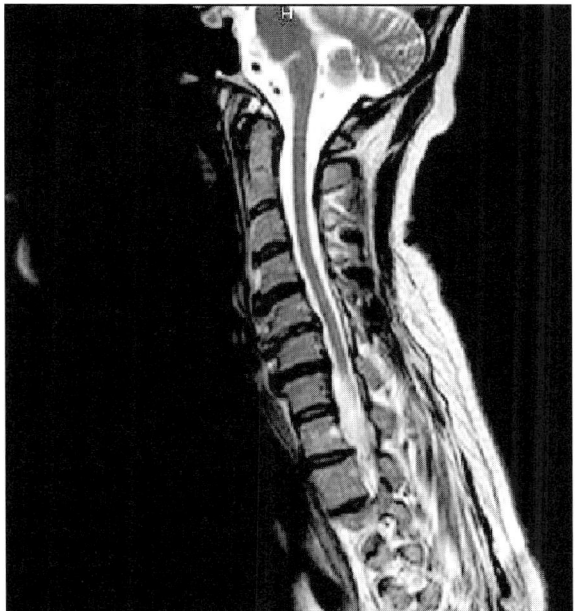

Figure 20.1 MRI of the spinal cord (cervical segments) in a patient presenting with Friedreich ataxia (T2-weighted image). Shrinkage of the spinal cord is visible. From: Manto and Jissendi, 2009. With permission.

Neuroimaging

MRI of the spinal cord demonstrates signal abnormalities in the posterior and lateral columns, with thinning of the spinal cord (Wessel et al., 1989; Riva & Bradac, 1995) (Figure 20.1). The brainstem and cerebellum are less affected, but have a smaller size as compared with those of control subjects (Junck et al., 1994). A mild cerebellar atrophy, especially of the vermis, may develop in advanced cases (Giroud et al., 1994). Voxel-based morphometry (VBM) shows a symmetrical volume loss in the dorsal medulla, inferomedial portions of the cerebellar hemispheres, rostral vermis, and dentate region (Della Nave et al., 2008). The atrophy of the cerebellum and medulla is correlated with the severity of the clinical deficit and disease duration. VBM analysis also confirms white matter atrophy in the posterior cingulate gyrus, paracentral lobule, and middle frontal gyrus (França et al., 2009). Hydrogen-1 magnetic resonance spectroscopy (MRS) suggests that neuronal dysfunction is more diffuse than clinically expected (França et al., 2009).

Single-photon emission CT (SPECT) shows a reduction of blood flow in the cerebellum (Giroud et al., 1994). Glucose metabolism evaluated by posi-

tron emission tomography (PET) is initially increased and decreases with time as the disease progresses and patients lose their ability to walk (Junck et al., 1994).

Molecular genetics

One form of Friedreich ataxia (FRDA1) is caused by a mutation in the gene encoding frataxin (FXN), which has been mapped to chromosome 9q (Campuzano et al., 1996). FRDA patients inherit a GAA expansion in the first intron of the FXN gene from both parents in 98% of cases. A small number of patients have an expanded allele and a second mutated allele with a point mutation leading to a premature stop codon (2%) (Bidichandani et al., 1997). Another locus for the disorder has been mapped to chromosome 9p (FRDA2) (Kostrzewa et al., 1997).

Normal individuals have 5 to 30 GAA repeat expansions. Patients have from 61 to 1700 GAA triplets (Al-Mahdawi et al., 2006). Patients show a marked reduction in the FXN mRNA amount, suggesting that the expansion is related to the FXN silencing. Long uninterrupted GAA tracts adopt triple helical structures, inhibiting transcription. The frataxin gene is involved in the regulation of mitochondrial iron content.

The relationship between trinucleotide (GAA) repeat length and clinical features in FRDA is an important aspect for evaluating and understanding FRDA phenotype severity. With GAA repeats greater than 500, the phenotype is more severe, with early-onset ataxia and increased incidences of diabetes, cardiomyopathy, and scoliosis (Filla et al., 1996).

Biochemical aspects

Several biochemical deficits are observed at the level of the mitochondria. In particular, reduction in the activity of the aconitase and the enzymes in the complexes I to III of the respiratory chain is found. These enzymes contain iron–sulfur groups. There is a consensus that frataxin is a ferrous iron chaperone, maintaining iron biologically unavailable to reactive oxygen species. The frataxin–iron link is probably a key aspect of the disease (Babcock et al., 1997).

Neuropathology

The neuropathology differs in patients with homozygous GAA trinucleotide expansions and in those with compound heterozygotes.

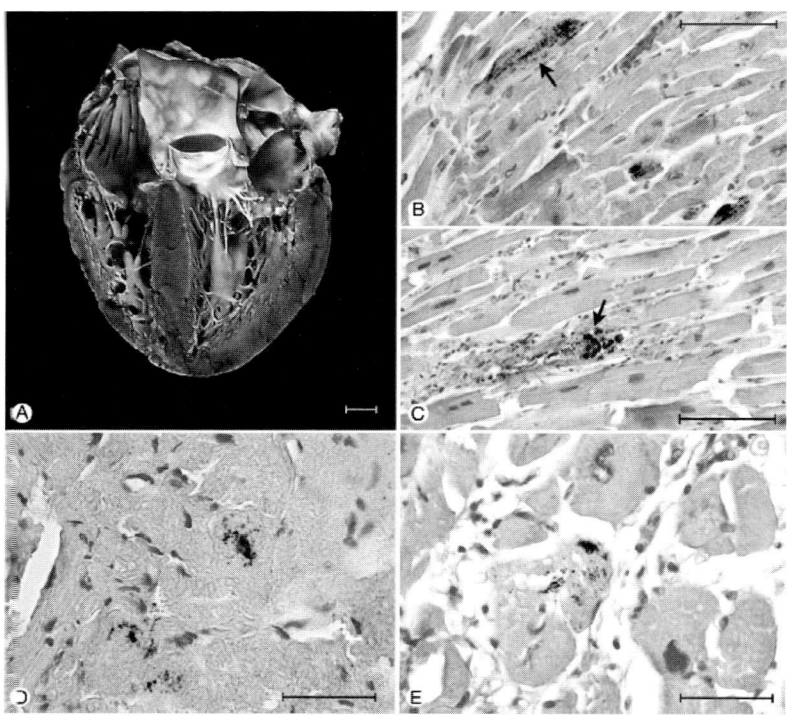

Figure 20.2 Gross pathology of a Friedreich (FRDA) heart and light microscopy of iron-reactive granules in sarcoplasm and endomysium. (A) Gross specimen. Left and right ventricular walls are greatly thickened. The myocardium is discolored, lacking the normal dark and homogeneous appearance of normal heart. (B–E) Iron histochemistry. The stain shows finely granular reaction products that lie parallel to the long axis of cardiomyocytes (arrow in B). A cluster of much larger iron-positive granules lies adjacent to or within a necrotic muscle fiber (arrow in C). (D, E) Iron histochemistry of an endocardial biopsy of an FRDA patient at the age of 9 years (D) and a section of the autopsy specimens at the age of 26 years (E). Both sections display iron-positive granules in cardiac muscle fibers, and the frequency of iron-reactive fibers among all cardiomyocytes is similar. Sections illustrated in B–E are counterstained with Brazilin. Markers: A, 1 cm; B, C, 100 mm; D, E, 50 mm. From: Michael et al., 2006. With permission. (See color section.)

The dorsal columns are invariably reduced in size, with reduced transverse and anteroposterior diameters. The dorsal columns often show a clear thinning, and the dorsal root ganglia a reduction in size. The dorsal spinocerebellar tract is often more affected than the ventral spinocerebellar tract. The nucleus dorsalis of Clarke is characterized by neuronal loss. The dorsal root ganglia show a paucity of nerve cells and an unusual abundance of the nodules of Nageotte. The fiber depletion of dorsal roots contrasts with the sparing of the anterior roots. Loss of large myelinated fibers is often obvious in peripheral sensory nerves, such as the sural nerve.

The cerebellar cortex is usually normal, although the dendritic arborization of Purkinje neurons may be abnormal. The dentate nuclei are commonly involved. The size of the nucleus is decreased due to a neuronal loss. Stainings for iron argue in favor of a decrease of iron accumulation in the dentate nuclei, unlike what is observed in MRI images (Waldvogel et al., 1999). The superior cerebellar peduncles may be thinned.

Pathology of the heart

Cardiomyopathy is characterized by a thickened ventricular wall and increased endomysial connective tissue, resulting in a wider space between cardiac fibers. The cellular nuclei are often enlarged, with inclusion bodies. Iron staining reveals fibers with granular reaction products near the nuclei (Figure 20.2).

Differential diagnosis of disorders associated with cerebral iron accumulation

FRDA should be distinguished first from other recessive ataxias. The following disorders are also associated with iron accumulation: pantothenate kinase–associated neurodegeneration (Hallervorden-Spatz disease, characterized by progressive extra-pyramidal dysfunction and dementia) due to mutation in the PANK2 gene (gene locus 20p13-p12.3), neuroferritinopathy (dominantly inherited, FTL gene: locus 19q13.3-q13.4; see Chapter 23), aceruloplasminemia (gene locus 3q23-q24; see section Aceruloplasminemia), and autosomal recessive Karak syndrome, characterized by early-onset cerebellar ataxia, dystonia, spasticity, and intellectual decline (Morita et al., 1995; Mubaidin et al., 2003; Maciel et al., 2005; Hartig et al., 2006). In the majority of cases, these different subtypes of neurodegeneration associated with brain iron accumulation can be distinguished with T2 and T2 fast-spin echo brain MRI (McNeill et al., 2008).

Prognosis

Over a few years, patients become wheelchair-bound in most cases, with a global worsening of neurological and extra-neurological deficits. Advent of new therapies (see next section) might change the prognosis.

Treatment

Therapeutic trials aim to counter the effects of FXN deficiency or to increase its expression (Tsou et al., 2009).

It is widely accepted that therapy should start as early as possible. Sensory deficits are established very early and might be difficult to counteract, but in theory early treatment might stop cerebellar and motor impairment. Symptomatic therapies are used for specific symptoms such as spasticity (baclofen).

The possible role of iron in the pathogenesis of the disease suggests that chelation therapy could provide benefits. Although desferrioxamine can reduce iron in the extracellular fluid and in the cytosol, the drug is not effective for removing iron directly from mitochondria. Moreover, there is no iron overload globally in the body. Deferiprone, an atypical iron chelator, might decrease build-up of toxic iron in the mitochondria. Attention should be paid to not fully deplete mitochondrial iron stores in order to avoid undesirable consequences (Goncalves et al., 2008).

Beta-blockers at high doses could provide benefits in patients with heart disease. Antioxidants are a second line of therapy. Coenzyme Q10 derivatives such as idebenone (up to 60 mg/kg per day) are still being evaluated. Although the neurological benefit is still a matter of debate (in particular for low doses in the range of 5 mg/kg per day), idebenone seems effective in reducing cardiomyopathy at an early stage of the disease (Schulz et al., 2009). Idebenone acts as both an antioxidant and an electron carrier, promoting adenosine triphosphate (ATP) synthesis in the mitochondria.

Other drugs are under investigation. Recent experimental data suggest that peroxisome proliferator–activated receptor-γ agonists and modulation of the transcriptional regulator PGC1α (a regulator of mitochondrial biogenesis) might be viable alternatives (Marmolino et al., 2009). Human recombinant erythropoietin increases levels of FXN protein in vitro and could exert neuroprotective effects. Human trials have started. Attempts to revert silent heterochromatin to active chromatin using histone deacetylase inhibitors are being carried out. Safety issues deserve special attention.

Ataxia-telangiectasia

Clinical description

Ataxia-telangiectasia (AT; Louis-Bar syndrome) is the more common autosomal recessive ataxia after Friedreich ataxia, with an estimated prevalence of 1 to 2.5 per 100 000 (Swift et al., 1986). AT is the most common recessive ataxia in children under 5 years of age. The disorder is seen among all races and is most prominent among ethnic groups with a high frequency of consanguinity. The disease commonly begins at the age of 2 to 4 years. AT is characterized by progressive cerebellar ataxia, oculomotor apraxia, and choreoathetosis/dystonia (Louis-Bar., 1941). Patients present with very suggestive oculocutaneous telangiectasia, appearing between the ages of 2 and 9 years. Oculomotor signs are present in almost all cases. Truncal ataxia precedes appendicular ataxia. A majority of patients show facial hypotonia and drooling. Tendon reflexes become diminished or absent by age 8. Mental retardation is absent, although some older patients have a loss of short-term memory. Posterior column sensory loss and Babinski sign reflect the diffuse spinal long tract demyelination in patients surviving beyond the second decade. Patients are at risk for recurrent sinopulmonary infections due to variable immunodeficiencies. Moreover, they have a high risk of malignancy, especially leukemia and lymphoma, but also solid tumors of other tissues. Other features of the disease include mild diabetes mellitus, premature graying of the hair, and delayed physical and sexual development.

Neurophysiological investigations

Decreased sensorimotor conduction velocities and amplitudes of responses are related to peripheral nerve degeneration.

Neuroimaging

MRI shows cerebellar atrophy. Atrophy can be restricted to the vermis, with an enlarged fourth ventricle and enlarged infracerebellar subarachnoid spaces (Sardanelli et al., 1995). Proton spectroscopy analysis of the cerebellum in adults shows significantly lower N-acetyl-aspartate (NAA)/choline (Cho) and higher Cho/creatine (Cr) ratios, but a normal NAA/Cr ratio (Wallis et al., 2007). These findings suggest increased Cho signal intensity in the cerebellum of AT patients. Conventional techniques with irradiation should be avoided.

Molecular genetics

The AT gene has been localized to 11q22-q23 (Gatti et al., 1988). Mutation analysis of the ataxia-telangiectasia mutated (ATM) gene has confirmed the genetic homogeneity of AT. The gene product defective in this syndrome normally recognizes DNA damage. More than 200 distinct mutations have been reported associated with AT. Mutations are usually truncating or splicing mutations. Approximately 10% are missense mutations (Chun & Gatti, 2004). Mutation analysis is useful not only to confirm the clinical diagnosis, but also for carrier detection, genetic counseling, and pre-natal diagnosis. Cytogenetic study shows a 7:14 translocation (t [7;14] [q11;q32]) in 5% to 15% of affected individuals.

Blood investigations

Levels of serum alpha-fetoprotein are elevated above 10 ng/mL in more than 90% of patients. Other liver enzymes may be raised. Serum immunoglobulin (Ig) G2 or IgA levels are diminished or absent in 80% and 60% of patients, respectively (Gatti et al., 1991). Levels of IgE/IgM levels may be reduced. Elevated IgM levels may also be found (Noordzij et al., 2009). Some patients develop a high blood viscosity syndrome. Lymphopenia is commonly encountered.

Sensitivity to ionizing radiation

AT cells are abnormally sensitive to ionizing radiation and abnormally resistant to inhibition of DNA synthesis by ionizing radiation. In vitro radiosensitivity is the basis of the colony survival assay performed on transformed lymphocytes (Huo et al., 1994).

Neuropathology

Neuropathologic studies show cerebellar atrophy, predominating in the cerebellar vermis. Purkinje cells are decreased in number, and their arborization is poor.

Thinning of the granular cell layer and minor changes in the dentate nuclei and inferior olivary complex are observed. Gliosis in basal ganglia is found in the oldest cases, with neurofibrillary tangles and lipofuscin granules possibly due to accelerated aging of the brain. Muscle biopsy shows a denervation pattern.

Differential diagnosis

Diagnosis of AT may be difficult before the appearance of telangiectases. AT must be distinguished from the following autosomal recessive cerebellar ataxias (ARCAs):

- Friedreich ataxia (see section Friedreich ataxia)
- Joubert syndrome (see Chapter 7)
- X-linked Pelizaeus-Merzbacher disease: this disorder is characterized by progressive psychomotor delay, spastic quadriplegia, and cerebellar ataxia. Brain MRI shows a severe leukoencephalopathy. The disorder is caused by mutations of the proteolipid protein 1 (PLP1) gene (chromosomal locus Xq22) encoding a structural component of myelin.
- Mre11 deficiency (AT-like disease): these patients have a milder phenotype (Stewart et al., 1999).
- The oculomotor apraxias 1 (AOA1, aprataxin deficiency) and 2 (AOA2, senataxin deficiency) (see section Ataxia with oculomotor apraxia [AOA1])
- The Nijmegen breakage syndrome (NBS; ataxia-telangiectasia variant v1-AT-v1): this disorder is due to mutations in the NBS1 gene, coding for nibrin. Patients present with microcephaly, bird-like facies, and mental retardation, without ataxia, apraxia, or telangiectasia. Serum levels of alpha-fetoprotein are normal, but immune deficits are found (lymphopenia, immunoglobulin deficiencies). The Berlin breakage syndrome (AT variant-2) is phenotypically indistinguishable from the Nijmegen breakage syndrome.
- Spinocerebellar ataxia with axonal neuropathy (SCAN): This disorder is discussed in section Spinocerebellar ataxia with axonal neuropathy.
- Cockayne syndrome: This disorder is a childhood-onset recessive disease characterized by sensorial loss with blindness (associated with cataracts and pigmentary retinopathy) and deafness. Patients present with microcephaly, cerebellar ataxia, pyramidal and extra-pyramidal

deficits, and seizures with possible status epilepticus. Facies is wizened, similar to progeria. Skin photosensitivity, systemic hypertension, and renal and hepatic dysfunction are found. The clinical variability is wide (Pasquier et al., 2006) The diagnosis should be suspected in cases of cerebellar ataxia occurring in a context of growth retardation, microcephaly, and blindness. Death in the second or third decade is common. Exceptionally, patients live until their forties in a cachectic state (Inoue et al., 1997). Cultured skin fibroblasts show abnormal ultraviolet (UV) sensitivity. Calcification of basal ganglia is detected by brain CT scanning, and white matter changes are observed on MRI. Mutations are found in the excision-repair cross-complementing group 8 gene (ERCC8) in type I or the excision-repair cross-complementing group 6 gene (ERCC6) in type II. Neuropathology shows a decreased brain weight and demonstrates white matter atrophy, tigroid leukodystrophy with string vessels, oligodendrocyte proliferation, bizarre reactive astrocytes, multifocal dystrophic calcification in the basal ganglia, advanced atherosclerosis, mixed demyelinating and axonal neuropathy, neurogenic muscular atrophy, and degeneration of the organ of Corti and the eyes (Lindenbaum et al., 2001; Rapin et al., 2006).

• Xeroderma pigmentosum (XP) is a genetically heterogenous autosomal recessive disorder. Prevalence is estimated at between 1 per 100 000 and 1 per 250 000. There are seven types, designated A through G (or I–VII). An eighth type of XP is called the "variant" type. XP shares similarities with Cockayne syndrome. Patients exhibit microcephaly, sensorineural deafness, cerebellar ataxia, chorea, axonal polyneuropathy in a context of cutaneous photosensitivity, and multiple cancers. Laboratory investigations show defective DNA repair after UV exposure. However, intra-cranial calcifications are absent. Treatment includes avoiding harmful exposure to UV radiation and management of tumors. Prognosis is poor.

Prognosis

Most patients need a wheelchair around the age of 12. Patients survive to more than 20 years of age.

Treatment

Patients should avoid excess sun exposure. Regular physical examinations and routine blood studies are recommended. Drooling may respond to anticholinergic agents.

Rapid treatment of infections and hygiene suggestions are important. Pulmonary rehabilitation is recommended for respiratory infections. Gammaglobulin injections every month are proposed to reduce recurrence of infections in susceptible individuals. Immunizations should preferentially be with killed vaccines.

Administration of oral betamethasone (0.1 mg/kg per day for 10 days) has been associated with improvement of neurological performance (Broccoletti et al., 2008). The clinical improvement is inversely correlated with the level of cerebellar atrophy. However, this improvement does not seem to persist after discontinuation of the drug.

Treatment of malignancies with conventional dosages of radiation can be fatal to AT patients. Protocols for chemotherapy should be adapted appropriately to reduce the risk of a second malignancy.

The case of a boy with AT treated with intracerebellar and intrathecal injection of human fetal neural stem cells has been reported (Amariglio et al., 2009). Four years after the first treatment, he was diagnosed with a multifocal brain tumor. This is the first report of a human brain tumor complicating neural stem cell therapy in AT.

Ataxia and isolated vitamin E deficiency

Clinical description

Ataxia and isolated vitamin E deficiency (AVED) is particularly frequent in countries from the Mediterranean basin, and most cases come from North African populations. AVED is characterized by a progressive sensory and cerebellar ataxia, usually beginning before the age of 18 years (Harding et al., 1985). Loss of vibration and joint position sense are usual. Dysdiadochokinesia, positive Romberg sign, tendon areflexia, and positive Babinski sign are commonly found. Most patients present with various levels of head titubation and decreased visual acuity. Patients may exhibit dystonia. Psychotic episodes and intellectual decline are relatively rare. Symptoms and disease severity can vary among siblings (Shorer et al., 1996).

The phenotype of AVED mimics the phenotype of Friedreich ataxia. However, cardiomyopathy and glucose intolerance are much less frequent than in Friedreich ataxia.

Blood studies

Diagnosis is based on the finding of low serum vitamin E values (<2.5 mg/L) in absence of gastrointestinal disease (such as cholestatic liver disease, cystic fibrosis, Crohn disease, and short bowel syndrome). Because of possible oxidation of α-tocopherol by air, precautions must be taken following collection of blood. Unlike in abetalipoproteinemia (see section Abetalipoproteinemia), lipidogram is normal in AVED, and acanthocytes are absent.

Neuroimaging

Cerebellar atrophy is reported in approximately half of patients (Mariotti et al., 2004). In some patients, small T2-weighted high-intensity lesions are found in the periventricular region and the deep white matter (Amiel et al., 1995, Usuki & Maruyama, 2000).

Neurophysiology

Electrophysiological studies show axonal sensory neuropathy and normal motor nerve conduction velocities (Zouari et al., 1998, Schuelke et al., 1999, Gabsi et al., 2001). Somatosensory evoked potentials may show increased central conduction times (increased conduction time between the N13 wave and the N20 wave). The P40 wave may be totally absent. Electroretinogram is often abnormal.

Neuropathology

Neuropathological studies show spinal sensory demyelination with neuronal atrophy and axonal spheroids, dying back–type degeneration of the posterior columns, and neuronal lipofuscin accumulation in the cerebral cortex, thalamus, and spinal horns (Larnaout et al., 1997, Yokota et al., 2000). There is a mild cellular loss of Purkinje neurons. Retina is atrophic.

Genetic and molecular aspects

Most individuals are homozygous or compound heterozygous for one of the mutations of the TTPA gene encoding the α-tocopherol transfer protein. The 744delA frameshift mutation is the most common in individuals of Mediterranean or North African descent and is distributed as a result of a founder effect. The 303T>G mutation (mainly described in Japanese subjects) is characterized by a late-onset disease (age >30 years) and a mild course. These patients have an increased risk for pigmentary retinopathy. AVED shows nearly complete penetrance in individuals who are homozygous or compound heterozygous for a TTPA mutation.

The TTPA gene encodes a 278–amino acid protein which is mainly expressed in liver cells (Sato et al., 1993), but also in the cerebellum (Copp et al., 1999) and in the placenta (Muller-Schmehl et al., 2004). Liver ATTP incorporates the α-tocopherol from the chylomicrons into very low density lipoproteins (VLDLs), which are then secreted into the circulation (Traber et al., 1990). In the absence of ATTP, α-tocopherol is lost in the urine.

Treatment

The treatment for AVED is lifelong high-dose oral vitamin E supplementation. Doses of vitamin E range from 800 to 1500 mg/day (or 40 mg/kg body weight in children) (Burck et al., 1981; Harding et al., 1985; Amiel et al., 1995). Ataxia decreases if the treatment is initiated early. Although disease progression can be stopped in older patients, the deficits in proprioception and gait ataxia remain (Gabsi et al., 2001, Mariotti et al., 2004). Plasma vitamin E levels should be monitored every 6 months, in particular in children. The plasma level of vitamin E should be maintained in the high normal range. Patients should avoid smoking because of the reduction of total radical-trapping antioxidant parameters of plasma (Sharpe et al., 1996).

Abetalipoproteinemia

Clinical description

Abetalipoproteinemia (ABL; Bassen-Kornzweig disease) is a rare metabolic disorder with a frequency <1 in 100 000. The association of peripheral blood acanthocytosis with retinitis pigmentosa and ataxia was first reported by Bassen and Kornzweig in 1950

(Bassen & Kornzweig, 1950). Homozygous dysfunctional mutations in apolipoprotein B cause a clinically similar disorder called homozygous hypobetalipoproteinemia.

The signs and symptoms of abetalipoproteinemia may appear in the first few months of life, but many ABL patients present in the second to fourth decades. Features include retinitis pigmentosa (most patients have loss of night vision early in the course of disease), progressive ataxia, demyelinating neuropathy, dystonia, extra-pyramidal signs, and spastic paraparesis secondary to defective intestinal absorption of lipids. Funduscopic examination reveals an atypical pigmentation of the retina characterized by small, irregularly distributed white spots. Patients present with steatorrhea and may have a previous history of diarrhea resolving upon fat restriction. Cirrhosis has been reported in a few cases, and one patient required transplantation for hepatic cirrhosis.

A possible association with certain cancers such as ileal adenocarcinoma and metastatic spinal cord glioblastoma has been reported (Al-Shali et al., 2003; Newman et al., 1984).

Blood studies

Serum cholesterol concentration is very low, and serum β-lipoproteins are absent. Low-density lipoproteins (LDLs) and VLDLs cannot be synthesized. Patients exhibit deficiencies of fat-soluble vitamins, including vitamin E (see section Ataxia and isolated vitamin E deficiency). Acanthocytosis is found on peripheral blood smear. Acanthocytes cause very low erythrocyte sedimentation rates. Anemia is due to deficiencies in iron, folate, and other nutrients secondary to fat malabsorption. Hemolysis may also contribute to anemia. Elevated prothrombin time and international normalized ratio due to vitamin K deficiency have been noted in several cases. Vitamin K deficiency may be associated with gastrointestinal bleeding in childhood. Hepatic manifestations include elevated serum transaminases with hepatomegaly due to hepatic steatosis (Collins et al., 1989).

Genetic and molecular aspects

Abetalipoproteinemia is caused by mutations in the gene MTP (chromosome 4q22-24), which encodes microsomal triglyceride transfer protein (Shoulders et al., 1993). The protein forms a heterodimer with the ubiquitous endoplasmic reticulum enzyme protein

disulfide isomerase (Narcisi et al., 1995). MTP acts as a chaperone which facilitates the transfer of lipids onto apolipoprotein B (Zamel et al., 2008). Hypobetalipoproteinemia is caused by mutations in the gene APOB, which encodes the protein apolipoprotein B.

Treatment

Patients are treated with high oral doses of fat soluble vitamins, including vitamin E. Treatment has a favorable impact on the course of the neuropathy (Zamel et al., 2008). A 12-year follow-up indicates that high-dose oral vitamin E (100 IU/kg) slows retinal degeneration (Runge et al., 1986). High doses of vitamin A (100–400 IU/kg per day) are required. The risk of papilledema should be kept in mind (Bishara et al., 1982). Vitamin D replacement (1000 mg daily) should be considered in all patients. Replacement of vitamin K is necessary (5 mg/day). Other supplementary nutrients like iron and folic acid can also be considered. A low-fat diet improves steatorrhea associated with fat malabsorption and allows absorption of other nutrients essential for growth and development (Zamel et al., 2008).

Autosomal recessive spastic ataxia of Charlevoix-Saguenay

Geographical distribution

Autosomal recessive spastic ataxia of Charlevoix-Saguenay (ARSACS) was first described among inhabitants of the Charlevoix-Saguenay region in northeastern Quebec, Canada (Bouchard et al., 1978). This disease has a high prevalence in two small regions of Quebec. The gene carrier prevalence is estimated to be 1 in 22 due to a relatively small founder population (De Braekeleer et al., 1993). Several families with SACS mutations have been reported in Italy, Spain, Tunisia, Turkey, and Japan. Thus ARSACS now "goes global" (Gomez, 2004; Takiyama, 2007).

Clinical description

Age of onset ranges from 1 to 14 years. ARSACS is characterized by early-onset spastic ataxia, axonal and demyelinating neuropathy, and hypermyelination of retinal nerve fibers. Pes cavus is common. Gait unsteadiness is the first symptom in most cases. A minority of patients develop seizures. Intelligence is usually normal. Non-Quebec patients show some

197

atypical features in comparison with Quebec patients. For instance, patients may lack spasticity in the lower limbs (Shimazaki et al., 2005). Intellectual impairment is sometimes found in non-Quebec patients. Although increased visibility of myelinated retinal nerve fibers is a hallmark of ARSACS in Quebec patients, there is a substantial number of non-Quebec patients without this characteristic sign. When retinal hypermyelination is absent, ARSACS is a differential diagnosis of early-onset cerebellar ataxia with retained tendon reflexes (EOCARR), Friedreich ataxia with retained reflexes (FARR, see section Friedreich ataxia), ataxia with oculomotor apraxia (AOA1 and AOA2, see section Ataxia with oculomotor apraxia [AOA1]), and several forms of hereditary spastic paraplegia. The disease has a progressive course. The mean age for patients becoming wheelchair-bound varies at between 30 and 41 years (Bouchard, 1991).

Neuroimaging

Brain MRI shows a cerebellar atrophy, especially in the upper vermis, sparing the brainstem. A mega-cisterna magna and a thin spinal cord in the cervical segment may be found in some cases. White matter appears normal.

SPECT of the brain shows a decreased blood flow in the upper cerebellar vermis (Shimazaki et al., 2007).

Neurophysiology

Peripheral nerve conduction studies show an axonal neuropathy with absent sensory action potentials and decreased motor conduction velocities (Peyronnard et al., 1979).

Neuropathology

The pathological features include atrophy of the upper cerebellar vermis, loss of Purkinje cells, and neuronal lipid accumulation (Bouchard et al., 2000). The dentate nuclei and inferior olives are spared. In sections of the medulla oblongata, the pyramids are slightly reduced in size. There is a severe bilateral symmetrical loss of myelin staining centered on the lateral corticospinal tracts at the spinal cord level. Sural nerve biopsy confirms severe axonal degeneration with loss of large myelinated fibers.

Genetic and molecular aspects

The gene, called SACS, maps to 13q12.12 (Engert et al., 2000). At least 28 mutations of the SACS gene

have been found in Quebec and non-Quebec patients, consisting of 8 missense, 5 nonsense, and 15 frameshift (11 deletion and 4 insertion) ones (Takiyama, 2007). Most of the SACS mutations are homozygous.

The final full-length version of human sacsin contains 4579 amino acids. Sacsin is expressed in a variety of tissues, including the brain (Engert et al., 2000). Sacsin might function in chaperone-mediated protein folding.

Differential diagnosis

Table 20.3 lists the main disorders presenting as recessive spastic ataxia syndromes. Friedreich ataxia and Marinesco-Sjögren syndrome are discussed elsewhere in this chapter.

Treatment

Patients exhibiting spasticity may benefit from stretching exercises and administration of baclofen (orally or by the intrathecal route). Orthesis may be useful. Arthrodesis may be considered in selected cases (Bouchard & Langlois, 1999). The most effective surgical procedures are triple arthrodesis with percutaneous lengthening of the Achilles tendon and adductor and psoas tenotomies combined with neurectomy of the obturator nerve. Urinary urgencies are managed with anticholinergic drugs. Seizures are controlled with conventional anti-epileptic agents.

Ataxia with oculomotor apraxia (AOA1)
Geographical distribution

Patients with ataxia with oculomotor apraxia (AOA1) have been identified worldwide. The estimated prevalence of AOA1 in Portugal is 55 per 1 000 000, representing the second most frequent recessive ataxia after Friedreich ataxia (Barbot et al., 2001). In Japan, AOA1, which represents the most frequent cause of autosomal recessive ataxia (Hirano et al., 2004), is often called early-onset ataxia with oculomotor apraxia and hypoalbuminemia.

Clinical description

Symptoms appear between 2 and 16 years of age (mean around 7 years). Onset at ages 28 and 29 years has been reported (Criscuolo et al., 2004). Patients exhibit a slowly progressive gait imbalance followed by dysarthria and upper-limb dysmetria with mild

Table 20.3 Recessive spastic ataxia syndromes

Disorder	Clinical features	Brain imaging	Gene locus
Karak syndrome (phospholipase A2) (Mubaidin et al., 2003)	Early onset Cerebellar ataxia Intellectual decline Dystonia Spasticity	"Eye-of-tiger" sign Cerebellar atrophy	22q13.1
Krabbe disease (Galactosylceramide lipoidosis; deficiency in beta-galactocerebrosidase)	Early infantile or late onset Mental retardation Irritability with excessive crying Optic atrophy Spasticity Hypertonia Seizures Ataxia Polyneuropathy	Corticospinal tract and periventricular demyelination	14q24.3-q32.1
Pelizaeus Merzbacher–like (PMLD; HLD2)	Impaired motor development Ataxia Choreoathetosis Spasticity Seizures Peripheral nerve neuropathy	Leukodystrophy (hypomyelination)	1q41-q42
Leukoencephalopathy with vanishing white matter	Onset variable Chronic progressive or episodic Ataxia Spasticity Optic atrophy Epilepsy Mental dysfunction	Cerebral hemispheric leukoencephalopathy Areas of abnormal white matter (high T2-weighted signal intensity like CSF)	1p34.1; 2p23.3; 3q27; 12, 14q24
Portneuf spastic ataxia with leukoencephalopathy (ARSAL; SPAX3) (Thiffault et al., 2006)	Onset: birth to 60 years Ataxia Spasticity Hyperreflexia Urinary urgency Scoliosis Dystonia Cognitive impairment Optic atrophy Cataract Hearing impairment	Cerebellar atrophy Cortical atrophy Leukoencephalopathy	2q33-34
SAX2	Childhood onset Ataxia Spasticity Extensor plantar reflexes Fasciculations	Normal brain MRI	17p13
SPG7[a]	Variable clinical presentation Optic atrophy	Cortical and cerebellar atrophy	16q24.3
SPG30	Onset: 12 to 21 years Spastic paraparesis Peripheral neuropathy Ataxia	Cerebellar atrophy	2q37.3
Hypomyelination and congenital cataract (Biancheri et al., 2007)	Congenital cataract Developmental delay Spasticity Ataxia Peripheral neuropathy	Supratentorial hypomyelination Cerebellar white matter hypomyelination	7p21.3-p15.3
Megalencephalic leukoencephalopathy with subcortical cysts (Van der Knapp disease)	Infantile onset Megalencephaly Ataxia Seizures Mild pyramidal signs Mental decline	Extensive white matter signal changes involving the corpus callosum and frontal/temporal subcortical cysts Cerebellar hemispheres mildly involved	22qtel

[a]The gene encodes paraplegin, a mitochondrial protein (adenosine triphosphate–dependent m-AAA protease) involved in ribosome assembly.

kinetic tremor. Oculomotor apraxia is present in 80% of individuals and is usually reported after the onset of ataxia. Patients have difficulties for ocular fixation and typically show difficulties in moving the eyes towards a fixed target. When the examiner blocks the head, movement of the eyes is often impossible. Slow eye movements occur on lateral and vertical gaze (in adults, this should not be confused with spinocerebellar ataxia type 2 [SCA2], see Chapter 23), and apraxia is followed by progressive external ophthalmoplegia. Oculocephalic reflexes are spared at the beginning. Tendon areflexia is common, as a result of peripheral nerve involvement. Vibration sense is usually preserved during the first years of the disease. Pes cavus is observed in 30% of cases, and therefore, AOA1 with peripheral neuropathy and pes cavus should be distinguished from Charcot-Marie-Tooth syndrome. Nearly half of patients will exhibit chorea or dystonia during the course of the disease. Different degrees of cognitive impairment have been reported (Tachi et al., 2000). Loss of independent walking occurs about a decade after onset of symptoms. Survival is long (Barbot et al., 2001).

Neuroimaging

Cerebellar atrophy is observed in all patients. A small percentage of patients present with concomitant brainstem atrophy.

Neurophysiology

Signs of axonal neuropathy are found in all patients, although needle electromyography studies and nerve conduction velocities may be normal at the very beginning.

Blood studies

Serum concentration of albumin is decreased below 3.8 g/L in about 80% of patients with disease duration of more than 10 years, and levels of cholesterol in blood are increased (>5.6 mmol) in about 70% of cases after several years of evolution.

Neuropathology

Axonal neuropathy is confirmed by sural nerve biopsy. A mild loss of large myelinated axons is found.

Genetic and molecular aspects

AOA1 is caused by a mutation in the APTX gene, located on chromosome 9p13.3. Sixteen different mutations have been identified so far. APTX encodes a ubiquitously expressed protein, called aprataxin. AOA1 is a novel type of DNA damage response-defective disease in which aprataxin may be associated with both the DNA single-strand and double-strand break repair machinery (Clements et al., 2004).

Management

Physical therapy is recommended. A wheelchair is usually necessary by the age of 15 to 20 years. A high-protein diet restores serum albumin concentration and prevents edema due to hypoalbuminemia. A low-cholesterol diet is also recommended.

Ataxia with oculomotor apraxia type 2 (AOA2)

Clinical description

Ataxia with oculomotor apraxia type 2 (AOA2; also called non-Friedreich spinocerebellar ataxia type 1 [SCAR1]) represents approximately 8% of non-Friedreich ARCAs (Le Ber et al., 2004). Onset is between 11 and 22 years in the majority of cases (extremes of 3–30 years). In addition to cerebellar ataxia and oculomotor apraxia (occurring in about 45% of cases and which may be accompanied by strabismus), patients exhibit choreoathetosis and dystonia. A clinical picture of writer's cramp may be present initially. Tendon areflexia is common. Mild cognitive impairment is present in some individuals. Deep sensory loss, extensor plantar reflexes, and sphincter disturbances are observed in some patients. Mean disease duration until wheelchair is about 15 to 20 years (Tazir et al., 2009).

Neuroimaging

Patients present with cerebellar atrophy on brain MRI (Duquette et al., 2005). Atrophy is more severe in the oldest patients.

Neurophysiology

Nerve conduction velocities show an absence of sensory potentials.

Blood studies

Values of gamma-globulins (IgG, IgA), alpha-fetoprotein, cholesterol, and creatine kinase (CK) are increased (Le Ber et al., 2004). However, serum alpha-fetoprotein concentrations are lower than that usually observed in ataxia-telangiectasia (Le Ber et al., 2004).

Neuropathology

Biopsy of sural nerve confirms the axonal neuropathy.

Genetic and molecular aspects

The causative gene has been mapped to chromosome 9q34. The gene encodes senataxin (SETX), a protein that contains a classic seven-motif domain found in the superfamily of helicases (Moreira et al., 2004). Senataxin is involved in DNA repair and also may be a nuclear RNA helicase with a role in the splicing machinery. Mutations in the SETX gene have also been identified in the autosomal dominant juvenile form of amyotrophic lateral sclerosis (Chen et al., 2004).

Management

Treatment remains supportive. A low-cholesterol diet is advised.

Cerebellar ataxia associated with coenzyme Q10 deficiency

Deficiency of coenzyme Q10 (CoQ10) in muscle has been associated with a spectrum of diseases, including infantile-onset multisystemic diseases, encephalomyopathies with recurrent myobinuria, cerebellar ataxia, and pure myopathy (Quinzii et al., 2007). CoQ10 deficiency predominantly affects children.

Phenotypes

Five phenotypes are associated with CoQ10 deficiencies:

- An ataxic form. This is the most common phenotype related to coenzyme Q (CoQ) deficiency and will be detailed in this chapter.
- A severe infantile syndrome presenting with nystagmus, myopia, retinitis pigmentosa, optic nerve atrophy, bilateral sensorineural deafness, progressive ataxia, dystonia, and nephritic syndrome causing renal failure (Rotig et al., 2000).

A neonatal form has also been described (Rahman et al., 2001).
- Leigh syndrome, a severe necrotizing encephalopathy (Leshinsky-Silver et al., 2003; Van Maldergem et al., 2002) (see also Chapter 21).
- A syndrome characterized by recurrent myoglobinuria, brain involvement, ragged-red fibers, and lipid storage associated with CoQ deficiency in muscle.
- A pure myopathic form (Horvath et al., 2006).

The ataxic form

Patients exhibit a cerebellar syndrome as the main deficit. Symptoms may start in infancy or in adulthood. Other features include seizures, developmental delay, mental retardation, pyramidal signs, and absence of tendon reflexes. A late-onset ataxia associated with hypergonadotrophic hypogonadism has been reported (Gironi et al., 2004).

Coenzyme Q10: biochemical aspects

CoQ10 is composed of a benzoquinone ring, synthesized from tyrosine, and a polyprenyl side chain, generated from acetyl-coenzyme A (Montero et al., 2007; Figure 20.3). The biosynthesis of CoQ is complex. Several enzymes are implicated. The polyprenyl side chain is composed of several isoprenoid units which are species-specific. Human CoQ contains 10 units.

CoQ10 is a key electron carrier in the mitochondrial respiratory chain (Montero et al., 2007). CoQ10 transfers electrons from complexes I and II to complex III (Crane et al., 1957) and contributes to the synthesis of ATP (Figure 20.4). Moreover, CoQ10 plays an antioxidant function in the membranes of the cell (Santos-Ocana et al., 1998) by preventing the progression of lipid peroxidation and by recycling vitamin E or ascorbate (Kagan et al., 1998; Villalba et al., 1995). Redox functions of CoQ10 are related to its ability to exchange two electrons in a redox cycle between the oxidized form (ubiquinone) and the reduced form (ubiquinol) (Kagan et al., 1998).

The hallmark of CoQ deficiency syndrome is a decreased CoQ concentration in muscle and/or fibroblasts. Other markers of mitochondrial dysfunction such as concentrations of lactate and pyruvate are normal (Gironi et al., 2004; Artuch et al., 2006). In some studies, biochemical investigations in cultured skin fibroblasts have found a defect in the transprenylation pathway or in the metabolic steps after condensation of

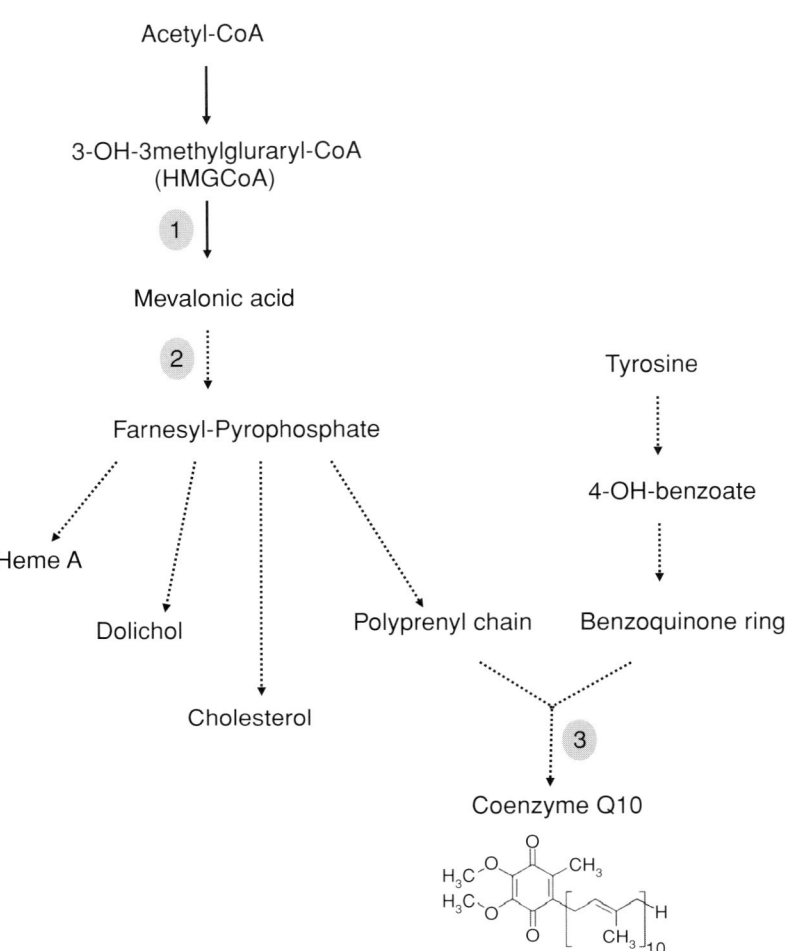

Figure 20.3 Synthesis of coenzyme Q10. Coenzyme Q10 is composed of a benzoquinone ring deriving from tyrosine and from a poly prenyl side chain synthesized from acetyl-CoA via the mevalonic acid pathway. (1) Site of action of the HMG-CoA reductase; (2) the deficit in mevalonate kinase causes mevalonic aciduria and decreased levels of cholesterol, dolichol, and coenzyme Q10; (3) deficit in parahydroxybenzoate-polyprenyl transferase (CoQ2) causes a deficiency in coenzyme Q10.

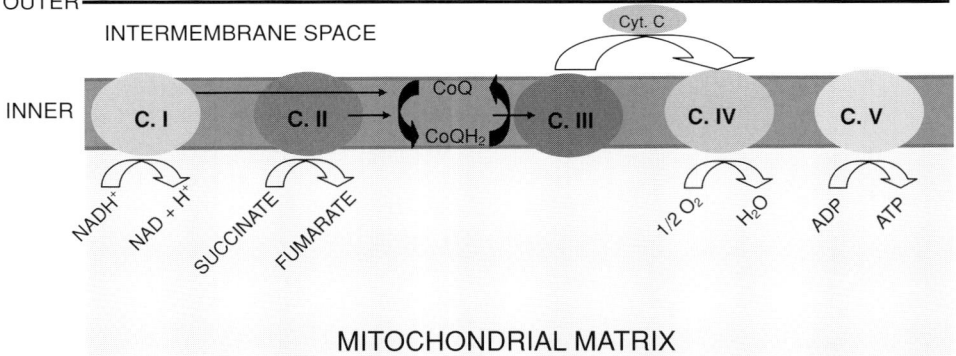

Figure 20.4 Illustration of the mitochondrial respiratory chain. Electrons are transferred from complex I (C. I) and II (C. II) to the oxidized form of coenzyme Q10 (CoQ). CoQ is reduced to $CoQH_2$, which transfers the electrons to Complex III (C. III). Other abbreviations: C. IV: complex IV; C. V: complex V; Cyt. C: cytochrome C. (See color section.)

4-hydroxybenzoate and the prenyl side chain of CoQ (Artuch et al., 2006). Oxidative phosphorylation dysfunction occurs in CoQ deficiency syndromes.

Genetic aspects

Mutations in genes required for the CoQ10 biosynthetic pathway have been identified only in patients with infantile-onset multisystemic diseases or isolated nephropathy (Lagier-Tourenne et al., 2008). Mutations in ADCK3 gene (chromosome 1q41) have recently been identified in patients with childhood-onset cerebellar ataxia and in a large consanguineous family (Lagier-Tourenne et al., 2008). The ADCK3 gene codes for a mitochondrial protein. Some patients have a low endogenous pool of CoQ10 in their fibroblasts or lymphoblasts and show impaired ubiquinone synthesis, indicating that ADCK3 is likely involved in CoQ10 biosynthesis.

Mutations in the aprataxin gene (APTX gene, see section Ataxia with oculomotor apraxia [AOA1]) have been associated with CoQ deficiency. Patients homozygous for the W279X mutation have lower values of muscle CoQ10 levels (Le Ber et al., 2007).

Treatment with CoQ10

Early diagnosis and treatment of the deficiency are very important in order to prevent progression of the disease (Montero et al., 2007). There is no general agreement on the dose which should be given. A clear improvement with low doses (100 mg/day) has been reported. Other authors suggest daily doses up to 3000 mg/day (Artuch et al., 2005), with a progressive reduction according to plasma CoQ monitoring and clinical evolution (Montero et al., 2007). Familial cases (Artuch et al., 2006) may show a very good response of ataxia, with improvement of dysarthria, tremor, ataxia, and nystagmus. Decreases in the International Cooperative Ataxia Rating Scale (ICARS) scores have been reported. However, other patients with ataxia do not show such amelioration after CoQ therapy (Hirano et al., 2006).

Marinesco-Sjögren syndrome

Clinical symptoms

Symptoms of Marinesco-Sjögren syndrome (MSS) start in infancy (Van Raamsdonk, 2006). Manifestations of MSS are cerebellar ataxia, congenital cataracts, retarded somatic and mental development, muscle weakness, hypotonia, and tendon areflexia. Some patients present with episodes of rhabdomyolysis with sustained or episodic increase of serum creatine kinase activity. Hypergonadotropic hypogonadism is not rare. Patients survive to old age, with varying disabilities.

Neuroimaging

Brain MRI shows a cerebellar atrophy involving in particular the vermis.

Neurophysiology

Nerve conduction studies show a demyelinating peripheral neuropathy.

Neuropathology

Muscle biopsies show myopathic changes with rimmed vacuoles.

Brain studies show cerebellar cortical atrophy with vacuolated or binuclear Purkinje cells.

Genetic aspects

A locus for classical MSS has recently been assigned to chromosome 5q31. Mutations have been identified in the SIL1 gene, which encodes a factor involved in protein folding (Lagier-Tourenne et al., 2003; Anttonen et al., 2005; Senderek et al., 2005). SIL1 is ubiquitously expressed.

Treatment

Cataracts often require surgical removal to maintain vision. Hypogonadism is treated with hormonal replacement therapy.

Cerebrotendinous xanthomatosis

Epidemiology

The prevalence of cerebrotendinous xanthomatosis (CTX) has been estimated at approximately 1 per 50 000 among Caucasians (Lorincz et al., 2005). The disease occurs worldwide.

Clinical symptoms

CTX is characterized by infantile-onset diarrhea, cataract, tendon xanthomas, and adult-onset progressive

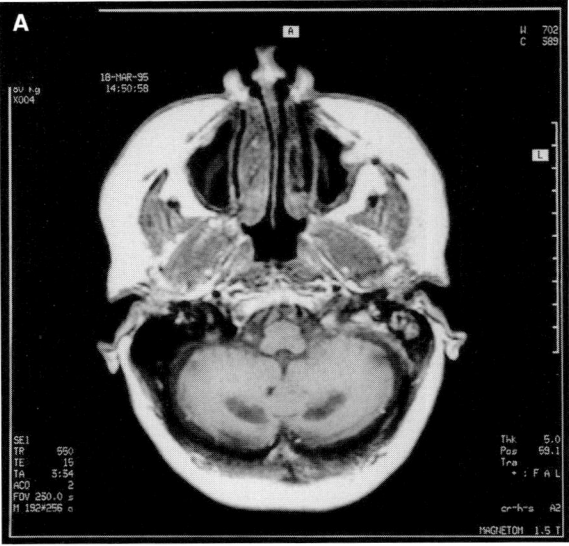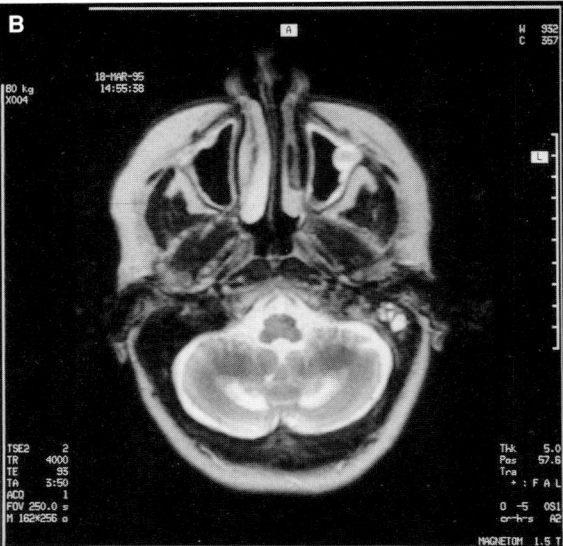

Figure 20.5 Cerebrotendinous xanthomatosis. T1-weighted image (A) shows low-intensity lesions in the cerebellar hemispheres. Lesions appear hyperintense on T2-weighted images (B). With permission from: De Michele and Filla, 2002.

neurological deficits. Patients exhibit combinations of dementia, psychiatric disturbances, pyramidal deficits, extra-pyramidal deficits (dystonia), cerebellar signs, seizures, and peripheral neuropathy. Neuropsychiatric symptoms such as behavioral changes, hallucinations, agitation, depression, and suicide attempts may be prominent. Intra-familial variability is noticeable (Verrips et al., 2000). Rarely, patients exhibit a spinal presentation with a predominant spastic paraparesis.

Xanthomas usually appear in the second or third decade. They are observed on the Achilles tendon, the extensor tendons of the elbow and hand, and the patellar tendon. Xanthomas have also been reported in the lungs and bones.

Premature atherosclerosis and coronary artery disease have been described (Valdivielso et al., 2004).

Neuroimaging

MRI shows bilateral hyperintensity of the dentate nuclei areas and cerebral/cerebellar white matter (De Michele & Filla, 2002; Figure 20.5). A diffuse brain atrophy may be observed.

MRS reveals decreased NAA levels and increased values for lactate, suggesting widespread brain mitochondrial dysfunction (De Stefano et al., 2001).

Neurophysiology

Nerve conduction velocities are decreased. Abnormalities in somatosensory, motor, brainstem, and visual evoked potentials are often found (Mondelli et al., 1992).

Neuropathology

Granulomatous and xanthomatous lesions are observed in the cerebellum and basal ganglia. Various degrees of demyelination and gliosis are observed in the spinal cord. Nerve biopsy reveals primary axonal degeneration, signs of demyelination, and remyelination.

Biochemical studies

CTX is caused by deficiency of the mitochondrial enzyme sterol 27-hydroxylase. Cholestanol concentrations are raised in blood (normal range 330±30 μg/dL). Plasma cholesterol concentration is normal or decreased. Levels of chenodeoxycholic acid are decreased due to impaired primary bile acid synthesis. Increased concentrations of cholestanol and apolipoprotein B are found in the cerebrospinal fluid (CSF). Concentrations of bile alcohols in urine are raised.

Enzyme assay

The activity of sterol 27-hydroxylase is decreased in fibroblasts, leukocytes, and liver.

Genetic aspects

CYP27A1 is the only gene known to be associated with CTX.

Treatment

Inhibitors of HMG-CoA reductase alone or in combination with chenodeoxycholic acid (750 mg/day in adults) are effective in decreasing cholestanol concentration and improving clinical signs as well as neurophysiological deficits. They may cause muscle cramps.

Symptomatic treatment is recommended for epilepsy, spasticity, and parkinsonism. Parkinsonism is usually poorly responsive to levodopa. Interestingly, patients may respond to an antihistamine drug, diphenylpyraline hydrochloride (Ohno et al., 2001).

Cataract extraction is often required in at least one eye by the age of 50 years.

Autosomal recessive cerebellar ataxia type 1

Clinical symptoms

Autosomal recessive cerebellar ataxia type 1 (ARCA-1) is a cerebellar ataxia with middle-age onset (mean 31.6 years; range 17–46 years) (Dupré et al., 2007). The disease has been reported in a cluster of French-Canadian families originating from the same region of Quebec.

Progression is slow, with moderate disability. Patients exhibit a significant dysarthria and mild oculomotor abnormalities and may also show brisk reflexes in the lower limbs.

Neuroimaging

Brain MRI shows diffuse cerebellar atrophy.

Neurophysiology

Nerve conduction velocities are normal.

Genetic aspects

Several mutations in synaptic nuclear envelope protein-1 (SYNE1), which participates in vesicular trafficking, have been identified. Despite the genotypic heterogeneity, the phenotype is relatively homogeneous. SYNE1 is the first gene responsible for a recessively inherited pure cerebellar ataxia (Gros-Louis et al., 2007).

Refsum disease (phytanic acid oxidase deficiency; heredopathia atactica polyneuritiformis)

Clinical description

The age of onset for Refsum disease varies from early childhood to 50 years of age. Most patients have suggestive symptoms before the age of 20 years. The main clinical features are retinitis pigmentosa, chronic polyneuropathy, and cerebellar ataxia. Most cases have anosmia, sensorineural deafness, cardiac arrhythmias, renal failure, and bony and skin abnormalities. Some individuals have shortened bones in their fingers or toes, or a visibly shortened fourth toe. The infantile Refsum disease manifests clinically with severe sensorineural deafness, atypical retinitis pigmentosa, mental and growth retardation, facial dysmorphism, peripheral neuropathy, cerebellar ataxia, high concentrations of protein in the CSF, and hepatomegaly (Dubois et al., 1991). Some cases presenting with atypical acute demyelinating polyneuropathy mimicking the familial Guillain-Barré syndrome have been reported (Verny et al., 2006).

Blood studies

Blood studies show increased levels of phytanic acid (normal values <6 µg/mL), a branched-chain fatty acid produced from phytol.

Genetic and molecular aspects

The PHYH (or PAHX) gene located on chromosome 10pter-p11.2 is responsible for the disorder in the majority of cases (Mihalik et al., 1997). The PHYH gene encodes for the phytanoyl-CoA hydroxylase (PhyH), catalyzing the first step in the alpha oxidation of phytanic acid. Degradation of phytanic acid normally takes place inside the peroxisome. A second locus involved in Refsum disease is the PEX7 gene (chromosome 6q21-q22.2) (Van den Brink et al., 2003). To date, only a few Refsum patients have been reported with mutations in this gene (Horn et al., 2007). Mutations in the PEX7 gene have been found

205

to be causative for other disorders, such as rhizomelic chondrodysplasia punctata (Braverman et al., 1997). PEX genes encode for peroxisomal assembly proteins called peroxins, which are required for the import of matrix proteins into peroxisomes.

Neuroimaging

Abnormal signals are observed in cerebral white matter using brain MRI. The infantile form is characterized by symmetrical signal changes involving the corticospinal tracts, cerebellar dentate nuclei, and corpus callosum (Cakirer & Savas, 2005).

Differential diagnosis

Other peroxisome biogenesis disorders associated with high levels of phytanic acid are Zellweger syndrome, neonatal adrenoleukodystrophy, infantile Refsum disease (a variant occurring in young children), and rhizomelic chondrodysplasia punctata (Palau & Espinós, 2006).

Neuropathology

Autopsy findings include mild diffuse reduction of axons and myelin within the corpus callosum, periventricular white matter, optic nerves, and corticospinal tracts. Lipid-laden macrophages are observed in the cerebral white matter. Severe hypoplasia of the cerebellar granule layer and ectopic Purkinje cells in the molecular layer are found (Torvik et al., 1988).

Treatment

Treatment of Refsum disease is based on dietary restriction of phytanic acid (contained in dairy products, beef and lamb, and fatty fish). Plasmapheresis may be helpful. With treatment, muscle weakness, numbness, and skin abnormalities generally improve. However, visual deficits, hearing problems, and loss of the sense of smell may persist. Cochlear implantation may be associated with good audiological outcomes (Raine et al., 2008). Orthotopic liver transplantation improves biochemical parameters in infantile Refsum disease type (Van Maldergem et al., 2005).

Infantile-onset spinocerebellar ataxia

Clinical description

Infantile-onset spinocerebellar ataxia (IOSCA) has been described in Finland. The disorder is characterized by a very early onset ataxia (between 1 and 2 years), athetosis, and tendon hyporeflexia. Ophthalmoplegia, hearing loss, and sensory neuropathy appear later in the disease course. Refractory status epilepticus, migraine-like headaches, and severe psychiatric symptoms are also suggestive (Lönnqvist et al., 2009). Female hypogonadism is a late manifestation. Some individuals show reduced mental capacity. Patients are usually wheelchair-bound by their teenage years. Some cases present with a severe early-onset encephalopathy and signs of liver involvement, a phenotype reminiscent of Alpers syndrome, an autosomal recessive hepatocerebral syndrome of early onset associated with mitochondrial DNA (mtDNA) depletion, and mutations in polymerase gamma gene (Hakonen et al., 2007; see also Chapter 21).

Neuroimaging

Brain MRI shows cerebellar atrophy extending to the brainstem and spinal cord. Stroke-like lesions may be observed, varying from small cortical to large hemispheric edematous lesions (Lönnqvist et al., 2009).

Neurophysiology

There is abnormal background activity in the electroencephalogram with advancing age (Koskinen et al., 1994). Epilepsia partialis continua may lead to life-threatening generalized epileptic statuses (Lönnqvist et al., 2009). Nerve conduction velocities show a sensory neuropathy.

Neuropathology

The most severe atrophic changes are observed in the spinal cord (Lönnqvist et al., 1998). The brainstem and cerebellum are also atrophic. Cerebellar peduncles, the inferior olives, the accessory cuneate nuclei, and the dentate nuclei appear small and present gliosis. The cerebellar cortex shows patchy atrophy. The ventral pontine nuclei and transverse fibers are slightly involved. Tegmental nuclei and tracts, especially sensory structures, are more severely affected. Sural nerve biopsy shows a progressive loss of myelinated fibers in the sural nerves. Overall, there are analogies with the neuropathological findings of Friedreich ataxia (see section Friedreich ataxia). Brain atrophy with focal laminar cortical necrosis and hippocampal damage are found.

Genetic and molecular aspects

IOSCA is caused by mutations in the C10orf2 gene (chromosome 10q22.3-q24.1) encoding Twinkle, a mitochondrial DNA-specific helicase, and a rarer splicing variant Twinky (Nikali et al., 2005). Mutations in this gene have also been reported in individuals with autosomal dominant progressive external ophthalmoplegia (Spelbrink et al., 2001).

Early-onset cerebellar ataxia with retained tendon reflexes

Epidemiology

Early-onset cerebellar ataxia with retained tendon reflexes (EOCARR; Harding ataxia) was originally described by Harding (Harding, 1981). EOCARR is among the most common autosomal recessive ataxias (after Friedreich ataxia and AT). The prevalence is estimated at 1 per 100 000 population. The consanguinity rate is between 15% and 40% according to the studies. About half of the patients present as sporadic cases and half have an affected sibling (De Michele & Filla, 2002).

Clinical description

EOCARR is characterized by ataxia starting in the first or second decade of life (peaks at 1–4 years, 9–12 years, and 17–20 years) with preservation of tendon reflexes (De Castro et al., 1999). Gait difficulties are usually the first manifestation. Gait is either ataxic or ataxospastic. Most patients exhibit a gaze-evoked nystagmus, a saccadic pursuit, and dysmetric saccades. A small percentage of patients complain of dysphagia. Knee jerks may be brisk. Ankle jerks vary from brisk to absent. Plantar reflexes are flexor in two-thirds of cases. About 60% of patients have diminished vibration sense in the lower limbs. Associated symptoms, such as muscle wasting, foot deformity, scoliosis, and electrocardiographic abnormalities, are encountered less frequently in EOCARR than in Friedreich ataxia (Klockgether et al., 1991). Echocardiographic signs of hypertrophic cardiomyopathy are absent. Diabetes is not encountered. Patients may present with various degrees of cognitive impairment and visuospatial deficits. Indi-

viduals with EOCARR have a better prognosis than those suffering from Friedreich ataxia. The survival rate is 77% after 20 years from onset (Chiò et al., 1993). Prognosis is worse for males.

Neuroimaging

Brain MRI shows cerebellar atrophy, often predominating in the vermis. One-third of patients have concomitant brainstem atrophy. SPECT (technetium-99 hexamethylpropyleneamine oxime) shows cerebellar hypoperfusion in two-thirds of cases. A cerebral cortical hypometabolism may also be detected with positron emission tomography (PET). This technique shows reduced cerebellar benzodiazepine receptor binding (Mielke et al., 1998). By comparison with age-matched control subjects, EOCARR is characterized by a global metabolic decline and predominant hypometabolism in the cerebellum and thalamus.

Neurophysiology

Peripheral neuropathy is detected in half of patients (Santoro et al., 1992). The electrophysiological findings point to axonal degeneration in the peripheral nerves, predominating in the sensory nerves. Somatosensory evoked potentials evoked from tibial nerves are abnormal in 80% of cases. Brainstem auditory evoked potentials show abnormalities in about 75% of cases (Santoro et al., 1992).

Neuropathology

The cerebellum is grossly atrophic. There is a loss of Purkinje neurons and granule cells. The dentate nuclei are also atrophic. The nuclei of the pons are thinned. The inferior olivary complex appears smaller. The spinal cord is spared. Sural nerve biopsies show a loss of large myelinated fibers.

Genetic and molecular aspects

A locus on chromosome 13q11-12 has been identified in a Tunisian family, in a position where ARSACS has also been mapped (see section Autosomal recessive spastic ataxia of Charlevoix-Saguenay). EOCARR might represent a group of genetically heterogeneous disorders with similar phenotypic manifestations.

Spinocerebellar ataxia with axonal neuropathy

Spinocerebellar ataxia with axonal neuropathy (SCAN1) is characterized by recessive ataxia with peripheral sensorimotor axonal neuropathy, distal muscular atrophy, and pes cavus with steppage during gait. The phenotype can mimic Charcot-Marie-Tooth disease. Patients have often a history of seizures. Brain MRI shows mild brain atrophy. Blood studies show mild hypercholesterolemia and moderate hypoalbuminemia. Genetic studies in a large Saudi Arabian family mapped the disease to chromosome 14q31 (Takashima et al., 2002). The mutation affects the gene encoding topoisomerase I (TDP1), an enzyme essential for preventing the formation of double-strand breaks.

Cerebellar ataxia and hypogonadism

Clinical description

Cerebellar ataxia and hypogonadism are mainly encountered in Boucher-Neuhäuser syndrome (BNS) and Holmes ataxia (this terminology has also been applied for dominant ataxias characterized by a cerebello-olivary degeneration, on the basis of the neuropathological similarities) (De Michele et al., 1993; Rump et al., 1997).

BNS is characterized by the triad of spinocerebellar ataxia, chorioretinal dystrophy, and hypogonadotropic hypogonadism. Puberty may be delayed. Primary amenorrhea, poor development of sexual organs, and sparse growth of secondary sexual hair suggest a diagnosis of hypogonadism. Patients present with a retinal pigment epithelium atrophy and degeneration in both fundi. Ophthalmological manifestations may be variable.

In Holmes ataxia, patients exhibit nystagmus, dysarthria, and brisk tendon reflexes and may also show mental deficiency and urinary incontinence. Skeletal deformities may be present.

Ophthalmologic investigations

In BNS, both fluorescein and indocyanine green angiography show choriocapillaris atrophy. Electroretinographic studies reveal absent or abnormal photopic or scotopic responses.

Blood studies

Luteinizing hormone and follicle-stimulating hormones are deficient. The absence of a response to luteinizing hormone-releasing hormone injections strongly suggests a disturbed pituitary function. Evidence of additional involvement of the hypothalamus may be present.

Neuroimaging

Brain MRI shows a cerebellar atrophy in BNS and Holmes ataxia. In some instances, involvement of either gray or white cerebral matter is found.

Neurophysiology

Axonal neuropathy is found in some patients with Holmes ataxia.

Neuropathology

Post-mortem studies in Holmes ataxia show atrophy of the cerebellum and inferior olives. Muscle biopsy may reveal a deficiency in cytochrome c oxidase (De Michele et al., 1993).

Genetic and molecular aspects

A mitochondrial respiratory chain complex I deficiency and a 5.5-kb mtDNA single deletion in skeletal muscle have been reported (Barrientos et al., 1997).

Differential diagnosis

IOSCA (see section Infantile-onset spinocerebellar ataxia) and Oliver-McFarlane syndrome should be distinguished from Holmes ataxia and BNS (see Table 20.4). Congenital disorders of glycosylation are recessive metabolic disorders described in Chapter 7.

The occurrence of retinal degeneration, hypogonadism, and cerebellar ataxia has been described in several syndromes with overlapping features, such as Laurence-Moon syndrome, Bardet-Biedl syndrome, Alström syndrome, and Usher syndrome. These syndromes are complicated by additional features like deafness, mental retardation, polydactyly, spastic paraplegia, various dysmorphic features, and glucose intolerance. Ataxia may have a prominent bilateral vestibular component, as in Usher syndrome (Möller et al., 1989). This syndrome is genetically heterogeneous. Type I patients are profoundly deaf, whereas type II patients are "hard of hearing." Type III patients have

Table 20.4 Differential diagnosis of Boucher-Neuhäuser syndrome (BNS)

Features	BNS	Holmes ataxia	IOSCA	Oliver-McFarlane syndrome
Cerebellar ataxia	+	+	+	Rare
Chorioretinal degeneration	+	Rare	−	+
Hypogonadotrophic hypogonadism	+	+	−	+
Hypergonadotrophic hypogonadism	−	+	+	−
Alopecia	−	−	−	+
Trichomegaly	−	−	−	+
Mental retardation	−	+	−	+
Pre-natal onset growth retardation	−	−	−	+

Modified from: Rump et al. (1997).

progressive hearing loss and usually normal vestibular responses. Type IC (Acadian variety) is caused by mutation in harmonin (11p15.1), and type ID and type IF are caused by a mutation in the cadherin-23 and protocadherin-15 genes, respectively. Both genes map to 10q21-q22. Type IG is caused by mutation in the SANS gene (17q24-q25). Type IE maps to 21q21, and type IH maps to 15q22-q23. Type IIA is caused by a mutation in the usherin gene on chromosome 1q41.

Treatment

Treatment includes hormone replacement therapy. Fertility can be restored by hormone substitution. Female patients with BNS may give birth to children.

Cerebellar ataxia and deafness

Several autosomal recessive ataxias are associated with deafness:

- Richards-Rundle syndrome: also called ataxia-deafness-retardation syndrome with ketoaciduria (Richards & Rundle, 1959). Patients may also present with underdevelopment of secondary sex characteristics due to hypogonadism (see also section Cerebellar ataxia and hypogonadism). Cochleovestibular investigation shows more or less severe forms of bulbopontine cochleovestibular dysfunction.
- Lichtenstein-Knorr syndrome: patients present with combinations of ataxia, hearing loss, and peripheral neuropathy in absence of mental retardation and cataract.
- Berman syndrome: characterized by mental retardation, progressive ataxia, sensorineural deafness, and signs of peripheral neuropathy. Growth deficit may be present.
- Koletzko syndrome: this syndrome resembles Berman syndrome. There is no growth deficiency (Koletzko et al., 1987).
- Jeune-Tommasi disease: the disorder is characterized by the triad of ataxia, deafness, and mental retardation (Jeune et al., 1963). Concomitant heart deficits may be present.
- Flynn and Aird syndrome: the absence of mental retardation and the presence of cataract allow the differential diagnosis with Berman syndrome. Transmission is autosomal dominant.

Cerebellar ataxia and ocular features

The main disorders with autosomal recessive inheritance and combining cerebellar ataxia with ocular features are listed in Table 20.5.

Wolfram syndrome is characterized by diabetes insipidus, juvenile diabetes mellitus, optic atrophy, and deafness (hence the acronym of DIDMOAD syndrome). Neurological deficits include ataxia, myoclonus, mental retardation, and peripheral neuropathy. Deficits appear in childhood. Reduced visual acuity is associated with bilateral optic atrophy and constriction of the peripheral visual field. Urinary tract disorders are common. Mutations in the WFS1 gene located in the 4p16.1 region have been identified (Inoue et al., 1998; Cano et al., 2007). WFS1 encodes wolframin, a polytopic membrane protein of the endoplasmic reticulum. Brain MRI shows atrophy of the cerebellum (Mathis et al., 2007). The brainstem may also appear atrophic.

Table 20.5 Disorders combining cerebellar ataxia and ocular features

Optic atrophy
  Wolfram syndrome
  Behr syndrome
  Arts syndrome (X-linked)
  Neuronal ceroid lipofuscinosis (see Chapter 17)

Retinitis pigmentosa
  Neuropathy, ataxia, and retinitis pigmentosa
  Kearns-Sayre syndrome
  Refsum disease
  Abetalipoproteinemia
  Ataxia and vitamin E deficiency
  Deficiency in coenzyme Q10
  Posterior column ataxia with retinitis pigmentosa

Cataract
  Progressive external ophthalmoplegia
  Cerebrotendinous xanthomatosis
  Marinesco-Sjögren syndrome
  Lichtenstein-Knorr syndrome
  Flynn and Aird syndrome
  Dysequilibrium syndrome (very low density lipoprotein
    receptor–associated cerebellar hypoplasia)

Aniridia
  Gillespie syndrome

Other disorders are associated with combinations of cerebellar ataxia and optic atrophy, such as Behr syndrome, which manifests in early childhood and is characterized by various degrees of pyramidal deficits like spasticity and mental retardation (Behr, 1909). Gait often appears spastic ataxic. Tendon reflexes are decreased in some patients. Brain MRI shows moderate to marked cerebellar atrophy (Pizzatto & Pascual-Castroviejo, 2001). Nerve biopsy shows signs of axonal degeneration, and muscle biopsy reveals multiple inclusions composed of spiral cylindrical structures (Thomas et al., 1984). Spasticity and muscle contractures of the hip adductors, hamstrings, and soleus may be treated with surgery or injections of botulinum toxin (Copeliovitch et al., 2001). Type III 3-methylglutaconic aciduria presents with a very similar clinical phenotype. Urinary levels of 3-methyglutaconic acid are increased. The disorder is most common in patients of Iraqi Jewish origin. Behr syndrome should be distinguished from the recessively inherited biotinidase deficiency (multiple carboxylase deficiency), a defect in the recycling of the vitamin biotin. Children present with seizures, optic atrophy, hearing loss, acute intermittent ataxia, skin rash, alopecia, infections, and lactic acidosis. Atypical neurological findings are myoclonic jerks, neuropathy, and spastic paraparesis. Urinary excretion of 3-hydroxyisovaleric acid and 3-hydroxypropionic acid is elevated. The disorder is associated with mutations at the BTD gene (chromosome 3q25). Patients respond both clinically and biochemically to biotin (10–20 mg/day) (de Parscau et al., 1989; Grünewald et al., 2004).

Arts syndrome is an X-linked disorder characterized by mental retardation, hypotonia, ataxia, delayed motor development, hearing impairment, and optic atrophy (Arts et al., 1993; de Brouwer et al., 2007). Later, the clinical picture is dominated by a flaccid tetraplegia and areflexia. These patients are susceptible to infections. The candidate gene phosphoribosyl pyrophosphate synthetase 1 (PRPS1) maps to Xq22.1-q24 (de Brouwer et al., 2007). The loss-of-function mutations of PRPS1 induce impaired purine biosynthesis. Hypoxanthine is not detected in urine, and uric acid levels are decreased in serum. Treatment with S-adenosylmethionine has been suggested to replenish low levels of purines (de Brouwer et al., 2007).

Posterior column ataxia and retinitis pigmentosa (PCARP) has been reported in an inbred family of Dutch-German ancestry belonging to a sectarian population that has been genetically semi-isolated from mainstream society for several centuries (Higgins et al., 1999). Another family has also been reported in Spain. Patients exhibit visual deficits (especially a concentric contraction of the visual fields), proprioceptive loss with sensory ataxia, and tendon areflexia. Individuals become blind by the third decade and develop achalasia and scoliosis. MRI showed hyperintense signals in the spinal cord. The locus (AXPC1) has been assigned to chromosome 1q31-q32 (Higgins et al., 2000). PCARP is distinct from Biemond ataxia (posterior column ataxia), which is characterized by a sensory ataxia due to degeneration in the posterior columns, starting from the first to third decade (Biemond, 1951; Singh et al., 1973). There is a progressive loss of vibration and postural sensibility and ataxia. Patients develop tendon areflexia, but pain and temperature sensations are preserved. Plantar reflexes are flexor. Individuals present with scoliosis. Degeneration of Purkinje neurons and dorsal root sensory ganglion neurons has been reported (Nachmanoff et al., 1997).

Gillespie syndrome is characterized by aniridia, cerebellar ataxia, and mental retardation. The typical presentation is based on fixed dilated pupils in a hypotonic child. Cognitive and behavioral assessments reveal a pattern of abnormalities that closely resembles the cerebellar cognitive and affective syndrome (Mariën et al., 2008). MRI shows global cerebral atrophy or a pattern of cerebellar atrophy suggestive of cerebellar hypoplasia. Abnormal signals in the white matter may be observed. Muscle biopsies and nerve conduction velocities are normal. A mutation of the PAX6 gene has been reported (Ticho et al., 2006; Graziano et al., 2007).

Dysequilibrium syndrome

The dysequilibrium syndrome (DES) is caused by a mutation in the VLDLR gene (chromosome 9p24) encoding the very low density lipoprotein receptor. Many patients who were initially reported came from one region of Sweden, with parental consanguinity. Several cases have been reported in the Dariusleut Hutterites and more recently in Turkey (Schurig et al., 1981). The social characteristics of the Hutterite population have resulted in virtual genetic isolation. DES is a form of congenital cerebral palsy characterized by mental retardation, impaired equilibrium, retarded motor development, muscular hypotonia, and tendon hyperreflexia (Hagberg et al., 1972; Sanner, 1973; Boycott et al., 2005). Some individuals prefer quadrupedal walking. Additional features include strabismus and pes planus in the majority of patients, seizures in 40% of patients, and short stature in 15% of patients (Boycott et al., 2005). Brain imaging shows cerebellar atrophy or hypoplasia, with absence of inferior portions of the cerebellum and vermis, a small pons, and a simplified cortical sulcation pattern (Boycott et al., 2009). The very low density lipoprotein receptor is part of the reelin signaling pathway, which guides neuroblast migration in the cerebral cortex and cerebellum (Tissir & Goffinet, 2003; see also Chapter 1). A second disorder involving the reelin signaling pathway is the congenital syndrome of autosomal recessive lissencephaly (lissencephaly is a brain malformation characterized by absence of gyral formation, causing a smooth brain surface) with cerebellar hypoplasia due to a mutation in the RELN gene (Hong et al., 2000; see also Chapter 7). Brain MRI shows moderate to marked lissencephaly and profound cerebellar hypoplasia. In addition to cerebellar ataxia, patients have severe epilepsy and mental retardation. This disorder is distinct from the autosomal recessive syndrome of familial lissencephaly, cleft palate, diffuse agyria, and severe cerebellar hypoplasia (Kerner et al., 1999).

Cayman ataxia

Clinical description

Autosomal recessive Cayman cerebellar ataxia has been reported in Grand Cayman Island (Johnson et al., 1978). Patients exhibit a congenital syndrome characterized by psychomotor retardation and non-progressive cerebellar dysfunction. Neurological examination shows nystagmus, dysarthria, kinetic tremor, and ataxic gait. Hypotonia is present from early childhood.

Neuroimaging

Imaging studies show cerebellar hypoplasia.

Genetic and molecular aspects

The gene ATCAY (chromosome 19p13.3) encodes a neuron-restricted protein called caytaxin (BNIP-H), which contains a CRAL-TRIO motif common to proteins that bind small lipophilic molecules (Bomar et al., 2003). Mutations interfere with normal splicing. Cayataxin binds to glutaminase, a neurotransmitter-producing enzyme, affecting its activity and intracellular localization (Buschdorf et al., 2008).

Wilson disease

Epidemiology

The worldwide prevalence of Wilson disease is estimated to be about 30 per 1 million. There is a higher prevalence in Sardinia. The heterozygote carrier frequency is 1 in 90 to 100.

Clinical description

Patients exhibit various combinations of neurological and extra-neurological deficits (Table 20.6). They show extra-pyramidal signs (which can mimic Parkinson disease), ataxia, and cognitive or neuropsychiatric deficits. Tremor is observed in about half of patients. Seizure is a late manifestation. Wilson disease rarely presents with polyneuropathy (Jung et al., 2005). Patients may complain of intermittent paresthesia and exhibit weakness in both hands and feet, but sensory examination is usually normal. The Kayser-Fleischer ring (a deep copper-colored ring at the periphery of the cornea, with color ranging from greenish gold to brown) is observed in up to 90% of individuals and is

Table 20.6 Clinical signs in Wilson disease

Parkinsonism

Tremor

Dystonia

Chorea

Ataxia

Neuropsychiatric features
  Emotional lability
  Disinhibition
  Self-injury

Extra-neurological
  Kayser-Fleischer ring
  Arthropathy
  Evidence of liver disease

almost invariably present in patients with neurological manifestations.

Patients with Wilson disease usually present with liver disease during the first two decades of life. Liver involvement can take the aspect of a chronic active hepatitis or a cirrhosis. Patients may develop fulminant hepatic failure, with age at diagnosis ranging from 11 to 54 years (Gow et al., 2000). Hypercalciuria and nephrocalcinosis are not uncommon (Wiebers et al., 1979). The risk of nephrolithiasis is increased. A Fanconi-like syndrome can evolve. Some individuals present with chondrocalcinosis and osteoarthritis due to copper accumulation. Hemolytic anemia is not rare.

Slit-lamp examination

Neuroophthalmologic slit-lamp assessment is highly recommended. A false-positive test may be found in chronic liver disorders.

Neuroimaging

Brain MRI shows atrophy of the cerebrum in 70% of cases, brainstem in 66% of cases, and cerebellum in 52% of cases (Sinha et al., 2006). Signal abnormalities are noted in the putamen, caudate, thalami, midbrain, pons, cerebral white matter, cortex, medulla, and cerebellum. A characteristic T2-weighted globus pallidal hypointensity is found in one-third of cases. The "face of the giant panda" sign is detected in about 10% of cases. Pronounced lesions in the dentate nuclei have been reported (Matsuura et al., 1998). MRI changes correlate with disease severity scores.

Neurophysiology

Auditory evoked potentials are disturbed in 70% of cases and somatosensory evoked potentials in 46%. Nerve conduction studies and sural nerve biopsy are consistent with a mixed demyelinating and axonal neuropathy (Jung et al., 2005).

Blood studies

Low ceruloplasmin levels are found in blood. A false-negative test may occur in patients with marked hepatic inflammation. Levels of total copper are decreased. Hemolytic anemia (Coombs-negative) occurs in 10% to 15% of cases.

Urinary studies

Classically, patients have high urinary copper (24-hour urinary copper >100 μg/day), but urinary excretion is normal in some patients. In presymptomatic cases, urinary copper excretion may be normal, but increases after D-penicillamine challenge.

Liver biopsy

Liver biopsy shows increased amounts of copper deposition (>250 μg/g dry weight; normal <50 μg/g dry weight). Lesions suggestive of a chronic liver disorder may be observed. There is evidence of severe mitochondrial dysfunction in the livers of patients with Wilson disease (Gu et al., 2000).

Genetic and molecular aspects

Wilson disease is due to mutations in the adenosine triphosphatase ATP7B gene (chromosome 13q14.3-q21.1; Bull et al., 1993). The most common mutation in patients from Europe is H1069Q. Mutation M645R is common in Spain, and R778L is common in eastern Asia (Ferenci, 2006). Given the difficulties in searching for mutations in a gene spanning more than 80 kb of genomic DNA, haplotyping is important as a guide to mutation detection.

Once a diagnosis of Wilson disease is made in a patient, an evaluation of the family is important. The likelihood of finding a homozygote among siblings is 25% and among children is 0.5%.

Pathogenesis

The major defect is decreased liver excretion of copper. The estimated total body copper content is lower than

100 mg, with an average daily intake of 1 to 2 mg. (See also next section.)

Treatment

Wilson disease is effectively treated with D-penicillamine (1–2 g/day), trientine (triethylene-tetramine dihydrochloride 15–20 mg/kg daily), or zinc acetate/sulfate (50–150 mg/day) (Brewer et al., 1987). Zinc induces hepatic metallothionein, which sequesters copper in a non-toxic pool. Some authors consider that penicillamine should not be used as the initial therapy (Brewer, 1999). Ammonium tetrathiomolybdate is an alternative (Brewer et al., 2006). Prophylactic treatment of asymptomatic patients with zinc results in decreased levels of urinary copper.

Fulminant Wilson disease is treated with orthotopic liver transplant (Sokol et al., 1985). Improvement in neurological function over a period of 3 or 4 months can be marked (Polson et al., 1987). Postoperative central pontine and extrapontine myelinolysis is a potential complication (Guarino et al., 1995).

Aceruloplasminemia

Epidemiology

Aceruloplasminemia is observed worldwide. The prevalence has been estimated to be approximately 1 per 2 000 000 in non-consanguineous marriages in Japan (Miyajima et al., 1999).

Clinical description

Symptoms usually appear between 30 and 50 years of age. The age at diagnosis ranges from 16 to 71 years. Complete ceruloplasmin deficiency presents with progressive confusion, dementia, extra-pyramidal deficits (blepharospasm, torticollis, chorea, cogwheel rigidity), and ataxia (Logan et al., 1994; Morita et al., 1992; Miyajima et al., 2003). Retinal degeneration is found in about 70% of cases. Funduscopy shows yellowish opacities and atrophy of the retinal pigmented epithelium. Patients often develop diabetes. Heterozygotes of ceruloplasmin gene mutations have hypoceruloplasminemia and may exhibit a mild ataxia (Miyajima et al., 2001)

Neuroimaging

The dentate nucleus, thalamus, putamen, caudate nucleus, and liver of patients show low signal intensities on T2-weighted MRI. In heterozygous cases, brain MRI can show an isolated cerebellar atrophy without hypointense signals in basal ganglia. PET studies can reveal a hypometabolism in the basal ganglia and thalamus. The hypometabolism extends to the cerebral and cerebellar cortices after several years.

Blood studies

Patients have absent or decreased levels of serum ceruloplasmin (see also preceding section), low serum iron, and increased serum ferritin concentrations. Microcytic anemia is common.

Liver biopsy

Liver biopsy confirms the presence of an excess of iron.

Neuropathology

Post-mortem study demonstrates excessive iron deposition in the brain, liver, and pancreas (Morita et al., 1992; Morita et al., 1995). Autopsy reveals severe destruction of the basal ganglia and dentate nucleus, with iron deposition in neuronal and glial cells. Many astrocytes are enlarged with abundant cytoplasm.

Genetic and molecular aspects

The locus is located at 3q23-q24. Intrafamilial phenotypic variations may occur (Fasano et al., 2008). The majority of mutations in the ceruloplasmin gene are truncated mutations leading to the formation of a premature stop codon. Due to the high number of mutations, genetic testing is not a first-line procedure.

Pathogenesis

Ceruloplasmin is mainly synthesized in hepatocytes and is also expressed in the CNS (Kono & Miyajima, 2006). In the brain, most of the ceruloplasmin is located on the surface of astrocytes. Under normal circumstances, circulating ceruloplasmin does not cross the blood–brain barrier. Ceruloplasmin functions in iron transport and storage. Ceruloplasmin catalyzes the oxidation of ferrous iron to ferric iron or the peroxidation of Fe(II) transferrin to form Fe(III) transferrin (Logan et al., 1994). Aceruloplasminemia can be considered as an autosomal recessive disorder of iron metabolism (see also section Friedreich ataxia). Iron accumulation generates oxidative stress and lipid

213

peroxidation. Deposits are typically observed in the pancreas, liver, and cerebral tissue.

Treatment

Favorable results have been reported with desferrioxamine (Miyajima et al., 1997). Some authors have observed a benefit on gait ataxia of the combination of fresh-frozen plasma (450 mL/week for 6 weeks) and desferrioxamine (recommended dose 500 mg intravenously twice a week). Beneficial treatment of oral zinc sulfate for heterozygous mutation of the ceruloplasmin gene has been reported (Kuhn et al., 2007).

Lysosomal storage diseases

Lysosomal storage diseases can be classified as follows:

- Lipid storage disorders, including sphingolipidoses
- Mucopolysaccharidoses
- Mucolipidoses
- Glycoprotein storage disorders

Table 20.7 lists the main lysosomal disorders associated with cerebellar ataxia. Most patients are clinically normal at birth but develop symptoms early in childhood (Meikle et al., 2006). Taken together, inborn errors of lysosomal metabolism occur in approximately 1 per 5000 live births.

Gangliosidoses

GM1 gangliosidosis is due to a deficiency of the beta-galactosidase enzyme. Three clinical forms of the disease are recognized: infantile onset, juvenile onset, and adult onset. The disease is lethal in the infantile and juvenile forms. The infantile form is characterized by psychomotor deterioration beginning within 6 months of birth, hepatosplenomegaly, facial dysmorphism, macular cherry-red spots, and skeletal dysplasia. The juvenile form is characterized by mental deterioration and progressive spastic, cerebellar, and extrapyramidal signs, without facial dysmorphisms and organomegaly. The adult/chronic form starts between 3 and 30 years and is characterized by skeletal involvement and localized CNS involvement. Patients exhibit dystonia and gait or speech disturbances. More than 100 mutations distributed along the beta-galactosidase gene (GLB1; 3p21.33) have been reported (Brunetti-Pierri & Scaglia, 2008).

Table 20.7 Lysosomal disorders associated with cerebellar ataxias

Gangliosidoses
  GM1 gangliosidosis
  GM2 gangliosidosis (Tay-Sachs disease, Sandhoff disease)

Sulfatidosis
  Multiple sulfatase deficiency
  Metachromatic leukodystrophy

Glucocerebroside lipoidosis
  Gaucher disease

Globotriaosylceramide lipidosis
  Fabry disease (see Chapter 8)

Galactosylceramide lipoidosis
  Krabbe disease

Sphingomyelinosis
  Niemann-Pick disease type C

Glycoproteinosis
  Alpha-mannosidosis
  Fucosidosis

Mucolipidosis
  Type I sialidosis (see Chapter 17)
  Infantile sialic acid storage disease
  Salla disease
  Cerebellar ataxia with elevated cerebrospinal free sialic acid

Cystinosis

Neuronal ceroid lipofuscinosis (see Chapter 17)

GM2 gangliosidosis type I (Tay-Sachs disease) is caused by mutation in the alpha subunit of the hexosaminidase A gene (HEXA; chromosome 15q23-24) and is 100 times more common in infants of Ashkenazi Jewish ancestry than in non-Jewish infants. Classically, the disease is characterized by the onset in infancy. Symptoms are developmental delay, dementia, startle, and blindness. Death occurs in the second or third year of life. A central cherry-red spot is a typical funduscopic finding. The thalamus and basal ganglia are principally involved on brain MRI. Late-onset Tay-Sachs disease is characterized by cerebellar dysfunction, tendon areflexia, proximal neurogenic muscle weakness, fasciculations, and psychiatric/behavioral deficits, including psychosis, mania, or depression. The late-onset form can present as a Friedreich ataxia phenotype or as an amyotrophic lateral sclerosis, or can mimic a Charcot-Marie-Tooth disease (Johnson, 1981; Willner et al., 1981). Cerebral cortical and cerebellar atrophy is marked on brain MRI (Hund et al., 1997). Neurophysiological studies show a predominantly axonal polyneuropathy affecting distal nerve segments in the lower and upper extremities (Shapiro et al., 2008).

GM2 gangliosidosis type II (Sandhoff disease) is often clinically indistinguishable from Tay-Sachs disease. In the classical infantile presentation, progressive psychomotor retardation is common, associated with a rapidly progressive spastic tetraparesis and seizures after a few months. Death occurs within the first years. The most common deficits of the juvenile presentation include cerebellar ataxia and speech abnormalities (Hendriksz et al., 2004). The cherry-red spot may be absent. Some patients develop early and severe sensory loss in addition to chronic motor neuron disease and cerebellar ataxia (Schnorf et al., 1995). Peripheral neuropathy may be predominantly sensory in the adult-onset form. Brain MRI shows signal changes in the periventricular white matter, pyramidal tract, basal ganglia, and cerebellar hemispheres. Cerebellar atrophy may be observed in the adult form. Accumulation of hexosamine-containing oligosaccharides may be detected by brain MRS (Wilken et al., 2008). The disease results from mutation in the beta subunit of the hexosaminidase A and B enzymes (chromosome 5q13).

Sulfatidoses

Multiple sulfatase deficiency is associated with deficiency of several sulfatases (Soong et al., 1988). The disorder affects at least seven members of the sulfatase family, a group of lysosomal enzymes specifically involved in the degradation of sulfated glycosaminoglycans, sulfolipids, or other sulfated molecules (Dierks et al., 2009). The phenotype combines features of mucopolysaccharidoses, metachromatic leukodystrophy (MLD), and X-linked ichthyosis. The clinical course ranges from severe neonatal to mild juvenile cases. Patients exhibit combinations of short stature, microcephaly, facial dysmorphism, limited joint mobility, retinal degeneration, and ataxia. The disorder is caused by mutations in the SUMF1 gene encoding the formylglycine-generating enzyme (FGE), which post-translationally activates sulfatases by generating formylglycine in their catalytic sites (Schlotawa et al., 2008; see also Chapter 23).

MLD is reported to occur in 1 per 40 000 to 1 per 160 000 individuals worldwide. MLD is due to a deficiency of the arylsulfatase A, which initiates the degradation of sulfatides. Accumulation occurs mainly in the nervous system, kidneys, and gallbladder. The disorder is classically divided into late infantile (onset <4 years), early juvenile (age 4–6 years), late juvenile (age 6–16 years), and adult forms (age >16 years). Juvenile and adult-onset MLD show a marked phenotypic heterogeneity. The arylsulfatase A gene (ARSA) is located at chromosome 22q13.31. The most common mutations are P426L and I179S. P426L homozygotes typically present with gait difficulties due to spastic paraparesis and cerebellar ataxia (Rauschka et al., 2006). Inappropriate behavior and social dysfunction are observed in compound heterozygotes for I179S. Patients may be misdiagnosed as schizophrenic. Demyelination in the nervous system is detected by brain MRI and neurophysiological studies showing a demyelinating polyneuropathy. This latter may precede the advent of brain MRI abnormalities (Haberlandt et al., 2009). Cerebrospinal fluid protein levels are often increased.

Gaucher disease

Gaucher disease (GD) is the most common lysosomal storage disorder, with an incidence around 1 per 40 000 to 1 per 60 000 inhabitants. GD is a common genetic disease in the Jewish population. The multisystem involvement is due to deficient activity of beta-glucocerebrosidase (Grabowski, 2008). The disorder is classically divided phenotypically into three main subtypes: non-neuronopathic type I, acute neuronopathic type II, and subacute neuronopathic type III. Type I is the most common form and lacks primary CNS involvement. It usually presents in childhood with hepatosplenomegaly, pancytopenia, and manifestations of bone marrow infiltration. Patients may develop severe orthopedic complications, including vertebral compression, necrosis of the femoral head, and pathologic fractures of long bones. Types II and III are associated with neurologic manifestations. The adult-onset form manifests with an akinetic-rigid syndrome poorly responsive to levodopa, supranuclear gaze palsy, myoclonus, seizure, cerebellar ataxia, and cognitive and psychotic disturbances. The intracellular accumulation of glucosylceramide affects primarily cells of mononuclear phagocyte origin, the so-called "Gaucher cells" identified in most tissues. GD is caused by a mutation in the glucocerebrosidase gene (GBA; chromosome 1q21). An atypical form is caused by a mutation in the gene encoding saposin C, an enzymatic activator.

Niemann-Pick disease type C

Niemann-Pick disease type C (NPC) has an estimated incidence in European countries of 1 per 120 000 to

1 per 150 000 live births (Vanier & Millat, 2003). The average age of diagnosis is 10 years, but the disorder can affect older patients up to the fifth decade (Sévin et al., 2007). NPC is characterized by accumulation of unesterified cholesterol and glycolipids. Clinically, patients present with neonatal jaundice, hepatosplenomegaly, pulmonary symptoms, vertical gaze palsy, cerebellar ataxia, dystonia, dysphagia, seizures, deafness, cataplexy, and neuropsychiatric symptoms usually consistent with psychosis, in a context of progressive neurodegeneration (Garver et al., 2007). Cerebellar ataxia affecting both the trunk and the limbs is the most common neurological manifestation in the adult form. An axonal sensorimotor polyneuropathy may be associated (Uc et al., 2000). Cognitive deficits range from a mild dysexecutive syndrome to severe dementia with mutism requiring institutionalization. NPC may be particularly challenging in terms of diagnosis when the disorder presents as a pure psychiatric disorder, as a frontal dementia, as a cerebellar syndrome, or as a dystonic phenotype (Sévin et al., 2007). Some patients are misdiagnosed with Gaucher disease (Uc et al., 2000). Brain MRI shows cortical atrophy predominating in the frontal lobes with variable atrophy of the corpus callosum and subcortical atrophy and may disclose a cerebellar atrophy extending to the brainstem. Functional imaging studies reveal more diffuse abnormalities. White matter high-intensity signals are common. About 95% of patients have mutations in the NPC1 gene (18q11) encoding a membrane glycoprotein. The remaining patients have mutations in the NPC2 gene (14q24.3) encoding a lysosomal protein binding cholesterol with high affinity. The two proteins function in tandem or in sequence to facilitate the intracellular transport of lipids from the lysosome to other cellular sites (Sleat et al., 2004).

Alpha-mannosidosis

The prevalence of alpha-mannosidosis is about 1 per 500 000. The disorder is characterized by immune deficits leading to recurrent infections, facioskeletal abnormalities (large head with prominent forehead, rounded eyebrows, macroglossia, prognathism, dysostosis multiplex, scoliosis, deformation of the sternum, genu valgus), sensorineural hearing loss, and mental retardation caused by deficiency in alpha-mannosidase (Malm & Nilssen, 2008). Three clinical types have been suggested:

- Type 1: mild form with very slow progression and affecting patients older than 10 years.
- Type 2 (the most common): moderate form with skeletal abnormalities and development of ataxia at age 20 to 30 years. Ataxia is slowly progressive.
- Type 3: severe form leading to early death due to primary CNS involvement or myopathy.

Brain MRI shows brachycephaly, thick calvaria, verticalization of the chiasmatic sulcus, low pneumatization of the sphenoid body, partial empty sella turcica, cerebellar atrophy, and white matter signal changes related to demyelination and associated gliosis (Dietemann et al., 1990). Mutations involve the MAN2B1 gene (chromosome 19p13.2-p13.11). More than 40 mutations have been identified, and there is no apparent correlation between the genotype and the phenotype (Berg et al., 1999).

Fucosidosis

Fucosidosis, a glycoproteinosis, is due to decreased amounts of alpha-L-fucosidase, causing progressive neurological deterioration that includes mental deficits and clumsiness, cardiomegaly, and dysostosis multiplex. Clusters occur in southern Italy, in the Mexican-Indian population of the western United States, and in Cuba. Type 1 presents early in infancy and is rapidly progressive to a decerebrate state and death before the age of 5 years. Children present with a mild hepatomegaly and splenomegaly. Type 2 starts at a late infantile stage. Patients present with confluent skin lesions called angiokeratoma corporis diffusum (see also Fabry disease, see Chapter 8). Most patients die before the age of 30 years. Brain MRI shows hyperintense areas on T2-weighted images in the periventricular areas. Hyperintense signal in T1-weighted images is found in the globus pallidus. These lesions appear hypointense on T2-weighted images (Provenzale et al., 1995). Cerebral and cerebellar atrophy is detected in advanced cases. Neuropathological studies show prominent neuronal loss in the gray matter structures, particularly in the thalamus, hypothalamus, cerebral cortex, Purkinje layer, and dentate nuclei (Durand et al., 1969). Cells appear vacuolated, and intracellular inclusion bodies can be detected. The disease is associated with mutations of the alpha-L-fucosidase (FUCA1) gene (Lin et al., 2007). All these mutations lead to nearly absent enzymatic activity (Willems et al., 1999).

Type I sialidosis

This disorder is discussed in Chapter 17.

Infantile sialic acid storage disease and Salla disease

These disorders are due to impaired function of sialin, a sialic acid transporter located at the lysosomal membrane. Infantile sialic acid storage disease is a severe form characterized by facial dysmorphism, developmental delay, hypotonia, and failure to thrive. Hepatosplenomegaly and cardiomegaly are relatively common. Death occurs usually within 2 years (Sagné & Gasnier, 2008). Salla disease is a less severe form, which occurs essentially in Finland and Sweden, although cases have been reported in the United Kingdom, Holland, Argentina, and France. The disease first manifests from infancy to childhood. The terminology relates to the geographic area in Finland where the first patients have been diagnosed. Hypotonia starts in the first year of life. Patients exhibit intellectual deficits, developmental delay, seizures, cerebellar ataxia, spasticity, and athetosis. Half of patients have a demyelinating peripheral neuropathy. Individuals usually survive into adulthood. Hypoplasia of the corpus callosum is a consistent finding on brain MRI, which shows also cerebellar atrophy and central hypomyelination (Parazzini et al., 2003). Diagnosis is confirmed by the measurement of free sialic acid excretion in the urine, abnormal lysosomes in skin biopsy, and DNA studies. Several mutations of the sialin gene SCL17A5 (localized on chromosome 6q14-q15) are known.

Cerebellar ataxia with elevated cerebrospinal free sialic acid

First symptoms appear between the ages of 10 and 24 years (Mochel et al., 2009). Patients exhibit cerebellar ataxia, with peripheral neuropathy (mainly of the axonal type) and cognitive deficits or behavioral abnormalities. There is no dysmorphism and no general sign of storage disease. Brain MRI shows mild to moderate cerebellar atrophy and hyperintense white matter lesions on T2-weighted sequence in the peridentate areas and periventricular zones. Aspect of peridentate regions is similar to the aspect observed in cerebrotendinous xanthomatosis (see section Cerebrotendinous xanthomatosis) or in some mitochondrial disorders. The corpus callosum appears normal.

Laboratory studies disclose hyposialylation of transferrin in the CSF, distinguishing this disorder from Salla disease. Moreover, the levels of free sialic acid are increased in CSF, but not in urine, plasma, or cultured skin fibroblasts.

Cystinosis

Cystinosis is a disorder of amino acid transport characterized by photosensitive dermatitis and initially intermittent neurological symptoms occurring in children or in adults. Ataxia, headache, personality disorders, and photophobia tend to occur periodically. A late-onset myopathy can develop. Generalized proximal tubular insufficiency causes massive urinary excretion of amino acids. Patients present with anorexia with vomiting contributing to growth retardation. Swallowing dysfunction presents a risk of fatal aspiration (Sonies et al., 2005). The disorder is caused by mutations in the CTNS gene (chromosome 17p13) coding for a cystine transporter in the lysosomal membrane called cystinosin (Town et al., 1998).

Diagnosis of a lysosomal storage disease

Assessment of enzymatic activities in leukocytes and cultured skin fibroblasts is completed by urine analysis (elevated urinary excretion) and genetic testing. Light or electron microscopy may show accumulation of material in bone marrow smears and lymphocytes from peripheral blood. Morphologic changes may be evident in rectal, muscle, or nerve biopsies. Brain imaging (MRI, MRS) and neurophysiological tests may be useful for both diagnosis and follow-up.

Differential diagnosis

Mevalonic aciduria can mimic a lysosomal storage disease. This autosomal recessive disorder is due to a defect in the biosynthesis of cholesterol as a consequence of a deficiency of mevalonate kinase. Symptoms usually start between the ages of 2 and 6 years. Affected children present with severe failure to thrive, developmental delay, dysmorphic facies, and hepatosplenomegaly with possible anemia and thrombocytopenia. Recurrent episodes of fever with inflammation and skin rash are common. Cerebellar ataxia can be a predominant neurological manifestation in patients who survive infancy (Gibson et al., 1988; Prietsch et al., 2003; Bretón Martínez et al., 2007). MRI shows cerebellar atrophy (Hoffmann et al., 1993;

Bretón Martínez et al., 2007). Important quantities of mevalonic acid are found in the urine. The activity of mevalonate kinase is severely deficient in fibroblasts and lymphocytes. Mevalonic aciduria is caused by mutation in the mevalonate kinase gene (locus 12q24). Allogeneic bone marrow transplantation has been associated with sustained remission of febrile attacks and inflammation (Neven et al., 2007). Deficiency of mevalonate kinase can also cause a hyperimmunoglobulinemia D syndrome (HIDS) manifesting with recurrent fever attacks (Haas & Hoffmann, 2006). A subgroup of patients with HIDS may develop neurological abnormalities, including mental retardation, ataxia, ocular deficits (retinal dystrophy), and seizures (Haas & Hoffmann, 2006; Simon et al., 2004). Increased levels of IgD and, in most patients, of IgA in combination with enhanced excretion of mevalonic acid provide strong evidence for HIDS (Haas & Hoffmann, 2006). The diagnosis is confirmed by low activity of mevalonate kinase or by demonstration of disease-causing mutations. Inhibitor of HMG-CoA reductase and anakinra, an interleukin-1 receptor antagonist, have beneficial effects in HIDS (van der Hilst et al., 2008; Cailliez et al., 2006).

Alexander disease is characterized by development of megalencephaly accompanied by progressive spasticity and dementia (Alexander, 1949). Based on age of onset, three forms are recognized: infantile, juvenile, and adult. The adult-onset form may present with palatal tremor, spastic paraparesis, signs of bulbar dysfunction (dysarthria, dysphonia, dysphagia), cerebellar ataxia, sleep disorders, and dysautonomia (Schwankhaus et al., 1995; Pareyson et al., 2008). Brain MRI shows leukodystrophy, preferentially affecting the frontal regions. Hypodense space-occupying lesions in the posterior fossa and mimicking a tumor may be observed (Duckett et al., 1992). Abnormalities tend to predominate in the brainstem–spinal cord junction in the adult-onset form, in the absence of cognitive impairment (Pareyson et al., 2008). Atrophy of the medulla oblongata extending caudally to the cervical spinal cord is suggestive of the disease. The diagnosis should be suspected in any adult presenting with a palatal tremor associated with brainstem signs and in whom MRI shows atrophy of the lower brainstem extending caudally. Histologically, Alexander disease is characterized by homogeneous eosinophilic masses called Rosenthal fibers, most numerous in the subpial, perivascular, and subependymal regions. These fibers are located in astrocytes. They are commonly found in astrocytomas (see Chapter 13) and in cases of chronic reactive gliosis. Demyelination is a prominent feature. Proton MRS studies are consistent with astrocytosis, demyelination, and neuroaxonal degeneration in the cerebral and cerebellar white matter (Brockmann et al., 2003). The disease is caused by mutation in the gene encoding glial fibrillary acidic protein (GFAP; gene locus 17q21), an intermediate filament of astrocytes, and is inherited in an autosomal dominant manner.

Treatment

Treatment is mainly symptomatic. Feeding difficulties often require gastrostomy. Patients may require splenectomy for management of thrombocytopenia and anemia. Skeletal deformities may be corrected by surgical intervention.

Bone marrow transplantation and enzyme replacement therapy may be successful in lysosomal disorders. Benefits of bone marrow transplantation are probably greater in younger patients before development of complications, hence the importance of an early diagnosis. However, the risks of the procedure should not be underestimated. Enzyme replacement therapy with intravenous imiglucerase (Cerezyme) is a therapeutic gold standard in Gaucher disease. Miglustat (N-butyldeoxynojirimycin), a small imino sugar inhibiting glycosphingolipid synthesis (substrate reduction therapy), is approved in Gaucher disease type I (200 mg/day). Miglustat does not appear to have significant benefits on the neurological manifestations of Gaucher disease type III (Schiffmann et al., 2008). The drug might have some beneficial effect on brain dysfunction, including on dysarthria and gait ataxia, in NPC (Galanaud et al., 2009; Santos et al., 2008). Cysteamine is an effective treatment for renal dysfunction associated with cystinosis (Gahl et al., 1987). However, renal transplantation may be required.

References

Ackroyd RS, Finnegan JA, Green SH. Friedreich ataxia. A clinical review with neurophysiological and echocardiographic findings. *Arch Dis Child* 1984;**59**:217–21.

Alboliras ET, Shub C, Gomez MR, et al. Spectrum of cardiac involvement in Friedreich ataxia: clinical, electrocardiographic and echocardiographic observations. *Am J Cardiol* 1986;**58**:518524.

Alexander WS. Progressive fibrinoid degeneration of fibrillary astrocytes associated with mental retardation in a hydrocephalic infant. *Brain* 1949;**72**:373–81.

Al-Mahdawi S, Pinto RM, Varshney D, et al. GAA repeat expansion mutation mouse models of Friedreich ataxia exhibit oxidative stress leading to progressive neuronal and cardiac pathology. *Genomics* 2006;**88**(5)580–90.

Al-Shali K, Wang J, Rosen F, Hegele RA. Ileal adenocarcinoma in a mild phenotype of abetalipoproteinemia. *Clin Genet* 2003;**63**:135–8.

Amariglio N, Hirshberg A, Scheithauer BW, et al. Donor-derived brain tumor following neural stem cell transplantation in an ataxia telangiectasia patient. *PLoS Med* 2009;**6**(2)e1000029.

Amiel J, Maziere JC, Beucler I, et al. Familial isolated vitamin E deficiency. Extensive study of a large family with a 5-year therapeutic follow-up. *J Inherit Metab Dis* 1995;**18**:333–40.

Anttonen AK, Mahjneh I, Hamalainen RH, et al. The gene disrupted in Marinesco-Sjogren syndrome encodes SIL1, an HSPA5 cochaperone. *Nat Genet* 2005;**37**:1309–11.

Arts WFM, Loonen MCB, Sengers RCA, Slooff JL. X-linked ataxia, weakness, deafness, and loss of vision in early childhood with a fatal course. *Ann Neurol* 1993;**33**:535–9.

Artuch R, Brea-Calvo G, Briones P, et al. Cerebellar ataxia with coenzyme Q10 deficiency: Diagnosis and follow-up after coenzyme Q10 supplementation. *J Neurol Sci* 2006;**246**:153–8.

Artuch R, Pineda M, Vilaseca MA, Sanchez-Alcazar JA, Navas P. Coenzyme Q10 deficiency and mitochondrial encephalomyopathies: Clinical, biochemical and molecular diagnosis. Ubiquinone-10 supplementation. In *New Frontiers in Mitochondrial Biogenesis and Disease*, ed. F. Villaroya. Kerala, India: Research Signpost, 2005, pp. 93–110.

Babcock M, de Silva D, Oaks R, et al. Regulation of mitochondrial iron accumulation by Yfh1, a putative homolog of frataxin. *Science* 1997;**276**: 1709–12.

Barbeau A. Friedreich's ataxia 1978: an overview. *Can J Neurol Sci* 1978;**5**:161–5.

Barbot C, Coutinho P, Chorao R, et al. Recessive ataxia with ocular apraxia: review of 22 Portuguese patients. *Arch Neurol* 2001;**58**:201–5.

Barrientos A, Casademont J, Genís D, et al. Sporadic heteroplasmic single 5.5 kb mitochondrial DNA deletion associated with cerebellar ataxia, hypogonadotropic hypogonadism, choroidal dystrophy, and mitochondrial respiratory chain complex I deficiency. *Hum Mutat* 1997;**10**(3)212–6.

Bassen FA, Kornzweig AL. Malformation of the erythrocytes in a case of atypical retinitis pigmentosa. *Blood* 1950;**5**:381–7.

Behr C. Die komplizierte, hereditaer-familiaere Optikusatrophie des Kindesalters: ein bisher nicht beschriebener Symptomenkomplex. *Klin Mbl Augenheilk* 1909;**47**:138–60.

Berg T, Riise HM, Hansen GM, et al. Spectrum of mutations in alpha-mannosidosis. *Am J Hum Genet* 1999;**64**(1)77–88.

Biancheri R, Zara F, Bruno C, et al. Phenotypic characterization of hypomyelination and congenital cataract. *Ann Neurol* 2007;**62**(2)121–7.

Bidichandani SI, Ashizawa T, Patel PI. Atypical Friedreich ataxia caused by compound heterozygosity for a novel missense mutation and the GAA triplet-repeat expansion. *Am J Hum Genet* 1997;**60**(5)1251–6.

Biemond A. Les degenerations spino-cerebelleuses. *Folia Psychiatr Neurol Neurochir Neerl* 1951;**54**:216–23.

Bishara S, Merin S, Cooper M, et al. Combined vitamin A and E therapy prevents retinal electrophysiological deterioration in abetalipoproteinaemia. *Br J Ophthalmol* 1982;**66**:767–70.

Bomar JM, Benke PJ, Slattery EL, et al. Mutations in a novel gene encoding a CRAL-TRIO domain cause human Cayman ataxia and ataxia/dystonia in the jittery mouse. *Nat Genet* 2003;**35**(3)264–9.

Bouchard JP. Recessive spastic ataxia of Charlevoix-Saguenay. In *Handbook of Clinical Neurology* (Chapter 16, Hereditary neuropathies and spinocerebellar degenerations), ed. J.M.B.V. de Jong. Amsterdam: Elsevier Science, 1991, pp. 451–9.

Bouchard JP, Barbeau A, Bouchard R, Bouchard RW. Autosomal recessive spastic ataxia of Charlevoix-Saguenay. *Can J Neurol Sci* 1978;**5**:61–9.

Bouchard JP, Richter A, Melancon SB, Mathieu J, Michaud J. Autosomal recessive spastic ataxia (Charlevoix-Saguenay). In *Handbook of Ataxia Disorders*, ed. T. Klockgether. New York: Marcel Dekker, 2000, pp. 311–24.

Bouchard M, Langlois G. Orthopedic management in autosomal recessive spastic ataxia of Charlevoix-Saguenay. *Can J Surg* 1999;**42**(6)440–4.

Boycott KM, Bonnemann C, Herz J, et al. Mutations in VLDLR as a cause for autosomal recessive cerebellar ataxia with mental retardation (dysequilibrium syndrome). *J Child Neurol* 2009 Mar 30 [Epub ahead of print].

Boycott KM, Flavelle S, Bureau A, et al. Homozygous deletion of the very low density lipoprotein receptor gene causes autosomal recessive cerebellar hypoplasia with cerebral gyral simplification. *Am J Hum Genet* 2005;**77**:477–83.

Boyer SH, Chisolm AW, McKusick VA. Cardiac aspects of Friedreich ataxia. *Circulation* 1962;**25**:493–505.

Braverman N, Steel G, Obie C, et al. Human PEX7 encodes the peroxisomal PTS2 receptor and is responsible for rhizomelic chondrodysplasia punctata. *Nat Genet* 1997;**15**:369–76.

Bretón Martínez JR, Cánovas Martínez A, Casaña Pérez S, Escribá Alepuz J, Giménez Vázquez F. Mevalonic aciduria: report of two cases. *J Inherit Metab Dis* 2007;**30**(5)829.

Bull PC, Thomas GR, Rommens JM, Forbes JR, Cox DW. The Wilson disease gene is a putative copper transporting P-type ATPase similar to the Menkes gene. *Nat Genet* 1993;**5**:327–37.

Buschdorf JP, Chew LL, Soh UJ, Liou YC, Low BC. Nerve growth factor stimulates interaction of Cayman ataxia protein BNIP-H/Caytaxin with peptidyl-prolyl isomerase Pin1 in differentiating neurons. *PLoS ONE* 2008;**3**(7)e2686.

Brewer GJ. Penicillamine should not be used as initial therapy in Wilson's disease. *Mov Disord* 1999;**14**:551–4.

Brewer GJ, Askari F, Lorincz MT, et al. Treatment of Wilson disease with ammonium tetrathiomolybdate: IV. Comparison of tetrathiomolybdate and trientine in a double-blind study of treatment of the neurologic presentation of Wilson disease. *Arch Neurol* 2006;**63**:521–7.

Brewer GJ, Yuzbasiyan-Gurkan V, Young AB. The treatment of Wilson's disease. *Semin Neurol* 1987;**7**:209–20.

Broccoletti T, Del Giudice E, Amorosi S, et al. Steroid-induced improvement of neurological signs in ataxia-telangiectasia patients. *Eur J Neurol* 2008;**15**(3)223–8.

Brockmann K, Dechent P, Meins M, et al. Cerebral proton magnetic resonance spectroscopy in infantile Alexander disease. *J Neurol* 2003;**250**(3)300–6.

Brunetti-Pierri N, Scaglia F. GM1 gangliosidosis: review of clinical, molecular, and therapeutic aspects. *Mol Genet Metab* 2008;**94**(4)391–6.

Burck U, Goebel HH, Kuhlendahl HD, Meier C, Goebel KM. Neuromyopathy and vitamin E deficiency in man. *Neuropediatrics* 1981;**12**:267–78.

Cailliez M, Garaix F, Rousset-Rouvière C, et al. Anakinra is safe and effective in controlling hyperimmunoglobulinaemia D syndrome-associated febrile crisis. *J Inherit Metab Dis* 2006;**29**(6)763.

Cakirer S, Savas MR. Infantile Refsum disease: serial evaluation with MRI. *Pediatr Radiol* 2005;**35**(2) 212–5.

Campanella G, Filla A, De Falco F, et al. Friedreich ataxia in the south of Italy: a clinical and biochemical survey of 23 patients. *Can J Neurol Sci* 1980;**7**:351–7.

Campuzano V, Montermini L, Moltò MD, et al. Friedreich's ataxia: autosomal recessive disease caused by an intronic GAA triplet repeat expansion. *Science* 1996;**271**(5254)1423–7.

Cano A, Rouzier C, Monnot S, et al; French Group of Wolfram Syndrome. Identification of novel mutations in WFS1 and genotype-phenotype correlation in Wolfram syndrome. *Am J Med Genet A* 2007;**143A**(14):1605–12.

Cassandro E, Mosca F, Sequino L, De Falco FA, Campanella G. Otoneurological findings in Friedreich ataxia and other inherited neuropathies. *Audiology* 1986;**25**:84–91.

Castelnovo G, Biolsi B, Barbaud A, et al. Isolated spastic paraparesis leading to diagnosis of Friedreich's ataxia. *J Neurol Neurosurg Psychiatry* 2000;**69**:693.

Chen YZ, Bennett CL, Huynh HM, et al. DNA/RNA helicase gene mutations in a form of juvenile amyotrophic lateral sclerosis (ALS4). *Am J Hum Genet* 2004;**74**:1128–35.

Chiò A, Orsi L, Mortara P, Schiffer D. Reduced life expectancy in 40 cases of early onset cerebellar ataxia with retained tendon reflexes: a population-based study. *Acta Neurol Scand* 1993;**88**(5)358–62.

Chun HH, Gatti RA. Ataxia-telangiectasia, an evolving phenotype. *DNA Repair (Amst)* 2004;**3**(8–9):1187–96.

Cisneros E, Braun CM. Vocal and respiratory diadochokinesia in Friedreich ataxia. Neuropathological correlations. *Rev Neurol (Paris)* 1995;**151**:113–23.

Clements PM, Breslin C, Deeks ED, et al. The ataxia-oculomotor apraxia 1 gene product has a role distinct from ATM and interacts with the DNA strand break repair proteins XRCC1 and XRCC4. *DNA Repair (Amst)* 2004;**3**:1493–502.

Collins JC, Scheinberg IH, Giblin DR, Sternlieb I. Hepatic peroxisomal abnormalities in abetalipoproteinemia. *Gastroenterology* 1989;**97**:766–70.

Copeliovitch L, Katz K, Arbel N, et al. Musculoskeletal deformities in Behr syndrome. *J Pediatr Orthop* 2001;**21**(4)512–4.

Copp RP, Wisniewski T, Hentati F, et al. Localization of alpha-tocopherol transfer protein in the brains of patients with ataxia with vitamin E deficiency and other oxidative stress related neurodegenerative disorders. *Brain Res* 1999;**822**:80–7.

Crane FL, Hatefi Y, Lester RL, Widmer C. Isolation of a quinone from beef heart mitochondria. *Biochim Biophys Acta* 1957;**25**:220–1.

Criscuolo C, Mancini P, Sacca F, et al. Ataxia with oculomotor apraxia type 1 in Southern Italy: late onset and variable phenotype. *Neurology* 2004;**63**:2173–5.

Dean G, Chamberlain S, Middleton L. Friedreich's ataxia in Kathikas-Arodhes, Cyprus (letter). *Lancet* 1988;**II**: 587.

De Braekeleer M, Giasson F, Mathieu J, et al. Genetic epidemiology of autosomal recessive spastic ataxia of Charlevoix-Saguenay in northeastern Quebec. *Genet Epidemiol* 1993;**10**:17–25.

de Brouwer APM, Williams KL, Duley JA, et al. Arts syndrome is caused by loss-of-function mutations in PRPS1. *Am J Hum Genet* 2007;**81**:507–18.

De Castro M, Cruz-Martinez A, Vilchez JJ, et al. Early onset cerebellar ataxia and preservation of tendon reflexes: clinical phenotypes associated with GAA trinucleotide repeat expanded and non-expanded genotypes. *J Peripher Nerv Syst* 1999;**4**:58–62.

Della Nave R, Ginestroni A, Giannelli M, et al. Brain structural damage in Friedreich's ataxia. *J Neurol Neurosurg Psychiatry* 2008;**79**(1)82–5.

De Michele G, Filla A. Early-onset inherited ataxias. In *The Cerebellum and Its Disorders*, ed. M. Manto and M. Pandolfo. Cambridge, UK: Cambridge University Press, 2002, pp. 519–30.

De Michele G, Filla A, Striano S, Rimoldi M, Campanella G. Heterogeneous findings in four cases of cerebellar ataxia associated with hypogonadism (Holmes' type ataxia). *Clin Neurol Neurosurg* 1993;**95**(1)23–8.

de Parscau L, Beaufrère B, Vianey-Liaud C, et al. Biotinidase deficiency: a disease with neurologic and cutaneous expression susceptible to biotin. *Pediatrie* 1989;**44**(5)383–6.

De Stefano N, Dotti MT, Mortilla M, Federico A. Magnetic resonance imaging and spectroscopic changes in brains of patients with cerebrotendinous xanthomatosis. *Brain* 2001;**124**(Pt 1)121–31.

Dierks T, Schlotawa L, Frese MA, et al. Molecular basis of multiple sulfatase deficiency, mucolipidosis II/III and Niemann-Pick C1 disease – Lysosomal storage disorders caused by defects of non-lysosomal proteins. *Biochim Biophys Acta* 2009;**1793**(4)710–25.

Dietemann JL, Filippi de la Palavesa MM, Tranchant C, Kastler B. MR findings in mannosidosis. *Neuroradiology.* 1990;**32**(6)485–7.

Dubois J, Sebag G, Argyropoulou M, Brunelle F. MR findings in infantile Refsum disease: case report of two family members *AJNR Am J Neuroradiol* 1991;**12**:1159–60.

Duckett S, Schwartzman RJ, Osterholm J, et al. Biopsy diagnosis of familial Alexander's disease. *Pediatr Neurosurg* 1992;**18**(3)134–8.

Dupré N, Gros-Louis F, Chrestian N, et al. Clinical and genetic study of autosomal recessive cerebellar ataxia type 1. *Ann Neurol* 2007;**62**(1)93–8.

Duquette A, Roddier K, McNabb-Baltar J, et al. Mutations in senataxin responsible for Quebec cluster of ataxia with neuropathy. *Ann Neurol* 2005;**57**:408–14.

Durand P, Borrone C, Della Cella G. Fucosidosis. *J Pediatr* 1969;**75**(4)665–74.

Elias G. Muscular subaortic stenosis and Friedreich's ataxia. *Am Heart J.* 1972;**84**:843.

Ell J, Prasher D, Rudge P. Neuro-otological abnormalities in Friedreich ataxia. *J Neurol Neurosurg Psychiatry* 1984;**47**:26–32.

Engert JC, Bérubé P, Mercier J, et al. ARSACS, a spastic ataxia common in northeastern Québec, is caused by mutations in a new gene encoding an 11.5-kb ORF. *Nat Genet* 2000;**24**:120–5.

Fasano A, Colosimo C, Miyajima H, et al. Aceruloplasminemia: a novel mutation in a family with marked phenotypic variability. *Mov Disord* 2008;**23**(5)751–5.

Ferenci P. Regional distribution of mutations in the ATP7B gene in patients with Wilson disease: impact on genetic testing. *Hum Genet* 2006;**120**:151–9.

Filla A, De Michele G, Cavalcanti F, et al. The relationship between trinucleotide (GAA) repeat length and clinical features in Friedreich ataxia. *Am J Hum Genet* 1996;**59**(3)554–60.

França MC Jr, D'Abreu A, Yasuda CL, et al. A combined voxel-based morphometry and (1)H-MRS study in patients with Friedreich's ataxia. *J Neurol* 2009 Mar 12 [Epub ahead of print].

Friedreich N. Ueber degenerative atrophie der spinalen hinterstränge. *Virchows Arch Pathol Anat Physiol Klein Med.* 1863a;**26**:391–419.

Friedreich N. Ueber degenerative atrophie der spinalen hinterstränge. *Virchows Arch Pathol Anat Physiol Klein Med* 1863b;**26**:433–459.

Friedreich N. Ueber degenerative atrophie der spinalen hinterstränge. *Virchows Arch Pathol Anat Physiol Klein Med* 1863c;**27**:1–26.

Gabsi S, Gouider-Khouja N, Belal S, et al. Effect of vitamin E supplementation in patients with ataxia with vitamin E deficiency. *Eur J Neurol* 2001;**8**:477–81.

Gahl WA, Reed GF, Thoene JG, et al. Cysteamine therapy for children with nephropathic cystinosis. *N Engl J Med* 1987;**316**(16)971–7.

Galanaud D, Tourbah A, Lehéricy S, et al. 24 month-treatment with miglustat of three patients with Niemann-Pick disease type C: follow up using brain spectroscopy. *Mol Genet Metab* 2009;**96**(2)55–8.

Garver WS, Francis GA, Jelinek D, et al. The National Niemann-Pick C1 disease database: report of clinical features and health problems. *Am J Med Genet A* 2007;**143A**(11):1204–11.

221

Gatti RA, Berkel I, Boder E, et al. Localization of an ataxia-telangiectasia gene to chromosome 11q22–23. *Nature* 1988;**336**: 577–80.

Gatti RA, Boder E, Vinters HV, et al. Ataxia-telangiectasia: an interdisciplinary approach to pathogenesis. *Medicine (Baltimore)* 1991;**70**(2)99–117.

Gentil M. Dysarthria in Friedreich disease. *Brain Lang* 1990;**38**:438–48.

Geoffroy G, Barbeau A, Breton G, et al. Clinical description and roentgenologic evaluation of patients with Friedreich ataxia. *Can J Neurol Sci* 1976;**3**:279–86.

Gibson KM, Hoffmann G, Nyhan WL, et al. Mevalonate kinase deficiency in a child with cerebellar ataxia, hypotonia and mevalonic aciduria. *Eur J Pediatr* 1988;**148**(3)250–2.

Gironi M, Lamperti C, Nemni R, et al. Late-onset cerebellar ataxia with hypogonadism and muscle coenzyme Q10 deficiency. *Neurology* 2004;**62**:818–20.

Giroud M, Septien L, Pelletier JL, Dueret N, Dumas R. Decrease in cerebellar blood flow in patients with Friedreich's ataxia: A TC-HMPAO SPECT study of three cases. *Neurol Res* 1994;**16**(5)342–4.

Gomez CM. ARSACS goes global. *Neurology* 2004;**62**:10–11.

Goncalves S, Paupe V, Dassa EP, Rustin P. Deferiprone targets aconitase: implication for Friedreich's ataxia treatment. *BMC Neurol* 2008;**8**:20

Gow PJ, Smallwood RA, Angus PW, et al. Diagnosis of Wilson's disease: an experience over three decades. *Gut* 2000;**46**:415–19.

Grabowski GA. Phenotype, diagnosis, and treatment of Gaucher's disease. *Lancet* 2008;**372**(9645)1263–71.

Graziano C, D'Elia AV, Mazzanti L, et al. A de novo nonsense mutation of PAX6 gene in a patient with aniridia, ataxia, and mental retardation. *Am J Med Genet A* 2007;**143A**(15):1802–5.

Gros-Louis F, Dupré N, Dion P, et al. Mutations in SYNE1 lead to a newly discovered form of autosomal recessive cerebellar ataxia. *Nat Genet* 2007;**39**(1)80–5.

Grünewald S, Champion MP, Leonard JV, Schaper J, Morris AA. Biotinidase deficiency: a treatable leukoencephalopathy. *Neuropediatrics* 2004;**35**(4)211–6.

Gu M, Cooper JM, Butler P, et al. Oxidative-phosphorylation defects in liver of patients with Wilson's disease. *Lancet* 2000;**356**:469–74.

Guarino M, Stracciari A, D'Alessandro R, Pazzaglia P. No neurological improvement after liver transplantation for Wilson's disease. *Acta Neurol Scand* 1995;**92**:405–8.

Haas D, Hoffmann GF. Mevalonate kinase deficiencies: from mevalonic aciduria to hyperimmunoglobulinemia D syndrome. *Orphanet J Rare Dis* 2006;**1**:13.

Haberlandt E, Scholl-Bürgi S, Neuberger J, et al. Peripheral neuropathy as the sole initial finding in three children with infantile metachromatic leukodystrophy. *Eur J Paediatr Neurol* 2009;**13**(3)257–60.

Hagberg B, Sanner G, Steen M. The dysequilibrium syndrome in cerebral palsy. Clinical aspects and treatment. *Acta Paediatr Scand* 1972;**61**(suppl 226):1–63.

Hakonen AH, Isohanni P, Paetau A, et al. Recessive Twinkle mutations in early onset encephalopathy with mtDNA depletion. *Brain* 2007;**130**(Pt 11)3032–40.

Hanna MG, Davis MB, Sweeney MG, et al. Generalized chorea in two patients harboring the Friedreich's ataxia gene trinucleotide repeat expansion. *Mov Disord* 1998;**13**:339–40.

Harding AE. Early onset cerebellar ataxia with retained tendon reflexes: a clinical and genetic study of a disorder distinct from Friedreich's ataxia. *J Neurol Neurosurg Psychiatry* 1981;**44**:503–8.

Harding AE. Friedreich's ataxia: a clinical and genetic study of 90 families with an analysis of early diagnostic criteria and intrafamilial clustering of clinical features. *Brain* 1981;**104**(3)589–620.

Harding AE, Matthews S, Jones S, et al. Spinocerebellar degeneration associated with a selective defect of vitamin E absorption. *N Engl J Med* 1985;**313**:32–5.

Hartig MB, Hortnagel K, Garavaglia B, et al. Genotypic and phenotypic spectrum of PANK2 mutations in patients with neurodegeneration with brain iron accumulation. *Ann Neurol* 2006;**59**:248–56.

Hendriksz CJ, Corry PC, Wraith JE, et al. Juvenile Sandhoff disease–nine new cases and a review of the literature. *J Inherit Metab Dis* 2004;**27**(2)241–9.

Higgins JJ, Kluetzman K, Berciano J, Combarros O, Loveless JM. Posterior column ataxia and retinitis pigmentosa: a distinct clinical and genetic disorder. *Mov Disord* 2000;**15**(3)575–8.

Higgins JJ, Morton DM, Loveless JM. Posterior column ataxia with retinitis pigmentosa (AXPC1) maps to chromosome 1q31-q32. *Neurology* 1999;**52**:146–50.

Hirano M, Furiya Y, Kariya S, Nishiwaki T, Ueno S. Loss of function mechanism in apratxin-related early-onset ataxia. *Biochem Biophys Res Commun* 2004;**322**(2)380–6.

Hirano M, Quinzii CM, DiMauro S. Restoring balance to ataxia with coenzyme Q10 deficiency. *J Neurol Sci* 2006;**246**:11–12.

Hoffmann GF, Charpentier C, Mayatepek E, et al. Clinical and biochemical phenotype in 11 patients with mevalonic aciduria. *Pediatrics* 1993;**91**(5)915–21.

Hong SE, Shugart YY, Huang DT, et al. Autosomal recessive lissencephaly with cerebellar hypoplasia is associated with human RELN mutations. *Nat Genet* 2000;**26**: 93–96.

Horn MA, Van Den Brink DM, Wanders RJ, et al. Phenotype of adult Refsum disease due to a defect in peroxin 7. *Neurology* 2007;**68**(9)698–700.

Horvath R, Schneiderat P, Schoser BGH, et al. Coenzyme Q10 deficiency and isolated myopathy. *Neurology* 2006;**66**:253–5.

Hund E, Grau A, Fogel W, et al. Progressive cerebellar ataxia, proximal neurogenic weakness and ocular motor disturbances: hexosaminidase A deficiency with late clinical onset in four siblings. *J Neurol Sci* 1997;**145**(1)25–31.

Huo YK, Wang Z, Hong JH, et al. Radiosensitivity of ataxia-telangiectasia, X-linked agammaglobulinemia, and related syndromes using a modified colony survival assay. *Cancer Res* 1994;**54**(10)2544–7.

Inoue H, Tanizawa Y, Wasson J, et al. A gene encoding a transmembrane protein is mutated in patients with diabetes mellitus and optic atrophy (Wolfram syndrome). *Nat Genet* 1998;**20**:143–8.

Inoue T, Sano N, Ito Y, et al. An adult case of Cockayne syndrome without sclerotic angiopathy. *Intern Med* 1997;**36**(8)565–70.

Jeune M, Tommassi M, Freycon F, Nivelon JL. Syndrome familial associant ataxie, surdité et oligophrénie. Sclérose myocardique d'evolution fatale chez l'un des enfants. *Soc Fr Pediatr* 1963;**18**:984–7.

Johnson WG. The clinical spectrum of hexosaminidase deficiency diseases. *Neurology* 1981;**31**(11)1453–6.

Johnson WG, Murphy M, Murphy WI, Bloom AD. Recessive congenital cerebellar disorder in a genetic isolate: CPD type VII? *Neurology* 1978;**28**:352–3.

Junck L, Gilman S, Gebarski SS, et al. Structural and functional brain imaging in Friedreich's ataxia. *Arch Neurol* 1994;**51**(4)349–55.

Jung K-H, Ahn T-B, Jeon BS. Wilson disease with an initial manifestation of polyneuropathy. *Arch Neurol* 2005;**62**:1628–31.

Kagan VE, Arroyo A, Tyurin VA, et al. Plasma membrane NADH-coenzyme Q0 reductase generates semiquinone radicals and recycles vitamin E homologue in a superoxide-dependent reaction. *FEBS Lett* 1998;**428**:43–6.

Kerner B, Graham JM Jr, Golden JA, Pepkowitz SH, Dobyns WB. Familial lissencephaly with cleft palate and severe cerebellar hypoplasia. *Am J Med Genet* 1999;**87**(5)440–5.

Klockgether T, Chamberlain S, Wullner U, et al. Late-onset Friedreich ataxia. Molecular genetics, clinical neurophysiology and magnetic resonance imaging. *Arch Neurol* 1993;**50**:803–6.

Klockgether T, Petersen D, Grodd W, Dichgans J. Early onset cerebellar ataxia with retained tendon reflexes. Clinical, electrophysiological and MRI observations in comparison with Friedreich's ataxia. *Brain* 1991;**114** (Pt 4):1559–73.

Koletzko S, Koletzko B, Lamprecht A, Lenard HG. Ataxia-deafness-retardation syndrome in three sisters. *Neuropediatrics* 1987;**18**:18–21.

Kono S, Miyajima H. Molecular and pathological basis of aceruloplasminemia. *Biol Res* 2006;**39**:15–23.

Koskinen T, Santavuori P, Sainio K, et al. Infantile onset spinocerebellar ataxia with sensory neuropathy: a new inherited disease. *J Neurol Sci* 1994;**121**:50–6.

Kostrzewa M, Klockgether T, Damian MS, Müller U. Locus heterogeneity in Friedreich ataxia. *Neurogenetics* 1997;**1**(1)43–7.

Kuhn J, Bewermeyer H, Miyajima H, et al. Treatment of symptomatic heterozygous aceruloplasminemia with oral zinc sulphate. *Brain Dev* 2007;**29**(7)450–3.

Lagier-Tourenne C, Tazir M, López LC, et al. ADCK3, an ancestral kinase, is mutated in a form of recessive ataxia associated with coenzyme Q10 deficiency. *Am J Hum Genet* 2008;**82**(3)661–72.

Lagier-Tourenne C, Tranebaerg L, Chaigne D, et al. Homozygosity mapping of Marinesco-Sjogren syndrome to 5q31. *Eur J Hum Genet* 2003;**11**:770–8.

Larnaout A, Belal S, Zouari M, et al. Friedreich's ataxia with isolated vitamin E deficiency: a neuropathological study of a Tunisian patient. *Acta Neuropathol (Berl)* 1997;**93**:633–7.

Le Ber I, Bouslam N, Rivaud-Pechoux S, et al. Frequency and phenotypic spectrum of ataxia with oculomotor apraxia 2: a clinical and genetic study in 18 patients. *Brain* 2004;**127**:759–67.

Le Ber I, Dubourg O, Benoist JF, et al. Muscle coenzyme Q10 deficiencies in ataxia with oculomotor apraxia 1. *Neurology* 2007;**68**(4)295–7.

Leshinsky-Silver E, Levine A, Nissenkorn A, et al. Neonatal liver failure and Leigh syndrome possibly due to CoQ-responsive OXPHOS syndrome. *Mol Gen Metab* 2003;**79**:288–93.

Lin SP, Chang JH, de la Cadena MP, Chang TF, Lee-Chen GJ. Mutation identification and characterization of a Taiwanese patient with fucosidosis. *J Hum Genet* 2007;**52**(6)553–6.

Lindenbaum Y, Dickson D, Rosenbaum P, et al. Xeroderma pigmentosum/cockayne syndrome complex: first neuropathological study and review of eight other cases. *Eur J Paediatr Neurol* 2001;**5**(6)225–42.

Livingstone IR, Mastaglia FL, Edis R, Howe JW. Visual involvement in Friedreich ataxia and hereditary spastic ataxia. A clinical and visual evoked response study. *Arch Neurol* 1981;**38**:75–79.

Logan JI, Harveyson KB, Wisdom GB, Hughes AE, Archbold GPR. Hereditary ceruloplasmin deficiency, dementia and diabetes mellitus. *Quart J Med* 1994;**87**:663–70.

Lönnqvist T, Paetau A, Nikali K, von Boguslawski K, Pihko H. Infantile onset spinocerebellar ataxia with sensory neuropathy (IOSCA): neuropathological features. *J Neurol Sci* 1998;**161**(1)57–65.

Lönnqvist T, Paetau A, Valanne L, Pihko H. Recessive twinkle mutations cause severe epileptic encephalopathy. *Brain* 2009 Mar 20 [Epub ahead of print].

Lorincz MT, Rainier S, Thomas D, Fink JK. Cerebrotendinous xanthomatosis: possible higher prevalence than previously recognized. *Arch Neurol* 2005;**62**(9)1459–63.

Louis-Bar D. Sur un syndrome progressif comprenant des télangiectasies capillares cutanées et conjonctivales symétriques, à disposition naevoïde et troubles cérébelleux. *Confin Neurol (Basel)* 1941;**4**:32–42.

Maciel P, Cruz VT, Constante M, et al. Neuroferritinopathy: missense mutation in FTL causing early-onset bilateral pallidal involvement. *Neurology* 2005;**65**:603–5.

Maione S, Giunta A, Filla A, et al. May age onset be relevant in the occurrence of left ventricular hypertrophy in Friedreich ataxia? *Clin Cardiol* 1997;**20**:141–5.

Malm D, Nilssen Ø. Alpha-mannosidosis. *Orphanet J Rare Dis* 2008; **3**:21.

Manto M, Jissendi P. Spinocerebellar atrophy. In *Encyclopedia of Neuroscience*, volume 9, ed. L.R. Squire. Oxford: Academic Press, 2009, pp. 337–49.

Mariën P, Brouns R, Engelborghs S, et al. Cerebellar cognitive affective syndrome without global mental retardation in two relatives with Gillespie syndrome. *Cortex* 2008;**44**(1)54–67.

Mariotti C, Gellera C, Rimoldi M, et al. Ataxia with isolated vitamin E deficiency: neurological phenotype, clinical follow-up and novel mutations in TTPA gene in Italian families. *Neurol Sci* 2004;**25**:130–7.

Marmolino D, Acquaviva F, Pinelli M, et al. PPAR-gamma agonist Azelaoyl PAF increases frataxin protein and mRNA expression: new implications for the Friedreich's ataxia therapy. *Cerebellum* 2009;**8**(2)98–103.

Mathis S, Paquis V, Mesnage V, et al. Wolfram's syndrome presenting as a cerebellar ataxia. *Rev Neurol (Paris)* 2007;**163**(2)197–204.

Matsuura T, Sasaki H, Tashiro K. Atypical MR findings in Wilson's disease: pronounced lesions in the dentate nucleus causing tremor. *J Neurol Neurosurg Psychiatry* 1998;**64**(2)161.

McLeod JG. An electrophysiological and pathological study of peripheral nerves in Friedreich ataxia. *J Neurol Sci* 1971;**12**:333–49.

McNeill A, Birchall D, Hayflick SJ, et al. T2∗ and FSE MRI distinguishes four subtypes of neurodegeneration with brain iron accumulation. *Neurology* 2008;**70**(18)1614–9.

Meikle PJ, Grasby DJ, Dean CJ, et al. Newborn screening for lysosomal storage disorders. *Mol Genet Metab* 2006;**88**(4)307–14.

Michael S, Petrocine SV, Qian J, et al. Iron and iron-responsive proteins in the cardiomyopathy of Friedreich's ataxia. *Cerebellum* 2006;**5**(4)257–67.

Mielke R, Hilker R, Weber-Luxenburger G, et al. Early-onset cerebellar ataxia (EOCA) with retained reflexes: reduced cerebellar benzodiazepine-receptor binding, progressive metabolic and cognitive impairment. *Mov Disord* 1998;**13**:739–45.

Mihalik SJ, Morrell JC, Kim D, et al. Identification of PAHX, a Refsum disease gene. *Nat Genet* 1997;**17**:185–9.

Miyajima H, Kohno S, Takahashi Y, Yonekawa O, Kanno T. Estimation of the gene frequency of aceruloplasminemia in Japan. *Neurology* 1999;**53**:617–9.

Miyajima H, Kono S, Takahashi T, et al. Cerebellar ataxia associated with heteroallelic ceruloplasmin gene mutation. *Neurology* 2001;**57**:2205–10.

Miyajima H, Takahashi Y, Kamata T, et al. Use of desferrioxamine in the treatment of aceruloplasminemia. *Ann Neurol* 1997;**41**:404–7.

Miyajima H, Takahashi Y, Kono S. Aceruloplasminemia, an inherited disorder of iron metabolism. *Biometals* 2003;**16**:205–13.

Mochel F, Sedel F, Vanderver A, et al. Cerebellar ataxia with elevated cerebrospinal free sialic acid (CAFSA). *Brain* 2009;**132**(pt 3)801–9.

Möller CG, Kimberling WJ, Davenport SL, et al. Usher syndrome: an otoneurologic study. *Laryngoscope* 1989;**99**(1)73–9.

Mondelli M, Rossi A, Scarpini C, Dotti MT, Federico A. Evoked potentials in cerebrotendinous xanthomatosis and effect induced by chenodeoxycholic acid. *Arch Neurol* 1992;**49**(5)469–75.

Montero R, Pineda M, Aracil A, et al. Clinical, biochemical and molecular aspects of cerebellar ataxia and Coenzyme Q10 deficiency. *Cerebellum* 2007;**6**:118–22.

Moreira MC, Klur S, Watanabe M, et al. Senataxin, the ortholog of a yeast RNA helicase, is mutant in ataxia-ocular apraxia 2. *Nat Genet* 2004;**36**: 225–7.

Morita H, Ikeda S, Yamamoto K, et al. Hereditary ceruloplasmin deficiency with hemosiderosis: a clinicopathological study of a Japanese family. *Ann Neurol* 1995;**37**:646–56.

Morita H, Inoue A, Yanagisawa N. A case with ceruloplasmin deficiency which showed dementia, ataxia and iron deposition in the brain. *Rinsho Shinkeigaku* 1992;**32**:483–7.

Morvan D, Komajda M, Doan LD, et al. Cardiomyopathy in Friedreich ataxia: a Doppler-echocardiographic study. *Eur Heart J* 1992;**13**:1393–8.

Mubaidin A, Roberts E, Hampshire D, et al. Karak syndrome: a novel degenerative disorder of the basal ganglia and cerebellum. *J Med Genet* 2003;**40**(7) 543–6.

Muller-Schmehl K, Beninde J, Finckh B, et al. Localization of alpha-tocopherol transfer protein in trophoblast, fetal capillaries' endothelium and amnion epithelium of human term placenta. *Free Radic Res* 2004;**38**:413–20.

Nachmanoff DB, Segal RA, Dawson DM, Brown RB, De Girolami U. Hereditary ataxia with sensory neuronopathy: Biemond's ataxia. *Neurology* 1997;**48**:273–5.

Narcisi TM, Shoulders CC, Chester SA, et al. Mutations of the microsomal triglyceride-transfer-protein gene in abetalipoproteinemia. *Am J Hum Genet* 1995;**57**:1298–1310.

Neven B, Valayannopoulos V, Quartier P, et al. Allogeneic bone marrow transplantation in mevalonic aciduria. *N Engl J Med* 2007;**356**(26)2700–3.

Newman RP, Schaefer EJ, Thomas CB, Oldfield EH. Abetalipoproteinemia and metastatic spinal cord glioblastoma. *Arch Neurol* 1984;**41**:554–6.

Nikali K, Suomalainen A, Saharinen J, et al. Infantile onset spinocerebellar ataxia is caused by recessive mutations in mitochondrial proteins Twinkle and Twinky. *Hum Mol Genet* 2005;**14**:2981–90.

Noordzij JG, Wulffraat N, Haraldsson A, et al. Ataxia-telangiectasia patients presenting with hyper-IgM syndrome. *Arch Dis Child* 2009;**94**:448–449.

Ohno T, Kobayashi S, Hayashi M, Sakurai M, Kanazawa I. Diphenylpyraline-responsive parkinsonism in cerebrotendinous xanthomatosis: long-term follow up of three patients. *J Neurol Sci* 2001;**182**(2)95–7.

Palau F, Espinós C. Autosomal recessive cerebellar ataxias. *Orphanet J Rare Dis* 2006;**17**:47.

Parazzini C, Arena S, Marchetti L, et al. Infantile sialic acid storage disease: serial ultrasound and magnetic resonance imaging features. *Am J Neuroradiol* 2003;**24**(3)398–400.

Pareyson D, Fancellu R, Mariotti C, et al. Adult-onset Alexander disease: a series of eleven unrelated cases with review of the literature. *Brain* 2008;**131**(Pt 9)2321–31.

Pasquier L, Laugel V, Lazaro L, et al. Wide clinical variability among 13 new Cockayne syndrome cases confirmed by biochemical assays. *Arch Dis Child* 2006;**91**(2)178–82.

Peyronnard JM, Charron L, Barbeau A. The neuropathy of Charlevoix-Saguenay ataxia: an electrophysiological and pathological study. *Can J Neurol Sci* 1979;**6**:199–203.

Pizzatto MR, Pascual-Castroviejo I. Sindrome de Behr. Presentacion de siete casos. *Rev Neurol* 2001;**32**: 721–4.

Polson RJ, Rolles K, Calne RY, Williams R, Marsden D. Reversal of severe neurological manifestations of Wilson's disease following orthotopic liver transplantation. *Quart J Med* 1987;**64**:685–91.

Pousset F, Kalotka H, Durr A, et al. Parasympathetic activity in Friedreich's ataxia. *Am J Cardiol* 1996;**78**:847–50.

Prietsch V, Mayatepek E, Krastel H, et al. Mevalonate kinase deficiency: enlarging the clinical and biochemical spectrum. *Pediatrics* 2003;**111**(2)258–61.

Provenzale JM, Barboriak DP, Sims K. Neuroradiologic findings in fucosidosis, a rare lysosomal storage disease. *AJNR Am J Neuroradiol* 1995;**16**(4 suppl)809–13.

Quinzii CM, Hirano M, DiMauro S. CoQ10 deficiency diseases in adults. *Mitochondrion* 2007;7(suppl):S122–6.

Rabiah PK, Bateman JB, Demer JL, Perlman S. Ophthalmologic findings in patients with ataxia. *Am J Ophthalmol* 1997;**123**:108–17.

Rahman S, Hargreaves I, Clayton P, Heales S. Neonatal presentation of coenzyme Q10 deficiency. *J Pediatr* 2001;**139**:456–8.

Raine CH, Kurukulasuriya MF, Bajaj Y, Strachan DR. Cochlear implantation in Refsum's disease. *Cochlear Implants Int* 2008;**9**(2)97–102.

Rapin I, Weidenheim K, Lindenbaum Y, et al. Cockayne syndrome in adults: review with clinical and pathologic study of a new case. *J Child Neurol* 2006;**21**(11)991–1006.

Rauschka H, Colsch B, Baumann N, et al. Late-onset metachromatic leukodystrophy: genotype strongly influences phenotype. *Neurology* 2006;**67**(5)859–63.

Richards BW, Rundle AT. A familial hormonal disorder associated with mental deficiency, deaf mutism and ataxia. *J Ment Defic Res* 1959;**3**:33–55.

Riva A, Bradac GB. Primary cerebellar and spinocerebellar ataxia: an MRI study on 63 cases. *J Neuroradiol* 1995;**22**:71–6.

Rotig A, Appelkvist EL, Geromel V, et al. Quinone-responsive multiple respiratory chain dysfunction due to widespread coenzyme Q10 deficiency. *Lancet* 2000;**356**:391–5.

Rump P, Hamel BCJ, Pinckers AJLG, van Dop PA. Two sibs with chorioretinal dystrophy, hypogonadotrophic hypogonadism, and cerebellar ataxia: Boucher-Neuhauser syndrome. *J Med Genet* 1997;**34**:767–71.

Runge P, Muller DP, McAllister J, et al. Oral vitamin E supplements can prevent the retinopathy of abetalipoproteinaemia. *Br J Ophthalmol* 1986;**70**:166–73.

Sagné C, Gasnier B. Molecular physiology and pathophysiology of lysosomal membrane transporters. *J Inherit Metab Dis* 2008 Apr 15 [Epub ahead of print].

Sanner G. The dysequilibrium syndrome: a genetic study. *Neuropaediatrie* 1973;**4**:403–13.

Santoro L, De Michele G, Perretti A, et al. Relation between GAA repeat length and sensory neuropathy in Friedreich ataxia. *J Neurol Neurosurg Psychiatry* 1999;**66**: 93–6.

Santoro L, Perretti A, Filla A, et al. Is early onset cerebellar ataxia with retained tendon reflexes identifiable by electrophysiologic and histologic profile? A comparison with Friedreich's ataxia. *J Neurol Sci* 1992;**113**(1):43–9.

Santos ML, Raskin S, Telles DS, et al. Treatment of a child diagnosed with Niemann-Pick disease type C with miglustat: a case report in Brazil. *J Inherit Metab Dis* 2008 Oct 21 [Epub ahead of print].

Santos-Ocana C, Villalba JM, Cordoba F, et al. Genetic evidence for coenzyme Q requirement in plasma membrane electron transport. *J Bioenerg Biomembr* 1998;**30**:465–75.

Sardanelli F, Parodi RC, Ottonello C, et al. Cranial MRI in ataxia-telangiectasia. *Neuroradiology* 1995;**37**(1)77–82.

Sato Y, Arai H, Miyata A, et al. Primary structure of alpha-tocopherol transfer protein from rat liver. Homology with cellular retinaldehyde-binding protein. *J Biol Chem* 1993;**268**(24)17705–10.

Schiffmann R, Fitzgibbon EJ, Harris C, et al. Randomized, controlled trial of miglustat in Gaucher's disease type 3. *Ann Neurol* 2008;**64**(5)514–22.

Schlotawa L, Steinfeld R, von Figura K, Dierks T, Gärtner J. Molecular analysis of SUMF1 mutations: stability and residual activity of mutant formylglycine-generating enzyme determine disease severity in multiple sulfatase deficiency. *Hum Mutat* 2008;**29**(1)205.

Schnorf H, Gitzelmann R, Bosshard NU, Spycher M, Waespe W. Early and severe sensory loss in three adult siblings with hexosaminidase A and B deficiency (Sandhoff disease). *J Neurol Neurosurg Psychiatry* 1995;**59**(5)520–3.

Schuelke M, Mayatepek E, Inter M, et al. Treatment of ataxia in isolated vitamin E deficiency caused by alpha-tocopherol transfer protein deficiency. *J Pediatr* 1999;**134**:240–4.

Schulz JB, Di Prospero NA, Fischbeck K. Clinical experience with high-dose idebenone in Friedreich ataxia. *J Neurol* 2009;**256**(suppl 1):42–5.

Schurig V, Van Orman A, Bowen P. Nonprogressive cerebellar disorder with mental retardation and autosomal recessive inheritance in Hutterites. *Am J Med Genet* 1981;**9**:43–53.

Schwankhaus JD, Parisi JE, Gulledge WR, Chin L, Currier RD. Hereditary adult-onset Alexander's disease with palatal myoclonus, spastic paraparesis, and cerebellar ataxia. *Neurology* 1995;**45**(12)2266–71.

Senderek J, Krieger M, Stendel C, et al. Mutations in SIL1 cause Marinesco-Sjogren syndrome, a cerebellar ataxia with cataract and myopathy. *Nat Genet* 2005;**37**:1312–4.

Sévin M, Lesca G, Baumann N, et al. The adult form of Niemann-Pick disease type C. *Brain* 2007;**130**(pt 1)120–33.

Shapiro BE, Logigian EL, Kolodny EH, Pastores GM. Late-onset Tay-Sachs disease: the spectrum of peripheral neuropathy in 30 affected patients. *Muscle Nerve* 2008;**38**(2)1012–5.

Sharpe PC, Duly EB, MacAuley D, et al. Total radical trapping antioxidant potential (TRAP) and exercise. *QJM* 1996;**89**:223–8.

Shimazaki H, Sakoe K, Niijima K, Nakano I, Takiyama Y. An unusual case of a spasticity-lacking phenotype with a novel SACS mutation. *J Neurol Sci* 2007;**255**:87–9.

Shimazaki H, Takiyama Y, Sakoe K, Ando Y, Nakano I. A phenotype without spasticity in sacsin-related ataxia. *Neurology* 2005;**64**:2129–31.

Shorer Z, Parvari R, Bril G, Sela BA, Moses S. Ataxia with isolated vitamin E deficiency in four siblings. *Pediatr Neurol* 1996;**15**:340–3.

Shoulders CC, Brett DJ, Bayliss JD, et al. Abetalipoproteinemia is caused by defects of the gene encoding the 97 kDa subunit of a microsomal triglyceride transfer protein. *Hum Mol Genet* 1993;**2**:2109–16.

Simon A, Kremer HP, Wevers RA, et al. Mevalonate kinase deficiency: Evidence for a phenotypic continuum. *Neurology* 2004;**62**(6)994–7.

Singh N, Mehta M, Roy S. Familial posterior column ataxia (Biemond's) with scoliosis. *Eur. Neurol* 1973;**10**:160–7.

Sinha S, Taly AB, Ravishankar S, et al. Wilson's disease: cranial MRI observations and clinical correlation. *Neuroradiology* 2006;**48**(9)613–21.

Sleat DE, Wiseman JA, El-Banna M, et al. Genetic evidence for nonredundant functional cooperativity between NPC1 and NPC2 in lipid transport. *Proc Natl Acad Sci USA* 2004;**101**(16)5886–91.

Sokol RJ, Francis PD, Gold SH, et al. Orthotopic liver transplantation for acute fulminant Wilson disease. *J Pediatr* 1985;**107**:549–52.

Sonies BC, Almajid P, Kleta R, Bernardini I, Gahl WA. Swallowing dysfunction in 101 patients with nephropathic cystinosis: benefit of long-term cysteamine therapy. *Medicine (Baltimore)* 2005;**84**(3) 137–46.

Soong BW, Casamassima AC, Fink JK, Constantopoulos G, Horwitz AL. Multiple sulfatase deficiency. *Neurology* 1988;**38**(8)1273–5.

Spelbrink JN, Li FY, Tiranti V, et al. Human mitochondrial DNA deletions associated with mutations in the gene encoding Twinkle, a phage T7 gene 4-like protein localized in mitochondria. *Nat Genet* 2001;**28**: 223–31.

Spieker S, Schulz JB, Petersen D, et al. Fixation instability and oculomotor abnormalities in Friedreich ataxia. *J Neurol* 1995;**242**:517–21.

Stewart GS, Maser RS, Stankovic T, et al. The DNA double-strand break repair gene hMRE11 is mutated in individuals with an ataxia-telangiectasia-like disorder. *Cell* 1999;**99**(6)577–87.

Swift M, Morrell D, Cromartie E, et al. The incidence and gene frequency of ataxia-telangiectasia in the United States. *Am J Hum Genet* 1986;**39**:573–83.

Tachi N, Kozuka N, Ohya K, Chiba S, Sasaki K. Hereditary cerebellar ataxia with peripheral neuropathy and mental retardation. *Eur Neurol* 2000;**43**:82–7.

Takashima H, Boerkoel CF, John J, et al. Mutation of TDP1, encoding a topoisomerase I-dependent DNA damage repair enzyme, in spinocerebellar ataxia with axonal neuropathy. *Nat Genet* 2002;**32**:267–72.

Takiyama Y. Sacsinopathies: sacsin-related ataxia. *Cerebellum* 2007;**6**:353–9.

Tazir M, Ali-Pacha L, M'Zahem A, et al. Ataxia with oculomotor apraxia type 2: a clinical and genetic study of 19 patients. *J Neurol Sci* 2009;**278**(1–2):77–81.

Thiffault I, Rioux MF, Tetreault M, et al. A new autosomal recessive spastic ataxia associated with frequent white matter changes maps to 2q33–34. *Brain* 2006;**129**:2332–40.

Thomas PK, Workman JM, Thage O. Behr's syndrome: a family exhibiting pseudodominant inheritance. *J Neurol Sci* 1984;**64**:137–48.

Ticho BH, Hilchie-Schmidt C, Egel RT, et al. Ocular findings in Gillespie-like syndrome: association with a new PAX6 mutation. *Ophthalmic Genet* 2006;**27**(4)145–9.

Tissir F, Goffinet AM. Reelin and brain development. *Nat Rev Neurosci* 2003;**4**:496–505.

Torvik A, Torp S, Kase BF, et al. Infantile Refsum disease: a generalized peroxisomal disorder: report of a case with postmortem examination. *J Neurol Sci* 1988;**85**:39–53.

Town M, Jean G, Cherqui S, et al. A novel gene encoding an integral membrane protein is mutated in nephropathic cystinosis. *Nat Genet* 1998;**18**(4)319–24.

Traber MG, Sokol RJ, Burton GW, et al. Impaired ability of patients with familial isolated vitamin E deficiency to incorporate alpha-tocopherol into lipoproteins secreted by the liver. *J Clin Invest* 1990;**85**:397–407.

Tsou AY, Friedman LS, Wilson RB, Lynch DR. Pharmacotherapy for Friedreich ataxia. *CNS Drugs* 2009;**23**(3)213–23.

Uc EY, Wenger DA, Jankovic J. Niemann-Pick disease type C: two cases and an update. *Mov Disord* 2000;**15**:1199–1203.

Usuki F, Maruyama K. Ataxia caused by mutations in the alpha-tocopherol transfer protein gene. *J Neurol Neurosurg Psychiatry* 2000;**69**:254–6.

Valdivielso P, Calandra S, Duran JC, et al. Coronary heart disease in a patient with cerebrotendinous xanthomatosis. *J Intern Med* 2004;**255**:680–3.

Van Den Brink DM, Brites P, Haasjes J, et al. Identification of PEX7 as the second gene involved in Refsum disease. *Am J Hum Genet* 2003;**72**:471–7.

Van Der Hilst JC, Bodar EJ, Barron KS, et al; International HIDS Study Group. Long-term follow-up, clinical features, and quality of life in a series of 103 patients with hyperimmunoglobulinemia D syndrome. *Medicine (Baltimore)* 2008;**87**(6)301–10.

Van Maldergem L, Moser AB, Vincent MF, et al. Orthotopic liver transplantation from a living-related donor in an infant with a peroxisome biogenesis defect of the infantile Refsum disease type. *J Inherit Metab Dis* 2005;**28**(4)593–600.

Van Maldergem L, Trijbels F, DiMauro S, et al. Coenzyme Q-responsive Leigh's encephalopathy in two sisters. *Ann Neurol* 2002;**52**:750–4.

Van Raamsdonk JM. Loss of function mutations in SIL1 cause Marinesco-Sjogren syndrome. *Clin Genet* 2006;**69**:399–400.

Vanier MT, Millat G. Niemann-Pick disease type C. *Clin Genet* 2003;**64**(4)269–81.

Verny C, Prundean A, Nicolas G, et al. Refsum's disease may mimic familial Guillain Barré syndrome. *Neuromuscul Disord* 2006;**16**(11)805–8.

Verrips A, Hoefsloot LH, Steenbergen GC, et al. Clinical and molecular genetic characteristics of patients with cerebrotendinous xanthomatosis. *Brain 123*. 2000;**5**:908–19.

Villalba JM, Navarro F, Cordoba F, et al. Coenzyme Q reductase from liver plasma membrane: purification and role in trans-plasma-membrane electron transport. *Proc Natl Acad Sci USA* 1995;**92**:4887–91.

Waldvogel D, van Gelderen P, Hallett M. Increased iron in the dentate nucleus of patients with Friedrich's ataxia. *Ann Neurol* 1999;**46**(1)123–5.

Wallis LI, Griffiths PD, Ritchie SJ, et al. Proton spectroscopy and imaging at 3T in ataxia-telangiectasia. *Am J Neuroradiol* 2007;**28**(1)79–83.

Wessel K, Schroth G, Diener HC, Muller-Forell W, Dichgans J. Significance of MRI-confirmed atrophy of the cranial spinal cord in Friedreich ataxia. *Eur Arch Psychiatry Neurol Sci* 1989;**238**:225–30.

Wiebers DO, Wilson DM, McLeod RA, Goldstein NP. Renal stones in Wilson's disease. *Am J Med* 1979;**67**:249–54.

Wilken B, Dechent P, Hanefeld F, Frahm J. Proton MRS of a child with Sandhoff disease reveals elevated brain hexosamine. *Eur J Paediatr Neurol* 2008;**12**(1)56–60.

Willems PJ, Seo HC, Coucke P, Tonlorenzi R, O'Brien JS. Spectrum of mutations in fucosidosis. *Eur J Hum Genet* 1999;**7**(1)60–7.

Willner JP, Grabowski GA, Gordon RE, Bender AN, Desnick RJ. Chronic GM2 gangliosidosis masquerading as atypical Friedreich ataxia: clinical, morphologic, and biochemical studies of nine cases. *Neurology* 1981;**31**(7)787–98.

Yokota T, Uchihara T, Kumagai J, et al. Postmortem study of ataxia with retinitis pigmentosa by mutation of the alpha-tocopherol transfer protein gene. *J Neurol Neurosurg Psychiatry* 2000;**68**:521–5.

Zamel R, Khan R, Pollex RL, Hegele RA. Abetalipoproteinemia: two case reports and literature review. *Orphanet J Rare Dis* 2008;**3**:19.

Zouari M, Feki M, Ben Hamida C, et al. Electrophysiology and nerve biopsy: comparative study in Friedreich's ataxia and Friedreich's ataxia phenotype with vitamin E deficiency. *Neuromuscul Disord* 1998;**8**:416–25.

Mitochondrial disorders

Introduction and classification

Mitochondrial disorders are characterized by deficits of the mitochondrial energy output (Zeviani et al., 2002). The terminology of mitochondrial disorders is applied to designate the clinical syndromes associated with abnormalities of the final steps of the mitochondrial energy metabolism which occur in the inner mitochondrial membrane (oxidative phosphorylation) (Zeviani & Antozzi, 1997).

Both the nuclear and the mitochondrial genomes contribute to the respiratory chain, hence the genetic diversity. The wide range of clinical presentations of mitochondrial disorders is also explained by the complexity of the biochemistry of the respiratory chain and the mitotic segregation (the relative proportion between wild-type and mutant genomes can vary among cells).

In most cases, tissues with high aerobic demands are the most severely involved, in particular, brain, skeletal muscle, and heart. However, virtually any tissue can be affected. Although each tissue can be affected separately (encephalopathies, myopathies, cardiomyopathies), combinations are common, especially encephalomyopathies and encephalocardiomyopathies. Table 21.1 lists the most common symptoms. Ataxia is a frequent symptom of CNS involvement in mitochondrial disorders, but is rarely isolated.

Table 21.1 Common symptoms in mitochondrial disorders

Limb weakness

Exercise intolerance

Progressive external ophthalmoplegia

Pigmentary retinopathy

Encephalopathic signs: dementia, seizures, myoclonus, ataxia, stroke-like deficits

Cardiac conduction defects

Mitochondrial disorders can be divided into three main groups (Table 21.2):
1. Deficits of the mitochondrial genome
2. Deficits of nucleo-mitochondrial signaling
3. Nuclear gene defects

Defects of mitochondrial DNA

From a genetic point of view, the two categories of mitochondrial DNA (mtDNA) mutations are large-scale rearrangements and point mutations. Large-scale rearrangements include partial mtDNA deletions and partial duplications. Both are heteroplasmic. Large-scale rearrangements are associated with sporadic disorders, while mtDNA point mutations are usually maternally inherited.

The most common syndromes involving the cerebellum in relationship with a mitochondrial mutation are Kearns-Sayre syndrome; mitochondrial encephalomyopathy, lactic acidosis, and stroke-like episodes (MELAS); myoclonic epilepsy with ragged-red fibers MEERF (see also Chapter 17); and the disorder combining neuropathy, ataxia, and retinitis pigmentosa NARP. Table 21.3 summarizes the main features of these syndromes. Cerebellar ataxia can be a prominent deficit and even the sole apparent deficit at the beginning of these diseases.

Deficits of nucleo-mitochondrial signaling

Autosomal dominant PEO is characterized by adult-onset progressive external ophthalmoplegia (thus the acronym "PEO"), muscle weakness, cerebellar ataxia, vestibular areflexia, peripheral neuropathy, and cataracts (Zeviani et al., 1989). The recessive form occurs in childhood and is characterized by severe

Table 21.2 Classification of mitochondrial disorders

Phenotype	Mutation	Gene location
1. Defects of the mitochondrial DNA (mtDNA)		
Kearns-Sayre syndrome KSS	Single deletion/duplication	
Progressive external ophthalmoplegia (PEO)	Point mutation	
Pearson syndrome	Point mutation	
Mitochondrial encephalomyopathy, lactic acidosis, and stroke-like episodes MELAS	Point mutation	
Myoclonic epilepsy with ragged-red fibers MEERF	Point mutation	
Neuropathy, ataxia, and retinitis pigmentosa NARP	Point mutation	
Bilateral striatal necrosis	Tandem duplication	
Mitochondrial myopathy	Point mutation	
Mitochondrial myopathy and cardiomyopathy	Point mutation	
Hypertrophic cardiomyopathy	Point mutation	
Leber hereditary optic neuropathy	Point mutation	
Dementia – chorea	Point mutation	
Diabetes – deafness	Point mutation	
Tubulopathy, diabetes, ataxia	Large-scale duplication/depletion, duplication	
Ataxia-leukodystrophy	Large-scale duplication	
Hearing loss, ataxia, myoclonus	Large-scale deletion	
Myoglobinuria	Point mutation	
Sensorineural deafness	Point mutation	
Aminoside-induced deafness	Microdeletion Point mutation	
2. Deficits of nucleo-mitochondrial signaling		
Autosomal dominant/recessive PEO	Multiple deletions	
Myopathy/encephalomyopathy	Multiple deletions	
Familial myoglobinuria	Multiple deletions	
Familial cardiomyopathy	Multiple deletions	
Sensory ataxic neuropathy/PEO	Multiple deletions	
Infantile hepatopathy	mtDNA depletion	
Encephalomyopathy	mtDNA depletion	
Infantile myopathy	mtDNA depletion	
Myopathy of childhood	mtDNA depletion	
3. Nuclear gene defects		
Leigh syndrome	GAA expansion	Complex I/II
Friedreich ataxia	Mutation	9q13
X-linked sideroblastic anemia and ataxia	Deletion	Xq13
X-linked deafness – dystonia		Xq22

Table 21.3 Main ataxias associated with a mitochondrial DNA (mtDNA) mutation

Disorder	Phenotype	Neuroimaging	Neuropathology
Kearns-Sayre syndrome KSS	Onset before age of 20 Progressive external ophthalmoplegia Pigmentary retinopathy Progressive cerebellar syndrome Poor growth Heart block Increased protein levels in CSF	Hyperintensities in the subcortical white matter of cerebral hemispheres Hyperintensities in dentate nuclei and superior cerebellar peduncles, basal ganglia, and thalami	Neuronal loss and gliosis in basal ganglia Spongy degeneration of white matter Decreased expression of mtDNA-encoded proteins in neurons of the dentate nuclei
Mitochondrial encephalomyopathy, lactic acidosis, and stroke-like episodes MELAS	Stroke-like episodes (lesions in particular in parieto-occipital lobes) Lactic acidosis Ragged-red fibers Dementia Headache Seizures Deafness Ataxia Vomiting	Lesions mainly affecting the posterior regions of cerebral hemispheres Hyperintensities in basal ganglia and cerebellum	Infarct-like lesions Gliosis Demyelination Spheroids Degeneration of the posterior columns and spinocerebellar tracts Accumulation of abnormal mitochondria in smooth muscles and endothelium of blood vessels
Myoclonic epilepsy with ragged-red fibers MEERF	Myoclonus Epilepsy Muscle weakness Cerebellar ataxia Deafness Dementia	Cerebral and cerebellar atrophy Calcifications in basal ganglia Hyperintensities in dentate nuclei, superior cerebellar peduncles, and inferior olives	Neuronal loss and gliosis in dentate nuclei, inferior olives, posterior columns, and spinocerebellar tracts
Neuropathy, ataxia, and retinitis pigmentosa NARP	Neuropathy Cerebellar ataxia Retinitis pigmentosa	Cerebral and cerebellar atrophy Lesions in basal ganglia	

cardiomyopathy. In both cases, multiple deletions are found.

MNGIE is the acronym for mitochondrial neurogastrointestinal encephalomyopathy. Patients present with ophthalmoparesis, deficits related to a leukoencephalopathy, peripheral neuropathy, and gastrointestinal symptoms such as dysmotility. About one in eight patients exhibits a cerebellar ataxia. Mutations in the gene encoding thymidine phosphorylase have been reported.

mtDNA depletions are associated with congenital myopathy, De Toni-Fanconi renal syndrome, and infantile hepatopathy leading to liver failure.

Nuclear gene defects

Friedreich ataxia is discussed in Chapter 20. Mutations in ABC7 are associated with X-linked sideroblastic anemia/ataxia (Allikmets et al., 1999). X-linked deafness-dystonia results from a mutation of the deafness-dystonia protein which is involved in the insertion of metabolite carriers into the inner mitochondrial membrane (Koehler et al., 1999).

Leigh syndrome (also termed subacute necrotizing encephalopathy) is one of the most common mitochondrial disorders in infancy and childhood (Finsterer, 2008). The estimated incidence of Leigh syndrome is 1 per 40 000 live births (Rahman et al., 1996), with symptoms starting in the first 2 years of life in most cases. Leigh syndrome is characterized by psychomotor deficits, seizures, hypotonia (floppy infant), optic atrophy, cerebellar ataxia, pyramidal signs, and dystonic movements. Some patients also present with peripheral nervous system involvement, including polyneuropathy or myopathy, and extra-neurological abnormalities, such as diabetes, short stature, hypertrichosis, cardiomyopathy, renal failure, vomiting, or diarrhea (Leigh-like syndrome). Acute respiratory failure is a frequent feature of Leigh syndrome, occurring in about two in three patients. Lactic acidosis of the blood, cerebrospinal fluid, or urine is common. In some patients, the lactate/pyruvate ratio is increased. Muscle enzymes, in particular creatine kinase, may be elevated, but ragged-red fibers are usually absent. Ultrastructural studies of muscle biopsies show lipid deposits in the mitochondria and myofibrillar disorganization. Cyclooxygenase (COX) activity may be diffusely reduced or totally absent. In individual patients, the biochemical defect, such as COX deficiency, may also be evident in cultured skin fibroblasts. Needle electromyography may show abnormal spontaneous activity, and nerve conduction studies may show electrophysiological evidence of polyneuropathy (Rossi et al., 2003). Visually evoked potentials may show prolongation or amplitude reduction of the P100 component or may be completely absent (Malfatti et al., 2007). Auditory evoked brainstem potentials may reveal prolonged latencies even before clinical onset (Yoshinaga et al., 2003). Abnormal brainstem function may also be assessed by recording somatosensory evoked potentials or blink reflexes. Polysomnography demonstrates disturbances of both the tonic and phasic components of REM sleep (Araki et al., 1997). Electroencephalography may reveal irregular basic activity and focal epileptic signs with secondary generalization and hypsarrhythmia (Horth et al., 2006). Leigh syndrome and Leigh-like syndrome are the mitochondrial disorders with the largest genetic heterogeneity. Mutations can occur in genes encoding different subunits of complex I, as well as complexes II (succinate dehydrogenase) and IV, in particular, cases related to a SURF-1 mutation (Surfeit Locus Protein 1 gene on chromosome 9q34.2). The product of SURF-1 is a component of the mitochondrial inner membrane (Zhu et al., 1998). Deficits in coenzyme Q10 and pyruvate dehydrogenase complex have been reported. Patients with primary coenzyme Q deficiency may present with adult Leigh syndrome with encephalopathy, growth retardation, ataxia, and deafness (Van Maldergem et al., 2002) (see also Chapter 20). The outcome of patients with Leigh syndrome is generally poor. In the majority of cases, patients die before the age of 5 years. About 40% of patients die of respiratory failure.

Polymerase gamma is a nuclear-encoded protein essential for replication of mitochondrial DNA (see also Chapter 5). Mutations are associated with several phenotypes, such as mitochondrial recessive ataxia syndrome; sensory ataxic neuropathy, dysarthria, and ophthalmoparesis; or Alpers syndrome. Muscle biopsy may demonstrate ragged-red fibers, multiple respiratory chain defects, and multiple mitochondrial DNA deletions.

Brain imaging

Brain MRI may demonstrate cerebellar atrophy or hyperintense areas in the white matter of the cerebellum. White matter lesions observed in MELAS are illustrated in Figure 21.1.

In Leigh syndrome, brain MRI shows symmetrical lesions in the medulla, pontine tegmentum, periaqueductal region, dentate nuclei, and surrounding white matter areas (Figure 21.2). Basal ganglia may be affected. Some patients may also exhibit unifocal or multifocal infarctions, or diffuse or focal cortical atrophy with ventricular enlargement. Some patients may develop predominant cerebellar atrophy (Scaglia et al., 2005). Hyperintensities may be noticeable in the cerebellar nuclei in Kearns-Sayre syndrome (Figure 21.3).

Peaks of lactate can be detected in the cerebellar parenchyma with proton magnetic resonance spectroscopy (Figure 21.4).

Differential diagnosis

Mitochondrial disorders can mimic in particular autosomal recessive ataxias (see Chapter 20), X-linked ataxias (see Chapter 12), and autosomal dominant spinocerebellar ataxias (SCAs; see Chapter 23) and can present as a progressive myoclonic epilepsy (see Chapter 17).

Treatment

Creatine may be effective in some patients (Zeviani & DiDonato, 2004). Vitamin supplements and antioxidants are often administered, although these treatments are largely empirical. Administration of idebenone and coenzyme Q10 is discussed in

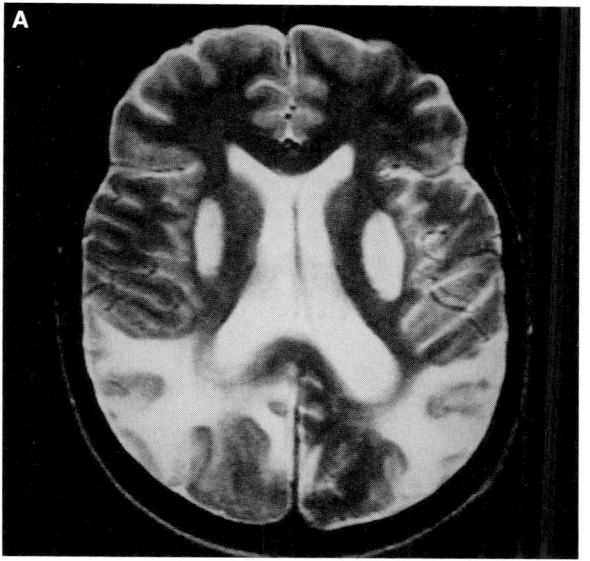
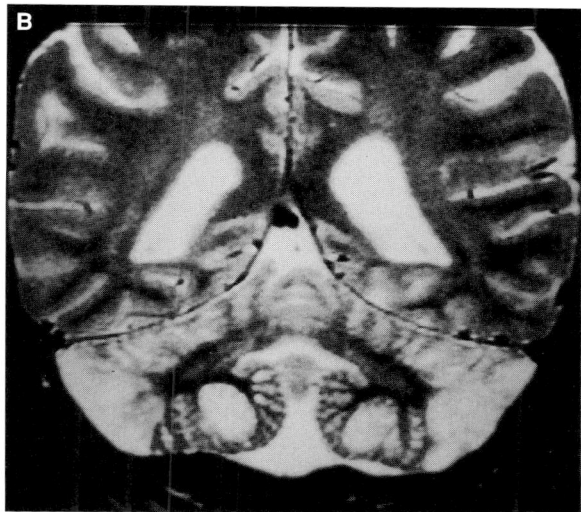

Figure 21.1 Mitochondrial encephalomyopathy, lactic acidosis, and stroke-like episodes (MELAS). (A) Axial T2-weighted image showing multiple lesions in the white matter. Lesions predominate in the posterior areas. Note the hypersignals in basal ganglia. (B) Coronal T2-weighted images showing hyperintensities in the cerebellum, especially in the lateral portions. With permission from: Zeviani et al., 2002.

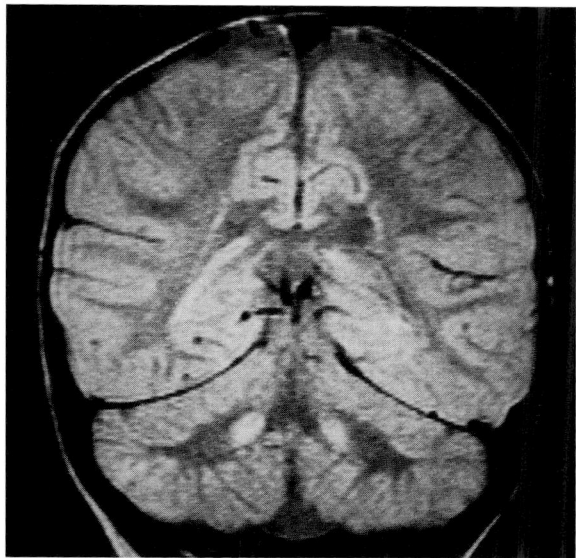

Figure 21.2 Top: Leigh syndrome. Coronal MRI (proton density image) showing hyperintensity of dentate nuclei. With permission from: Zeviani et al., 2002.

Chapter 20. In a study of 65 patients with Leigh syndrome, clinical improvement after the administration of L-carnitine, coenzyme Q, or thiamin was observed in only 8% of patients (Yang et al., 2006). In a patient with a NDUFV1 mutation, a ketogenic diet improved external ophthalmoplegia, but has not reduced cerebellar ataxia, spasticity, or dystonia (Laugel et al., 2007). Pyruvate has been proposed recently (Tanaka et al., 2007).

Epilepsy is managed with conventional drugs, keeping in mind that valproic acid should be used cautiously in mitochondrial disorders due to an inhibition of carnitine uptake (Di Mauro et al., 2004). Myoclonus can respond to clonazepam, high doses of piracetam or levetiracetam, zonisamide, and topiramate (Mancuso et al., 2006). The reader is also referred to Chapter 17.

So far, gene therapy has not shown a favorable effect on clinical deficits. Experimental investigations are ongoing.

Supportive measures such as surgical correction of ptosis and treatment of acidosis improve quality of life for patients (Zeviani & Di Donato, 2004). Aerobic exercise and physical therapy might improve exercise tolerance (Di Mauro et al., 2004).

Endocrine functions should be monitored.

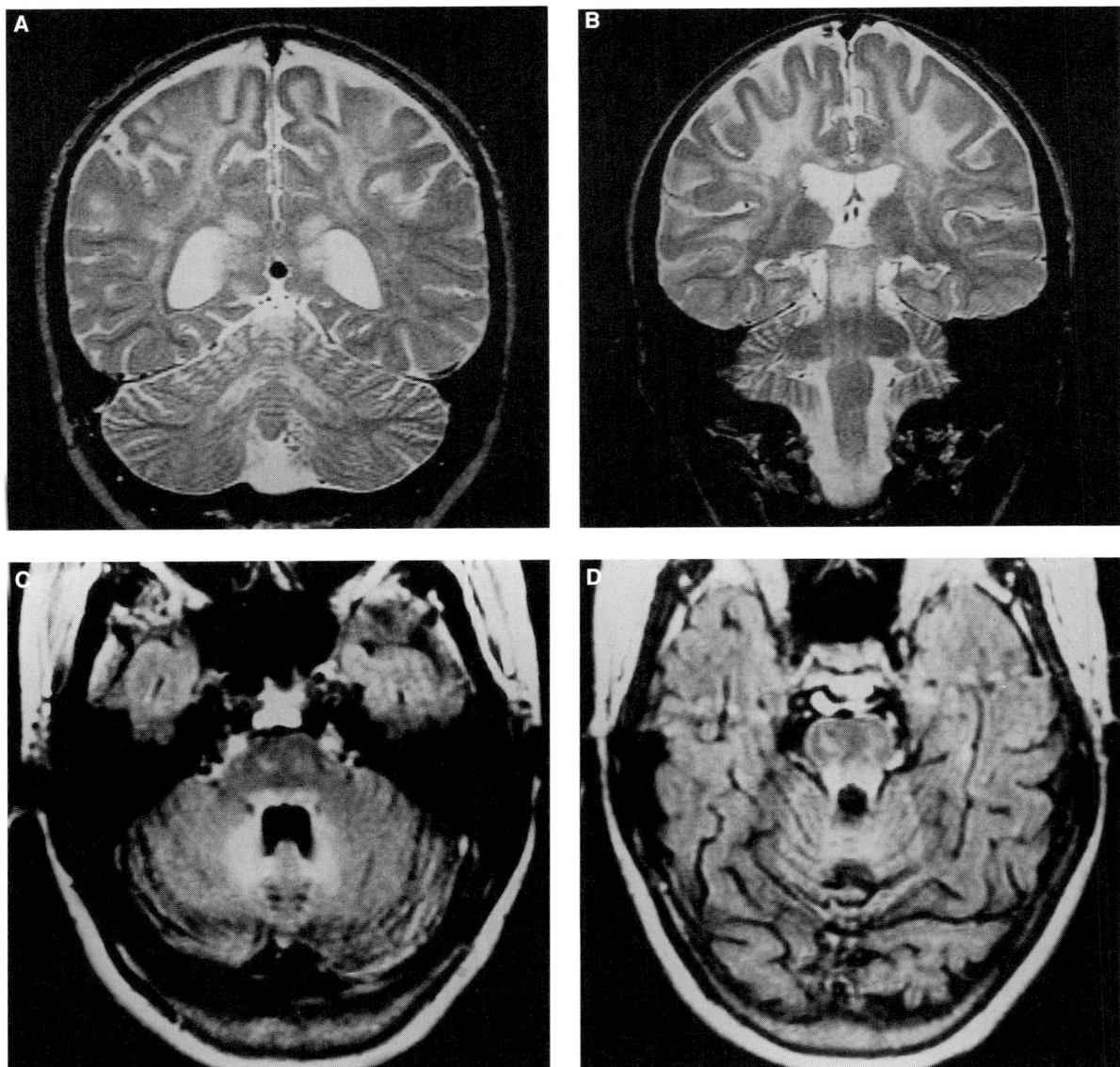

Figure 21.3 Kearns-Sayre syndrome. (A, B) T2-weighted image showing hyperintensities in the dentate nuclei and subcortical white matter. (C, D) Axial flair images showing hyperintensities in the dentate nuclei and superior cerebellar peduncles. With permission from: Zeviani et al., 2002.

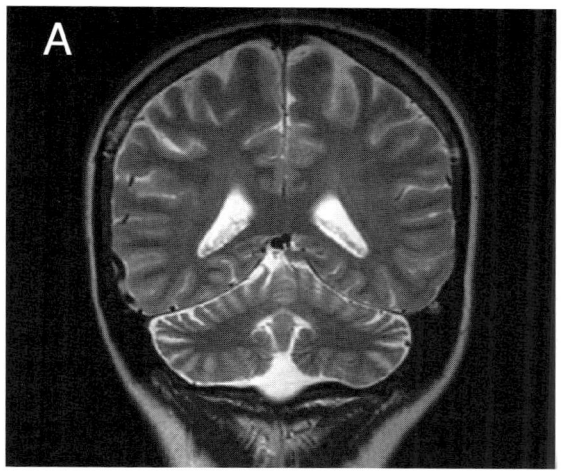
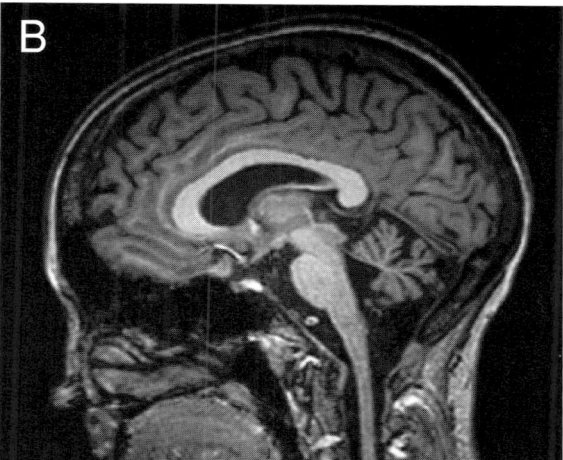
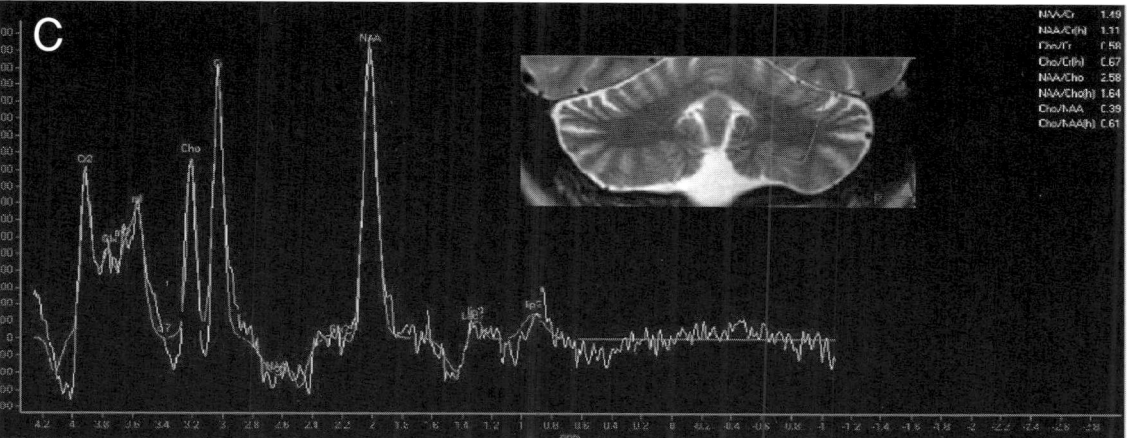

Figure 21.4 Brain MRI and magnetic resonance spectroscopy (MRS) in a patient with a mitochondrial disease. (A) Coronal T2-weighted sequence; (B) sagittal T1-weighted image demonstrating atrophy of the vermis; (C) a peak of lactate in the cerebellar parenchyma is detected on MRS. (See color section.)

References

Allikmets R, Raskind WH, Hutchinson A, et al. Mutation of a putative mitochondrial iron transporter gene (ABC7) in X-linked sideroblastic anemia and ataxia (KLSA/A). *Hum Molec Genet* 1999;**8**:743–9.

Araki S, Hayashi M, Yasaka A, Maruki K. Electrophysiological brainstem dysfunction in a child with Leigh disease. *Pediatr Neurol* 1997;**16**: 329–33.

Di Mauro S, Mancuso M, Naini A. Mitochondrial encephalomyopathies: therapeutic approach. *Ann N Y Acad Sci* 2004;**1011**:232–45.

Finsterer J. Leigh and Leigh-like syndrome in children and adults. *Pediatr Neurol* 2008;**39**:223–35.

Horváth R, Abicht A, Holinski-Feder E, et al. Leigh syndrome caused by mutations in the flavoprotein (Fp) subunit of succinate dehydrogenase (SDHA). *J Neurol Neurosurg Psychiatry* 2006;**77**:74–6.

Koehler CM, Leuenberger D, Merchant S, et al. Human deafness dystonia syndrome is a mitochondrial disease. *Proc Natl Acad Sci USA* 1999;**96**:2141–6.

Laugel V, This-Bernd V, Cormier-Daire V, et al. Early-onset ophthalmoplegia in Leigh-like syndrome due to NDUFV1 mutations. *Pediatr Neurol* 2007;**36**: 54–7.

Malfatti E, Bugiani M, Invernizzi F, et al. Novel mutations of ND genes in complex I deficiency associated with mitochondrial encephalopathy. *Brain* 2007;**130**:1894–904.

Mancuso M, Galli R, Pizzanelli C, et al. Antimyoclonic effect of levetiracetam in MERRF syndrome. *J Neurol Sci* 2006;**243**(1–2):97–9.

Rahman S, Blok RB, Dahl HH, et al. Leigh syndrome: Clinical features and biochemical and DNA abnormalities. *Ann Neurol* 1996;**39**:343–51.

Rossi A, Biancheri R, Bruno C, et al. Leigh syndrome with COX deficiency and SURF1 gene mutations: MR imaging findings. *AJNR Am J Neuroradiol* 2003;**24**:1188–91.

Scaglia F, Wong LJ, Vladutiu GD, Hunter JV. Predominant cerebellar volume loss as a neuroradiologic feature of pediatric respiratory chain defects. *AJNR Am J Neuroradiol* 2005;**26**:1675–80.

Tanaka M, Nishigaki Y, Fuku N, et al. Therapeutic potential of pyruvate therapy for mitochondrial diseases. *Mitochondrion* 2007;**7**(6):399–401.

Van Maldergem L, Trijbels F, DiMauro S, et al. Coenzyme Q-responsive Leigh's encephalopathy in two sisters. *Ann Neurol* 2002;**52**:750–4.

Yang YL, Sun F, Zhang Y, et al. Clinical and laboratory survey of 65 Chinese patients with Leigh syndrome. *Chin Med J* 2006;**119**:373–7.

Yoshinaga H, Ogino T, Endo F, et al. Longitudinal study of auditory brainstem response in Leigh syndrome. *Neuropediatrics* 2003;**34**:81–6.

Zeviani M, Antozzi C. Mitochondrial disorders. *Mol Hum Reprod* 1997;**3**:133–48.

Zeviani M, Antozzi C, Savoiardo M, Bertini E. Ataxia in mitochondrial disorders. In *The Cerebellum and Its Disorders*, ed. M. Manto and M. Pandolfo. Cambridge, UK: Cambridge University Press, 2002, pp. 548–61.

Zeviani M, Di Donato S. Mitochondrial disorders. *Brain* 2004;**127**(Pt 10):2153–72.

Zeviani M, Servidei S, Gellera C, et al. An autosomal dominant disorder with multiple deletions of mitochondrial DNA starting at the D-loop region. *Nature* 1989;**339**:309–11.

Zhu Z, Yao J, Johns T, et al. Surf1, a factor involved in the biogenesis of cytochrome C oxidase, is mutated in Leigh syndrome. *Nat Genet* 1998;**20**:337–43.

X-linked ataxias

Introduction

X-linked inheritance should be considered in any disorder affecting only males in one or more generations in the maternal line. Table 22.1 lists the disorders grouped under the terminology of X-linked ataxias (Spira et al., 1979; Aalfs et al., 1995; Guo et al., 2006; de Brouwer et al., 2007; Debray et al., 2008).

Table 22.2 shows the age of onset and the main clinical/paraclinical clues of the most common X-linked ataxias.

In X-linked adrenoleukodystrophy, impaired adrenocortical function and subtle to marked cognitive decline are present. In some patients, a progressive spastic paraparesis predominates. White matter lesions are observed, in particular, in the parietooccipital region. Blood studies show increased levels of very long chain fatty acids. Mutations affect the adenosine triphosphate–binding cassette (ABC), subfamily D gene (ABCD-1 gene; Xq28).

Differential diagnosis and treatment of deficit in pyruvate dehydrogenase E1-α

Deficit in pyruvate dehydrogenase E1-α (PDAH1) shares similarities with the pyruvate carboxylase (PC) deficiency (autosomal recessive inheritance; gene locus 11q13.4-q13.5), which usually presents in the neonatal period with severe lactic acidosis or in early infancy with features similar to PDAH1, including psychomotor retardation, hypotonia, and seizures. PC deficiency type A is found in North American Indians, type B is found in France and the United Kingdom and is associated with hyperammonemia (see also Chapter 23), and type C manifests with relatively benign intermittent ataxia.

PDAH1 should be distinguished from recessively inherited defects affecting mitochondrial beta-oxidation (such as carnitine palmitoyltransferase-1 deficiency or very long-chain acyl-CoA dehydrogenase deficiency) which cause intermittent episodes of neurological symptoms such as paresis, cerebellar ataxia, or coma. Symptoms may be triggered by prolonged fasting. Plasma carnitine levels are decreased in many fatty acid oxidation disorders. Carnitine supplementation (50–100 mg/kg per day), appropriate caloric intake (glucose), and substitution of dietary fat with medium-chain triglycerides are useful.

Treatment of PDAH1 includes thiamin supplementation in high doses (5–20 mg/kg per day up to 100 mg/d in the acute stage), which may be effective in the thiamin-responsive form. Some patients benefit from a ketogenic diet. Lactic acidosis may be treated with dichloroacetate (50 mg/kg body weight).

Table 22.1 X-linked ataxias

Fragile X tremor ataxia syndrome (FXTAS)

Arts syndrome (see also Chapter 20)

X-linked adrenoleukodystrophy (X-ALD)

Congenital ataxia

  Mental retardation with epilepsy and cerebellar hypoplasia (oligophrenin 1 [OPHN1]; Xq12)
  Congenital X-linked ataxia (Xq23)
  Congenital X-linked ataxia (SCAX1; Xp11.21-q21.3)
  Congenital ataxia with extra-pyramidal involvement (SCAX2)
  Ataxia-deafness syndrome (SCAX3)
  X-linked congenital ataxia (SCAX5; Xq25)
  Hoyeraal-Freidarsson syndrome (cerebellar hypoplasia with pancytopenia)
  Cataracts, ataxia, short stature, and mental retardation (CASM)

Mental retardation, microcephaly, epilepsy, and ataxia (Angelman-like syndrome; Xq24-q27.3)

Pelizaeus-Merzbacher allelic variant (SPG2; Xq22)

Rett syndrome (see Chapter 16)

Ataxia-dementia (SCAX4)

Sideroblastic anemia and spinocerebellar ataxia (XLSAA; adenosine triphosphate–binding cassette 7 transporter; Xq13)

Deficit in pyruvate dehydrogenase E1-α (PDHA1; Xp22.2-p22.1).

Table 22.2 Clues for X-linked ataxias

Onset of symptoms	Clinical/paraclinical deficits	Disorder
Birth – Neonatal	Slow eye movements, motor delay	SCAX1, SCAX5
	Microcephaly	Hoyeraal-Hreidarsson syndrome
	Cerebellar hypoplasia	
	Pancytopenia	
	Dyskeratosis congenita	
	Congenital cataract	CASM
	Short stature	
	Mental retardation	
	Cerebellar ataxia	
Early childhood	Optic atrophy, spastic paraparesis	SPG2
	Delayed walking, pyramidal deficits	SCAX4
	Pyramidal deficits	XLSA
	Anemia	
	Increased protoporphyrin levels in erythrocytes	
	Ring sideroblasts in bone marrow	
	Anemia	
	Seizures	PDHA1
	Episodic ataxia	
	Choreoathetosis	
	Recurrent dystonia	
	Hyperventilation	
	Lactic acidosis	
	Increased pyruvic acid and alanine levels in serum	
	Decreased levels of E1-α protein in serum	
	Mental retardation	
	Seizures	
	Grinding of teeth	Rett syndrome
	Loss of purposeful hand skills	
	Deafness	
	Hypoxanthine undetectable in urine	
	Death before the age of 6 years	Arts syndrome
Infancy	Deafness	SCAX3
	Optic atrophy	
Adulthood (> 50 years)	Cognitive deficits	FXTAS
	Parkinsonism	
	Dysautonomia	
	Peripheral neuropathy	

Fragile X tremor ataxia syndrome

Clinical presentation

Fragile X tremor ataxia syndrome (FXTAS) usually develops between the ages of 50 and 80 years. Patients exhibit a progressive syndrome involving the central and peripheral nervous systems and characterized by kinetic tremor, parkinsonism, cognitive decline, and autonomic dysfunction (see Table 22.3) (Hagerman et al., 2001; Jacquemont et al., 2003). Peripheral neuropathy usually develops after the sixth decade. Male premutation carriers have increased postural and kinetic tremor and limb ataxia (Berry-Kravis et al., 2003). Diagnostic criteria have been proposed (Table 22.4).

Individuals with FXTAS may be misdiagnosed with other conditions, including Parkinson disease, multiple system atrophy, Alzheimer disease, stroke, and peripheral neuropathy. Diagnosis should be considered in men over age 50 years with unexplained cerebellar ataxia and in men over age 50 with action tremor, parkinsonism, or dementia who also have a family history of developmental delay, autism, mental retardation, or premature ovarian failure (Hall et al., 2005; Table 22.4).

Neuroimaging

Symmetrical areas of increased T2-weighted signal intensity in the middle cerebellar peduncles and

Table 22.3 Clinical deficits in FXTAS

Cerebellar deficits
  Kinetic tremor
  Nystagmus
  Dysarthria
  Limb ataxia
  Gait ataxia

Parkinsonism
  Rigidity
  Dystonic posture

Cognitive deficits
  Short-term memory loss
  Impaired executive functions
  Attentional deficit
  Cognitive decline
  Frontal-subcortical dementia

Behavioral deficits
  Agitation
  Disinhibition
  Irritability
  Depression
  Apathy
  Reclusive behavior

Pyramidal deficits
  Spastic paraparesis
  Tendon hyperreflexia

Autonomic dysfunction
  Impotence
  Urinary disturbances
  Bowel incontinence
  Syncope

Peripheral neuropathy
  Distal sensory loss (vibration and pin)

Table 22.4 Diagnostic criteria of FXTAS (required: FMR1 allele size of 55–200 repeats)

1. Definite:
   A. One clinical major criterion (kinetic tremor and ataxic gait; minor criterion: parkinsonism) *and*
   B. One radiological major criterion (symmetrical white matter lesions at the level of the middle cerebellar peduncles; minor criterion: white matter lesions in cerebral white matter, moderate or severe generalized atrophy) *or*
   C. Presence of intra-nuclear inclusions on post-mortem brain tissue

2. Probable:
   A. Two clinical major criteria *or*
   B. One major radiological criterion *and*
   C. One clinical minor criterion

3. Possible:
   A. One clinical major criterion *and*
   B. One radiological minor criterion

adjacent cerebellar white matter are considered to be highly sensitive for FXTAS (Figure 22.1).

Females with FXTAS have less pronounced reductions in middle cerebellar peduncle volumes as compared with males with FXTAS (Adams et al., 2007). Older male premutation carriers have significantly reduced volumes of cerebrum, cerebellum, and cerebral cortex as compared with age-matched controls (Loesch et al., 2005). Total brain volumes are inversely related to the number of CGG repeats in the FMR1 gene (see below). Decreased cerebellar volume is associated with increased length of the repeat. Premutation carriers have increased hippocampal volumes, suggestive of a neurodevelopmental change.

Neurophysiology

Upper limb tremor has a frequency of 3 to 6 Hz and may be asymmetrical.

Peripheral nerve conduction velocities in motor and sensory nerves are mildly decreased, with a correlation between longer CGG repeat number and slowing of the conduction velocity (Soontarapornchai et al., 2008). Amplitudes of compound muscle action potentials and sensory nerve action potentials are moderately reduced.

Gait is ataxic, with impaired body sway (Figure 22.1). There is a correlation between the severity of posterior fossa lesions on brain MRI and the impairment of body sway.

Genetic and molecular aspects

FXTAS is caused by an expanded trinucleotide repeat in the FMR1 gene (Xq27.3). Premutations are characterized by expanded repeats ranging in size from 55 to 200 repeats. Full-repeat expansions with greater than 200 repeats result in FXTAS.

The penetrance of FXTAS in male carriers aged 50 years and over is at least 33% (Hagerman & Hagerman, 2004). The penetrance in female carriers is approximately 5% to 10% (Greco et al., 2008).

Molecular findings include increased mRNA and low-normal or mildly decreased levels of FMR1 protein. FXTAS results from a toxic gain of function of FMR1 RNA, whereas fragile X syndrome is due to a loss of FMR1 function.

Neuropathology

Post-mortem studies show significant cerebral and cerebellar white matter disease (Greco et al., 2006). Microscopic examination shows a spongiosis in the middle cerebellar peduncles, Purkinje cell loss, and

239

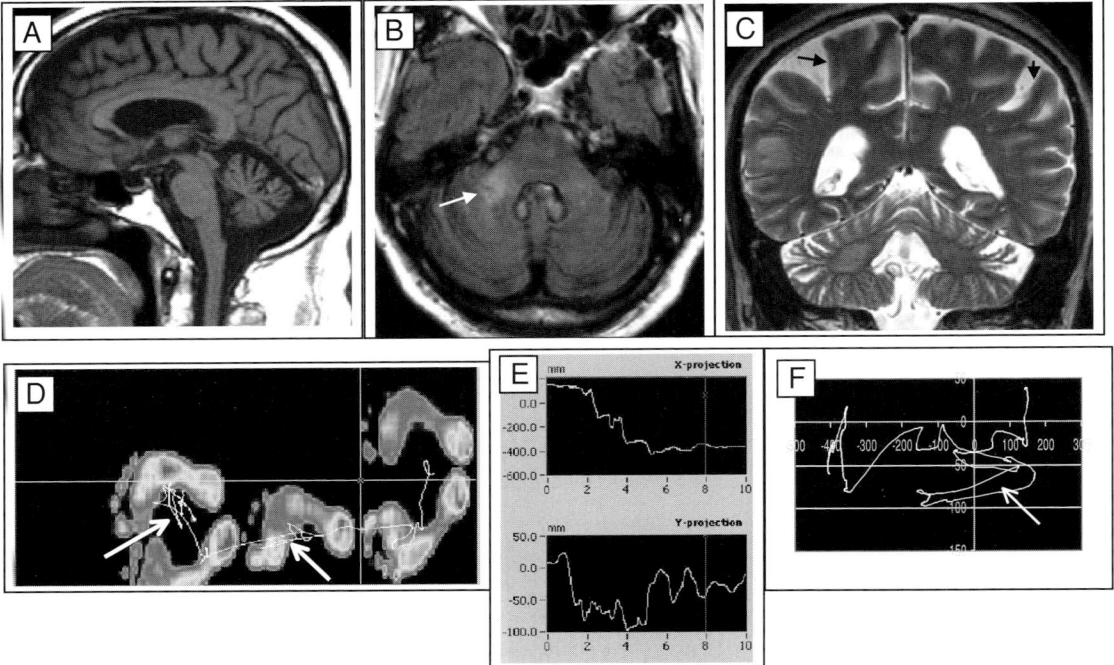

Figure 22.1 Brain MRI and gait analysis in a patient with fragile X tremor ataxia syndrome (FXTAS). (A) Sagittal T1-weighted image showing a moderate atrophy of the vermis; (B) hyperintense signals in the middle cerebellar peduncles on a T1-weighted axial image; (C) atrophy of the cerebellar cortex and cerebral sulci (arrows; T2-weighted image). (D–F) Analysis of tandem gait. The path of the center of pressure is dysmetric (arrows in D and F). (E) Representation of the displacements of the center of pressure in orthogonal planes X and Y. Reproduced in part from: Manto and Jissendi, 2009. With permission.

torpedoes. Intranuclear neuronal and astrocytic inclusions are observed. The inclusions are identified in the ganglion cells of the adrenal medulla, dorsal root ganglia, paraspinal sympathetic ganglia, myenteric ganglia of the stomach, and subepicardial autonomic ganglion of the heart (Gokden et al., 2009). These inclusions contain FMR1 mRNA, lamin A/C, neurofilaments, and ubiquitin. There is a correlation between the number of CGG repeats in the FMR1 gene and the number of intra-nuclear inclusions.

Treatment

There is currently no cure for FXTAS. Tremor may respond to primidone, beta-blockers, benzodiazepines, or memantine (Hagerman et al., 2008). Parkinsonism may respond to carbidopa/levodopa or dopaminergic agonists such as pramipexole. Although deep brain stimulation may be effective for tremor reduction, the usefulness of this procedure is limited by worsening of ataxia and cognitive effects (Leehey et al., 2003; Peters et al., 2006; Hagerman et al.,

2008). Treatment of cognitive impairment is based on off-label application of dementia treatments conventionally used in Alzheimer disease (Hagerman et al., 2008). Depression can be treated with selective serotonin reuptake inhibitors. Hyperactive detrusor activity may respond to muscarinic receptor antagonists. Cystoscopy under local anesthetic with injections of botulin toxin into the submucosal lining of the bladder is a secondary choice (Hagerman et al., 2008). Midodrine and fludrocortisone are administered for orthostatic hypotension.

Neuropathic pain is managed with antidepressants, anti-epileptics, and topical analgesics. Patients usually respond to gabapentin or pregabalin. In addition, application of lidocaine in patches can provide symptomatic relief.

Endocrine tests should be assessed regularly, especially for thyroid function.

Surgical procedures should be avoided if possible, because patients are at risk for deterioration of neurological status following general anesthesia.

Regular physical exercise is recommended.

References

Aalfs CM, Van Den Berg H, Barth PG, Hennekam RCM. The Hoyeraal-Hreidarsson syndrome: the fourth case of a separate entity with prenatal growth retardation, progressive pancytopenia and cerebellar hypoplasia. *Eur J Pediatr* 1995;**154**:304–8.

Adams JS, Adams PE, Nguyen D, et al. Volumetric brain changes in females with fragile X-associated tremor/ataxia syndrome (FXTAS). *Neurology* 2007;**69**:851–9.

Berry-Kravis E, Lewin F, Wuu J, et al. Tremor and ataxia in fragile X premutation carriers: blinded videotape study. *Ann Neurol* 2003;**53**:616–23.

de Brouwer AP, Williams KL, Duley JA, et al. Arts syndrome is caused by loss-of-function mutations in PRPS1. *Am J Hum Genet* 2007;**81**(3): 507–18.

Debray FG, Lambert M, Gagne R, et al. Pyruvate dehydrogenase deficiency presenting as intermittent isolated acute ataxia. *Neuropediatrics* 2008;**39**(1): 20–3.

Gokden M, Al-Hinti JT, Harik SI. Peripheral nervous system pathology in fragile X tremor/ataxia syndrome (FXTAS). *Neuropathology* 2009;**29**(3):280–4.

Greco CM, Berman RF, Martin RM, et al. Neuropathology of fragile X-associated tremor/ataxia syndrome (FXTAS). *Brain* 2006;**129**:243–55.

Greco CM, Tassone F, Garcia-Arocena D, et al. Clinical and neuropathologic findings in a woman with the FMR1 premutation and multiple sclerosis. *Arch Neurol* 2008;**65**:1114–6.

Guo X, Shen H, Xiao X, et al. Cataracts, ataxia, short stature, and mental retardation in a Chinese family mapped to Xpter-q13.1. *J Hum Genet* 2006;**51**: 695–700.

Hall DA, Berry-Kravis E, Jacquemont S, et al. Initial diagnoses given to persons with the fragile X associated tremor/ataxia syndrome (FXTAS). *Neurology* 2005;**65**:299–301.

Hagerman PJ, Hagerman RJ. The fragile-X premutation: a maturing perspective. *Am J Hum Genet* 2004;**74**:805–16.

Hagerman RJ, Hall DA, Coffey S, et al. Treatment of fragile X-associated tremor ataxia syndrome (FXTAS) and related neurological problems. *Clin Interv Aging* 2008;**3**(2):251–62.

Hagerman RJ, Leehey M, Heinrichs W, et al. Intention tremor, parkinsonism, and generalized brain atrophy in male carriers of fragile X. *Neurology* 2001;**57**:127–30.

Jacquemont S, Hagerman RJ, Leehey M, et al. Fragile X premutation tremor/ataxia syndrome: molecular, clinical, and neuroimaging correlates. *Am J Hum Genet* 2003;**72**:869–78.

Leehey MA, Munhoz RP, Lang AE, et al. The fragile X premutation presenting as essential tremor. *Arch Neurol* 2003;**60**:117–21.

Loesch DZ, Litewka L, Brotchie P, et al. Magnetic resonance imaging study in older fragile X premutation male carriers. *Ann Neurol* 2005;**58**(2):326–30.

Manto M, Jissendi P. *Spinocerebellar Atrophy*. In *Encyclopedia of Neuroscience, volume 9*, ed. L.R. Squire LR. Oxford, UK: Academic Press, pp. 337–49, 2009.

Peters N, Kamm C, Asmus F, et al. Intrafamilial variability in fragile X-associated tremor/ataxia syndrome. *Mov Disord* 2006;**21**:98–102.

Soontarapornchai K, Maselli R, Fenton-Farrell G, et al. Abnormal nerve conduction features in fragile X premutation carriers. *Arch Neurol* 2008;**65**:495–8.

Spira PJ, McLeod JG, Evans WA. A spinocerebellar degeneration with X-linked inheritance. *Brain.* 1979;**102**:27–41.

Dominant ataxias

An overview of spinocerebellar ataxias

The spinocerebellar ataxias (SCAs) are a group of genetically and clinically heterogeneous autosomal dominant progressive ataxic diseases (Schöls et al., 2004). Epidemiological studies conducted in various European areas have found prevalence rates of SCAs ranging from 0.9 to 3.0 per 100 000 (van de Warrenburg et al., 2002; Klockgether, 2008). However, due to founder effects, the prevalence is higher in some geographically isolated areas. This is the case for SCA2 in Cuba and SCA3 in the Azores. SCA1, 2, 3, and 6 are the most common SCAs worldwide (Figure 23.1). Dentatorubral-pallidoluysian atrophy (DRPLA) has a relatively high prevalence in Japan.

Harding has suggested a classification according to the mode of inheritance and the clinical signs (autosomal dominant cerebellar ataxia [ADCA] I–III) (Harding, 1982). Current molecular classification corresponds to the order of gene description. Almost 30 different gene loci have been identified. SCA1, 2, 3, 6, 7, and 17 are translated CAG repeat expansions coding for an elongated polyglutamine tract within the respective proteins (polyglutaminopathies, a group which includes also Huntington disease, DRPLA, and spinobulbar muscular atrophy). SCA8, 10, and 12 are due to untranslated repeat expansions in non-coding regions of the genes. Point mutations are associated with SCA5, SCA13, SCA14, SCA27, and 16q22-linked SCA. SCA4 and 16q22-linked SCA have been mapped to the same chromosomal region, but no mutations have been found in the original SCA4 family.

The occurrence of autosomal dominant ataxia in subsequent generations is highly suggestive of an SCA when the disease is transmitted by both sexes. Research of mutations is recommended in these patients. It should be kept in mind that a negative family history does not rule out an SCA. Indeed, affected parents might have died before onset of symptoms, especially in SCAs with a late-onset presentation,

such as SCA6 (Schöls et al., 1998). Moreover, relatives who carry the mutation may appear clinically unaffected due to a milder phenotype in elderly generations (anticipation) or due to a reduced penetrance. Furthermore, patients might present a de novo mutation. In addition, family history might appear negative due to false paternity. The frequency of positive genetic tests in apparently sporadic ataxia patients ranges from 2% to 22% (Schöls et al., 2000; Pujana et al., 1999).

The principal clues which guide the clinician for the diagnosis of a given SCA are summarized in Table 23.1. Average age at onset of SCAs is in the third decade, with large variations between subtypes. Patients usually exhibit a slowly progressive cerebellar syndrome with various combinations of oculomotor disorders, dysarthria, dysmetria/kinetic tremor, and/or ataxic gait (Manto, 2005). They can also present with pigmentary retinopathy, extra-pyramidal movement disorders (parkinsonism, dyskinesias, dystonia, chorea), pyramidal signs, cortical symptoms (seizures, cognitive impairment/behavioral symptoms), and peripheral neuropathy (Table 23.2). The clinical diagnosis of subtypes of SCAs is complicated by the salient overlap of the phenotypes between genetic subtypes. The following clinical features have some specific values for predicting a gene defect: slowing of saccades in SCA2; ophthalmoplegia in SCA1, SCA2, and SCA3; pigmentary retinopathy in SCA7; spasticity in SCA3;

Table 23.1 Main clues for diagnosis of a dominant spinocerebellar ataxia

Age of onset
Gender
Family history
Ethnic and geographical background
Presence of extra-cerebellar deficits
Findings of brain MRI

Table 23.2 Clinical presentations of spinocerebellar ataxias (SCAs)

Pure cerebellar syndrome	SCA5, SCA6, SCA11, SCA26		
Cerebellar ataxia plus	Cognitive impairment/behavioral symptoms		SCA1, SCA2, SCA3, SCA10, SCA12, SCA13, SCA14, SCA17, SCA19, SCA21 SCA27-FGF14, DRPLA
	Seizures		SCA10, SCA17, DRPLA
	Eyes/oculomotor deficits	Slow saccades	SCA1, SCA2, SCA3, SCA7, SCA28
		Down-beat nystagmus	SCA6
		Ophtalmoparesia	SCA1, SCA2, SCA3, SCA28, SCA30
		Ocular dyskinesia	SCA10
		Pigmentary retinopathy	SCA7
	Movement disorders	Parkinsonism	SCA1, SCA2, SCA3, SCA12, SCA17, SCA21
		Dystonia	SCA3, SCA14, SCA17
		Tremor	SCA8, SCA12, SCA16, SCA19, SCA20
		Dyskinesias	SCA27-FGF14
		Myoclonus	SCA2, SCA14, SCA19, DRPLA
		Chorea	SCA1, SCA17, DRPLA
		Myokymia	SCA5
	Pyramidal signs		SCA1, SCA2, SCA3, SCA4, SCA7, SCA8, SCA10, SCA11, SCA12, SCA13, SCA14, SCA15, SCA28, SCA30
	Peripheral neuropathy		SCA1, SCA2, SCA3, SCA4, SCA6, SCA8, SCA27-FGF14, SCA12, SCA18, SCA22, SCA25

dyskinesias associated with a mutation in the fibroblast growth factor 14 (FGF14) gene and cognitive impairment/behavioral symptoms in SCA17 and DRPLA; seizures in SCA10, SCA17, and DRPLA; and peripheral neuropathy in SCA1, SCA2, SCA3, SCA4, SCA8, SCA18, and SCA25.

Anticipation is a main feature of SCAs, due to instability of expanded alleles. Anticipation may be particularly prominent in SCA7. Several SCAs are associated with trinucleotide repeat extensions, and there is a correlation between the size of this expansion, the age of onset, and the severity of the disorder.

This explains the phenomenon of anticipation: instability of larger repeats cause further expansions in consecutive generations, hence the earlier onset and the greater severity of symptoms.

Three patterns of atrophy can be identified on brain MRI: a pure cerebellar atrophy, a pattern of olivopontocerebellar atrophy, and a pattern of global brain atrophy. A remarkable observation is the presence of dentate nuclei calcifications in SCA20, resulting in a low signal on brain MRI sequences. Most of the SCAs start with a cerebellar atrophy which progresses subsequently to involve extra-cerebellar structures.

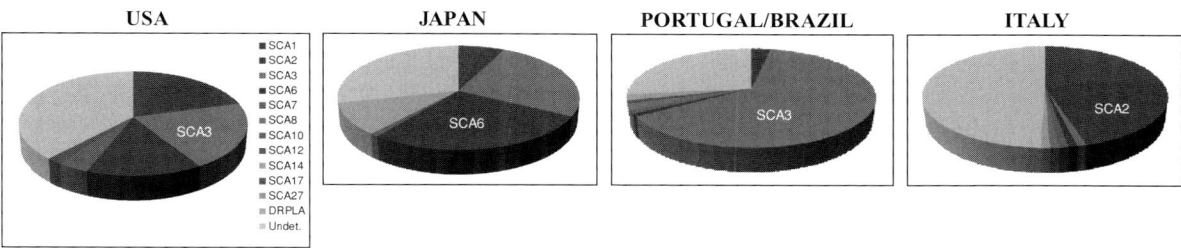

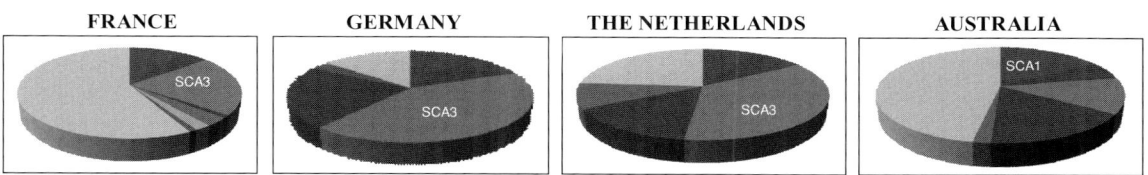

Figure 23.1 Relative frequencies of spinocerebellar ataxias (SCAs). The SCA with highest frequency is indicated in each pie. (See color section.)

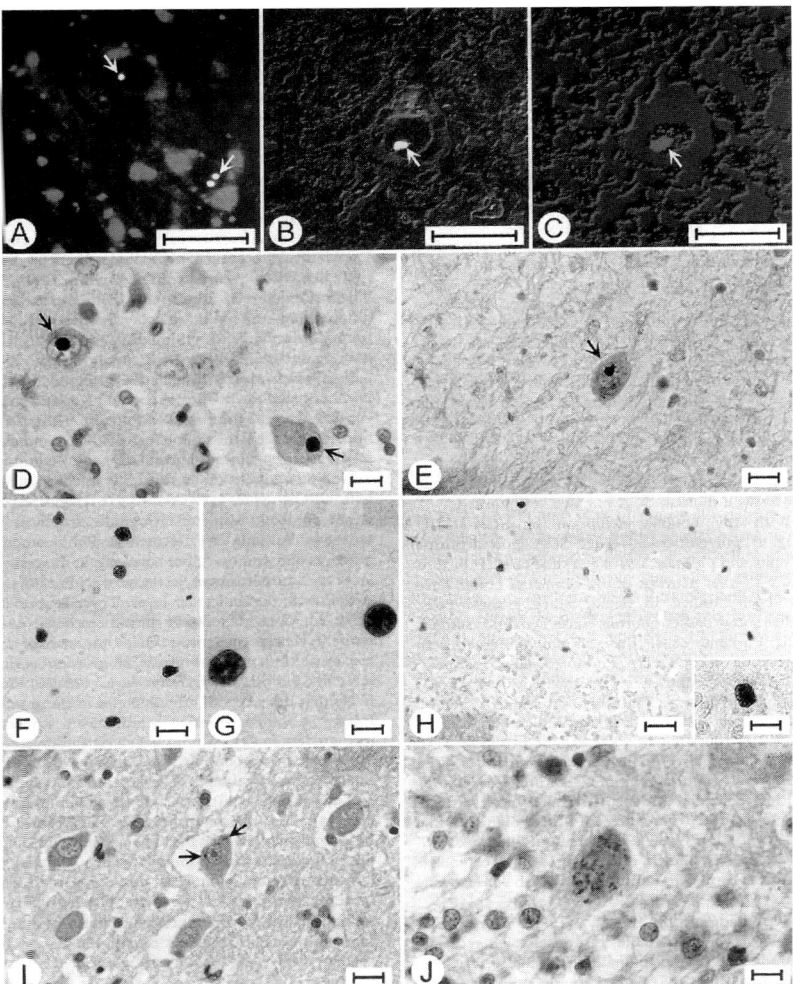

Figure 23.2 Inclusions in spinocerebellar ataxias (SCAs). Inclusion bodies in selected SCAs. (A–C) SCA-3/Machado-Joseph disease (MJD), anti-ataxin-3 (A and B), anti-ubiquitin (C): confocal fluorescence microscopy shows multiple small nucleoliform ataxin-3-reactive intranuclear inclusions in neurons of the basis pontis (arrows in A; fluorescein isothiocyanate [FITC]). Ataxin-3 reaction product in B (FITC) colocalizes with ubiquitin in C (Quantum Red) (arrows). The images were processed to reduce lipofuscin fluorescence. (D) SCA1, anti-polyglutamine: Positive-contrast reaction product is present in large intranuclear inclusions (arrows). (E) SCA-2, anti-polyglutamine: the intranuclear inclusion body (arrow) is relatively small compared with those in SCA-1 (D). (F–H) SCA-17, anti-polyglutamine (F and H), TATA-binding protein (G): neurons of the basis pontis reveal pan-nuclear reaction product (F, G). In the cerebellar cortex, pan-nuclear inclusions are present in the basket and stellate cells (H). The inset shows an intranuclear inclusion in a surviving Purkinje cell. (I, J) SCA-6, anti-polyglutamine: pontine neurons show small intracytoplasmic inclusions (I, arrows). A Purkinje cell contains multiple cytoplasmic inclusion bodies (J). Magnification markers: A–C, F, and H, 25 mm; D–E, G, J, and inset in H, 10 mm; I, 15.9 mm. From: Koeppen, 2005. With permission. (See color section.)

From the neuropathological point of view, SCA1, 2, and 7 are prototypes of a degeneration pattern previously designated as olivopontocerebellar atrophy with degeneration of the cerebellar cortex, pontine nuclei, and inferior olives (Koeppen, 2005). In polyglutaminopathies due to CAG trinucleotide repeats, characteristic nuclear inclusions are found in neurons (Figure 23.2). These inclusions result from aggregated disease proteins. They contain other proteins, such as chaperones, proteasomal subunits, and transcription factors (Schmidt et al., 2002). Degeneration of neurons in basal ganglia, cerebral cortex, spinal cord, and peripheral nerves is not exceptional in SCAs.

The differential diagnosis of SCAs includes episodic ataxias (EA), hereditary spastic paraplegias (HSP), Huntington disease, essential tremor (see Chapter 19), hereditary sensorimotor neuropathies, and Gerstmann-Sträussler-Scheinker disease (see Chapter 11), a dominantly inherited transmissible spongiform encephalopathy (Schöls et al., 2004). Autosomal recessive disorders, mitochondrial diseases, X-linked diseases, or even sporadic diseases can also mimic the phenotype of SCAs. In particular, leukodystrophies, mitochondrial cytopathies (Kearns-Sayre syndrome; myoclonic epilepsy with ragged-red fibers; mitochondrial encephalomyopathy, lactic acidosis, and stroke-like episodes; neuropathy, ataxia, and retinitis pigmentosa; Leigh syndrome), Friedreich ataxia, fragile X syndrome, progressive myoclonic epilepsies, or multiple system atrophy should be considered.

Trinucleotide repeat expansions may occur in coding and noncoding DNA regions (Figure 23.3). Therefore, the repeats will exert their detrimental effects through different molecular mechanisms, which may overlap.

Figure 23.4 shows the mechanisms of the various SCAs put in the global context of cerebellar ataxias. Disorders of unstable repeat expansions have been divided into four groups: (1) diseases caused by expansions of coding repeats which result in altered protein function, (2) diseases caused by expansions of non-coding repeats which result in loss of protein function (see also Chapter 20), (3) diseases caused by expansions of non-coding repeats which result in impaired RNA function (see also fragile X tremor ataxia syndrome in Chapter 22), and (4) diseases of unknown pathogenesis.

Polyglutamine expansions are associated with transcriptional dysregulation. Polyglutamine tracts interact closely with well-defined transcriptional regulators such as cAMP-responsive element-binding protein. For instance, the SCA7 gene product, ataxin 7, is part of a transcriptional coactivator complex (STAGA), which has histone acetyltransferase activity. In SCA17, the CAG repeat expansion occurs in TATA-binding protein (TBP), a transcription factor. Altered protein conformation leads to protein accumulation and a cascade of aberrant protein–protein interactions, which will lead to cell death. Chaperones and proteasomes are used to refold or dispose polyglutamine-containing fragments in order to prevent further aggregation. Aggregates sequester other proteins and protein complexes, including proteasomes and transcription factors, leading to inclusion bodies.

Genetic testing for diagnosis, prenatal evaluation, and predictive testing is discussed in Chapter 5.

Spinocerebellar ataxia type 1

Clinical presentation

Symptoms of spinocerebellar ataxia type 1 (SCA1) usually start in the third or fourth decade. Anticipation is classical: successive generations tend to have an earlier onset and more severe manifestations (Orr et al., 1993; Lin et al., 2002). The core of neurological symptoms is made of a combination of cerebellar and brainstem-related symptoms (Table 23.3). Patients often exhibit extra-pyramidal signs and peripheral

Table 23.3 Clinical deficits in SCA1

Cerebellar symptoms

Brainstem deficits
 Dysphagia
 Facial weakness
 Ophthalmoparesis

Extra-pyramidal deficits
 Blepharospasm
 Dystonia
 Choreiform or athetoid movements

Peripheral neuropathy
 Loss of tendon reflexes
 Loss of proprioception/vibration sense
 Amyotrophy
 Fasciculations

Cognitive deficits
 Inappropriate laughing
 Emotional lability
 Memory loss

Sphincter disturbances
 Urinary urgency

neuropathy. Usually the initial symptoms are gait and limb incoordination and slurred speech. Oculomotor deficits include dysmetria of saccades and nystagmus. Patients may also exhibit eyelid retraction, blepharospasm, and impaired vestibuloocular reflex (VOR)/optokinetic nystagmus. The disease typically progresses over 10 to 15 years, with a gradual increase of ataxia. Signs of bulbar dysfunction include dysphagia, accompanied by progressive tongue atrophy. Facial weakness becomes evident after a few years. Therefore, patients are at risk of pneumonia, which is a common cause of death.

Neuroimaging

Brain CT scan and MRI demonstrate pontocerebellar atrophy, with enlargement of the fourth ventricle (Figure 23.5). In general, on T2-weighted images, no signal abnormalities are reported in the basal ganglia and the posterior fossa (Döhlinger et al., 2008). A midline hyperintensity of the pontine base, which is not identical to "cross" sign (see Chapter 18), has been reported on T2-weighted changes (Adachi et al., 2006).

Positron emission tomography (PET) shows decreased glucose metabolism in the cerebellar cortex, brainstem, basal ganglia, thalamic nuclei, and cerebral cortex.

Figure 23.3 Trinucleotide repeat expansions in coding and noncoding DNA regions (the CAG expansions in Huntington disease are not illustrated). Abbreviations: SCA: spinocerebellar ataxia; FXTAS: fragile X tremor ataxia syndrome; FA: Friedreich ataxia; DRPLA: dentatorubral-pallidoluysian atrophy; SBMA: spinal and bulbar muscular atrophy; FGF: fibroblast growth factor; ORF: open reading frame; UTR: untranslated region.

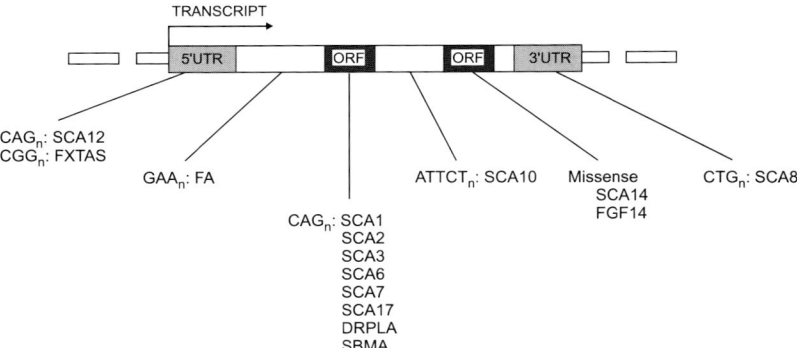

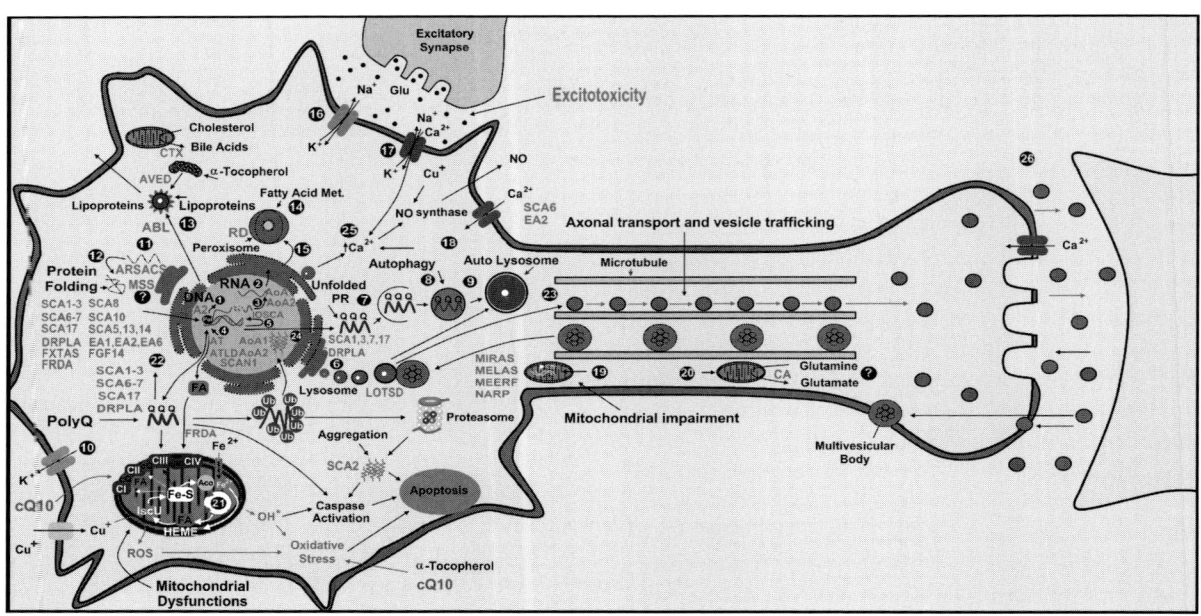

Figure 23.4 Illustration of the mechanisms of cerebellar ataxias at the cellular level. 1, transcription; 2, DNA repair; 3, transport; 4, processing; 5, replication; 6, glycosphingolipid metabolism; 7, isolation membrane; 8, autophagy; 9, autolysosome; 10, Ca2+ activated voltage-gated K+ channel; 11, translation; 12, protein folding; 13, lipoprotein assembly; 14, fatty acid metabolism; 15, protein import; 16, non-NMDA receptor; 17, NMDA receptor; 18, voltage-gated Ca2+ channels; 19, DNA repair/replication; 20, mitochondrial impairment; 21, Krebs cycle; 22, chaperones; 23, axonal transport and vesicle trafficking; 24, aggregation; 25 Ca2+ homeostasis; 26, synaptic function. Abbreviations: Ca2+: Calcium Ions; ER: endoplasmic reticulum; Glu: glutamate; K+: potassium ions; Na+: sodium ions; Q: glutamine; Ub: ubiquitin; CI: respiratory chain complex I; CII: respiratory chain complex II; CIII: respiratory chain complex III; CIV: respiratory chain complex IV; cQ: coenzyme Q; cytC: cytochrome C; ACO: aconitase; HEME; Fe2+: ferrous iron; IscU: iron-sulphur cluster scaffold protein; ROS: reactive oxygen species; RNA: ribonucleic acid; OH∗: hydroxyl radical; Fe-S: iron-sulfur cluster; Vitamin E; cQ10: coenzyme Q10; Cu+: copper; SCA (1–17): spinocerebellar ataxia (Type 1–17); DRPLA: dentatorubral-pallidoluysian atrophy; EA (Type 1–6): episodic ataxia (Type 1–6); FGF14: fibroblast growth factor 14; FXTAS: fragile X tremor/ataxia syndrome; FA: Friedreich ataxia; AOA (type 1–2): ataxia with oculomotor apraxia (Type 1–2); IOSCA: infantile-onset spinocerebellar ataxia; AT: ataxia telangiectasia; SCAN1: spinocerebellar ataxia with axonal neuropathy; LOTSD: late-onset Tay-Sachs disease; RD: Refsum disease; ARSACS: autosomal recessive ataxia of Charlevoix-Saguenay; MSS: Marinesco-Sjögren syndrome; ABL: abetalipoproteinemia; CTX: cerebrotendinous xanthomatosis; AVED: ataxia with vitamin E deficiency; CA: Cayman ataxia; MIRAS: mitochondrial recessive ataxia syndrome; MELAS: mitochondrial myopathy, encephalopathy, lactic acidosis, and stroke; MERRF: myoclonus epilepsy associated with ragged-red fibers; NARP: neuropathy, ataxia, and retinitis pigmentosa. From: Manto and Marmolino, 2009. With permission. (See color section.)

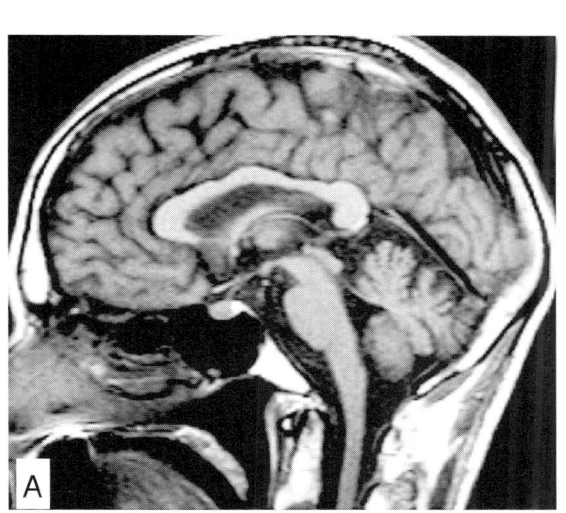
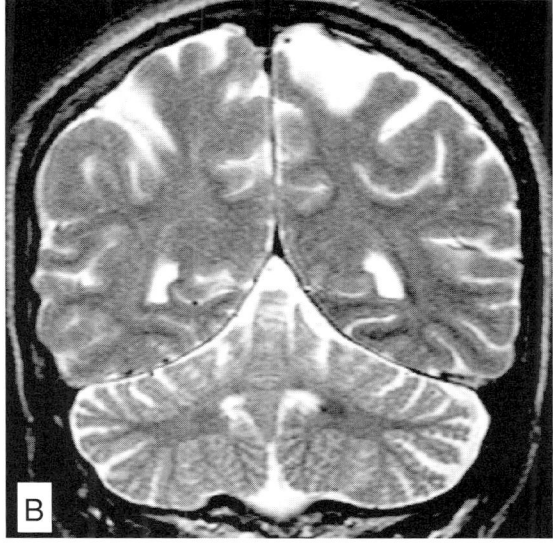

C   BODY SWAY-CENTER OF PRESSURE

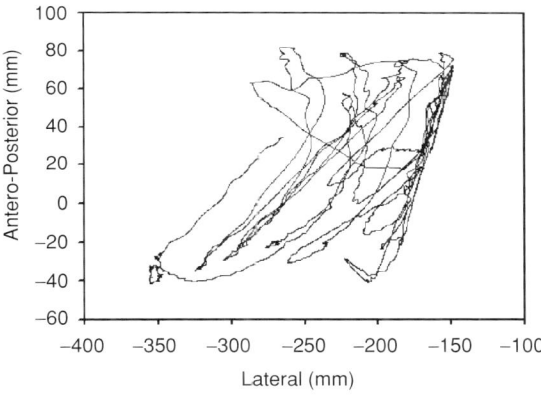

Figure 23.5 (A, B) Brain MRI of a patient with SCA1. Sagittal T1-weighted image (A) and coronal T2-weighted image (B). The images show vermian and cerebellar atrophy characterized by the enlargement of the fissures and the absence of pontine atrophy. Notice the atrophy of the supratentorial structures. (C) Illustration of the displacements of the center of pressure during standing. There is a marked body sway, in both the lateral and anterior-posterior axis. Reproduced in part from: Manto and Jissendi, 2009. With permission.

Neurophysiology

Nerve conduction velocities show a mild slowing of motor and sensory nerves (Schöls et al., 2008). On visual evoked potentials, the P100 wave is delayed in up to 75% of the patients. Auditory evoked potentials are abnormal in half of patients. Somatosensory evoked potentials show a loss of the P40 wave in many patients. Central motor conduction time is prolonged in 75% of cases.

Genetic and molecular aspects

The number of CAG repeats in the SCA1 gene (locus 6p23) is highly polymorphic in the general population, ranging from 6 to 44 (Lin et al., 2002). SCA1 patients typically have expansions between 39 and 82 repeats (Orr et al., 1993; Goldfarb et al., 1996). Normal alleles with 21 or more CAG repeats are interrupted with 1 to 4 CAT repeats (encoding histidine), whereas SCA1 alleles contain only uninterrupted CAG repeat tracts (Quan et al., 1995).

The CAG repeat in the SCA1 gene encodes a polyglutamine tract. Both SCA1 mRNA and the protein ataxin-1 are ubiquitously expressed. This protein is localized mainly in the nuclei of Purkinje and brainstem neurons. Ataxin-1 is also present in peripheral tissues, but its expression is lower.

There is a correlation between the length of the repeat, the age of onset, and the severity of the disease: for longer repeats, the onset occurs earlier and the phenotype is more severe. This is due to the dynamic aspect of the mutation during transmission and is especially evident for paternal transmission (see discussion of anticipation in section An overview of spinocerebellar ataxias).

Neuropathology

The overall size of the cerebellum is decreased, with a dilatation of the fourth ventricle. The cerebellar cortex is characterized by a loss of Purkinje cells or reduced arborization, preservation of parallel fibers, empty baskets, and torpedoes in the granular layer. Neuronal loss in the dentate nuclei and inferior olivary nuclei are common. Severe loss in the gray matter of the basis pontis is found.

Lessons from the animal models of SCA1

SCA1 pathogenesis is due to a gain of toxic function as a result of the accumulation of the polyglutamine tract. SCA1 null mice develop no ataxia, but exhibit spatial and motor learning deficits (Matilla et al., 1998). Transgenic mice expressing expanded polyglutamine tracts have been generated. These mice show impaired dendritic arborization of Purkinje cells, heterotopic Purkinje cells, and atrophy of the molecular layer. Nuclear aggregates are found in Purkinje cells. There is a positive ubiquitin immunoreactivity of the nuclear aggregates, suggesting a protein misfolding or impaired proteasomal degradation. Selective loss of Purkinje cells and brainstem neurons is likely the result of the protein interactions of the polyglutamine expansion, with consequent perturbation of nuclear events, in particular, gene transcription and mRNA processing (Lin et al., 2000).

Table 23.4 Clinical deficits in SCA2

Cerebellar syndrome
Reduced saccadic velocity
Myoclonus

Extra-pyramidal deficits
  Dystonia
  Chorea

Cognitive deficits
  Frontal executive dysfunction
  Dementia

Pyramidal involvement

Peripheral neuropathy
  Loss of tendon reflexes
  Loss of proprioception/vibration sense
  Amyotrophy
  Fasciculations

Spinocerebellar ataxia type 2

Clinical presentation

The clinical symptoms of spinocerebellar ataxia type 2 (SCA2) are summarized in Table 23.4 (Orozco et al., 1990). Cerebellar ataxia is present in all patients. One of the clinical hallmarks is the reduced velocity of saccades, which is found in up to 90% of patients. Square wave jerks and gaze-evoked nystagmus are usually absent. Myoclonus occurs in about 40% of patients. The size of the triplet expansion is usually larger in patients exhibiting dystonia or myoclonus. In a few patients, in particular those with smaller CAG repeat expansions, SCA2 may present as "pure" familial parkinsonism. Neuropathy may remain subclinical. Tendon hyperreflexia due to pyramidal tract involvement is usually followed by hyporeflexia as a result of peripheral neuropathy. Cognitive dysfunction manifests usually with frontoexecutive deficits, and about one in four patients will develop dementia (Storey et al., 1999).

Neuroimaging

On brain MRI, cerebellar and brainstem atrophy is usually more severe as compared with SCA1 and SCA3 (Klockgether et al., 1998). A flattening of the inferior part of the pons on midsagittal images is often observed. In some patients, signal hyperintensities are observed in the basal ganglia or posterior fossa, resembling those seen in multiple system atrophy C type (Figure 23.6; Burk et al., 2001; see Chapter 18).

Figure 23.6 Severe atrophy of the cerebellum and brainstem in a patient with SCA2. Axial T2-weighted images show a small mesencephalon with widened cerebellar sulci (A, B). Note the altered signal in the brainstem. The middle cerebellar peduncles are markedly atrophic (arrow, C). The inferior portions of the hemispheres are also involved (D).

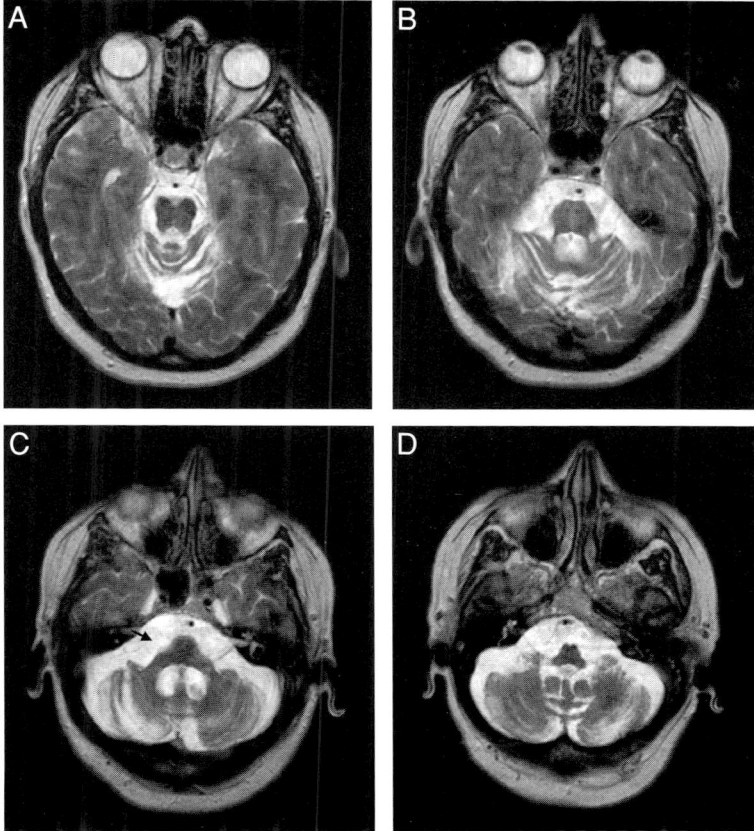

Voxel-based morphometry (VBM) reveals volume loss in the cerebellar hemispheres, vermis, pons, mesencephalon, thalamus, and distinct cortical areas (Guerrini et al., 2004). Clinical deficits are correlated with atrophy of the pons and cerebellum (Ying et al., 2006). Proton MRS may demonstrate decreased N-acetylaspartate/creatine ratios in patients with a mild cerebellar syndrome (Figure 23.7).

Neurophysiology

Electrooculography confirms the severe saccadic slowing. Saccadic speed is significantly lower as compared with that of SCA1 and SCA3 (Buttner et al., 1998). Values range from 80 to 300 degrees/sec (normal >390 degrees/sec). Nerve conduction velocities show an axonal sensory neuropathy. On visual evoked potentials, the P100 wave is delayed in 36% of patients and lost in 9% (Schöls et al., 2008). Auditory evoked potentials are abnormal in about 40% of cases. Somatosensory evoked potentials show a loss of the P40 wave in half of patients. Central motor conduction time is prolonged in a minority of cases. Polysomnography reveals REM sleep without atonia or an absence of REM sleep.

Genetic aspects

SCA2 is caused by an expansion of an unstable CAG repeat in the ataxin-2 gene (12q24.1). The CAG trinucleotide repeat is not highly polymorphic in normal individuals. The alleles of 22 and 23 repeats account for 95% of the alleles (Pulst et al., 1996). Normal alleles range from 15 to 32 repeats. The expansions are usually smaller than those occurring in SCA1 or SCA3. A number of 33 CAG repeats is sufficient to cause the disease (Fernandez et al., 2000). As for SCA1, there is a clear correlation between the length of the repeat and the age of onset.

Neuropathology

The gross appearance of the brain is characterized by cerebellar and pontine atrophy, with dilatation of the

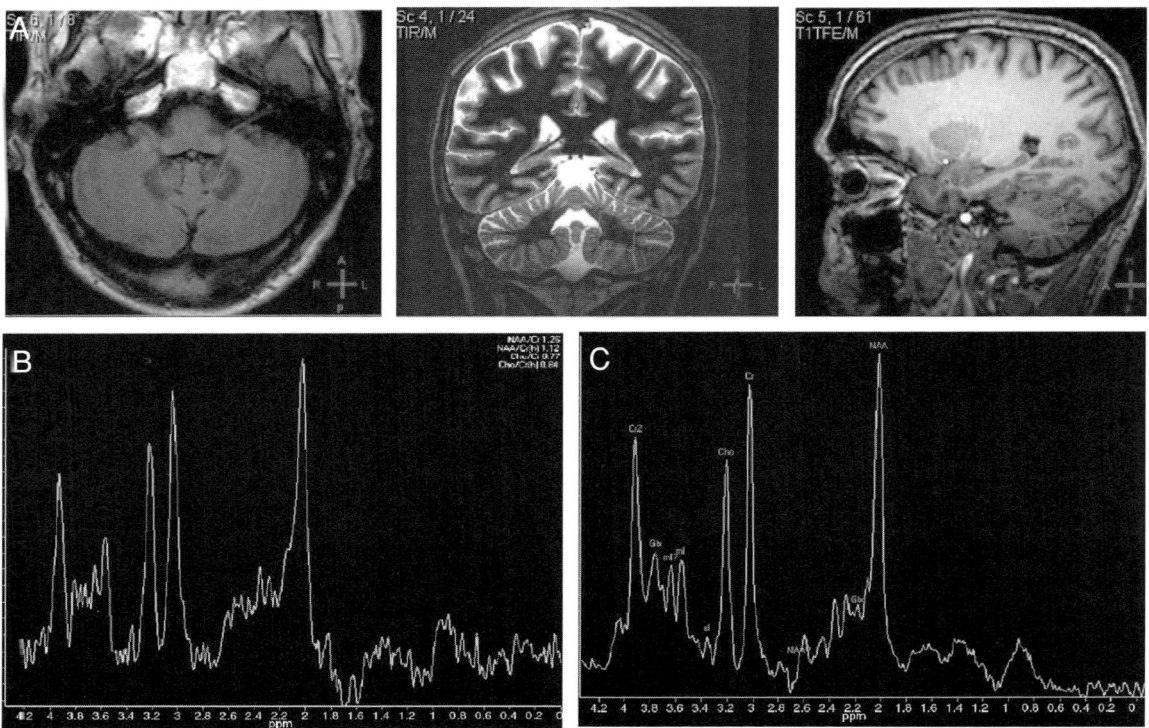

Figure 23.7 Brain MRI and H1 magnetic resonance spectroscopy of a patient with SCA2 exhibiting a slight cerebellar syndrome: (A) MRI used to plan the single voxel acquisition; (B) spectrum acquired in the deep left cerebellum of patient; (C) spectrum acquired in the deep left cerebellum of age- and sex-matched control. The images in (A), axial fluid-attenuated inversion recovery, coronal T2-weighted, and sagittal T1-weighted (from left to right), show global atrophy in the posterior fossa as well as in the supratentorium. The spectrum in (B) shows a decrease of the N-acetyl-aspartate/creatine ratio (1.26) compared with the control (1.53). From: Manto and Jissendi, 2009. With permission. (See color section.)

fourth ventricle (Orozco et al., 1990; Estrada et al., 1999). Lesions are usually more severe as compared with SCA1, especially in the inferior olivary complex. There is a marked loss of Purkinje cells. Torpedoes are common. Although the morphology of cell bodies of stellate and basket cells is affected, most of these cell populations survive. This is also the case for granule cells. Neuronal loss and dendritic atrophy occur in the dentate nuclei. Substantia nigra is characterized by a marked neuronal loss. Demyelination in the posterior columns of the spinal cord and to a lesser extent in the spinocerebellar tracts may develop. In some cases, atrophy of the frontotemporal lobes is observed.

Spinocerebellar ataxia type 3

Clinical presentation

In several studies, spinocerebellar ataxia type 3 (SCA3, or Machado-Joseph disease [MJD]) represents the

main cause of dominant ataxia worldwide. Prevalence among SCAs varies from 20% to 50% (Moseley et al., 1998; Schöls et al., 1995).

MJD was originally described in emigrants from the Azorean islands Sao Miguel (Machado family) and Flores (Joseph family) (Nakano et al., 1972). MJD is thought to have originated from founders in the Iberia Peninsula who moved to the Azores and then to several other countries. However, on the basis of haplotype studies characterizing polymorphisms flanking the MJD1 gene, there is strong evidence for independent and multiple origins of MJD/SCA3 in different populations (Iughetti et al., 1996).

The age of onset varies from childhood to late adult life. In most cases, symptoms start between 20 and 45 years of age. As with SCA1 and SCA2, patients exhibit combinations of cerebellar and extra-cerebellar deficits (Table 23.5). Four distinct subphenotypes of SCA3 have been suggested (Coutinho & Andrade, 1978):

Table 23.5 Clinical deficits in SCA3

Cerebellar syndrome
Ophtalmoparesia
Dysphagia
Upper/lower motor neuron signs (faciolingual fasciculations)
Sensory deficits
Pyramidal deficits   Spasticity

Extra-pyramidal deficits
   Dystonia
   Bradykinesia

Sleep disturbances, restless leg syndrome
Autonomic disturbances
Weight loss with preservation of appetite
Cognitive deficits

- Type 1: extra-pyramidal (especially dystonic) and pyramidal deficits; early onset (10–30 years)
- Type 2: pyramidal and cerebellar deficits; intermediate onset (20–50 years)
- Type 3: cerebellar deficits and peripheral neuropathy; late onset (40–75 years)
- Type 4: peripheral neuropathy and parkinsonism; variable onset.

The first symptoms are usually gait difficulties, slurred speech, and visual blurring. Saccades become slower with time, although the velocities remain higher as compared with SCA2, and patients develop supra-nuclear ophthalmoplegia (limitation of upward gaze). Lid retraction is not rare. Facial muscles often become atrophic, and the tongue may show fasciculations. Brisk tendon reflexes tend to attenuate with time. Extra-pyramidal signs may be initially dopa-responsive (Tuite et al., 1995). Some patients exhibit a dysautonomia. Abnormalities of visual attention are common.

Death is caused by loss of mobility and respiratory difficulties in a context of nutritional problems.

Neuroimaging

Structural MRI shows an enlargement of the fourth ventricle and moderate shrinkage of the cerebellar vermis and hemispheres, as well as pontine atrophy (Figure 23.8). Volumetric analysis demonstrates putaminal and caudate atrophy in SCA3 (Klockgether et al., 1998). Atrophy of the superior cerebellar peduncles, atrophy in the frontal and temporal lobes, and diminished transverse diameter of the pallidum have also been reported (Murata et al., 1998). On T2-weighted and/or proton density–weighted axial MRI, a hyperintense signal in the transverse pontine fibers has been observed in 14 out of 31 SCA3 patients, as well as in 1 post-mortem–confirmed case (Döhlinger et al., 2008)

^{18}F-fluorodeoxyglucose PET may reveal early presymptomatic changes in SCA3 (Soong & Liu, 1998). Dopamine transporter studies show decreased binding in the striatum similar to Parkinson disease (Wüllner et al., 2005).

Neurophysiology

Electrooculography shows a mild saccadic slowing with a prominent gaze-evoked nystagmus. Patients present with sensorimotor axonal neuropathy detected by needle electromyelography (EMG) studies/conduction velocity tests. On visual evoked potentials, the P100 wave is delayed in 25% of the patients and lost in 6% (Schöls et al., 2008). Auditory evoked potentials are abnormal in two-thirds of

Figure 23.8 Brain MRI of a patient presenting with SCA-3. Sagittal T1- (A) and axial T2-weighted (B) images show enlargement of the cisterns in the posterior fossa with global cerebellar atrophy; an involvement of the brainstem is visible at the level of the medulla. From: Manto and Jissendi, 2009. With permission.

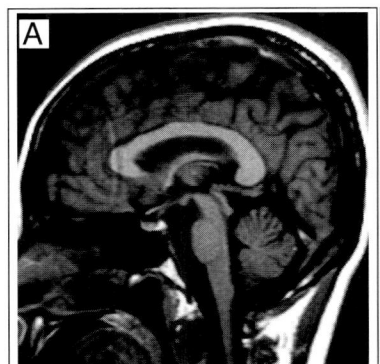
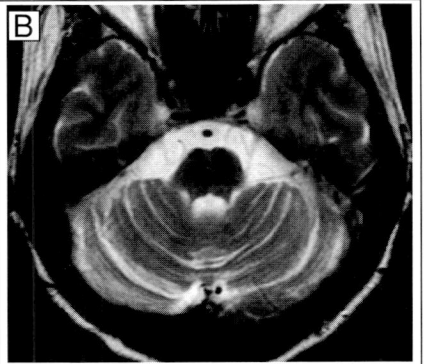

patients. Somatosensory evoked potentials show a loss of the P40 wave in 27% of cases and a delayed P40 wave in 60%. Central motor conduction time is prolonged in 28% of patients. Polysomnography reveals periodic leg movements in sleep or an REM sleep behavior disorder.

Genetic and molecular aspects

The MJD1 gene of 1776 bp maps to the 14q32.1 region (Kawaguchi et al., 1994). The genomic sequence of the MJD1 gene spans about 48 kb and contains up to 11 exons. The gene is ubiquitously expressed in humans, with multiple alternative spliced transcripts. In the brain, MJD1 is preferentially transcribed in neurons, although low levels are also present in glial cells (Nishiyama et al., 1996).

The normal range of CAG repeats in the MJD1 gene is up to 47. The expanded repeat size is more than 44 (Padiath et al., 2005), with 86 being the largest expanded repeat reported. There is an overlap of normal repeat sizes (up to 47), with the smallest expanded repeat of 45 CAGs. Individuals with a repeat length in the overlapping region do not always present with the disease (reduced penetrance) (Riess et al., 2008). It should be noted that variant CAA (third and sixth positions) and AGG (fourth position) triplets are found in the normal alleles (Kawaguchi et al., 1994).

The expanded CAG repeat is widely unstable, especially during paternal transmission. Thus there is a higher risk for earlier symptoms in children from affected fathers. A combination of paternal transmission and expanded (CAG)n-CGG/normal (CAG)n-GGG haplotypes is associated with a 75-fold increased relative risk compared with that of maternal transmission and expanded (CAG)n-CGG/normal(CAG)n-CGG or expanded (CAG)n-GGG/normal(CAG)n-GGG haplotypes, indicating interallelic effects on CAG repeat stability (Matsumura et al., 1996a; Matsumura et al., 1996b). There is a somatic mosaicism of the expanded allele. Smaller expanded repeat sizes may be found in the cerebellar cortex as compared with other brain regions, such as the frontal cortex (Hashida et al., 1997). Regarding the age of onset of MJD, the triplet repeat length does not account for all of the variations observed. Among the additional factors are homozygosity of the expanded CAG repeat, which predisposes to earlier age at onset (Lang et al., 1994), sex (the symptoms appear later in females), and probably lifestyle. Repeats of more than 73 CAG motifs are commonly associated with a pyramidal phenotype, whereas patients with fewer than 73 repeats more often develop peripheral neuropathy (Schöls et al., 1996).

The protein ataxin-3 has an approximate molecular weight of 42 kDa in healthy individuals. The molecular weight is larger in affected patients due to the polyglutamine disorders (polyQ) stretch. Several isoforms have been described (Schmidt et al., 1998). The exact functions of ataxin-3 are under investigation. Ataxin-3 might be a ubiquitin-binding protein (Hofmann & Falquet, 2001) and could participate in proteasomal protein degradation (Wang et al., 2000).

Neuropathology

Macroscopic examination shows a depigmentation of the substantia nigra, cerebellar atrophy, and atrophy of the pons and medulla oblongata, as well as atrophy of cranial nerves III to XII (Rüb et al., 2006). Recent studies have demonstrated widespread damage to the cerebellum, thalamus, midbrain, pons, medulla oblongata, and spinal cord. The cerebellar dentate nucleus, the substantia nigra, and a subset of vestibular, oculomotor, and precerebellar nuclei are the early targets of the degenerative process of SCA3, while the thalamus, ingestion-related brainstem nuclei, and the rest of the cranial nerve and precerebellar nuclei are affected only later during the course of the disease (Riess et al., 2008).

Like in most polyglutamine diseases, intranuclear aggregates and neuronal cell loss are found in selected areas of the brain.

Animal models of SCA3

Mice transgenic for the CAG repeat expansion show neurodegeneration (Ikeda et al., 1996). *Drosophila* models overexpressing mutant ataxin-3 mimic some of the features of SCA3 in humans, such as intranuclear inclusions and late-onset neurodegeneration (Warrick et al., 1998).

Spinocerebellar ataxia type 4

Clinical presentation

Spinocerebellar ataxia type 4 (SCA4; also known as hereditary ataxia with sensory neuropathy) has been reported in a pedigree of Scandinavian origin. Onset of SCA4 is usually in the fourth or fifth decade, with a range from 19 to 61 years (Flanigan et al., 1996;

Hellenbroich et al., 2003). Ataxia progresses over decades and leads to wheelchair dependence in most cases. The phenotype includes ataxia with a prominent axonal sensory neuropathy. The earliest symptoms are usually composed of difficulties of gait and fine motor tasks, as well as speech difficulties. All patients have loss of vibratory and joint position sense. Pinprick sensation is commonly impaired. Tendon reflexes are abolished at the ankles. A majority of patients also have decreased or absent knee reflexes. Full tendon areflexia occurs in 25% of cases. Babinski sign is observed in up to 20% of cases.

A possibly related endemic cerebellar syndrome (see also SCA type 31 in page 268) has been reported in the Nagano area of Japan (Shimizu et al., 2004; Ishikawa et al., 2005; Yoshida et al., 2009). The frequency of this ataxia is much higher than in the other areas of Japan. This autosomal dominant cerebellar ataxia (ADCA) might be the third most common form in Japan, after MJD and spinocerebellar ataxia type 6 (SCA6) (Ouyang et al., 2006). Age of onset is 30 to 78 years in the series of Yoshida et al. (2009). Patients show a relatively pure cerebellar ataxia of late onset, similarly to SCA6. However, dementia and hearing impairment have been reported in patients over 65 years of age.

Electrophysiology

Sural sensory nerve action potentials are absent in the majority of cases.

There is audiological evidence of mild to moderate bilateral sensorineural hearing loss in Japanese 16q-ADCA.

Genetic and molecular aspects

SCA4 maps to chromosome 16q22.1 (Flanigan et al., 1996). This locus overlaps with the 16q-ADCA described in Japan. A single nucleotide substitution ($-16C>T$) in the 5′ untranslated region of the gene encoding puratrophin-1 is a specific marker for 16q-ADCA (Ishikawa et al., 2005). This specific substitution has been found exclusively in the Japanese population (Wieczorek et al., 2006).

Neuropathology

Neuropathological studies show widespread cerebellar and brainstem neurodegeneration with marked neuronal loss (Hellenbroich et al., 2006). Severe neuronal

loss is found in the Purkinje cell layer of the cerebellum and in the cerebellar nuclei. Degeneration of the posterior columns and roots of the spinal cord is observed. Immunocytochemical analysis using the anti-polyglutamine antibody 1C2 does not detect any polyglutamine-related immunoreactivity, supporting the hypothesis that SCA4 is not a member of the CAG-repeat or polyglutamine diseases (Hellenbroich et al., 2006).

Purkinje cell degeneration is the most prominent pathological finding in the 16q-ADCA in the endemic Nagano area (Owada et al., 2005).

Spinocerebellar ataxia type 5

Clinical presentation

Spinocerebellar ataxia type 5 (SCA5) has been initially reported in an American kindred descending from President Abraham Lincoln. Onset of the disease varies from 10 to 68 years, with most cases starting in the third or fourth decade (Ranum et al., 1994). The disease is characterized by anticipation in most individuals. Juvenile cases (onset between 10 and 18 years) are maternally inherited. The overall clinical phenotype is a slowly progressive cerebellar syndrome resembling the phenotype of SCA6, with patients remaining ambulatory after 25 to 30 years of progression. Nystagmus is a consistent feature (Burk et al., 2004). Other common features include impaired smooth pursuit, ataxia of stance and gait, limb ataxia, dysarthria, and kinetic tremor. There is no sign of bulbar paralysis in most cases, although some bulbar involvement may develop in juvenile patients. Mild sensory impairment is noted in one-third of cases. Tendon hyporeflexia or hyperreflexia has been reported.

Neuroimaging

MRI shows atrophy of the cerebellar vermis and hemispheres. There is a relative sparing in the inferior vermis. Mild brainstem atrophy may be detected at a late stage.

Genetic and molecular aspects

SCA5 maps to chromosome 11q13. Deletions and missense mutations in the beta-III spectrin gene (STBN2) cause SCA5. Spectrin mutations affect glutamate signaling. Beta-3 spectrin is highly expressed in Purkinje cells and stabilizes the glutamate transporter EAAT4 at the surface of the cell membrane. Cell culture studies show that mutant beta-III spectrin fails to stabilize EAAT4 at the cell membrane (Ikeda et al., 2006).

Neuropathology

SCA5 appears mainly as cerebellar degeneration mainly affecting the cortex.

Spinocerebellar ataxia type 6

Clinical presentation

Early signs of spinocerebellar ataxia type 6 (SCA6) are often insidious. The age at onset ranges from 19 to 73 years, with average age at onset of 45 years (Ishikawa et al., 1997; Schöls et al., 1998). Anticipation of age of onset occurs over successive generations. The course is slowly progressive in most cases, although a rapid course has been described (Watanabe et al., 1998). Lifespan usually appears normal. Gait ataxia is the initial symptom in most cases and usually remains the chief symptom throughout the clinical course. Patients often complain of vertigo, oscillopsia, or blurred vision (Jen et al., 1998). At the beginning of the disease, symptoms may be intermittent. Patients present with cerebellar dysarthria, limb ataxia, decreased muscle tone, and horizontal/vertical gaze nystagmus. Tendon reflexes are normal or slightly increased. Proprioceptive sensory loss is found in some patients. Pyramidal or extra-pyramidal tract signs or ophthalmoparesis is usually absent, although reported in rare cases.

There is an overlap between SCA6, episodic ataxia type 2 (EA2, see section Episodic ataxias), and familial hemiplegic migraine (Sinke et al., 2001).

Neuroimaging

Atrophy of the vermis is moderate to severe on brain MRI. There is a mild atrophy of the cerebellar hemispheres and usually no atrophy of the middle cerebellar peduncles, pons, or other posterior fossa structures (Schöls et al., 1998; Satoh et al., 1998). Size reduction of the anterior-posterior diameter of the pons has been reported (Murata et al., 1998). Red nucleus may be slightly atrophied. In general, there are no signal abnormalities on T2-weighted and/or proton-weighted axial MRI in SCA6 patients (Murata et al., 1998; Döhlinger et al., 2008).

PET using labeled glucose shows a significant hypometabolism in SCA6 patients, ranging from 63% to 78% of control values, in the brainstem, cerebellar hemisphere, basal ganglia, and various areas of the cortex (Soong et al., 2001).

Electrophysiology

Electrooculography shows normal saccadic velocity with a gaze-evoked nystagmus. A down-beat nystagmus may be recorded. Saccades are dysmetric. Reduced gain for pursuit tracking may be detected in presymptomatic cases. The VOR is hyperactive. Early functional oculomotor impairments in SCA6 are caused by neuronal dysfunction and/or loss in the posterior cerebellar vermis and flocculus (Christova et al., 2008). Some patients present with a mild sensorimotor axonal neuropathy. Visual evoked potentials are normal. Auditory evoked potentials are abnormal in two-thirds of patients. Somatosensory evoked potentials show a delayed P40 wave in one-third of patients. Central motor conduction time is normal. Polysomnography reveals periodic leg movements in sleep in some patients.

Genetic and molecular aspects

SCA6 is associated with an expansion of a CAG repeat in the human alpha-1A-voltage-dependent Ca(2+) channel gene CACNA1A which maps to 19p13 (Zhuchenko et al., 1997). SCA6 can thus be classified among channelopathies. Normal alleles range from 4 to 18 units, with expanding alleles ranging from 20 to 30 repeats. This number is relatively small as compared with polyglutamine disorders. There is an inverse correlation between the age at onset and the length of the expanded allele and also between the age at onset and the sum of CAG repeats in the normal and the expanded alleles (Takahashi et al., 2004). Homozygous patients show a slightly earlier onset and a more rapid course as compared with heterozygous patients (Takiyama et al., 1998).

Using reverse-transcriptase polymerase chain reaction and in situ hybridization, Ishikawa et al. have demonstrated that the calcium channel mRNA/protein containing the CAG repeat/polyglutamine tract is most intensely expressed in Purkinje cells of normal human brains (Ishikawa et al., 1999).

Whereas SCA6 is due to an expansion of a repeat sequence, EA2 and familial hemiplegic migraine are associated with point mutations or missense mutations.

Figure 23.9 Purkinje cell atrophy in SCA-6. (A) and (B): Immunofluorescence with anti-calbindin-1. (A) SCA-6; (B) normal. The fluorescent reaction product shows the reduction in the size of Purkinje cell bodies and the simplification of the dendritic tree in SCA-6. Magnification markers: 50 μm. From: Koeppen, 2005. With permission.

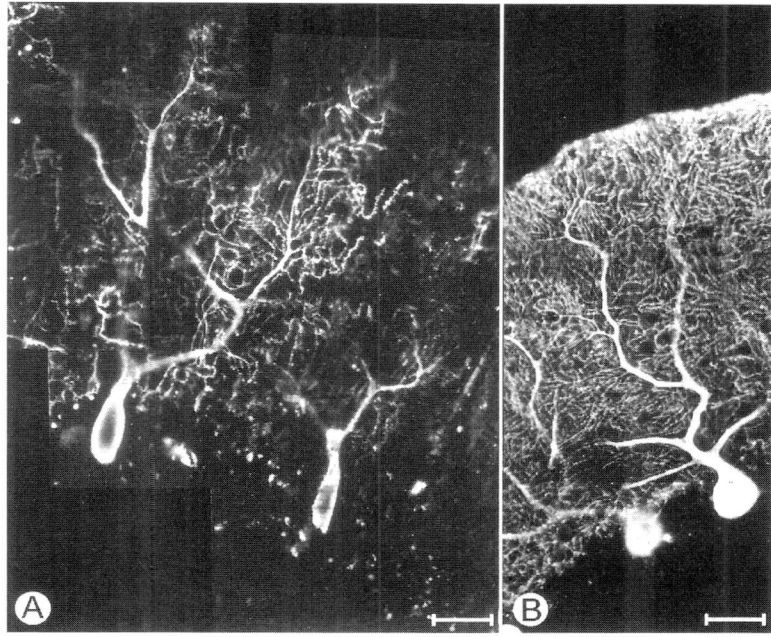

Neuropathology

The loss of Purkinje neurons is extensive (Figure 23.9), with proliferation of Bergmann glia. Granule cell loss is less severe. Reduced neuronal cell population occurs in the inferior olivary complex. This is interpreted as a change secondary to the cerebellar cortical lesion. Atrophy of the brainstem has occasionally been reported (Zhuchenko et al., 1997). Numerous oval or rod-shaped aggregates are observed exclusively in the cytoplasm of Purkinje cells. These cytoplasmic inclusions are not ubiquitinated, in contrast with the neuronal intranuclear inclusions of other CAG repeat/polyglutamine diseases.

Spinocerebellar ataxia type 7

Clinical presentation

Clinical severity in spinocerebellar ataxia type 7 (SCA7) ranges from infantile onset with early death to elderly presentations of slowly progressive ataxia. Cerebellar ataxia, which presents with walking difficulties, limb clumsiness, and speech deficits, is the most common clinical feature of SCA7. SCA7 patients may develop dysarthria, dysphagia, hypoacusis, and eye movement deficits (slowing of saccades; staring) which can evolve into ophthalmoplegia. Involvement of the corticospinal tracts cause exaggerated deep ten-don reflexes, spasticity, and extensor plantar reflexes (Giunti et al., 1999).

Neuroimaging

Brain MRI shows a marked atrophy of the cerebellum and pons. In some patients, a high T2-weighted signal intensity is observed in transverse pontine fibers. Volumetric analysis shows a greater pontine atrophy as compared with other SCAs. Volume loss might occur in the pons prior to the development of cerebellar atrophy, indicating that the primary site of disease onset could be the brainstem (Bang et al., 2004).

Neurophysiology

Loss of the P100 wave on visual evoked potentials occurs in all patients. Auditory evoked potentials are abnormal in most cases. Nerve conduction velocities are normal.

Genetic and molecular aspects

Localization of the gene responsible for the SCA7 phenotype showed linkage to chromosome 3p12-21.1 (Benomar et al., 1995). The gene codes for a protein called ataxin-7 (David et al., 1997). Healthy individuals possess ataxin-7 repeats ranging in size from 7 to 34 CAGs. Expansions beyond 37 CAGs cause the

SCA7 phenotype. There is a correlation between repeat length and the type of clinical presentation in SCA7. Repeat mutations with less than 59 CAGs are often associated with initial cerebellar findings, whereas those with more than 59 CAGs typically induce visual impairment as the first symptom (Johansson et al., 1998). Anticipation is marked in SCA7. When very long repeats are inherited, patients exhibit an early-onset rapidly progressive juvenile form or even a severe infantile form characterized by a widespread disease pathology including extra-neurological involvement (Benton et al., 1998).

Expansion of the polyQ tract leads to accumulation of the mutant protein in nuclear inclusions and to selective neuronal and photoreceptor degeneration. Mutant ataxin-7 has been localized to nuclear inclusions, together with a host of other proteins, including ubiquitin-proteasome components (Holmberg et al., 1998). Ataxin-7 is expressed throughout the CNS and in many extra-neurological organs. Ataxin-7 is a component of a transcription coactivator complex called STAGA, which mediates interactions between upstream transcription activators and the RNA polymerase II transcription complex (Conaway et al., 2005).

Neuropathology

Patients with SCA7 develop atrophy of the cerebellar cortex, dentate nuclei, inferior olivary complex and olivocerebellar tract, spinocerebellar tract, subthalamic nucleus, and pyramidal tracts (Michalik et al., 2004). Loss of Purkinje neurons is extensive and contrasts with the mild neuronal loss in the cerebellar granule layer. Marked neuronal loss with gliosis may occur in the inferior olive. Neuronal loss is also found in the motor nuclei of cranial nerves (III, IV, and XII), spinal motor neurons, and substantia nigra. Demyelination of the pyramidal tracts and of the posterior columns of the spinal cord is found. As for other polyQ-expanded proteins, nuclear inclusions are commonly observed.

Dentatorubral-pallidoluysian atrophy

Epidemiology

The terminology of dentatorubral-pallidoluysian atrophy (DRPLA) was originally coined by Smith et al. to report the severe cell loss in the dentatorubral and pallidoluysian systems in a sporadic case (Smith et al., 1958). Familial cases were first reported by Naito and Oyanagi (1982). DRPLA occurs mainly in Japan (Sasaki et al., 2003), although cases are reported in other ethnic groups in European and North American families (Farmer et al., 1989; Connarty et al., 1996). The prevalence of DRPLA in Japan has been estimated at 0.2 to 0.7 per 100 000.

Clinical presentation

The onset of DRPLA ranges from childhood to late adulthood (range 1–62 years; mean 30 years). Patients exhibit various combinations of cerebellar ataxia, choreoathetosis, epilepsy, myoclonus, dementia, and psychiatric symptoms (Naito & Oyanagi, 1982). A main feature of DRPLA is the substantial clinical heterogeneity. The juvenile form (onset before the age of 20 years) is characterized by progressive myoclonus epilepsy (PME; tonic, clonic, tonic-clonic, absent, or atonic seizures) with intellectual deterioration (see Chapter 17 for the differential diagnosis of PMEs). In patients with onset between 20 and 40 years, the occurrence of seizures decreases. These latter are relatively rare when the disease presents after the age of 40. When the disease presents after the age of 20, the main phenotype is composed of cerebellar ataxia, choreoathetosis, and dementia, mimicking Huntington disease or other ADCAs. Cervical dystonia was the presenting feature in one family (Hatano et al., 2003). Corneal endothelial degeneration has been reported (Ito et al., 2002).

Neuroimaging

Atrophic changes in the cerebellum and brainstem, in particular, the pontomesencephalic tegmentum, are the typical MRI findings. Areas of increased intensity signals on T2-weighted images and fluid-attenuated inversion recovery images are commonly found in the cerebral white matter (Yoshii et al., 1998). Exceptionally, the appearance of the pons is reminiscent of a central pontine myelinolysis, with low-intensity signal on T1-weighted sequence and high-intensity signal on T2-weighted sequence (Kobayashi et al., 2009).

A genotype-phenotype correlation exists on brain MRI (Koide et al., 1997). There is a marked inverse correlation between the areas of the cerebellum and brainstem and the length of the expanded CAG repeat, when large expansions (>66) are considered.

Neurophysiology

Electroencephalogram (EEG) recordings show features suggestive of a PME (see Chapter 17). Partial seizures are persistently recorded throughout the clinical course in juvenile cases (Egawa et al., 2008). Brief generalized seizures (atypical absence and myoclonic seizure) are observed in about 50% of patients at the early stage, whereas generalized tonic-clonic seizures occur in advanced-stage patients.

Genetic and molecular aspects

DRPLA is characterized by a prominent anticipation (Koide et al., 1994). Anticipation is more severe with paternal transmission (26–29 years/generation) than with maternal transmission (14–15 years/generation).

The gene has been mapped to 12p13.31 (Takano et al., 1998). In normal individuals, the size of the CAG repeat is 6 to 35 (Koide et al., 1994). The size of the expansion is 48 to 93 repeat units in patients with DRPLA. Analysis of the distribution of normal DRPLA alleles by size has shown that CAG repeats larger than 17 repeats are significantly more frequent in the Japanese population than in Caucasian populations (Burke et al., 1994; Takano et al., 1998). The transcript is widely expressed in various tissues, without predilection for regions exhibiting neurodegeneration (Onodera et al., 1995). The CAG repeat expansion does not impair transcription or translation efficiency of the mutant DRPLA gene (Tsuji, 2002). Mutant proteins are neurotoxic (gain of toxicity).

Neuropathology

The major neuropathologic changes detected by conventional neuropathologic observations mainly consist of combined degeneration of the dentatorubral and pallidoluysian systems. Autopsy studies of white matter lesions show diffuse myelin pallor and reactive astrogliosis in the cerebral white matter, with only mild atherosclerotic changes (Munoz et al., 2004). Neuronal intranuclear inclusions are found (Hayashi et al., 1998, Igarashi et al., 1998). Accumulation of mutant DRPLA protein (atrophin-1) in the neuronal nuclei is detected as a diffuse nuclear staining by the antibody specifically detecting expanded polyglutamine stretches.

Spinocerebellar ataxia type 8

Clinical presentation

Onset of symptoms for spinocerebellar ataxia type 8 (SCA8) ranges from age 18 to 72 years, with a mean in the fourth or fifth decade (Koob et al., 1999; Ikeda et al., 2000). Dysarthria and gait instability are the initial symptoms in many cases. Dysarthria has ataxic and spastic components (Day et al., 2000). Patients exhibit nystagmus, limb and gait ataxia, limb spasticity, and diminished vibration perception. Tendon hyperreflexia is common. Babinski sign is noted in severely affected individuals (Juvonen et al., 2000). Occasionally, intermittent low-amplitude myoclonic jerks in the fingers and arms and athetotic movements of extended fingers are observed (Ikeda et al., 2008). Patients may exhibit a rapidly progressive parkinsonism-plus syndrome resembling corticobasal degeneration (Baba et al., 2005; see Chapter 12).

Progression is generally slow, but severely affected individuals become nonambulatory by the fourth to fifth decade. The need for mobility aids usually occurs approximately 20 years after the presentation of initial symptoms. Disease severity appears to correlate with repeat length and age.

Neuroimaging

MRI shows pancerebellar atrophy. There is little or no involvement of the brainstem, basal ganglia, and cerebral hemispheres. Progression of cerebellar atrophy follows the slowly clinical worsening (Day et al., 2000). In some cases, cerebellar atrophy evolves over a relatively short period of time (Zeman et al., 2004).

Genetic and molecular aspects

The mutation for SCA8 was initially characterized as a dominantly inherited ataxia with a CTG repeat expansion mutation in the non-coding region of the SCA8 gene (see also non-coding mutations in SCA10 and SCA12).

The SCA8 gene is located on chromosome 13q21. The expanded alleles range from 89 to 155 repeats (normal range 15 to 34 repeats). In humans, there are three different genes: ATXN8, ATXN8OS (previously known as SCA8 or KLHL1AS), and Kelch-like 1 (KLHL1, encoding an actin-binding protein expressed in the CNS and with no overlap with the repeat located in close proximity). The SCA8 expansion is expressed in both directions (CUG and CAG). The gene expressed in the CAG direction encodes a pure polyglutamine expansion protein (ataxin 8). The expression of non-coding (CUG)n expansion transcripts (ataxin 8 opposite strand; expression of a non-coding CUG expansion RNA) suggests that SCA8 pathogenesis may involve a toxic gain-of-function mechanism at both the protein and RNA levels.

Expansion carriers may be clinically unaffected at the time of evaluation (Ikeda et al., 2008). The repeat lengths among these asymptomatic carriers are significantly shorter than those of affected individuals, indicating that disease penetrance is influenced by CTG-CAG repeat length. SCA8 expansions found among ataxia patients vary in size, and SCA8 expansions cannot be used to predict whether or not asymptomatic carriers will develop a cerebellar syndrome (Ikeda et al., 2004). While the linkage and size-dependent penetrance of the SCA8 CTG • CAG expansion argue that the SCA8 expansion causes ataxia, the reduced penetrance in some SCA8 families and the discovery of expansions in the general population have led to a controversy regarding the pathogenic aspect of the SCA8 expansion. In a patient with cerebellar deficits and dysautonomia, and in whom MRI showed cerebellar and pontine atrophy, molecular analysis demonstrated an expansion of 145 CTA-CTG repeats in one allele and 28 repeats in the other allele. This was consistent with SCA8. However, post-mortem examination showed findings of multiple-system atrophy (Factor et al., 2005). Therefore, testing sporadic cases with late-onset ataxia may lead to a misdiagnosis of SCA8. SCA8 expansions have also been reported in individuals with positive gene tests for SCA1, SCA6, Friedreich ataxia, Alzheimer disease, and Parkinson disease (Sobrido et al., 2001; Ikeda et al., 2008).

Neuropathology

Post-mortem examination shows cerebellar atrophy with severe loss of Purkinje neurons and mild granule cell loss (Ito et al., 2006). The inferior olives also show neuronal loss, but the dentate nucleus is relatively preserved. There is extensive gliosis in the periaqueductal gray matter. Substantia nigra appears depigmented.

Animal models

A *Drosophila* model in which human SCA8 cDNA transcripts (ATXN8OS) are overexpressed in photoreceptor neurons has been generated (Mutsuddi et al., 2004). Transcripts containing either the CUG expansion or the normal length repeat induce a late-onset, neurodegenerative phenotype.

A mouse model with SCA8 expansion develops a progressive neurological phenotype, arguing for the pathogenicity of the (CTG • CAG)n expansion. These mice show a loss of cerebellar GABAergic inhibition and, similar to human patients, have positive intranuclear inclusions in Purkinje cells and other neurons. Mice that are either homozygous or heterozygous for the KLHL1 gene deletion have significant gait abnormalities at an early age and develop a significant loss of motor coordination, suggesting that loss of KLHL1 activity is likely to play a significant part in the pathophysiology of SCA8 (He et al., 2006).

Spinocerebellar ataxia type 10

Geographical distribution

All the spinocerebellar ataxia type 10 (SCA10) families are from Latin America, including Mexican families and Brazilian families. SCA10 is the second most common SCA in these populations, secondary to SCA2 in Mexico and SCA3 in Brazil.

Clinical presentation

The course is progressive, often resulting in severe disability. SCA10 patients exhibit a cerebellar syndrome (Matsuura et al., 1999). Ocular abnormalities include ocular dysmetria, most commonly presenting as intrusions of hypometric saccade during pursuit, which may progress to overt ocular flutter with brief conjugate oscillations of the eyes during attempted fixation or movement (Lin & Ashizawa, 2005). Gaze-evoked nystagmus may be observed in some patients. Irregularity in ocular pursuit is often seen in early stages of the disease. Speech is slurred or scanning. Patients also exhibit a wide-based ataxic gait with impaired tandem test, dysdiadochokinesia, kinetic tremor, and dysmetria. Seizures are variably associated with SCA10. Seizures are present only in families of Mexican origin, and the prevalence between families is also significantly different, ranging from 25% to 80% (Lin & Ashizawa, 2005). Patients present with generalized motor seizure and/or complex partial seizures. Status epilepticus has occurred in a few patients. Some SCA10 patients of Mexican origin have additional deficits beyond cerebellar degeneration.

Deficits include pyramidal signs (hyperreflexia, spasticity, Babinski sign) and mild sensory loss in distal lower extremities. Individuals may have low IQ and may present with depressive, aggressive, and/or irritable traits (Lin & Ashizawa, 2005). In one family, hepatic, cardiac, and hematological abnormalities have been reported.

Neuroimaging

Brain MRI or CT shows pancerebellar atrophy. Other brain structures, such as the brainstem or cerebral cortex, are only minimally involved.

Neurophysiology

Interictal EEG is abnormal in many SCA10 patients with epilepsy and in some individuals without seizures. The most common findings are diffuse cortical dysfunction with slow, fused, and disorganized activities. Focal cortical irritability or slow activity may be observed. Nerve conduction studies may confirm the presence of a peripheral neuropathy.

Genetic and molecular aspects

SCA10 is caused by a microsatellite repeat expansion primarily composed of ATTCT pentanucleotide repeats. It is localized in intron 9 of a gene on chromosome 22q13.3 designated as ATXN10 (previously known as E46L). SCA10 is the only known human disease caused by an expansion of pentanucleotide repeats (Matsuura et al., 2000). The number of the ATTCT repeat units is polymorphic and ranges from 10 to 29 in the normal population. The expanded allele ranges from 800 to 4500, one of the largest microsatellite repeat expansions in the human genome. The size of the expanded repeat shows an inverse correlation with the age of onset. The repeats are highly unstable during paternal transmission. By contrast, maternal transmission is relatively stable. Sperm DNA has a marked heterogeneity in the size of the expanded allele, contributing to the high degree of instability in the male germline. The inter-tissue variability in terms of ATTCT repeats raises the issue of DNA sampling, which is routinely collected from peripheral blood leukocytes (Lin & Ashizawa, 2005). Precautions should be taken for diagnosis and counseling when the repeat length derived from peripheral blood leukocyte DNA is used to correlate with pathology in the CNS and age of onset (Lin & Ashizawa, 2005).

ATTCT repeats are characterized by the high content of A-T, a feature of DNA sequences that form unpaired structures when under torsional stress, called DNA unwinding elements (Potaman et al., 2003). Expansion of ATTCT repeats facilitates DNA unwinding, resulting in aberrant replication initiation (Lin & Ashizawa, 2005).

The SCA10 gene encodes a protein of 475 amino acids, called ataxin-10. "Knock-down" of SCA10 in primary cerebellar and cortical neurons in culture by small interfering RNAs (siRNAs) induces apoptosis (Marz et al., 2004). Cerebellar neurons are significantly more sensitive to reduced levels of ataxin-10. It is likely that RNA gain-of-function is an integral part of SCA10 pathogenesis (Lin & Ashizawa, 2005).

Spinocerebellar ataxia type 11
Clinical presentation

The mean age of onset for spinocerebellar ataxia type 11 (SCA11) is 24.2±8.4 years, ranging from 15 to 43 years (Worth et al., 1999; Johnson et al., 2008). The disease has a relatively slow progressive course. Life expectancy is normal (mean age at death 69.7±13.1 years). Patients exhibit a relatively pure cerebellar syndrome, with dysarthria, oculomotor ataxia (jerky pursuit, horizontal or vertical nystagmus), limb ataxia, and truncal ataxia. Although some patients present with tendon hyperreflexia, there is no Babinski sign.

Neuroimaging

Brain MRI shows a marked atrophy restricted to the cerebellar hemispheres.

Genetic aspects

The locus is at chromosome 15q14-q21.3 (Worth et al., 1999). Insertion of one base and a frameshift deletion of two bases have been reported in the gene encoding tau tubulin kinase-2 (TTBK2) (Houlden et al., 2007). TTBK2 encodes a member of the casein kinase (CK1) group of protein kinases.

Neuropathology

Gross examination shows atrophy of the cerebellum without brainstem involvement (Johnson et al., 2008). Examination of the cerebellum demonstrates a severe loss in the Purkinje cell layer with empty "baskets." There is a proliferation of Bergmann glial cells and cerebellar astroglial cells that have their somas in the Purkinje cell layer. No intranuclear inclusions are found. There is evidence that the medulla is atrophic. A tangle pathology is not excluded.

Spinocerebellar ataxia type 12

Clinical presentation

Spinocerebellar ataxia type 12 (SCA12) is a rare SCA described in European-American and Asian (Indian) pedigrees (Holmes et al., 1999; Cholfin et al., 2001). Age of onset ranges from 8 to 55 years. Clinically, the distinguishing feature is an early and prominent action tremor, with variability in other signs. Tremor typically begins in the fourth decade, progressing over several decades to include head tremor, gait ataxia, limb dysmetria, dysdiadochokinesia, tendon hyperreflexia, oculomotor deficits, and dementia in advanced cases. Extra-pyramidal features and pyramidal deficits are less commonly observed. Psychiatric symptoms, including depression, anxiety, or delusions, are present in some affected family members (O'Hearn et al., 2001).

Neuroimaging

MRI or CT scans show both cortical and cerebellar atrophy. White matter hyperintensities are commonly observed.

Electrophysiology

A peripheral neuropathy is detected in about 25% of patients. Signs of autonomic dysfunction are found in about one-third of cases.

Genetic and molecular aspects

SCA12 is caused by CAG repeat expansion in the noncoding region of the PPP2R2B gene, which has been mapped to 5q31-q33. The repeat size ranges from 55 to 78 triplets in the mutant allele of affected individuals and from 9 to 28 triplets in normal alleles (Holmes et al., 1999). Homozygosity is not associated with a more severe course. The PPP2R2B gene encodes Bbeta1 and Bbeta2, alternatively spliced and neuron-specific regulatory subunits of the protein phosphatase 2A (PP2A) holoenzyme. The expansion might predispose to neuronal death by promoting mitochondrial division (Dagda et al., 2008).

Spinocerebellar ataxia type 13

Clinical presentation

Spinocerebellar ataxia type 13 (SCA13) was originally described in a four-generation French family, but has now also been reported in a large Filipino pedigree (Waters & Pulst, 2008). These two families represent the only well-characterized genotype-phenotype correlations so far. A striking feature in the French family is the childhood onset with minimal progression of disease. Patients exhibit a typical cerebellar syndrome. Absence seizures (with typical 3-Hz spike and wave complexes on EEG recordings) have been reported. A mild to moderate global cognitive impairment is found, with IQ between 62 and 76. The Filipino pedigree is characterized by an adult-onset dominant ataxia with prominent cerebellar signs. Some patients exhibit a mild hyperreflexia without a Babinski sign.

Neuroimaging

Cerebral MRI performed on one patient with a disease duration of 3 years has shown a cerebellar atrophy restricted to the vermis, with enlargement of the fourth ventricle and a slight atrophy of the pons and the medulla (Stevanin et al., 2005).

Genetic and functional aspects

Heterozygous mutations are detected in the affected members. Mutations in the voltage-gated potassium channel KCNC3 (chromosome 19q13.3-q13.4) are responsible for SCA13 (Herman-Bert et al., 2000). Sequence analysis of KCNC3 shows mutations 1639C→A (F448L) in the French and 1554G→A (R420H) in the Filipino pedigrees. In the Filipino pedigree, the G→A transition in exon 2 causes an arginine-to-histidine substitution (R420H) in the S4 transmembrane functional segment, which is the principal voltage-sensing element of the protein.

The functional properties of KCNC3 channels are unique among voltage-gated K+ channels. These channels activate in a more depolarized range and close more rapidly than other Kv channels, facilitating high-frequency firing of action potentials. This is a characteristic of burst neuron populations found in the mammalian neocortex, hippocampus, auditory nuclei, substantia nigra, and cerebellum (Rudy & McBain, 2001; Martina et al., 2003). KCNC3 is expressed in Purkinje cells, cerebellar granule cells, and cerebellar neurons. It forms heteromultimeric channels by coassembly with KCNC1 and/or KCNC4. Initial characterization of KCNC3 expression detected the highest levels of messenger ribonucleic acid (mRNA) expression in the cerebellar cortex, inferior colliculus, hindbrain, and spinal cord. There is a particular mRNA enrichment in terminally differentiated Purkinje cells and deep cerebellar nuclei (Weiser et al., 1994).

SCA13 mutations not only impair the firing properties of fast-spiking cerebellar neurons and influence neuronal function, but also interfere with the capacity of cerebellar neurons to handle oxidative stress (Duprat, 1995; Waters et al., 2006).

Spinocerebellar ataxia type 14

Clinical presentation

Spinocerebellar ataxia type 14 (SCA14) has been discovered in a Japanese family with an autosomal dominant neurodegenerative disorder characterized by cerebellar ataxia and intermittent axial myoclonus. Other families have been reported in Europe (van de Warrenburg et al., 2003). Age of onset ranges from childhood to age 60 years (Stevanin et al., 2004). Ataxia is frequently associated with brisk reflexes. A cognitive impairment may be present, and myoclonic jerks may also be observed in limbs. Some patients exhibit dystonia, and others have reduced vibration sense in lower limbs.

Neuroimaging

Brain MRI shows pure cerebellar atrophy.

Genetic and functional aspects

SCA14 is caused by missense mutations in the protein kinase C gamma (PRKCG) gene in chromosome 19q13.4-qter (Brkanac et al., 2002; Yabe et al., 2003). In-frame deletion and a possible splice site mutation have been reported (Chen et al., 2005).

Expression of the protein is high in the brain, especially in the cerebellar cortex. Mutations increase the intrinsic activity of PRKCG. The mutant protein translocates more rapidly to selected regions of the plasma membrane in response to Ca2+ influx (Verbeek et al., 2005). Mutant proteins tend to aggregate in the cytoplasm (Seki et al., 2005).

Spinocerebellar ataxia type 15–type 16

Clinical presentation

Spinocerebellar ataxia type 15 (SCA15) has been originally described in an Australian kindred with a dominantly inherited pure cerebellar ataxia (Gardner et al., 2005). Ataxia has a slow progression. A mild degree of gait ataxia after three or more decades of disease duration has been observed. Some patients have evidence of mental impairment. Japanese families exhibiting ataxia and postural/action tremor have been reported. This syndrome was initially called spinocerebellar ataxia type 16 (SCA16) (Iwaki et al., 2008). Age at onset ranges from 20 to 66 years. Additional families have been reported to link to the SCA15 locus.

Neuroimaging

Brain MRI shows pure cerebellar atrophy, particularly in the vermis.

Genetic and functional aspects

SCA15 and SCA16 are associated with deletions of the inositol 1,4,5-triphosphate receptor (ITPR1) gene (Knight et al., 2003; van de Leemput et al., 2007). IPTR1 mediates calcium release from the endoplasmic reticulum in various neurons, in particular, the Purkinje neurons (Hartmann & Konnerth, 2005). The disease locus maps to chromosome 3p24.2-3pter. Deletions identified in the SCA15 families also include the neighboring sulfatase modifying factor 1 (SUMF1) gene, a causative gene for multiple sulfatase deficiency (Hara et al., 2008; see also Chapter 20). This autosomal recessive disorder presents with mental retardation, seizure, and leukodystrophy (Cosma et al., 2003). Individuals with heterozygous mutations in the SUMF1 gene are asymptomatic.

Spinocerebellar ataxia type 17 (Huntington disease–like 4 [HDL4])

Epidemiology

The minimal prevalence of spinocerebellar ataxia type 17 (SCA17) has been estimated at 0.16 per 100 000 in the northeast of England (Craig et al., 2005). Most families are from Japan (n517 families) (Nakamura et al., 2001) and Germany (Rolfs et al., 2003). Other families are from Italy, Taiwan, England, France, Belgium,

Table 23.6 Clinical symptoms in SCA17

Cerebellar ataxia (gait ataxia, dysarthria, dysmetria)

Dementia

Psychiatric symptoms
    Behavioral changes
    Psychosis
    Depression

Pyramidal signs

Dystonia, chorea, choreoathetosis

Parkinsonism

Epilepsy

the United States, and Portugal (Stevanin & Brice, 2008). Several cases with de novo expansions have been reported.

Clinical presentation

SCA17 has a progressive course. Mean age at onset is 35 years, with a range from 3 to 75 years. Mean disease duration is 19 ± 9 years (Stevanin & Brice, 2008). Mean age of death is 40 ± 20 years. SCA17 is clinically heterogeneous. The most common symptoms are gait difficulties, extra-pyramidal signs, psychiatric disturbances, and dementia (see Table 23.6; Fujigasaki et al., 2001; Stevanin et al., 2003). Cerebellar deficits include ataxia of stance/gait, limb dysmetria, and dysarthria. Gaze-evoked nystagmus and deficits in saccades are uncommon. Dementia affects up to 75% of patients, whereas early dementia is relatively rare in ADCA, with the exception of DRPLA. Prior to the molecular genetic diagnosis, several patients had been diagnosed as having Huntington disease. Patients with a progressive cerebellar syndrome exhibiting dementia and extra-pyramidal signs should be screened for SCA17. Hypogonadotropic hypogonadism has been reported in monozygotic twins (Rolfs et al., 2003). Parkinson disease–like, Creutzfeldt-Jakob disease–like, and Alzheimer disease–like phenotypes have also been reported with small SCA17 expansions.

Differential diagnosis

Differential diagnosis includes Huntington disease–like 2 (HDL2), familial prion disease (Wild & Tabrizi, 2007; see Chapter 11), and neuroferritinopathy (Burn & Chinnery, 2006). HDL2 is a neurodegenerative disorder found in people of African ancestry with clinical, radiological, and neuropathological manifestations similar to Huntington disease. HDL2 is caused

by a pathological expansion of CAG/CTG triplets in exon 2A of the junctophilin JPH3 gene at chromosome 16. Neuroferritinopathy (also called hereditary ferritinopathy and neurodegeneration with brain iron accumulation type 2 [NBIA2]) is an autosomal dominant disorder caused by a mutation in the ferritin light chain gene (FTL). Age of onset ranges from 13 to 63 years. The main presentation is a movement disorder suggestive of a basal ganglia dysfunction: dystonia, chorea, and dyskinesia (Burn & Chinnery, 2006). A cerebellar phenotype associated with cerebellar atrophy and cerebellar hypometabolism has been reported (Ory-Magne et al., 2009). Cognitive deficits are usually subtle. Serum level of ferritin is normal or decreased. Brain MRI shows iron deposits in the brain, especially in the globus pallidus. Pathological deposits are found in the liver, kidney, muscle, and skin.

Neuroimaging

Brain MRI may be normal when the first symptoms appear. Patients may also present with moderate global atrophy or focal cerebellar atrophy. After several years, the atrophy is always pronounced in the cerebellum. There is a relative sparing of the brainstem. The cerebral cortex and caudate nuclei become atrophic with time. Putaminal rim hyperintensities have been described (Loy et al., 2005). VBM confirms the degeneration of the gray matter centered around medial cerebellar structures, occipitoparietal structures, the anterior putamen, the thalamus, and other parts of the motor network, reflecting the cerebellar, pyramidal, and extra-pyramidal signs (Lasek et al., 2006). There is a significant correlation between the Mini-Mental State Examination scores and atrophy of the nucleus accumbens (Lasek et al., 2006). Dopamine transporter (putamen) and glucose metabolism (putamen, cerebellum, and caudate nucleus) is reduced in SCA17 patients (Minnerop et al., 2005). Hypometabolism predominates in the putamen, caudate nucleus, cerebellum, and inferior and superior parietal cortex.

Neurophysiology

EEG monitoring ranges from normal to diffuse slowing and epileptic discharges. In the majority of cases, visual and motor evoked potentials are normal. By contrast, somatosensory and brainstem auditory evoked potentials are often abnormal (Bruni et al., 2004). Some cases with mild sensorimotor

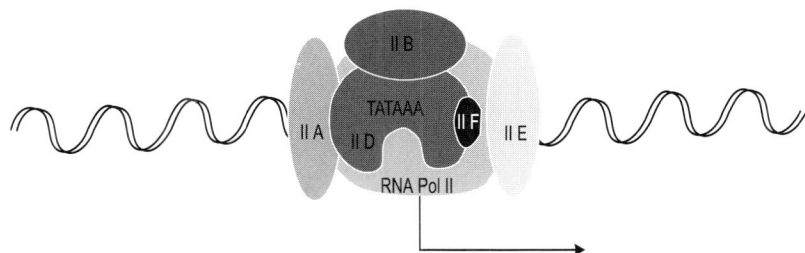

Figure 23.10 The transcription initiation complex. The initiation of the RNA synthesis by RNA polymerase II requires the transcription factors TFIIA, B, D, E, and F. TFIID (TBP: TATA-box binding protein) binds to the TATA-box (TATAAA). TBP has a variable size depending on the number of glutamine residues (25–42 in normal condition). Arrow corresponds to the transcription start site. Adapted from: Zühlke and Bürk, 2007. (See color section.)

axonal neuropathy in lower limbs have been reported (Maltecca et al., 2003).

Genetic and molecular aspects

SCA17 is due to an expanded CAG repeat in the TATA-box binding protein (TBP) (Figure 23.10). TBP is a transcription factor ubiquitously expressed from a single gene on chromosome 6q27. TBP is a component of the transcription initiation complexes of the 3 RNA polymerases (Rigby, 1993; Lescure et al., 1994). The TBP protein is the DNA-binding subunit of the RNA polymerase II transcription factor D (TFIID) implicated in mRNA transcription. A complete loss of normal TBP function is not compatible with life.

The glutamine tract is polymorphic in the normal population. The allelic distribution varies slightly according to ethnic/geographical origins (Rubinsztein et al., 1996). Population studies have shown that the normal range is between 25 and 42 residues. Most alleles contain between 32 and 39 repeats (Koide et al., 1999; Imbert et al., 1994). The threshold for pathological expansions varies from 43 to 45 repeats. The mean size of the repeat is above the pathological threshold of most polyglutamine diseases. Determination of the pathological threshold is complicated by the incomplete penetrance. Elongation of repeated CAG elements, alone or following the loss of CAA interruptions, is the main mechanism of elongated SCA17 repeats. In some cases, the expanded repeat results from a partial duplication or insertion of repeats into the CAG-CAA stretch. The result is a complex composition of CAG and CAA triplets. A majority of pathological alleles contain interspersed CAA CAG CAA elements separating the (CAG)n sequence in two parts. Expanded glutamine stretch may result from intragenic duplications (Koide et al., 1999), which is unusual in SCAs.

By comparison with other polyglutaminopathies, the SCA17 mutation is relatively stable during parent–child transmission (Stevanin & Brice, 2008). Although

there is a correlation between the age at onset and the size of the repeat, it is not as strong as in other ADCAs. Clinical deficits and age at onset may be variable within the same family members who carry the same number of repeats.

The size of the glutamine stretch inside full-length TBP increases its insolubility and aggregation. Given the role of TBP in anchoring the transcription machinery to the DNA, it is hypothesized that alteration of the tertiary structure of this protein causes an alteration of its binding to the DNA and/or activation or binding function of other TFIID components (Stevanin & Brice, 2008).

Neuropathology

The brain shows mild global atrophy, with predominance in the cerebellum. There is a severe loss of Purkinje neurons associated with Bergmann gliosis. Neuronal loss is usually mild in the granular layer and the dentate nuclei. The pontine nuclei are globally spared. However, the locus coeruleus and the substantia nigra are mildly affected. The caudate nuclei may show marked atrophy (Toyoshima et al., 2004). Atrophy of the cerebral cortex is more severe in the motor cortex and visual areas (Bruni et al., 2004).

As in several other ADCAs, the pathological hallmarks of this disease are the presence of neuronal intranuclear inclusions containing the pathological proteins, as well as heat shock proteins and ubiquitin, although with a lower frequency (Stevanin & Brice, 2008). There is an inverse correlation between the severity of atrophy and the presence of nuclear inclusions. For instance, inclusions are not found in the Purkinje and granule cell layers.

Spinocerebellar ataxia type 18

Clinical presentation

Spinocerebellar ataxia type 18 (SCA18), also called sensorimotor neuropathy with ataxia, has been

263

reported in a five-generation American family of Irish ancestry (Brkanac et al., 2002). Age of onset is in the second and third decades. The first symptom is usually a gait disturbance. Patients exhibit limb dysmetria, tendon hyporeflexia/areflexia, and muscle weakness and atrophy, as well as decreased vibratory and proprioceptive sense. Some patients show extensor plantar reflexes. There is no cognitive deficit. Affected members may present with pes cavus.

Neuroimaging
Brain MRI shows mild cerebellar atrophy.

Neurophysiology
Nerve conduction studies show evidence of sensory axonal neuropathy, confirmed by muscle biopsy revealing a neurogenic atrophy.

Genetic aspects
Gene maps to locus 7q22-q32.

Spinocerebellar ataxia types 19 and 22

Clinical presentation
The features of spinocerebellar ataxia type 19 (SCA19) were reported in a large ADCA Dutch family in 2001 (Schelhaas et al., 2001). In 2003, a similar family was found in China and showed linkage to the same locus (Chung et al., 2003). The candidate disease locus in the Chinese patients was called spinocerebellar ataxia type 22 (SCA22), but these disorders could represent the same SCA subtype (Schelhaas et al., 2004).

The age at onset ranges from 10 to 45 years in the Dutch family, but the clinical features seem to occur at a younger age in successive generations. However, this is not accompanied by an increase in the severity of the disorder. Anticipation is not demonstrated yet. The SCA19 phenotype is characterized by a very slowly progressive cerebellar syndrome which does not impact on life expectancy. Patients exhibit oculomotor deficits (horizontal nystagmus, saccadic eye movements), cerebellar dysarthria, and gait imbalance. Ataxia of the upper extremities is a relatively late symptom. Additional neurological features include mood disturbances, impulsive behavior, irregular postural head tremor, myoclonic jerks, and tendon hypo/areflexia. Cogwheel rigidity, akine-

sia, myoclonus, or cognitive impairment is absent in the Chinese family.

Neuropsychological findings
Cognitive impairment has been noted in several patients with low verbal IQ. Patients present a fronto-executive dysfunction. In particular, affected individuals have poor performance on the Wisconsin Card Sorting Test, which suggests damage to the dorsolateral prefrontal cortex or its connection to subcortical structures (see Chapter 2 and Chapter 3).

Neuroimaging
Brain MRI shows cerebellar atrophy involving the vermis and the hemispheres. In some patients, the pattern of atrophy also involves the cerebral cortex.

Neurophysiology
EEG recordings show a normal alpha rhythm background, associated with paroxysmal rhythmic theta activity over the temporal and parietal lobes. This paroxysmal activity might be related to cortical myoclonus.

Transcranial magnetic stimulation shows mildly increased central conduction times in patients exhibiting pyramidal deficits.

Peripheral nerve studies are consistent with length-dependent axonal neuropathy. Needle EMG studies show neurogenic changes that are more pronounced in the distal muscles of the lower extremities (Schelhaas & Van De Warrenburg, 2005). Nerve conduction studies show slightly reduced sensorimotor nerve conduction velocities, with reduced compound muscle action potentials in a minority of patients.

Genetic aspects
The SCA19 locus is located on chromosome 1p21-q21 (Dutch family) and 1p21-q23 (Chinese family).

Spinocerebellar ataxia type 20

Clinical presentation
SCA20 has been reported in an Australian pedigree of Anglo-Celtic origin (Knight et al., 2004). The mean age of onset is 46.5 years (range 19–64 years), with an

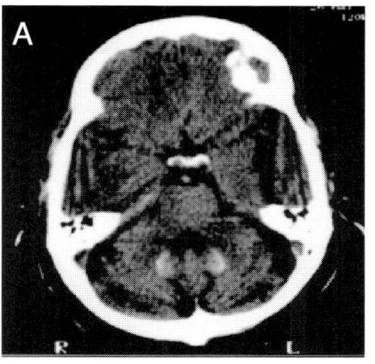
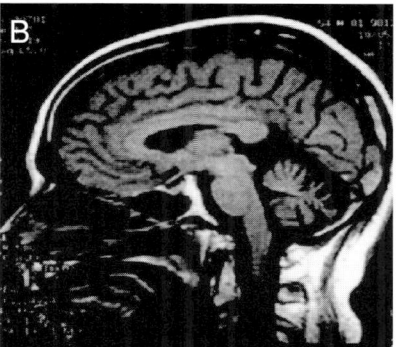
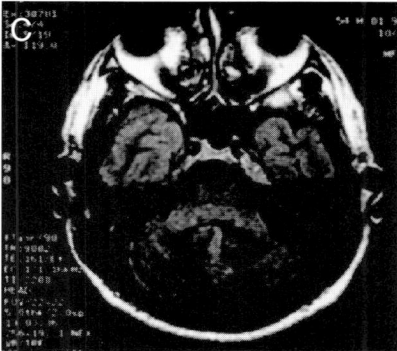

Figure 23.11 Brain MRI in SCA20. (A) CT brain scan showing striking calcification of the dentate nucleus of the cerebellum, but no other brain calcification. (B, C) MRI scans showing vermal atrophy (B) and low signal from the dentate nucleus (C). From: Storey et al., 2005. With permission.

average 10-year earlier onset in the children of affected parents. Progression is relatively slow over several decades. The initial symptom is dysarthria without gait ataxia in the majority of the cases. In some patients, onset of speech difficulties is sudden. Gait ataxia follows from 3 months to 25 years later. Other presentations are dysarthria combined with gait ataxia, isolated gait ataxia, and head tremor with upper limb action tremor. A distinctive feature is the concurrence of dysphonia with cerebellar dysarthria. Dysphonia mimics adductor spasmodic dysphonia (Storey et al., 2005). Ocular saccades are dysmetric. A majority of patients exhibit a palatal tremor, which may be subtle in some individuals. Mild pyramidal features (abnormally brisk knee jerks, crossed adductor spread) are found in some patients, but spasticity is absent, and extensor plantar responses are equivocal. Sensory testing is essentially unremarkable.

A probably similar disorder has been reported in Portugal (Coutinho et al., 2006). Patients exhibit paroxysmal coughing attacks starting at 25 to 55 years of age. Cerebellar ataxia develops later at 40 to 65 years of age. The coughing presents in bursts, without clear precipitating factors, and lasts several minutes. The coughing episodes decrease in frequency and severity with age. Patients with long-standing disease may show nystagmus.

SCA20 is distinct from familial progressive ataxia and palatal tremor, which combines progressive cerebellar deficits and corticospinal signs (Samuel et al., 2004). Brain MRI shows marked brainstem and cervical cord atrophy, without hypertrophic olivary appearance on MRI.

Neuroimaging

Neuroimaging provides important clues for the diagnosis. Brain CT scan shows dentate calcifications (Figure 23.11). These calcifications might be an early feature of the disease. Concomitant pallidal calcifications are seen in a few patients, in the absence of disorders of calcium metabolism (Storey et al., 2005). Brain MRI shows mild to moderate pancerebellar atrophy with dentate calcifications. The cerebral hemispheres appear normal. Inferior olivary pseudohypertrophy is observed in association with palatal tremor.

Neurophysiology

Lower limb motor and sensory nerve conduction studies are normal (Storey et al., 2005).

Genetic aspects

SCA20 is associated with a duplication at chromosome 11q22.2-11q12.3 (Knight et al., 2008). It has been suggested that the mutation causes a disruption of the diacylglycerol lipase alpha subunit, a neural stem cell–derived dendrite regulator which contributes to the modulation of parallel fiber–Purkinje cell synapses (Yoshida et al., 2006). The gene locus overlaps that of SCA5, but the phenotypes are different (see section Spinocerebellar ataxia type 5).

Spinocerebellar ataxia type 21

Clinical presentation

Spinocerebellar ataxia type 21 (SCA21) has been reported in a large French ADCA family (Devos et al., 2001). Age of onset is 1 to 30 years (mean 16.5±7.2 years). The disease does not seem to affect life expectancy. SCA21 is characterized by a slowly progressive cerebellar syndrome associated with extrapyramidal deficits (Delplanque et al., 2008). Patients exhibit moderate gait and limb ataxia variably associated with akinesia, tremor, rigidity, hyporeflexia, and mild cognitive impairment. Response to levodopa is mild or absent. The ophthalmologic examination shows intermittent microsaccadic pursuit and square wave jerks without ophthalmoplegia. The Mini-Mental State Examination and Mattis Dementia Rating Scale scores are below the normal values in several members of this family. Verbal IQ may be under the lower limit. Some patients show decreased tendon reflexes and hypopallesthesia of the lower limbs. However, others show mild hyperreflexia, in the absence of extensor plantar reflexes. None of the patients have fasciculations. Patients remain ambulant without external aid.

Neuroimaging

Brain MRI shows isolated cerebellar atrophy.

Neurophysiology

EEG, motor, visual, and brainstem auditory evoked potentials are normal.

Genetic aspects

The gene has been assigned on chromosome 7p21.3-p15.1. In 16 informative parent–child pairs, the mean apparent anticipation was 10.2±5.2 years, ranging from 4 to 18 years (Delplanque et al., 2008).

Neuropathology

Grossly, the brain and cerebellum are not atrophic. A very mild decrease of neuron density in the Purkinje cell layer of the vermis is found. The immunohistochemical study (using antibodies directed against ubiquitin, cystatin, synuclein, tau, neurofilaments, and beta-amyloid peptide) does not show any intracellular inclusion or extracellular deposit (Delplanque et al., 2008).

Spinocerebellar ataxia type 23

Clinical presentation

In 2004, Verbeek et al. described a two-generation Dutch ADCA family with a slowly progressive ataxia (Verbeek et al., 2004). Mean age of onset for spinocerebellar ataxia type 23 (SCA23) is 50.4 years (range 43–56 years). Progression is relatively slow, and the disease severity correlates with the duration of the disease (Verbeek, 2009). All patients show a slowly evolving cerebellar syndrome without cognitive deterioration, epilepsy, or extra-pyramidal features. Mild slowing of saccades, decreased vibration sense below the knee, and pyramidal signs have been noted in a few cases.

Genetic aspects

The disease locus on chromosome 20p13-12.3 spans a region of approximately 6 Mb of genomic DNA, containing 97 known or predicted genes.

Neuropathology

Macroscopic examination of the brain of one SCA23 patient showed marked atrophy of the frontotemporal region and vermis of the cerebellum, the basis pontis, and the spinal cord (Verbeek, 2009). There is a marked neuronal loss in the Purkinje cell layer of the rostral vermis, the dentate nuclei, and the inferior olives, resembling the autopsy findings of SCA6. The surrounding white matter shows myelin loss and gliosis. Cerebellopontine tracts are relatively small. Ubiquitin-positive neural inclusions (2–5 μm in diameter) are detected in some nigral neurons, but these inclusions are distinct from the aggregates observed in polyglutaminopathies and are considered to be Marinesco bodies (Verbeek, 2009).

Spinocerebellar ataxia type 25

Clinical presentation

Spinocerebellar ataxia type 25 (SCA25) is a rare SCA for which the age at onset ranges from 17 months to 39 years, without evidence of anticipation. Disease severity varies among affected patients. Cerebellar ataxia is present in all patients (Stevanin et al., 2005). However, cerebellar ataxia may not be the predominant sign. SCA25 is unusual because it is associated with severe sensory neuropathy, as observed in some mitochondrial diseases (see Chapter 21). Vibration sense at ankles is decreased or abolished. Most patients have decreased sensation for light touch and pain. Tendon reflexes are absent in the lower limbs in all patients. Patients also exhibit scoliosis and pes cavus. Extensor plantar reflexes, facial tics and myokymia, instability of central fixation, strabismus, and urinary urgencies are occasionally observed. Vomiting and gastrointestinal pain are described as the initial symptoms in some patients.

Neuroimaging

Cerebral MRI is characterized by global cerebellar atrophy, sparing the brainstem (Stevanin et al., 2004). The mesencephalon can have a molar-like appearance.

Neurophysiology

Studies of nerve conduction velocities show sensory neuropathy.

Genetic aspects

SCA25 maps to chromosome 2p15-p21 (Stevanin et al., 2004). SCA25 is associated with reduced penetrance.

Neuropathology

Sural nerve biopsy shows massive loss of myelinated fibers without myelin proliferation (Stevanin et al., 2005).

Spinocerebellar ataxia type 26

Clinical presentation

Spinocerebellar ataxia type 26 (SCA26) has been reported in a family of Norwegian ancestry who immigrated to the United States (Yu et al., 2005). Patients present with autosomal dominant pure cerebellar ataxia. Age at onset ranges from 26 to 60 years (mean 42 years), in absence of anticipation. Patients exhibit dysarthria, saccadic ocular pursuit, upper limb ataxia, and a slowly progressive gait ataxia. Intelligence is normal.

Neuroimaging

MRI shows atrophy of the cerebellum sparing the brainstem.

Genetic aspects

The candidate disease locus is located on chromosome 19p13.3, adjacent to the genes of Cayman ataxia and SCA6 (see Chapter 20 and section Spinocerebellar ataxia type 6 in this chapter).

Spinocerebellar ataxia type 27

Clinical presentation

Spinocerebellar ataxia type 27 (SCA27) has been reported in a Dutch family (van Swieten et al., 2003). Patients present with a tremor of both hands starting in childhood. Tremor has a high frequency and small amplitude and is increased by emotional stress and physical exercise. Mild unsteadiness and ataxia of the upper limbs begins between 15 and 20 years of age. Patients exhibit dysmetric saccades, impaired ocular pursuit, gaze-evoked nystagmus, and cerebellar dysarthria. Head tremor and subtle orofacial dyskinesias are observed in some patients. Severe limb and gait ataxia occurs in the oldest patients. Aggressive outbursts and depression are reported. Neuropsychological testing confirms deficits in memory and executive functioning. Some patients do not complete primary education due to mild mental retardation (IQ around 70). Pes cavus may occur (Dalski et al., 2005).

Neuroimaging

Brain MRI shows moderate cerebellar atrophy.

Functional imaging supports the hypothesis of basal ganglia involvement to explain the dyskinesias (Brusse et al., 2006).

Neurophysiology

Nerve conduction studies show a mild axonal sensory neuropathy in some cases.

Genetic aspects

SCA27 is caused by a missense mutation (F145S) in the gene encoding fibroblast growth factor-14 (FGF14) on chromosome 13q34.

Animal models

FGF14 knockout mice exhibit ataxia and paroxysmal dyskinesia (Wang et al., 2002). FGF14 belongs to the intracellular FGF homologous factor subfamily of FGF proteins (iFGFs). The iFGFs interact with the pore-forming (alpha) subunits of voltage-gated Na+ (Na[v]) channels. The expression of FGF14(F145S) reduces Na(v) alpha subunit expression at the axon initial segment, reduces Na(v) channel currents, and decreases the excitability of neurons (Laezza et al., 2007). FGF14 might play a role in spatial

Table 23.7 Clinical deficits in SCA28

Gait ataxia
Limb ataxia
Dysarthria
Ophthalmoparesis
Slow saccades
Ptosis
Gaze-evoked nystagmus
Increased tendon reflexes
Babinski sign
Increased muscle tone

learning functions and synaptic plasticity (Wozniak et al., 2007).

Spinocerebellar ataxia type 28

Clinical presentation

Spinocerebellar ataxia type 28 (SCA28) was initially reported in a four-generation Italian family with an inherited form of slowly progressive cerebellar ataxia (Cagnoli et al., 2006). Affected members show a relatively homogeneous phenotype. The mean age at onset is 19.5 years (range 12–36 years). There is no evidence of anticipation. Unbalanced standing and gait difficulties are the initial symptoms. Table 23.7 summarizes the clinical deficits. Most patients remain ambulant in their late sixties (Mariotti et al., 2008). There is no clinical evidence of sensory involvement. No cognitive impairment is observed at neuropsychological examination.

Neuroimaging

Brain MRI shows isolated cerebellar atrophy predominating in the superior vermis.

Neurophysiology

Nerve conduction studies and visual, auditory, somatosensory, and motor evoked potentials are normal.

Genetic aspects

The disease locus on chromosome 18p11.22-q11.2 spans a region of 7.9 Mb of genomic DNA (Cagnoli et al., 2006). Direct sequencing of candidate genes within the critical interval has led to the identification of a heterozygous point mutation in one of them.

Biochemical assays

Biochemical assays on muscle homogenates demonstrate normal activities of the respiratory chain enzymes (complexes I–V), and Southern blot analyses have excluded the presence of mitochondrial DNA deletions. The hypothesis of a mitochondrial disorder transmitted in an autosomal dominant fashion is also ruled out by normal morphologic results of muscle biopsies (Cagnoli et al., 2006).

Spinocerebellar ataxia type 30

Clinical presentation

Spinocerebellar ataxia type 30 (SCA30) has been reported in an Australian family of Anglo-Celtic ethnicity (Storey et al., 2009). Patients exhibit a relatively pure, slowly progressive ataxia developing in mid to late life. Saccades are hypermetric. Gain of the VOR is normal. Gaze-evoked nystagmus may be observed. Patients show minor pyramidal signs and no evidence of neuropathy.

Spinocerebellar ataxia type 31

The disorder has been discussed in page 253 (see also SCA type 4).

Neuroimaging

Brain MRI shows cerebellar atrophy, with sparing of the brainstem.

Genetic aspects

Linkage analysis has excluded currently known SCAs. Chromosome 4q34.3-q35.1 is the candidate region for the locus. The gene ODZ3 might be involved.

Therapies of SCAs

General recommendations

Logopedic rehabilitation and regular physiotherapy are recommended. Intensive coordinative training (3 sessions of 1 hour per week) improves motor performance and enable the patients to achieve personal goals for daily activities (IIg et al., 2009). Most patients will have some improvements with the use of orthoses, sticks, or strollers.

Seizures are managed with standard anti-epileptic drugs. Appropriate psychotropic medications are given for the psychiatric manifestations.

Table 23.8 Therapeutic strategies under investigation in SCAs

Strategies	Experimental observations and results
Reducing the oxidative stress	Increased aggregation and cell death under oxidative stress in human mutant ataxin-1 expressing cells (Kim et al., 2003). Antioxidants show some benefit in mouse models of Huntington disease (Beal & Ferrante, 2004).
Acting on the excitotoxic cascade	NMDA receptor antagonists improve survival in mouse models of Huntington disease (Ferrante et al., 2002).
Silencing gene expression via RNA interference	Reduction of aggregates and phenotypic improvements in mouse models of SCA1 (Zu et al., 2004; Xia et al., 2004)
Enhancing the clearance of the mutant protein	Rescue in cell, fly, and mouse models of Huntington disease (Ravikumar et al., 2004)
Targeting the toxicity of the protein via modulation of phosphorylation	Favorable effect on ataxia in SCA1 mice (Kaytor et al., 2005; Emamian et al., 2003)
Acting on chaperones	Overexpression of HSP70 decreases the toxicity of ataxin 1 in cells, flies, and mice (Cummings et al., 2001).
Inhibition of transglutaminases	Cystamine decreases toxicity in cell models of DRPLA and mouse models of Huntington disease (Karpuj et al., 2002)
Acting on transcriptional regulation	Mutant polyglutamine-expanded ataxin 7 inhibits the histone acetyltransferase function (Palhan et al., 2005). Improved neuropathology and motor phenotypes in fly and mouse models of Huntington disease treated with histone deacetylase inhibitors
Inhibition of caspase activation	Favorable effects of caspase inhibitors in mouse models of Huntington disease (Chen et al., 2000)
Transplantation	Graft survival and behavioral improvements in SCA-1 transgenic mice (Kaemmerer & Low, 1999)

Abbreviations: DRPLA: dentatorubral-pallidoluysian atrophy; NMDA: N-methyl-D-aspartic acid.

Adaptation of environment is recommended in case of cognitive deficit.

The reader is also referred to Chapter 6.

Clinical trials and observations

Trials have limited implications because of the small size of samples, the short time periods to evaluate treatment, the selection of advanced cases, and the fact that the agents used do not target a deleterious pathway involved in the pathogenesis of the disease. The absence of biomarkers is another source of difficulties for the evaluation of patients (Underwood & Rubinsztein, 2008).

Regarding ataxic symptoms, several drugs have been assessed, especially in SCA3 and SCA6. Sulfamethoxazole-trimethoprim has shown contradictory results in SCA3 (Correia et al., 1995; Schulte et al., 2001). Some positive results have also been observed in SCA3 with tetrahydrobiopterin, taltirelin, and tandospirone (Sakai et al., 1996; Takei et al., 2004). Buspirone may slightly improve the ataxia of stance. Acetazolamide has also been associated with improvement of ataxia in SCA6 (Yabe et al., 2001). The drug can reduce frequency, duration, and severity of ataxic episodes at the beginning of the disease (Jen et al., 1998). This feature is shared with episodic ataxia type 2 (EA2, see section Episodic ataxias). Deep brain stimulation has been shown to improve tremor in SCA2 (Pirker et al., 2003). Amantadine/levodopa/dopamine agonists may provide some motor improvements in patients with SCA2 and SCA3 presenting extra-pyramidal deficits. Amantadine might be useful for dystonia and bradykinesia in SCA3 (Woods & Schaumburg, 1972). Dyskinesias are treated symptomatically. Muscle cramps are usually disabling in SCA3 and may subside with magnesium, quinine, and mexiletine (Kanai et al., 2003). Dopaminergic agents or tilidine may improve restless leg symptoms. Baclofen/tizanidine may reduce spasticity. Botulinum toxin should be used cautiously.

Therapies of polyglutamine repeat disorders under investigation

The new strategies of treatment of SCAs associated with an expanded CAG trinucleotide repeat which are being assessed in transgenic models are summarized in Table 23.8. Several of these therapies have been successful in models of Huntington disease. Given the similarities between this disease and the SCAs caused by CAG repeats, they are being considered for polyglutamine repeat disorders (Underwood & Rubinsztein, 2008). The phenotype in the polyglutaminopathies has been widely considered to be due to a toxic gain-of-function in the mutant protein, although some loss-of-function might also contribute to pathology. Because of the similarity in the fundamental genetic mutation and the consequences at a cellular level, such as the formation of aggregates, some treatments may generalize to all polyglutamine diseases (Underwood & Rubinsztein, 2008).

The objective of RNA interference (RNAi) therapies is to inhibit polyglutamine-induced neurodegeneration and the associated cascade of neurotoxic events. RNAi use in humans remains hampered by difficulties for delivering RNAi and the absence of data regarding long-term safety. In particular, RNAi might block other genes such as tumor suppression genes. Moreover, loss of the wild-type allele product might be problematic.

Increasing the clearance of unwanted proteins is another approach. Cellular mechanisms for degrading proteins include the ubiquitin-proteasome system and autophagy (Ravikumar et al., 2003). Experimental data show that upregulation of autophagy rescues toxicity in models of Huntington disease. However, autophagy is primarily a cytosolic process. Therefore, if aggregates are largely restricted to the nucleus (e.g. in SCA1, SCA7, and SCA17), the beneficial effects might be light.

Attempts to decrease protein toxicity are being evaluated. One way to achieve this goal is to modulate the phosphorylation of proteins. Prevention of protein misfolding and aggregation by overexpressing chaperones (chaperones are proteins which promote normal protein folding), such as heat shock protein HSP70 or DNAJ1, and application of histone deacetylase inhibitors, which are capable of reversing heterochromatin formation (see also Chapter 20), are being assessed. Acetylation of histones increases transcription by allowing transcription factors to access packed DNA. Histone acetyltransferases and acetylate histones therefore influence the process of transcription. Polyglutamine expanded proteins may induce apoptosis by activating caspases or even by failing to sequester proteins activating caspases (Sanchez et al., 1999). Transplantation of stem cells has shown benefits in animal models, but their poten-

tial application in cerebellar ataxias remains poorly defined.

Episodic ataxias

Clinical presentation

Hereditary episodic ataxias (EAs) represent a group of monogenic channelopathies characterized by recurrent episodes of vertigo and ataxia, variably associated with progressive ataxia (Jen, 2008). Onset of EAs occurs in childhood or early adulthood in most cases. Attacks include oculomotor disturbances, impaired speech, and lack of coordination. Some patients may also complain of headache. Episodes last from minutes to hours. A main historical feature is discrete attacks of ataxia usually without impairment of consciousness. One distinction between EA and other types of ataxia in general is that patients with EA typically report clear onset and clear resolution rather than waxing and waning of their symptoms (Jen, 2008). The number of phenotypes and genotypes is continuously expanding (Table 23.9).

EA2 is the most common EA. EA2 is allelic with familial hemiplegic migraine type 1 (FHM1), characterized by complicated migraine with hemiplegia, interictal nystagmus, and progressive ataxia (Ducros et al., 2001) and SCA6 (see section Spinocerebellar ataxia type 6). The attacks are variably associated with nausea or vomiting, headaches, fluctuating weakness, seizures, and dystonia (Jen et al., 2004). Attacks are typically brief (seconds to minutes) in EA1 and more prolonged in EA2 or in EA7 (lasting hours to days) (Kerber et al., 2007; Riant et al., 2008). Movement-induced (kinesigenic) attacks of ataxia provoked by exercise, emotions, change of position, and startle are characteristic of EA1. The clinical spectrum of EA6 includes mild forms without attacks of hemiplegia (de Vries et al., 2009). A new phenotype with late onset between 48 and 56 years has been reported recently (Damak et al., 2009). Severity and duration of symptoms are heterogeneous. The most affected patients have daily attacks of ataxia and do not respond to acetazolamide.

Neuroimaging

Brain MRI can be normal at the beginning of the manifestations. Progressive cerebellar atrophy develops with time. Atrophy can predominate in the vermis.

Table 23.9 Characteristics of main episodic ataxias (EAs)

EA	Phenotype	Onset	Triggering	Mutation/locus
EA1	Interictal myokymia Muscle cramps	Early childhood	Physical exertion Emotional stress Startle	KCNA1 (12q13)

EA2	Interictal nystagmus
	Migraine
	Interictal cerebellar signs (nystagmus,
	  limb ataxia)
		Childhood or adolescence
		Rarely in adulthood (up to 5th decade)
			Exertion
			Stress
			Alcohol,
			  Caffeine
			Phenytoin
				CACNA1A (19p13)

EA3	Episodic vertigo, tinnitus, and ataxia No baseline deficit			Linked to 1q42
EA4	Episodic vertigo Interictal nystagmus No response to acetazolamide	Late onset		
EA5	Similar to EA2			CACNB4 (2q22-q23)
EA6	Attacks of hemiplegia and migraine Seizures			SLC1A3 (5p13)
EA7	Seizures Attacks of vertigo, weakness, and slurring	Before the age of 20	Exertion Excitement	19q13

Neurophysiology

In EA1, myokymia is associated with continuous muscle unit activity. An EMG pattern of repeated doublets and multiplets is detected in facial muscles and hand muscles.

Genetic aspects

Spontaneous mutations have been reported for EA1, EA2, and EA6. Therefore, the lack of a family history does not rule out the diagnosis. Nearly all EA mutations identified so far occur in individuals with onset early in life. Mutations have been identified in four genes, all coding for membrane proteins including ion channels and transporters, underlining the important roles of ion channels and transporters in cerebellar function (Jen, 2008). EA1 is caused by mutations in the potassium channel Kv1.1-encoding gene KCNA1, which renders neurons hyperexcitable. EA2 is due to mutations in the gene CACNA1A encoding the pore-forming and voltage-sensing subunit of Cav2.1, the P/Qtype voltage-gated calcium channel highly expressed in the cerebellum and the neuromuscular junction (Mori et al., 1991). EA3 was recently found to be linked to chromosome 1q42.12 (Cader et al., 2005). EA5 is associated with mutations in the gene CACNB4, which encodes an auxiliary β4 subunit of Cav2.1. (Escayg et al., 2000). EA6 is associated with mutations in the gene SLC1A3, which encodes a glial glutamate transporter EAAT1(Jen et al., 2005)

Another heterozygous mutation in SLC1A3 has been recently found in a family with clinical features similar to EA2, but without mutations in the EA2 gene (de Vries et al., 2009). Another family with EA has been mapped to chromosome 19q13 and designated EA7 (Kerber et al., 2007).

Differential diagnosis

Differential diagnosis of EA includes inborn errors of metabolism (congenital, autosomal recessive, or X linked), mitochondrial diseases, and migraine. Recessive metabolic disorders with intermittent ataxia are given in Table 23.10 (Baron et al., 1956; DiDonato et al., 1979; Bindu et al., 2007). Hartnup disease has an incidence of 1 in 30 000. It results from impaired transport of neutral amino acids (primarily tryptophan) across epithelial cells (Kleta et al., 2004). The sodium-dependent neutral amino acid transporter SLC6A19 is defective. Sunlight exposure, emotional stress, fasting, and sulfonamides may precipitate the attacks. The disorder is treated with nicotinamide (25 mg/day). Maple syrup urine disease, caused by a deficiency in activity of the branched-chain alpha-keto acid dehydrogenase, is treated with protein restriction/removal of accumulated branched-chain amino acids (leucine, isoleucine, valine) and thiamin supplementation. Intermittent ataxia is often triggered by protein loads in hyperammonemias associated with deficiencies in urea cycle enzymes. Hyperammonemia states may present from

Table 23.10 Metabolic disorders with intermittent ataxia

Disorder	Clinical features	Brain imaging	Gene locus
Carnitine acetyltransferase deficiency	Onset: childhood or infancy Oculomotor palsy Hypotonia Impaired consciousness Fatal course		9q34.1
Hartnup disease	Photosensitivity (pellagra-like rash) Emotional instability Psychotic manifestations Seizures Dystonia Aminoaciduria	Diffuse atrophy	SLC6A19 gene – 5p15.33
Maple syrup urine disease	Onset: neonatal, infancy, early adulthood Burnt sugar odor Drowsiness, lethargy Seizures Mental retardation Dystonia Athetosis Limb weakness Hearing loss Axonal neuropathy	Brain edema Lesions of the white matter, thalami, globus pallidus, brainstem, cerebellum Brain atrophy	19q13.2, 7q31

Hyperammonemias
  Argininosuccinic academia
  Carbamoyl-phosphate
  Synthetase I (CPSI)
	Coma
	Seizures
	Mental retardation
	Respiratory alkalosis
			7q21.3-q22
			2q33-q36
			9q34

Citrullinemia Ornithine carbamoyltransferase			Xp21.1

the neonatal period to adulthood. Hyperammonemia can be triggered or exacerbated by valproate (Batshaw & Brusilow, 1982). Treatment includes low-protein diet, supplements of arginine, and administration of sodium benzoate. Deficiency in pyruvate dehydrogenase E1-α, pyruvate carboxylase deficiency, and biotinidase deficiency have been discussed in Chapter 20 and Chapter 22. Alternating hemiplegia of childhood is a differential diagnosis of SCA6. Diagnostic criteria are given in Table 23.11. Paroxysmal eye movements occurring in the first 3 months of life, hemiplegic attacks, and episodes of impaired consciousness are very suggestive (Sweney et al., 2009). Attacks can be triggered by environmental stress, water exposure, physical activity, lighting, or foods. Ataxia and cognitive deficits are found in a majority of children. Brain MRI is usually normal, although generalized cortical atrophy or isolated cerebellar atrophy can be observed. In the majority of cases, EEG recordings show an absence of epileptiform discharges during plegic or dystonic episodes (Sweney et al., 2009). Clinical outcome is frequently poor.

Table 23.11 Diagnostic criteria of alternating hemiplegia of childhood

Symptoms starting before the age of 18 months
Attacks of hemiplegia involving either side

Other paroxysmal disturbances
  Tonic or dystonic spells
  Oculomotor deficits (nystagmus, esotropia/exotropia)
  Autonomic symptoms

Episodes of bilateral hemiplegia or quadriplegia   as generalization of a hemiplegic episode or bilateral from the start
Disappearance of symptoms upon sleeping
Developmental delay

Neurological deficits
  Choreoathetosis
  Dystonia
  Cerebellar ataxia

CAPOS syndrome is the acronym for cerebellar ataxia (episodic ataxia with fever starting before the age of 5), areflexia without polyneuropathy, pes cavus, optic atrophy, and sensorineural hearing loss

Table 23.12 Dominantly inherited spastic ataxia syndromes

Disorder	Clinical features	Imaging	Neuropathology
Spastic paraplegia, ataxia, mental retardation	Onset: 15–36 years Spastic paraplegia Ataxia Dystonia Mental retardation	Atrophy of the spinal cord Possible cerebellar atrophy	
Lipodystrophy with spastic ataxia and congenital cataract[a]	Congenital Lipodystrophy Retinitis pigmentosa Cataract Spastic paraplegia Ataxia Orthostatic hypotension	Hypersignal in the spinal cord (T2-weighted sequence)	
Ataxia, spasticity, with congenital miosis	Impaired pupillary reaction to light Disorder of conjugate eye movements Ataxia Pyramidal deficits		
Branchial myoclonus with spastic paraparesis and cerebellar ataxia	Onset: 40–50 years Branchial myoclonus Spastic paraparesis Ataxia	Mild atrophy of the cerebral and cerebellar cortex Severe atrophy of the medulla and spinal cord Basal ganglia calcification	Myelin loss and presence of Rosenthal fibers
DYT9 (gene locus: 1p)	Onset: 2–15 years Paroxysmal choreoathetosis Dystonia Episodic ataxia Spastic paraplegia		
Cerebellar ataxia, deafness, and narcolepsy	Ataxia Sensorineural deafness Narcolepsy Optic atrophy Psychiatric symptoms Sensorimotor polyneuropathy Diabetes mellitus	Cerebral and cerebellar atrophy Enlargement of the third ventricle Loss of the olivary bulges, Disappearance of cortical–white matter differentiation	Increased iron content in the basal ganglia and thalami Neuronal loss in the brainstem and cerebellum
Myelocerebellar syndrome (ataxia-pancytopenia syndrome)	Onset: early childhood–young adult Ataxia Peripheral neuropathy Pancytopenia Hypoplastic anemia Myelodysplastic syndrome Acute myeloid leukemia	Cerebellar atrophy	

[a] High serum cholesterol and elevated vitamin E levels.
From: Hedera et al., 2002; Berger et al., 2002; Dick et al., 1983; de Yebenes et al., 1988; Howard et al., 1993; Auburger et al., 1996; Melberg et al., 1999; Gonzalez-del Angel et al., 2000.

(Nicolaides et al., 1996). Autosomal dominant versus maternal mitochondrial inheritance has been proposed.

Treatments

Acetazolamide, a carbonic anhydrase inhibitor, remains the mainstay of treatment for EAs, especially for EA2 (Jen, 2008). Doses vary from 125 to 500 mg twice daily as needed or as tolerated. Side effects include tingling and numbness, impaired appetite, and concentration difficulties. Patients should be asked to maintain adequate hydration because of the risk of nephrolithiasis. An alternative is the use of 4-aminopyridine 15 mg/day. Some patients report benefit with carbamazepine. Phenytoin may provide benefits in EA1, but carries the risk of cerebellar long-term toxicity (see Chapter 15). Anxiety and panic attacks should be treated specifically if necessary. Moderate exercise, healthy diet, and adequate sleep might decrease the number of attacks of ataxias. Some patients report a benefit following vestibular rehabilitation.

Dominantly inherited spastic ataxia syndromes

Most patients with dominantly inherited spastic ataxia syndromes exhibit lower limb spasticity, extensor plantar responses, bladder dysfunction, and reduced sensations in the lower extremities. Gait is spastic and ataxic. Table 23.12 summarizes the main features of these disorders. Spinocerebellar ataxias SCA3 and SCA7 and DRPLA can also present as a dominantly inherited spastic ataxia (see sections Spinocerebellar ataxia type 3, Spinocerebellar ataxia type 7, and Dentatorubral-pallidoluysian atrophy).

Differential diagnosis includes hereditary spastic paraplegias (HSP) with dominant transmission (SPG3–4, SPG6, SPG8–10, SPG12–13, SPG17–19). SPG4, the most common HSP, presents as a relatively pure spastic paraplegia. Cerebellar ataxia is rarely reported (Nielsen et al., 2004), although brain MRI may reveal cerebellar atrophy (Orlacchio et al., 2004). SPG2 presents with a spastic paraplegia evident in the first 2 years of life. Cognitive deficiencies, optic atrophy, and cerebellar ataxia are also found. Transmission is X linked. The hereditary neuronal intranuclear inclusion disease with autonomic failure and cerebellar degeneration (neuronal intranuclear inclusion disease) is dominantly inherited or is sporadic. Symptoms start in childhood and are associated typically with an autonomic failure such as incontinence, postural hypotension, hypohidrosis, or intestinal pseudo-obstruction (Zannolli et al., 2002). Rectal biopsy reveals suggestive eosinophilic inclusions. Brain MRI shows cerebellar atrophy.

Treatment remains symptom-directed. Multidisciplinary evaluation is recommended. Baclofen, tizanidine, benzodiazepines, and dantrolene are helpful for spasticity. Intrathecal administration of baclofen and botulinum toxin injections may improve mobility. Blocking antibodies may develop with time. Orthotics and physical therapy help maintain joint mobility. Patients with neurogenic bladder may benefit from anticholinergic agents (see also Chapter 20).

References

Adachi M, Kawanami T, Ohshima H, Hosoya T. Characteristic signal changes in the pontine base on T2-and multishot diffusion-weighted images in spinocerebellar ataxia type 1. *Neuroradiology* 2006;**48**:8–13.

Auburger G, Ratzlaff T, Lunkes A, et al. A gene for autosomal dominant paroxysmal choreoathetosis/spasticity (CSE) maps to the vicinity of a potassium channel gene cluster on chromosome 1p, probably within 2 cM between D1S443 and D1S197. *Genomics* 1996;**31**:90–4.

Baba Y, Uitti RJ, Farrer MJ, Wszolek ZK. Sporadic SCA8 mutation resembling corticobasal degeneration. *Parkinsonism Relat Disord* 2005;**11**(3)147–50.

Bang OY, Lee PH, Kim SY, Kim HJ, Huh K. Pontine atrophy precedes cerebellar degeneration in spinocerebellar ataxia 7: MRI-based volumetric analysis. *J Neurol Neurosurg Psychiatry* 2004;**75**:1452–6.

Baron DN, Dent CE, Harris H, Hart EW, Jepson JB. Hereditary pellagra-like skin rash with temporary cerebellar ataxia, constant renal amino-aciduria and other bizarre biochemical features. *Lancet* 1956;**268**:421–8.

Batshaw ML, Brusilow SW. Valproate-induced hyperammonemia. *Ann Neurol* 1982;**11**:319–21.

Beal MF, Ferrante RJ. Experimental therapeutics in transgenic mouse models of Huntington's disease. *Nat Rev Neurosci* 2004;**5**:373–84.

Benomar A, Krols L, Stevanin G, et al. The gene for autosomal dominant cerebellar ataxia with pigmentary macular dystrophy maps to chromosome 3p12-p21.1. *Nat Genet* 1995;**10**:84–8.

Benton CS, de Silva R, Rutledge SL, et al. Molecular and clinical studies in SCA-7 define a broad clinical spectrum and the infantile phenotype. *Neurology* 1998;**51**:1081–6.

Berger JR, Oral EA, Taylor SI. Familial lipodystrophy associated with neurodegeneration and congenital cataracts. *Neurology* 2002;**58**:43–7.

Bindu PS, Shehanaz KE, Christopher R, Pal PK, Ravishankar S. Intermediate maple syrup urine disease: neuroimaging observations in 3 patients from South India. *J Child Neurol* 2007;**22**(7)911–3.

Brkanac Z, Bylenok L, Fernandez M, et al. A new dominant spinocerebellar ataxia linked to chromosome 19q13.4-qter. *Arch Neurol* 2002;**59**:1291–5.

Brkanac Z, Fernandez M, Matsushita M, et al. Autosomal dominant sensory/motor neuropathy with Ataxia (SMNA):Linkage to chromosome 7q22–q32. *Am J Med Genet* 2002;**114**:450–7.

Bruni AC, Takahashi-Fujigasaki J, Maltecca F, et al. Behavioral disorder, dementia, ataxia, and rigidity in a large family with TATA box-binding protein mutation. *Arch Neurol* 2004;**61**(8)1314–20.

Brusse E, de Koning I, Maat-Kievit A, et al. Spinocerebellar ataxia associated with a mutation in the fibroblast growth factor 14 gene (SCA27): A new phenotype. *Mov Disord* 2006;**21**(3)396–401.

Burk K, Skalej M, Dichgans J. Pontine MRI hyperintensities ('the cross sign') are not pathognomonic for multiple system atrophy (MSA). *Mov Disord* 2001;**16**:535.

Burk K, Zuhlke C, Konig IR, et al. Spinocerebellar ataxia type 5: clinical and molecular genetic features of a German kindred. *Neurology* 2004;**62**:327–9.

Burke JR, Wingfield MS, Lewis KE, et al. The Haw River syndrome: dentatorubropallidoluysian atrophy (DRPLA) in an African-American family. *Nat Genet.* 1994;**7**:521–4.

Burn J, Chinnery PF. Neuroferritinopathy.*Semin Pediatr Neurol* 2006;**13**(3)176–81.

Buttner N, Geschwind D, Jen JC, et al. Oculomotor phenotypes in autosomal dominant ataxias. *Arch Neurol* 1998;**55**:1353–7.

Cader MZ, Steckley JL, Dyment DA, et al. A genome-wide screen and linkage mapping for a large pedigree with episodic ataxia. *Neurology* 2005;**65**:156–8.

Cagnoli C, Mariotti C, Taroni F, et al. SCA28, a novel form of autosomal dominant cerebellar ataxia on chromosome 18p11.22-q11.2. *Brain* 2006;**129**: 235–42.

Chen DH, Cimino PJ, Ranum LP, et al. The clinical and genetic spectrum of spinocerebellar ataxia 14. *Neurology* 2005;**64**(7)1258–60.

Chen M, Ona VO, Li M, et al. Minocycline inhibits caspase-1 and caspase-3 expression and delays mortality in a transgenic mouse model of Huntington disease. *Nat Med* 2000;**6**:797–801.

Cholfin JA, Sobrido M-J, Perlman S, Pulst SM, Geschwind DH. The SCA12 mutation as a rare cause of spinocerebellar ataxia. *Arch Neurol* 2001;**58**:1833–5.

Christova P, Anderson JH, Gomez CM. Impaired eye movements in presymptomatic spinocerebellar ataxia type 6. *Arch Neurol* 2008;**65**:530–6.

Chung MY, Lu YC, Cheng NC, Soong BW. A novel autosomal dominant spinocerebellar ataxia (SCA22) linked to chromosome 1p21-q23. *Brain* 2003;**126**:1293–9.

Conaway JW, Florens L, Sato S, et al. The mammalian Mediator complex. *FEBS Lett* 2005;**579**:904–8.

Connarty M, Dennis NR, Patch C, Macpherson JN, Harvey JF. Molecular re-investigation of patients with Huntington's disease in Wessex reveals a family with dentatorubral and pallidoluysian atrophy. *Hum Genet* 1996;**97**:76–8.

Correia M, Coutinho P, Silva MC, et al. Evaluation of the effect of sulphametoxazole and trimethoprim in patients with Machado-Joseph disease. *Rev Neurol* 1995;**23**(121)632–4.

Cosma MP, Pepe S, Annunziata I, et al. The multiple sulfatase deficiency gene encodes an essential and limiting factor for the activity of sulfatases. *Cell* 2003;**113**(4)445–56.

Coutinho P, Andrade C. Autosomal dominant system degeneration in Portuguese families of the Azores Islands. A new genetic disorder involving cerebellar, pyramidal, extrapyramidal and spinal cord motor functions. *Neurology* 1978;**28**:703–9.

Coutinho P, Cruz VT, Tuna A, Silva SE, Guimaraes J. Cerebellar ataxia with spasmodic cough: a new form of dominant ataxia. *Arch Neurol* 2006;**63**:553–5.

Craig K, Keers SM, Walls TJ, Curtis A, Chinnery PF. Minimum prevalence of spinocerebellar ataxia 17 in the north east of England. *J Neurol Sci* 2005;**239**: 105–9.

Cummings C, Sun Y, Opal P, et al. Over-expression of inducible HSP70 chaperone suppresses neuropathology and improves motor function in SCA1 mice. *Hum Mol Genet* 2001;**10**:1511–8.

Dagda RK, Merrill RA, Cribbs JT, et al. The spinocerebellar ataxia 12 gene product and protein phosphatase 2A regulatory subunit Bbeta2 antagonizes neuronal survival by promoting mitochondrial fission. *J Biol Chem* 2008;**283**(52)36241–8.

Dalski A, Atici J, Kreuz FR, et al. Mutation analysis in the fibroblast growth factor 14 gene: frameshift mutation and polymorphisms in patients with inherited ataxias. *Eur J Hum Genet* 2005;**13**:118–120.

Damak M, Riant F, Boukobza M, et al. Late onset hereditary episodic ataxia. *J Neurol Neurosurg Psychiatry* 2009;**80**(5)566–8.

David G, Abbas N, Stevanin G, et al. Cloning of the SCA7 gene reveals a highly unstable CAG repeat expansion. *Nat Genet* 1997;**17**:65–70.

Day JW, Schut LJ, Moseley ML, Durand AC, Ranum LPW. Spinocerebellar ataxia type 8: clinical features in a large family. *Neurology* 2000;**55**:649–57.

de Vries B, Mamsa H, Stam AH, et al. Episodic ataxia associated with EAAT1 mutation C186S affecting glutamate reuptake. *Arch Neurol* 2009;**66**(1) 97–101.

de Yebenes JG, Vazquez A, Rabano J, et al. Hereditary branchial myoclonus with spastic paraparesis and cerebellar ataxia: a new autosomal dominant disorder. *Neurology* 1988;**38**:569–72.

Delplanque J, Devos D, Vuillaume I, et al. Slowly progressive spinocerebellar ataxia with extrapyramidal signs and mild cognitive impairment (SCA21). *Cerebellum* 2008;7:179–183.

Devos D, Schraen-Maschke S, Vuillaume I, et al. Clinical features and genetic analysis of a new form of spinocerebellar ataxia. *Neurology* 2001;**56**:234–8.

Dick DJ, Newman PK, Cleland PG. Hereditary spastic ataxia with congenital miosis: four cases in one family. *Br J Ophthal* 1983;**67**:97–101.

DiDonato S, Rimoldi M, Moise A, Bertagnoglio B, Uziel G. Fatal ataxic encephalopathy and carnitine acetyltransferase deficiency: a functional defect of pyruvate oxidation? *Neurology* 1979;**29**:1578–83.

Döhlinger S, Hauser T-K, Borkert J, Luft AR, Schulz J. Magnetic resonance imaging in spinocerebellar ataxias. *Cerebellum* 2008;7:204–214.

Ducros A, Denier C, Joutel A, et al. The clinical spectrum of familial hemiplegic migraine associated with mutations in a neuronal calcium channel. *N Engl J Med* 2001;**345**:17–24.

Duprat F. Susceptibility of cloned K+ channels to reactive oxygen species. *Proc Natl Acad Sci USA* 1995;**92**:11796–800.

Egawa K, Takahashi Y, Kubota Y, et al. Electroclinical features of epilepsy in patients with juvenile type dentatorubral-pallidoluysian atrophy. *Epilepsia* 2008;**49**(12)2041–9.

Emamian ES, Kaytor MD, Duvick LA, et al. Serine 776 of ataxin-1 is crucial for polyglutamine induced disease in SCA1 transgenic mice. *Neuron* 2003;**38**:375–87.

Escayg A, DeWaard M, Lee DD, et al. Coding and noncoding variation of the human calcium channel beta4-subunit gene CACNB4 in patients with idiopathic generalized epilepsy and episodic ataxia. *Am J Hum Genet* 2000;**66**:1531–9.

Estrada R, Galarraga J, Orozco G, et al. Spinocerebellar ataxia 2 (SCA2): morphometric analyses in 11 autopsies. *Acta Neuropathol (Berl)* 1999;**97**:306–10.

Factor SA, Qian J, Lava NS, Hubbard JD, Payami H. False-positive SCA8 gene test in a patient with pathologically proven multiple system atrophy. *Ann Neurol* 2005;**57**:462–3.

Farmer TW, Wingfield MS, Lynch SA, et al. Ataxia, chorea, seizures, and dementia. Pathologic features of a newly defined familial disorder. *Arch Neurol* 1989;**46**(7)774–9.

Fernandez M, McClain ME, Martinez RA, et al. Late-onset SCA2: 33 CAG repeats are sufficient to cause disease. *Neurology* 2000;**55**:569–72.

Ferrante RJ, Andreassen OA, Dedeoglu A, et al. Therapeutic effects of coenzyme q10 and remacemide in transgenic mouse models of Huntington's disease. *J Neurosci* 2002;**22**:1592–9.

Flanigan K, Gardner K, Alderson K, et al. Autosomal dominant spinocerebellar ataxia with sensory axonal neuropathy (SCA4): clinical description and genetic localization to chromosome 16q22.1. *Am J Hum Genet* 1996;**59**:392–9.

Fujigasaki H, Martin JJ, De Deyn PP, et al. CAG repeat expansion in the TATA boxbinding protein gene causes autosomal dominant cerebellar ataxia. *Brain* 2001;**124**:1939–47.

Gardner RJ, Knight MA, Hara K, et al. Spinocerebellar ataxia type 15. *Cerebellum* 2005;**4**(1)47–50.

Giunti P, Stevanin G, Worth PF, et al. Molecular and clinical study of 18 families with ADCA type II: evidence for genetic heterogeneity and de novo mutation. *Am J Hum Genet* 1999;**64**:1594–603.

Goldfarb LG, Vasconcelos O, Platonov FA, et al. Unstable triplet repeat and phenotypic variability of spinocerebellar ataxia type 1. *Ann Neurol* 1996;**39**(4)500–6.

Gonzalez-del Angel A, Cervera M, Gomez L, et al. Ataxia-pancytopenia syndrome. *Am J Med Genet* 2000;**90**:252–4.

Guerrini L, Lolli F, Ginestroni A, et al. Brainstem neurodegeneration correlates with clinical dysfunction in SCA1 but not in SCA2. A quantitative volumetric, diffusion and proton spectroscopy MR study. *Brain* 2004;**127**:1785–95.

Hara K, Shiga A, Nozaki H, et al. Total deletion and a missense mutation of ITPR1 in Japanese SCA15 families. *Neurology* 2008;**71**(8)547–51.

Harding AE. The clinical features and classification of the late onset autosomal dominant cerebellar ataxias. A study of 11 families, including descendants of the 'the Drew family of Walworth'. *Brain* 1982;**105**:1–28.

Hartmann J, Konnerth A. Determinants of postsynaptic Ca2+ signaling in Purkinje neurons. *Cell Calcium* 2005;**37**(5)459–66.

Hashida H, Goto J, Kurisaki H, Mizusawa H, Kanazawa I. Brain regional differences in the expansion of a CAG repeat in the spinocerebellar ataxias: Dentatorubral-pallidoluysian atrophy, Machado-Joseph disease, and spinocerebellar ataxia type 1. *Ann Neurol* 1997;**41**:505–11.

Hatano T, Okuma Y, Iijima M, et al. Cervical dystonia in dentatorubral-pallidoluysian atrophy. *Acta Neurol Scand* 2003;**108**:287–9.

Hayashi Y, Kakita A, Yamada M, et al. Hereditary dentatorubral-pallidoluysian atrophy: ubiquitinated filamentous inclusions in the cerebellar dentate nucleus neurons. *Acta Neuropathol (Berl)* 1998;**95**:479–82.

He Y, Zu T, Benzow KA, et al. Targeted deletion of a single Sca8 ataxia locus allele in mice causes abnormal gait, progressive loss of motor coordination, and Purkinje cell dendritic deficits. *J Neurosci* 2006;**26**:9975–82.

Hedera P, Rainier S, Zhao XP, et al. Spastic paraplegia, ataxia, mental retardation (SPAR): a novel genetic disorder. *Neurology* 2002;**58**:411–6.

Hellenbroich Y, Bubel S, Pawlack H, et al. Refinement of the spinocerebellar ataxia type 4 locus in a large German family and exclusion of CAG repeat expansions in this region. *J Neurol* 2003;**250**:668–71.

Hellenbroich Y, Gierga K, Reusche E, et al. Spinocerebellar ataxia type 4 (SCA4): Initial pathoanatomical study reveals widespread cerebellar and brainstem degeneration. *J Neural Transm* 2006;**113**(7)829–43.

Herman-Bert A, Stevanin G, Netter J, et al. Mapping of spinocerebellar ataxia 13 to chromosome 19q13.3-q13.4 in a family with autosomal dominant cerebellar ataxia and mental retardation. *Am J Hum Genet* 2000;**67**:229–35.

Hofmann K, Falquet L. A ubiquitin-interacting motif conserved in components of the proteasomal and lysosomal protein degradation systems. *Trends Biochem Sci* 2001;**26**:347–50.

Holmberg M, Duyckaerts C, Durr A, et al. Spinocerebellar ataxia type 7 (SCA7): a neurodegenerative disorder with neuronal intranuclear inclusions. *Hum Mol Genet* 1998;**7**:913–8.

Holmes SE, O'Hearn EE, McInnis MG, et al. Expansion of a novel CAG trinucleotide repeat in the 5' region of PPP2R2B is associated with SCA12. *Nat Genet* 1999;**23**(4)391–2.

Houlden H, Johnson J, Gardner-Thorpe C, et al. Mutations in TTBK2, encoding a kinase implicated in tau phosphorylation, segregate with spinocerebellar ataxia type 11. *Nat Genet* 2007;**39**:1434–6.

Howard RS, Greenwood R, Gawler J, et al. A familial disorder associated with palatal myoclonus, other brainstem signs, tetraparesis, ataxia and Rosenthal fibre formation. *J Neurol Neurosurg Psychiatry* 1993;**56**:977–81.

Igarashi S, Koide R, Shimohata T, et al. Suppression of aggregate formation and apoptosis by transglutaminase inhibitors in cells expressing truncated DRPLA protein with an expanded polyglutamine stretch. *Nat Genet* 1998;**18**:111–7.

IIg W, Synofzik M, Brötz D, Burkard S, Giese MA, Schöls L. Intensive coordinative training improves motor performance in degenerative cerebellar disease. *Neurology* 2009;**73**:1823–1830.

Ikeda Y, Dalton JC, Moseley ML, et al. Spinocerebellar ataxia type 8: molecular genetic comparisons and haplotype analysis of 37 families with ataxia. *Am J Hum Genet* 2004;**75**:3–16.

Ikeda Y, Daughters Rs, Ranum Lp. Bidirectional expression of the SCA8 expansion mutation: One mutation, two genes. *Cerebellum* 2008;**7**:150–8.

Ikeda Y, Dick KA, Weatherspoon MR, et al. Spectrin mutations cause spinocerebellar ataxia type 5. *Nat Genet* 2006;**38**:184–90.

Ikeda Y, Shizuka M, Watanabe M, Okamoto K, Shoji M. Molecular and clinical analyses of spinocerebellar ataxia type 8 in Japan. *Neurology* 2000;**54**:950–5.

Ikeda H, Yamaguchi M, Sugai S, et al. Expanded polyglutamine in the Machado-Joseph disease protein induces cell death in vitro and in vivo. *Nat Genet* 1996;**13**:196–202.

Imbert G, Trottier Y, Beckmann J, Mandel JL. The gene for the TATA binding protein (TBP) that contains a highly polymorphic protein coding CAG repeat maps to 6q27. *Genomics* 1994;**21**:667–8.

Ishikawa K, Fujigasaki H, Saegusa H, et al. Abundant expression and cytoplasmic aggregations of alpha-1A voltage-dependent calcium channel protein associated with neurodegeneration in spinocerebellar ataxia type 6. *Hum Mol Genet* 1999;**8**:1185–93.

Ishikawa K, Tanaka H, Saito M, et al. Japanese families with autosomal dominant pure cerebellar ataxia map to chromosome 19p13.1-p13.2 and are strongly associated with mild CAG expansions in the spinocerebellar ataxia type 6 gene in chromosome 19p13.1. *Am J Hum Genet* 1997;**61**:336–46.

Ishikawa K, Toru S, Tsunemi T, et al. An autosomal dominant cerebellar ataxia linked to chromosome 16q22.1 is associated with a single-nucleotide substitution in the 5′ untranslated region of the gene encoding a protein with spectrin repeat and rho guanine-nucleotide exchange factor domains. *Am J Hum Genet* 2005;**77**:280–96.

Ito H, Kawakami H, Wate R, et al. Clinicopathologic investigation of a family with expanded SCA8 CTA/CTG repeats. *Neurology* 2006;**67**:1479–81.

Ito D, Yamada M, Kawai M, et al. Corneal endothelial degeneration in dentatorubral-pallidoluysian atrophy. *Arch Neurol* 2002;**59**(2)289–91.

Iughetti P, Zatz M, Bueno MR, Marie SK. Different origins of mutations at the Machado-Joseph locus (MJD1). *J Med Genet* 1996;**33**:439.

Iwaki A, Kawano Y, Miura S, et al. Heterozygous deletion of ITPR1, but not SUMF1, in spinocerebellar ataxia type 16. *J Med Genet* 2008;**45**:32–5.

Jen JC. Hereditary episodic ataxias. *Ann NY Acad Sci* 2008;**1142**:250–3.

Jen J, Kim GW, Baloh RW. Clinical spectrum of episodic ataxia type 2. *Neurology* 2004;**62**:17–22.

Jen JC, Wan J, Palos TP, et al. Mutation in the glutamate transporter EAAT1 causes episodic ataxia, hemiplegia, and seizures. *Neurology* 2005;**65**: 529–34.

Jen JC, Yue Q, Karrim J, Nelson SF, Baloh RW. Spinocerebellar ataxia type 6 with positional vertigo and acetazolamide responsive episodic ataxia. *J Neurol Neurosurg Psychiatry* 1998;**65**:565–8.

Johansson J, Forsgren L, Sandgren O, et al. Expanded CAG repeats in Swedish spinocerebellar ataxia type 7 (SCA7) patients: effect of CAG repeat length on the clinical manifestation. *Hum Mol Genet* 1998;**7**: 171–6.

Johnson J, Wood N, Giunti P, Houlden H. Clinical and genetic analysis of spinocerebellar ataxia type 11. *Cerebellum* 2008;**7**:159–64.

Juvonen V, Hietala M, Paivarinta M, et al. Clinical and genetic findings in Finnish ataxia patients with the spinocerebellar ataxia 8 repeat expansion. *Ann Neurol* 2000;**48**:354–61.

Kaemmerer W, Low W. Cerebellar allografts survive and transiently alleviate ataxia in a transgenic model of spinocerebellar ataxia type-1. *Exp Neurol* 1999;**158**:301–11.

Kanai K, Kuwabara S, Arai K, et al. Muscle cramp in Machado-Joseph disease: altered motor axonal excitability properties and mexiletine treatment. *Brain* 2003;**126**(pt 4)965–73.

Karpuj MV, Becher MW, Springer JE, et al. Prolonged survival and decreased abnormal movements in a transgenic model of Huntington disease, with administration of the transglutaminase inhibitor cystamine. *Nat Med* 2002;**8**:143–9.

Kawaguchi Y, Okamoto T, Taniwaki M, et al. CAG expansions in a novel gene for Machado-Joseph disease at chromosome 14q32.1. *Nat Genet* 1994;**8**: 221–8.

Kaytor MD, Byam CE, Tousey SK, et al. A cell-based screen for modulators of ataxin-1 phosphorylation. *Hum Mol Genet* 2005;**14**:1095–105.

Kerber KA, Jen JC, Lee H, Nelson SF, Baloh RW. A new episodic ataxia syndrome with linkage to chromosome 19q13. *Arch Neurol* 2007;**64**:749–52.

Kim SJ, Kim TS, Hong S, et al. Oxidative stimuli affect polyglutamine aggregation and cell death in human mutant ataxin-1 expressing cells. *Neurosci Lett* 2003;**348**:21–4.

Kleta R, Romeo E, Ristic Z, et al. Mutations in SLC6A19, encoding B0AT1, cause Hartnup disorder. *Nat Genet* 2004;**36**(9)999–1002.

Klockgether T. The clinical diagnosis of autosomal dominant spinocerebellar ataxias. *Cerebellum* 2008;**7**:101–5.

Klockgether T, Skalej M, Wedekind D, et al. Autosomal dominant cerebellar ataxia type 1. MRI-based volumetry of posterior fossa structures and basal ganglia in spinocerebellar ataxia type 1,2 and 3. *Brain* 1998;**121**:1687–93.

Knight MA, Gardner RJM, Bahlo M, et al. Dominantly inherited ataxia and dysphonia with dentate calcification: spinocerebellar ataxia type 20. *Brain* 2004;**127**:1172–81.

Knight MA, Hernandez D, Diede SJ, et al. A duplication at chromosome 11q12.2–11q12.3 is associated with spinocerebellar ataxia type 20. *Hum Mol Genet* 2008;**17**(24)3847–53.

Knight MA, Kennerson ML, Anney RJ, et al. Spinocerebellar ataxia type 15 (SCA15) maps to 3p24.2–3pter: exclusion of the ITPR1 gene, the human orthologue of an ataxic mouse mutant. *Neurobiol Dis* 2003;**13**:147–57.

Kobayashi J, Nagao M, Kawata A, Matsubara S. A case of late adult-onset dentatorubral-pallidoluysian atrophy mimicking central pontine myelinolysis. *J Neurol* 2009 Apr 24 [Epub ahead of print].

Koeppen AH. The pathogenesis of spinocerebellar ataxia. *Cerebellum* 2005;**4**:62–73.

Koide R, Ikeuchi T, Onodera O, et al. Unstable expansion of CAG repeat in hereditary dentatorubral-pallidoluysian atrophy (DRPLA). *Nat Genet* 1994;**6**(1):9–13.

Koide R, Kobayashi S, Shimohata T, et al. A neurological disease caused by an expanded CAG trinucleotide repeat in the TATA-binding protein gene: a new polyglutamine disease? *Hum Mol Genet* 1999;**8**(11)2047–53.

Koide R, Onodera O, Ikeuchi T, et al. Atrophy of the cerebellum and brainstem in dentatorubral pallidoluysian atrophy. Influence of CAG repeat size on MRI findings. *Neurology* 1997;**49**:1605–12.

Koob MD, Moseley ML, Schut LJ, et al. An untranslated CTG expansion causes a novel form of spinocerebellar ataxia (SCA8). *Nat Genet* 1999;**21**:379–84.

Laezza F, Gerber BR, Lou JY, et al. The FGF14(F145S) mutation disrupts the interaction of FGF14 with voltage-gated Na+ channels and impairs neuronal excitability. *J Neurosci* 2007;**27**(44)12033–44.

Lang AE, Rogaeva EA, Tsuda T, Hutterer J, George-Hyslop P. Homozygous inheritance of the Machado-Joseph disease gene. *Ann Neurol* 1994;**36**:443–7.

Lasek K, Lencer R, Gaser C, et al. Morphological basis for the spectrum of clinical deficits in spinocerebellar ataxia 17 (SCA17). *Brain* 2006;**129**:2341–52.

Lescure A, Lutz Y, Eberhard D, et al. The N-terminal domain of the human TATA-binding protein plays a role in transcription from TATA-containing RNA polymerase II and III promoters. *EMBO J* 1994;**13**:1166–75.

Lin X, Antalffy B, Kang D, Orr HT, Zoghbi HY. Polyglutamine expansion down-regulates specific neuronal genes before pathologic changes in SCA1. *Nat Neurosci* 2000;**3**(2)157–63.

Lin X, Ashizawa T. Recent progress in spinocerebellar ataxia type-10 (SCA10). *Cerebellum* 2005;**4**:37–42.

Lin X, Orr HT, Zoghbi H. Spinocerebellar ataxia type 1. In *The Cerebellum and Its Disorders*. Cambridge, UK: Cambridge University Press, 2002, pp. 409–18.

Loy CT, Sweeney MG, Davis MB, et al. Spinocerebellar ataxia type 17: extension of phenotype with putaminal rim hyperintensity on magnetic resonance imaging. *Mov Disord* 2005;**20**:1521–3.

Maltecca F, Filla A, Castaldo I, et al. Intergenerational instability and marked anticipation in SCA-17. *Neurology* 2003;**61**(10)1441–3.

Manto M. The wide spectrum of spinocerebellar ataxias. *Cerebellum* 2005;**4**:2–6

Manto M, Jissendi P. Spinocerebellar Atrophy. In *Encyclopedia of Neuroscience*, volume 9, ed. L.R. Squire LR. Oxford, UK: Academic Press, 2009, pp. 337–49.

Manto M, Marmolino D. Cerebellar ataxias. *Curr Opin Neurol* 2009;**22**:419–29.

Mariotti C, Brusco A, Di Bella D, et al. Spinocerebellar ataxia type 28: A novel autosomal dominant cerebellar ataxia characterized by slow progression and ophthalmoparesis. *Cerebellum* 2008;**7**:184–208.

Martina M, Yao GL, Bean BP. Properties and functional role of voltage-dependent potassium channels in dendrites of rat cerebellar Purkinje neurons. *J Neurosci* 2003;**23**:5698–707.

Marz P, Probst A, Lang S, et al. Ataxin-10, the spinocerebellar ataxia type 10 neurodegenerative disorder protein, is essential for survival of cerebellar neurons. *J Biol Chem* 2004;**279**(34):35542–50.

Matilla A, Roberson ED, Banfi S, et al. Mice lacking ataxin-1 display learning deficits and decreased hippocampal paired-pulse facilitation. *J Neurosci* 1998;**18**:5508–16.

Matsumura R, Takayanagi T, Fujimoto Y, et al. The relationship between trinucleotide repeat length and phenotypic variation in Machado-Joseph disease. *J Neurol Sci* 1996a;**139**(1):52–7.

Matsumura R, Takayanagi T, Murata K, et al. Relationship of (CAG)nC configuration to repeat instability of the Machado-Joseph disease gene. *Hum Genet* 1996b;**98**(6):643–5.

Matsuura T, Achari M, Khajavi M, et al. Mapping of the gene for a novel spinocerebellar ataxia with pure cerebellar signs and epilepsy. *Ann Neurol* 1999;**45**(3)407–11.

Matsuura T, Yamagata T, Burgess DL, et al. Large expansion of the ATTCT pentanucleotide repeat in spinocerebellar ataxia type 10. *Nat Genet* 2000;**26**(2)191–4.

Melberg A, Dahl N, Hetta J, et al. Neuroimaging study in autosomal dominant cerebellar ataxia, deafness, and narcolepsy. *Neurology* 1999;**53**: 2190–2.

Michalik A, Martin JJ, Van Broeckhoven C. Spinocerebellar ataxia type 7 associated with pigmentary retinal dystrophy. *Eur J Hum Genet* 2004;**12**:2–15.

Minnerop M, Joe A, Lutz M, et al. Putamen dopamine transporter and glucose metabolism are reduced in SCA17. *Ann Neurol* 2005;**58**:490–1.

Mori Y, Friedrich T, Kim MS, et al. Primary structure and functional expression from complementary DNA of a brain calcium channel. *Nature* 1991;**350**:398–402.

Moseley ML, Benzow KA, Schut LJ, et al. Incidence of dominant spinocerebellar and Friedreich triplet repeats among 361 ataxia families. *Neurology* 1998;**51**:1666–71.

Munoz E, Campdelacreu J, Ferrer I, et al. Severe cerebral white matter involvement in a case of dentatorubropallidoluysian atrophy studied at autopsy. *Arch Neurol* 2004;**61**:946–9.

Murata Y, Kawakami H, Yamaguchi S, et al. Characteristic magnetic resonance imaging findings in spinocerebellar ataxia 6. *Arch Neurol* 1998;**55**(10)1348–52.

Murata Y, Yamaguchi S, Kawakami H, et al. Characteristic magnetic resonance imaging findings in Machado-Joseph disease. *Arch Neurol* 1998;**55**(1)33–7.

Mutsuddi M, Marshall CM, Benzow KA, Koob MD, Rebay I. The spinocerebellar ataxia 8 noncoding RNA causes neurodegeneration and associates with staufen in Drosophila. *Curr Biol* 2004;**14**:302–8.

Naito H, Oyanagi S. Familial myoclonus epilepsy and choreoathetosis: hereditary dentatorubral-pallidoluysian atrophy. *Neurology* 1982;**32**:798–807.

Nakamura K, Jeong SY, Uchihara T, et al. SCA17, a novel autosomal dominant cerebellar ataxia caused by an expanded polyglutamine in TATA-binding protein. *Hum Mol Genet* 2001;**10**:1441–8.

Nakano KK, Dawson DM, Spence A. Machado disease. A hereditary ataxia in Portuguese emigrants to Massachusetts. *Neurology* 1972;**22**:49–55.

Nicolaides P, Appleton RE, Fryer A. Cerebellar ataxia, areflexia, pes cavus, optic atrophy, and sensorineural hearing loss (CAPOS): a new syndrome. *J Med Genet* 1996;**33**:419–21.

Nielsen JE, Johnsen B, Koefoed P, et al. Hereditary spastic paraplegia with cerebellar ataxia: a complex phenotype associated with a new SPG4 gene mutation. *Eur J Neurol* 2004;**11**(12)817–24.

Nishiyama K, Murayama S, Goto J, et al. Regional and cellular expression of the Machado-Joseph disease gene in brains of normal and affected individuals. *Ann Neurol* 1996;**40**:776–81.

O'Hearn E, Holmes SE, Calvert PC, Ross CA, Margolis RL. SCA-12: Tremor with cerebellar and cortical atrophy is associated with a CAG repeat expansion. *Neurology* 2001;**56**:299–303.

Onodera O, Oyake M, Takano H, Ikeuchi T, Igarashi S, Tsuji S. Molecular cloning of a full-length cDNA for dentatorubral-pallidoluysian atrophy and regional expressions of the expanded alleles in the CNS. *Am J Hum Genet* 1995;**57**:1050–60.

Orlacchio A, Kawarai T, Totaro A, et al. Hereditary spastic paraplegia: clinical genetic study of 15 families. *Arch Neurol* 2004;**61**(6)849–55.

Orozco G, Fleites A, Cordoves Sagaz R, et al. Autosomal dominant cerebellar ataxia: clinical analysis of 263 patients from a homogeneous population in Holguin, Cuba. *Neurology* 1990;**40**:1369–75.

Orr HT, Chung M, Banfi S, et al. Expansion of an unstable trinucleotide CAG repeat in spinocerebellar ataxia type 1. *Nat Genet* 1993;**4**:221–6.

Ory-Magne F, Brefel-Courbon C, Payoux P, et al. Clinical phenotype and neuroimaging findings in a French family with hereditary ferritinopathy (FTL498–499InsTC). *Mov Disord* 2009 Jun 9 [Epub ahead of print].

Ouyang Y, Sakoe K, Shimazaki H, et al. 16q-linked autosomal dominant cerebellar ataxia: a clinical and genetic study. *J Neurol Sci* 2006;**247**:180–6.

Owada K, Ishikawa K, Toru S, et al. A clinical, genetic, and neuropathologic study in a family with 16q-linked ADCA type III. *Neurology* 2005;**65**:629–32.

Padiath QS, Srivastava AK, Roy S, Jain S, Brahmachari SK. Identification of a novel 45 repeat unstable allele associated with a disease phenotype at the MJD1/SCA3 locus. *Am J Med Genet B Neuropsychiatr Genet* 2005;**133**:124–6.

Palhan VB, Chen S, Peng GH, et al. Polyglutamine-expanded ataxin-7 inhibits STAGA histone acetyltransferase activity to produce retinal degeneration. *Proc Natl Acad Sci USA* 2005;**102**(24)8472–7.

Pirker W, Back C, Gerschlager W, Laccone F, Alesch F. Chronic thalamic stimulation in a patient with spinocerebellar ataxia type 2. *Mov Disord* 2003;**18**: 222–5.

Potaman VN, Bissler JJ, Hashem VI, et al. Unpaired structures in SCA10 (ATTCT)n.(AGAAT)n repeats. *J Mol Biol* 2003;**326**(4)1095–111.

Pujana MA, Corral J, Gratacos M, et al. Spinocerebellar ataxias in Spanish patients: Genetic analysis of familial and sporadic cases. The Ataxia Study Group. *Hum Genet* 1999;**104**:516–22.

Pulst S, Nechiporuk A, Nechiporuk T, et al. Moderate expansion of a normally biallelic trinucleotide repeat in spinocerebellar ataxia type 2. *Nat Genet* 1996;**14**:269–76.

Quan F, Janas J, Popovich BW. A novel CAG repeat configuration in the SCA1 gene: implications for the molecular diagnostics of spinocerebellar ataxia type 1. *Hum Mol Genet* 1995;**4**(12)2411–3.

Ranum LPW, Schut LJ, Lundgren JK, Orr HT, Livingston DM. Spinocerebellar ataxia type 5 in a family descended from the grandparents of President Lincoln maps to chromosome 11. *Nat Genet* 1994;**8**:280–4.

Ravikumar B, Sarkar S, Berger Z, Rubinsztein DC. The roles of the ubiquitin proteasome and autophagy-lysosome pathways in Huntington's disease and related conditions. *Clin Neurosci Res* 2003;**3**:141–8.

Ravikumar B, Vacher C, Berger Z, et al. Inhibition of mTOR induces autophagy and reduces toxicity of polyglutamine expansions in fly and mouse models of Huntington's disease. *Nat Genet* 2004;**6**:585–95.

Riant F, Mourtada R, Saugier-Veber P, Tournier-Lasserve E. Large CACNA1A deletion in a family with episodic ataxia type 2. *Arch Neurol* 2008;**65**:817–20.

Riess O, Rub U, Pastore A, Bauer P, Schöls P. SCA3: Neurological features, pathogenesis and animal models. *Cerebellum* 2008;**7**:125–7.

Rigby PW. Three in one and one in three: it all depends on TBP. *Cell* 1993;**72**:7–10.

Rolfs A, Koeppen AH, Bauer I, et al. Clinical features and neuropathology of autosomal dominant spinocerebellar ataxia (SCA17). *Ann Neurol* 2003;**54**:367–75.

Rüb U, de Vos RA, Brunt ER, Sebesteny T, Schöls L, et al. Spinocerebellar ataxia type 3 (SCA3): thalamic neurodegeneration occurs independently from thalamic ataxin-3 immunopositive neuronal intranuclear inclusions. *Brain Pathol* 2006;**16**:218–27.

Rubinsztein DC, Leggo J, Crow TJ, et al. Analysis of polyglutamine-coding repeats in the TATA-binding protein in different human populations and in patients with schizophrenia and bipolar affective disorder. *Am J Med Genet* 1996;**67**:495–8.

Rudy B, McBain CJ. Kv3 channels: voltage-gated K+ channels designed for high-frequency repetitive firing. *Trends Neurosci* 2001;**9**:517–26.

Sakai T, Yasunobu A, Matsuishi T, Iwashita H. Tetrahydrobiopterin double-blind, crossover trial in Machado-Joseph disease. *J Neurolog Sci* 1996;**136**:71–2.

Samuel M, Torun N, Tuite PJ, Sharpe JA, Lang AE. Progressive ataxia and palatal tremor (PAPT): clinical and MRI assessment with review of palatal tremors. *Brain* 2004;**127**(pt 6)1252–68.

Sanchez C, Xu P, Juo A, et al. Caspase-8 is required for cell death induced by expanded polyglutamine repeats. *Neuron* 1999;**22**:623–33.

Sasaki H, Yabe I, Tashiro K. The hereditary spinocerebellar ataxias in Japan. *Cytogenet Genome Res* 2003;**100**:198–205.

Satoh JI, Tokumoto H, Yukitake M, et al. Spinocerebellar ataxia type 6: MRI of three Japanese patients. *Neuroradiology* 1998;**40**:222–7.

Schelhaas HJ, Ippel PF, Hageman G, et al. Clinical and genetic analysis of a four generation family with a distinct autosomal dominant cerebellar ataxia. *J Neurol* 2001;**248**:113–20.

Schelhaas HJ, Van De Warrenburg BPC. Clinical, psychological, and genetic characteristics of spinocerebellar ataxia type 19 (SCA19). *Cerebellum* 2005;**4**:51–4.

Schelhaas HJ, Verbeek DS, van de Warrenburg BP, Sinke RJ. SCA19 and SCA22: Evidence for one locus with a worldwide distribution. *Brain* 2004;**127**(pt 1)E6.

Schmidt T, Landwehrmeyer GB, Schmitt I, et al. An isoform of ataxin-3 accumulates in the nucleus of neuronal cells in affected brain regions of SCA3 patients. *Brain Pathol* 1998;**8**:669–79.

Schmidt T, Lindenberg KS, Krebs A, et al. Protein surveillance machinery in brains with spinocerebellar ataxia type 3: Redistribution and differential recruitment of 26S proteasome subunits and chaperones to neuronal intranuclear inclusions. *Ann Neurol* 2002;**51**: 302–10.

Schöls L, Amoiridis G, Epplen JT, et al. Relations between genotype and phenotype in German patients with the Machado-Joseph disease mutation. *J Neurol Neurosurg Psychiatry* 1996;**61**:466–70.

Schöls L, Amoiridis G, Langkafel M, et al. Machado-Joseph disease mutation as the genetic basis of most spinocerebellar ataxias in Germany. *J Neurol Neurosurg Psychiatry* 1995;**59**:449–50.

Schöls L, Bauer P, Schmidt T, Schulte T, Riess O. Autosomal dominant cerebellar ataxias: Clinical features, genetics, and pathogenesis. *Lancet Neurol* 2004;**3**:291–304.

Schöls L, Krüger R, Amoiridis G, et al. Spinocerebellar ataxia type 6: Genotype and phenotype in German kindreds. *J Neurol Neurosurg Psychiatry* 1998;**64**:67–73.

Schöls L, Linnemann C, Globas C. Electrophysiology in spinocerebellar ataxias: Spread of disease and characteristic findings. *Cerebellum* 2008;**7**:198–203.

Schöls L, Szymanski S, Peters S, et al. Genetic background of apparently idiopathic sporadic cerebellar ataxia. *Hum Genet* 2000;**107**:132–7.

Schulte T, Mattern R, Berger K, et al. Double-blind crossover trial of trimethoprim-sulfamethoxazole in spinocerebellar ataxia type 3. *Arch Neurol* 2001;**58**:1451–7.

Seki T, Adachi N, Ono Y, et al. Mutant protein kinase Cgamma found in spinocerebellar ataxia type 14 is susceptible to aggregation and causes cell death. *J Biol Chem* 2005;**280**(32)29096–106.

Shimizu Y, Yoshida K, Okano T, et al. Regional features of autosomal dominant cerebellar ataxia in Nagano: clinical and molecular genetic analysis of 86 families. *J Hum Genet* 2004;**49**:610–6.

Sinke RJ, Ippel EF, Diepstraten CM, et al. Clinical and molecular correlations in spinocerebellar ataxia type 6: a study of 24 Dutch families. *Arch Neurol* 2001;**58**:1839–44.

Smith JK, Gonda VE, Malamud N. Unusual form of cerebellar ataxia: combined dentato-rubral and pallido-luysian degeneration. *Neurology* 1958;**8**:205–9.

Sobrido MJ, Cholfin JA, Perlman S, Pulst SM, Geschwind DH. SCA8 repeat expansions in ataxia: a controversial association. *Neurology* 2001;**57**:1310–2.

Soong B, Liu R, Wu L, Lu Y, Lee H. Metabolic characterization of spinocerebellar ataxia type 6. *Arch Neurol* 2001;**58**:300–4.

Soong BW, Liu RS. Positron emission tomography in asymptomatic gene carriers of Machado-Joseph disease. *J Neurol Neurosurg Psychiatry* 1998;**64**:499–504.

Stevanin G, Bouslam N, Thobois S, et al. Spinocerebellar ataxia with sensory neuropathy maps to the SCA25 locus on chromosome 2. *Ann Neurol* 2004;**55**:97–104.

Stevanin G, Brice A. Spinocerebellar ataxia 17 (SCA17) and Huntington's disease-like 4 (HDL4). *Cerebellum* 2008;**7**:170–8.

Stevanin G, Broussolle E, Streichenberger N, et al. Spinocerebellar ataxia with sensory neuropathy (SCA25). *Cerebellum* 2005;**4**:58–61.

Stevanin G, Durr A, Benammar N, Brice A. Spinocerebellar ataxia with mental retardation (SCA13). *Cerebellum* 2005;**4**:43–6.

Stevanin G, Fujigasaki H, Lebre AS, et al. Huntington's disease-like phenotype due to trinucleotide repeat expansions in the TBP and JPH3 genes. *Brain* 2003;**126**:1599–603.

Stevanin G, Hahn V, Lohmann E, et al. Mutation in the catalytic domain of protein kinase C gamma and extension of the phenotype associated with spinocerebellar ataxia type 14. *Arch Neurol* 2004;**61**(8)1242–8.

Storey E, Bahlo M, Fahey M, et al. A new dominantly inherited pure cerebellar ataxia, SCA 30. *J Neurol Neurosurg Psychiatry* 2009;**80**(4)408–11.

Storey E, Forrest SM, Shaw JH, et al. Spinocerebellar ataxia type 2: clinical features of a pedigree displaying prominent fronto-executive dysfunction. *Arch Neurol* 1999;**56**:43–50.

Storey E, Knight MA, Forrest SM, Mckinlay Gardner RJ. Spinocerebellar ataxia type 20. *Cerebellum* 2005;**4**:55–7.

Sweney MT, Silver K, Gerard-Blanluet M, et al. Alternating hemiplegia of childhood: early characteristics and evolution of a neurodevelopmental syndrome. *Pediatrics* 2009;**123**(3)e534–41.

Takahashi H, Ishikawa K, Tsutsumi T, et al. A clinical and genetic study in a large cohort of patients with spinocerebellar ataxia type 6. *J Hum Genet* 2004;**49**:256–64.

Takano H, Cancel G, Ikeuchi T, et al. Close associations between prevalences of dominantly inherited spinocerebellar ataxias with CAG-repeat expansions and frequencies of large normal CAG alleles in Japanese and Caucasian populations. *Am J Hum Genet* 1998;**63**:1060–6.

Takei A, Fukazawa T, Hamada T, et al. Effects of tandospirone on '5-HT1A receptor associated symptoms' in patients with Machado-Joseph disease: An open label study. *Clin Neuropharmacol* 2004;**27**:9–13.

Takiyama Y, Sakoe K, Namekawa M, et al. A Japanese family with spinocerebellar ataxia type 6 which includes three individuals homozygous for an expanded CAG repeat in the SCA6/CACNL1A4 gene. *J Neurol Sci* 1998;**158**(2)141–7.

Toyoshima Y, Yamada M, Onodera O, et al. SCA17 homozygote showing Huntington's disease-like phenotype. *Ann Neurol* 2004;**55**:281–6.

Tsuji S. Dentatorubral-pallidoluysian atrophy. In *The Cerebellum and Its Disorders*, ed. M. Manto and M. Pandolfo. Cambridge, UK: Cambridge University Press, 2002, pp. 481–90.

Tuite PJ, Rogaeva EA, George-Hyslop PH, Lang AE. Dopa-responsive parkinsonism phenotype of Machado-Joseph disease: Confirmation of 14q CAG expansion. *Ann Neurol* 1995;**38**:684–7.

Underwood BR, Rubinsztein DC. Spinocerebellar ataxias caused by polyglutamine expansions: A review of therapeutic strategies. *Cerebellum* 2008;215–21.

van de Leemput J, Chandran J, Knight MA, et al. Deletion at ITPR1 underlies ataxia in mice and spinocerebellar ataxia 15 in humans. *PLoS Genet* 2007;**3**(6)e108.

van de Warrenburg BP, Sinke RJ, Verschuuren-Bemelmans CC, et al. Spinocerebellar ataxias in the Netherlands: prevalence and age at onset variance analysis. *Neurology* 2002;**58**:702–08.

van de Warrenburg BP, Verbeek DS, Piersma SJ, et al. Identification of a novel SCA14 mutation in a Dutch autosomal dominant cerebellar ataxia family. *Neurology* 2003;**61**(12)1760–5.

van Swieten JC, Brusse E, de Graaf BM, et al. A mutation in the fibroblast growth factor 14 gene is associated with autosomal dominant cerebral (sic) ataxia. *Am J Hum Genet* 2003;**72**:191–9.

Verbeek DS. Spinocerebellar ataxia type 23: A genetic update. *Cerebellum* 2009;**8**:104–7.

Verbeek DS, Knight MA, Harmison GG, Fischbeck KH, Howell BW. Protein kinase C gamma mutations in spinocerebellar ataxia 14 increase kinase activity and alter membrane targeting. *Brain* 2005;**128**(pt 2) 436–42.

Verbeek DS, van de Warrenburg BP, Wesseling P, et al. Mapping of the SCA23 locus involved in autosomal dominant cerebellar ataxia to chromosome region 20p13–12.3. *Brain* 2004;**127**(Pt 11):2551–7.

Wang Q, Bardgett ME, Wong M, et al. Ataxia and paroxysmal dyskinesia in mice lacking axonally transported FGF14. *Neuron* 2002;**35**(1)25–38.

Wang G, Sawai N, Kotliarova S, Kanazawa I, Nukina N. Ataxin-3, the MJD1 gene product, interacts with the two human homologs of yeast DNA repair protein RAD23, HHR23A and HHR23B. *Hum Mol Genet* 2000;**9**:1795–803.

Warrick JM, Paulson HL, Gray-Board, et al. Expanded polyglutamine protein forms nuclear inclusions and causes neural degeneration in Drosophila. *Cell* 1998;**93**:939–49.

Watanabe H, Tanaka F, Matsumoto M, et al. Frequency analysis of autosomal dominant ataxias in Japanese patients and clinical characterization of spinocerebellar ataxia type 6. *Clin Genet* 1998;**53**:13–9.

Waters M, Minassian N, Stevanin G, et al. Mutations in voltage-gated potassium channel KCNC3 cause degenerative and developmental central nervous system phenotypes." *Nat Genet* 2006;**38**(4):447–51.

Waters MF, Pulst SM. SCA13. *Cerebellum* 2008;**7**:165–9.

Weiser M, Vega-Saenz de Miera E, et al. Differential expression of Shaw-related K+ channels in the rat central nervous system. *J Neurosci* 1994;**14**:949–72.

Wieczorek S, Arning L, Alheite I, Epplen JT. Mutations of the puratrophin-1 (PLEKHG4) gene on chromosome 16q22.1 are not a common genetic cause of cerebellar ataxia in a European population. *J Hum Genet* 2006;**51**:363–7.

Wild EJ, Tabrizi SJ. Huntington's disease phenocopy syndromes. *Curr Opin Neurol* 2007;**20**:681–7.

Woods BT, Schaumburg HH. Nigro-spino-dentatal degeneration with nuclear ophthalmoplegia. A unique and partially treatable clinico-pathological entity. *J Neurol Sci* 1972;**17**(2)149–66.

Worth PF, Giunti P, Gardner-Thorpe C, et al. Autosomal dominant cerebellar ataxia type III: linkage in a large British family to a 7.6-cM region on chromosome 15q14–21.3. *Am J Hum Genet* 1999;**65**:420–6.

Wozniak DF, Xiao M, Xu L, Yamada KA, Ornitz DM. Impaired spatial learning and defective theta burst induced LTP in mice lacking fibroblast growth factor 14. *Neurobiol Dis* 2007;**26**(1)14–26.

Wüllner U, Reimold M, Abele M, et al. Dopamine transporter positron emission tomography in spinocerebellar ataxias type 1, 2, 3, and 6. *Arch Neurol* 2005;**62**:1280–5.

Xia H, Mao Q, Eliason SL, et al. RNAi suppresses polyglutamine-induced neurodegenerations in a model of spinocerebellar ataxia. *Nat Med* 2004; **10**:816–20.

Yabe I, Sasaki H, Chen DH, et al. Spinocerebellar ataxia type 14 caused by a mutation in protein kinase C gamma. *Arch Neurol* 2003;**60**(12)1749–51.

Yabe I, Sasaki H, Yamashita I, Takei A, Tashiro K. Clinical trial of acetazolamide in SCA6, with assessment using the ataxia rating scale and body stabilometry. *Acta Neurol Scand* 2001;**104**:44–7.

Ying SH, Choi SI, Perlman SL, et al. Pontine and cerebellar atrophy correlate with clinical disability in SCA2. *Neurology* 2006;**66**:424–6.

Yoshida T, Fukaya M, Uchigashima M, et al. Localization of diacylglycerol lipase-alpha around postsynaptic spine suggests close proximity between production site of an endocannabinoid, 2-arachidonoyl-glycerol, and presynaptic cannabinoid CB1 receptor. *J Neurosci* 2006;**26**(18)4740–51.

Yoshida K, Shimizu Y, Morita H, et al. Severity and progression rate of cerebellar ataxia in 16q-linked autosomal dominant cerebellar ataxia (16q-ADCA) in the endemic Nagano Area of Japan. *Cerebellum* 2009;**8**(1)46–51.

Yoshii F, Tomiyasu H, Shinohara Y. Fluid attenuation inversion recovery (FLAIR) images of dentatorubropallidoluysian atrophy: case report. *J Neurol Neurosurg Psychiatry* 1998;**65**(3)396–9.

Yu G-Y, Howell MJ, Roller MJ, Xie T-D, Gomez CM. Spinocerebellar ataxia type 26 maps to chromosome 19p13.*3 adjacent to SCA6. Ann Neurol* 2005;**57**:349–54.

Zannolli R, Gilman S, Rossi S, et al. Hereditary neuronal intranuclear inclusion disease with autonomic failure and cerebellar degeneration. *Arch Neurol* 2002;**59**:1319–26.

Zeman A, Stone J, Porteous M, et al. Spinocerebellar ataxia type 8 in Scotland: genetic and clinical features in seven unrelated cases and a review of published reports. *J Neurol Neurosurg Psychiatry* 2004;**75**:459–65.

Zhuchenko O, Bailey J, Bonnen P, et al. Autosomal dominant cerebellar ataxia (SCA6) associated with small polyglutamine expansions in the alpha(1A)-voltage-dependent calcium channel. *Nat Genet* 1997;**15**:62–9.

Zu T, Duvick LA, Kaytor MD, et al. Recovery from polyglutamine-induced neurodegeneration in conditional SCA1 transgenic mice. *J Neurosci* 2004;**24**(40)8853–61.

Zühlke C, Bürk K. Spinocerebellar ataxia type 17 is caused by mutations in the TATA-box binding protein. *Cerebellum* 2007;**19**:1–8.

Index

(lateral posterior inferior cerebellar artery), 88

(5-fluorouracil), 162

abetalipoproteinemia (Bassen-Kornzweig disease; ABL)
  blood studies, 197
  clinical description, 196–7
  genetic and molecular aspects, 197
  treatment, 197

abscesses, cerebellar, 119

aceruloplasminemia
  blood studies, 213
  clinical description, 213
  epidemiology, 213
  genetic and molecular aspects, 213
  liver biopsy, 213
  neuroimaging, 213
  neuropathology, 213
  pathogenesis, 213–14
  treatment, 214

acetazolamide, 269, 273

acoustic afferents, 13

acoustic artery, 3

action tremor, 41–3, 65

acute diffuse encephalomyelitis (ADEM), 122

adaptive filters, 30

ADEM (acute diffuse encephalomyelitis), 122

adenosine triphosphate (ATP), 19

ADHD (attention deficit hyperactivity disorder), 48

adiadochokinesia, 37

afferences, 7–8

age, diagnosis of cerebellar disorders as function of
  ataxia in elderly, 71–3
  ataxias in young adults, 71
  blood studies, 70

congenital and childhood disorders, 70–1
  cutoff for age, 70
  genetic testing, 73
  obtaining detailed genealogy, 69
  role of brain imaging, 69

agranular endoplasmic reticulum, 8

AHC (alternating hemiplegia of childhood), 272

AICA (anterior inferior cerebellar artery), 88, 89, 94, 95

Aicardi syndrome, 85

alcohol, cerebellar toxicity of
  blood studies, 158
  cerebellar atrophy, 157–8
  clinical findings, 157
  neuropathology, 158
  overview, 157
  pathogenesis, 158–9
  posture and gait studies, 158
  prognosis, 159–60
  treatment, 159

Alexander disease, 218

alien hand syndrome, 133

alpha-mannosidosis, 216

alternating hemiplegia of childhood (AHC), 272

aminergic inputs to cerebellum, 14

aminergic pathways, 14

aminopyridines, 75

amiodarone, 162

anatomy
  afferences, 7–8
  cerebellar circuitry, 8
  cerebellar cortex
    Bergmann glial cells, 10
    granule cells, 8–10
    inhibitory interneurons, 10
    Purkinje neurons, 8
    unipolar brush cells, 10
  cerebellar nuclei
    acoustic, visual, and trigeminal afferents, 13

aminergic and cholinergic inputs to cerebellum, 14
  autonomic centers, 15
  connections with limbic system, 15
  inferior olivary complex, 11
  neurosteroids, 19
  neurotransmitters, 15–19
  overview, 10–11
  pontine nuclei, 14
  reticular nuclei, 13–14
  spinocerebellar tracts, 11–13
  thalamocortical projections, 14
  vestibular afferents, 13
  nomenclature, 5–7

aneurysms, 96
  saccular, 96
  treatment of, 99

Angelman syndrome, 172

angiography, for diagnosis of cerebellar stroke, 98

animal-related cerebellar toxicity, 166

anterior inferior cerebellar artery (AICA), 88, 89, 94, 95

antibiotics
  for treatment of cerebellar abscesses, 119
  for treatment of infectious diseases, 124–5

anticonvulsivants
  carbamazepine, 161
  gabapentin, 161
  lamotrigine, 161
  phenobarbital, 161
  phenytoin, 160–1
  vigabatrin, 161

anti-GAD antibodies (GAD-Ab), ataxia with
  blood studies, 106
  clinical presentation, 106
  neuroimaging, 106
  neuropathology, 106
  overview, 106
  treatment, 106

antineoplastics
    5-FU (5-fluorouracil), 162
    Ara-C (cytosine arabinoside), 162
    cisplatin, 162
    methotrexate, 162
    oxaliplatin, 162
    taxol, 162

anti-Ri syndrome, 145

AOA1. *See* ataxia with oculomotor
    apraxia type 1

AOA2. *See* ataxia with oculomotor
    apraxia type 2

apolipoprotein E receptor type 2
    (ApoER2), 4

APS (autoimmune polyglandular
    syndromes), 108–9

Ara-C (cytosine arabinoside), 162

arachnoid cysts, 84

ARCAs. *See* autosomal recessive
    cerebellar ataxias

arrhythmokinesis (dysrythmokinesia),
    44

ARSACS. *See* autosomal recessive
    spastic ataxia of
    Charlevoix-Saguenay

Arts syndrome, 210

AS20 (ataxia scale on 20 points)
    global disability score, 57
    overview, 56
    visual analog scale, 57

Asperger syndrome, 171

aspergillosis, 96

aspiration, for treatment of cerebellar
    abscesses, 119

assistive therapy, 76–7

astrocytomas, cerebellar, 136

asynergia, 37

AT. *See* ataxia-telangiectasia

AT variant-2 (Berlin breakage
    syndrome), 194

ataxia. *See also* autosomal recessive
    cerebellar ataxias (ARCAs);
    FARS (Friedreich ataxia rating
    scale); SARA (scale for
    assessment and rating of
    ataxia); spinocerebellar ataxias
    (SCAs)
    adult-onset
      laboratory investigations in, 73
      secondary investigations in, 73
    with anti-GAD antibodies

blood studies, 106
clinical presentation, 106
neuroimaging, 106
neuropathology, 106
overview, 106
treatment, 106
associated with CoQ10 deficiency
    ataxic form, 201
    coenzyme Q10, 201–3
    genetic aspects, 203
    overview, 201
    phenotypes, 201
    treatment with CoQ10, 203
and autism spectrum disorders
    brain imaging, 171
    description and clinical features,
      171
    genetic studies, 172
    neuropathology, 171
    neurophysiology, 171
    pathogenesis of autism, 172
    phenotypic overlap with other
      disorders, 172
celiac disease and gluten ataxia
    blood studies, 107
    clinical presentation, 106–7
    neuroimaging, 107
    overview, 106
    pathogenesis, 107
    small bowel biopsy, 107
    treatment, 107
defined, 37
and diabetes, 116
differential diagnosis in young
    adults, 72
drugs for, 76, 77
in elderly, 71–3
environmental causes of
    carbon monoxide, 165
    chemical weapons, 165
    consumption of edible morels,
      166
    cyanide, 165
    eucalyptus oil, 166
    heavy metals, 164
    hyperthermia, 164–5
    insecticides, herbicides, 165
    polychlorinated biphenyls
      (PCBs), 165–6
    saxitoxin (shellfish poisoning),
      166
    toluene benzene derivatives, 164
Hashimoto's ataxia, 113–14
hereditary, cognitive deficits in, 47
and ocular features, 211
sensory, causes of, 46
in young adults, 71

ataxia and isolated vitamin E
    deficiency (AVED)

blood studies, 196
clinical description, 195–6
genetic and molecular aspects,
    196
neuroimaging, 196
neuropathology, 196
neurophysiology, 196
treatment, 196

ataxia with oculomotor apraxia
    (AOA1)
    blood studies, 200
    clinical description, 198–200
    genetic and molecular aspects, 200
    geographical distribution, 198
    management, 200
    neuroimaging, 200
    neuropathology, 200
    neurophysiology, 200

ataxia with oculomotor apraxia
    (AOA2; non-Friedreich
    spinocerebellar ataxia type 1 –
    SCAR1)
    blood studies, 201
    clinical description, 200
    genetic and molecular aspects, 201
    management, 201
    neuroimaging, 200
    neuropathology, 201
    neurophysiology, 200

ataxia scale on 20 points. *See* AS20

ataxia with vitamin E deficiency
    (AVED), 70–1

ataxia-telangiectasia (AT; Louise-Bar
    syndrome), 70
    blood investigations, 194
    clinical description, 193
    differential diagnosis, 194–5
    molecular genetics, 194
    neuroimaging, 193–4
    neuropathology, 194
    neurophysiological investigations,
      193
    prognosis, 195
    sensitivity to ionizing radiation (IR),
      194
    treatment, 195

ataxia-telangiectasia variant v1-AT-v1
    (Nijmegen breakage
    syndrome), 194

atherosclerosis, 95

ATP (adenosine triphosphate), 19

attention deficit hyperactivity
    disorder (ADHD), 48

autism spectrum disorders and ataxia
    brain imaging, 171

description and clinical features,
171
genetic studies, 172
neuropathology, 171
neurophysiology, 171
pathogenesis of autism, 172
phenotypic overlap with other
disorders, 172
autoimmune polyglandular syndromes
(APS), 108–9
autonomic centers, 15
autonomic signs, 46
autosomal recessive cerebellar ataxias
(ARCAs), 190
abetalipoproteinemia (ABL)
blood studies, 197
clinical description, 196–7
genetic and molecular aspects,
197
treatment, 197
aceruloplasminemia
blood studies, 213
clinical description, 213
epidemiology, 213
genetic and molecular aspects,
213
liver biopsy, 213
neuroimaging, 213
neuropathology, 213
pathogenesis, 213–14
treatment, 214
associated with coenzyme Q10
deficiency
ataxic form, 201
coenzyme Q10: biochemical
aspects, 201–3
genetic aspects, 203
overview, 201
phenotypes, 201
treatment with CoQ10, 203
ataxia and isolated vitamin E
deficiency (AVED)
blood studies, 196
clinical description, 195–6
genetic and molecular aspects,
196
neuroimaging, 196
neuropathology, 196
neurophysiology, 196
treatment, 196
ataxia-telangiectasia (AT)
blood investigations, 194
clinical description, 193
differential diagnosis, 194–5
molecular genetics, 194
neuroimaging, 193–4
neuropathology, 194

neurophysiological investigations,
193
prognosis, 195
sensitivity to ionizing radiation
(IR), 194
treatment, 195
Cayman ataxia
clinical description, 211
genetic and molecular aspects,
211
neuroimaging, 211
cerebrotendinous xanthomatosis
(CTX)
biochemical studies, 204
clinical symptoms, 203–4
enzyme assay, 205
epidemiology, 203
genetic aspects, 205
neuroimaging, 204
neuropathology, 204
neurophysiology, 204
treatment, 205
of Charlevoix-Saguenay (ARSACS)
clinical description, 197–8
differential diagnosis, 198
genetic and molecular aspects,
198
geographical distribution, 197
neuroimaging, 198
neuropathology, 198
neurophysiology, 198
treatment, 198
and deafness, 209
dysequilibrium syndrome (DES),
211
early onset, with retained tendon
reflexes (EOCARR)
clinical description, 207
epidemiology, 207
genetic and molecular aspects,
207
neuroimaging, 207
neuropathology, 207
neurophysiology, 207
Friedreich ataxia (FRDA)
biochemical aspects, 191
clinical description, 189–90
differential diagnosis of disorders
associated with cerebral iron
accumulation, 192–3
molecular genetics, 191
neuroimaging, 191
neuropathology, 191–2
neurophysiological investigations,
190
pathology of heart, 192
prognosis, 193
treatment, 193
and hypogonadism

blood studies, 208
clinical description, 208
differential diagnosis, 208–9
genetic and molecular aspects,
208
neuroimaging, 208
neuropathology, 208
neurophysiology, 208
ophtalmologic investigations, 208
treatment, 209
infantile-onset spinocerebellar
ataxia (IOSCA)
clinical description, 206
genetic and molecular aspects,
207
neuroimaging, 206
neuropathology, 206–7
neurophysiology, 206
lysosomal storage diseases
alpha-mannosidosis, 216
cerebellar ataxia with elevated
cerebrospinal free sialic acid
(CAFSA), 217
cystinosis, 217
diagnosis of lysosomal storage
disease, 217
differential diagnosis, 217–18
fucosidosis, 216
gangliosidoses, 214–15
Gaucher disease (GD), 215
infantile sialic acid storage disease
(ISSD) and Salla disease, 217
Niemann-Pick disease type C
(NPC), 215–16
overview, 214
sulfatidoses, 215
treatment, 218
Type I sialidosis, 217
Marinesco-Sjögren syndrome (MSS)
clinical symptoms, 203
genetic aspects, 203
neuroimaging, 203
neuropathology, 203
neurophysiology, 203
treatment, 203
ocular features, 211
with oculomotor apraxia (AOA1)
blood studies, 200
clinical description, 198–200
genetic and molecular aspects,
200
geographical distribution, 198
management, 200
neuroimaging, 200
neuropathology, 200
neurophysiology, 200
with oculomotor apraxia (AOA2)
blood studies, 201
clinical description, 200

autosomal recessive cerebellar ataxias (ARCAs), (cont.)
  with oculomotor apraxia (AOA2) (cont.) 201
    genetic and molecular aspects, management, 201
    neuroimaging, 200
    neuropathology, 201
    neurophysiology, 200
  overview, 189
  Refsum disease
    blood studies, 205
    clinical description, 205
    differential diagnosis, 206
    genetic and molecular aspects, 205–6
    neuroimaging, 206
    neuropathology, 206
    treatment, 206
  spinocerebellar ataxia with axonal neuropathy (SCAN1), 208
  type 1 (ARCA-1)
    clinical symptoms, 205
    genetic aspects, 205
    neuroimaging, 205
    neurophysiology, 205
  Wilson disease
    blood studies, 212
    clinical description, 211–12
    epidemiology, 211
    genetic and molecular aspects, 212
    liver biopsy, 212
    neuroimaging, 212
    neurophysiology, 212
    pathogenesis, 212–13
    slit-lamp examination, 212
    treatment, 213
    urinary studies, 212
autosomal recessive spastic ataxia of Charlevoix-Saguenay (ARSACS)
  clinical description, 197–8
  differential diagnosis, 198
  genetic and molecular aspects, 198
  geographical distribution, 197
  neuroimaging, 198
  neuropathology, 198
  neurophysiology, 198
  treatment, 198
AVED. See ataxia and isolated vitamin E deficiency

baclofen, 106
bacterial infections
  clinical presentation, 120
  differential diagnosis, 122–4
  infectious agents, 120
  investigations, 121–2
  neuroimaging, 118–19
  overview, 118
  pathogenesis, 120–1
  prognosis, 125
  treatment of cerebellar abscesses, 119
  treatment of cerebellitis, 124–5
Barany's test, for deficits in limb movements, 40–1
Bassen-Kornzweig disease. See abetalipoproteinemia
BARs scale (brief ataxia rating scale)
BCAs (beta-carboline alkaloids), 185
BDNF (brain-derived neurotrophic factor), 5
Behçet disease, 108
Behr syndrome, 210
benzodiazepines, 185
Bergmann glia cells, 2, 4, 10
Berlin breakage syndrome (AT variant-2), 194
Berman syndrome, 209
beta-blockers, 185, 193
beta-carboline alkaloids (BCAs), 185
beta-interferons, 105
betamethasone, 195
Bickerstaff encephalitis, 121–2
biomechanical loading, for treatment of essential tremor, 187
Blake pouch cyst (retrocerebellar arachnoid cyst), 84
BMPs (bone morphogenetic proteins), 4
BNS (Boucher-Neuhäuser syndrome), 208, 209
body sway
  in Ataxia Scale on 20 points, 56
  in Unified Multiple System Atrophy Rating Scale, 65
bone morphogenetic proteins (BMPs), 4
border zone infarctions (watershed), 92
botulinum toxin injections, 185
Boucher-Neuhäuser syndrome (BNS), 208, 209
brachium conjunctivum (superior cerebellar peduncle), 7
brachium pontis (middle cerebellar peduncle), 7
brain imaging, 69
brain-derived neurotrophic factor (BDNF), 5
brainstem gliomas, 136–8
brimonidine tartrate, 163
buspirone, 269

CAH (congenital adrenal hyperplasia), 103
calcineurin inhibitors, 163
cannabinoid receptors (CB1Rs), 17
cannabinoid receptors type 1 (CB1Rs), 17
capecitabine, 162
carbamazepine, 161
carbon monoxide, 165
cataract, 71, 205
Cayman ataxia
  clinical description, 211
  genetic and molecular aspects, 211
  neuroimaging, 211
CB1Rs (cannabinoid receptors type 1), 17
CB1Rs (Cayman ataxia), 17
CBD. See corticobasal ganglionic degeneration
CCAS (cerebellar cognitive affective syndrome), 46, 48
CCFS (Composite Cerebellar Functional Severity) score, 59
CCT (cuneocerebellar tract), 13
CDG. See congenital disorders of glycosylation
celiac disease, and gluten ataxia
  blood studies, 107
  clinical presentation, 106–7
  neuroimaging, 107
  overview, 106
  pathogenesis, 107
  small bowel biopsy, 107
  treatment, 107
cell formation, 2
cerebellar circuitry, 8
cerebellar cognitive affective syndrome (CCAS), 46, 48
cerebellar cortex
  Bergmann glial cells, 10

granule cells, 8–10
inhibitory interneurons, 10
Purkinje neurons, 8
unipolar brush cells, 10

cerebellar cortical degeneration, 49

cerebellar neurons, generation of, 2

cerebellar nuclei
acoustic, visual, and trigeminal
afferents, 13
activities in, 23–4
aminergic and cholinergic inputs to
cerebellum, 14
autonomic centers, 15
connections with limbic system, 15
inferior olivary complex, 11
neurosteroids, 19
neurotransmitters, 15–19
overview, 10–11
pontine nuclei, 14
reticular nuclei, 13–14
spinocerebellar tracts, 11–13
thalamocortical projections, 14
vestibular afferents, 13

cerebellar presentation (cMSA), 71

cerebellar stroke. See stroke

cerebellar vein thrombosis. See vein
thrombosis, cerebellar

cerebellitis, 121, 123
clinical presentation of, 120
differential diagnosis of, 124
infections and vaccinations
associated with, 121

cerebellum. See also cerebellar cortex;
cerebellar nuclei
development of, 3–4
illustration of, 6
malformations affecting, 82–3
origin of, 2
physiology of
activities in cerebellar nuclei,
23–4
activities of inferior olivary
complex, 25
activities of Purkinje neurons,
24–5
cerebellum and cognitive
operations, 31
cerebellum and timing, 29
computational models of
cerebellar function, 29–31
control of eye movements, 25
control of limb movements, 26
control of speech, 25–6
functional divisions, 23
learning, 27–8
mood and depression, 32

overview, 23
posture and gait, 26–7
sensory processing, 29
vessels, anatomy of, 88–9

cerebral folate deficiency (CFD), 71

cerebrospinal fluid (CSF) studies,
104

cerebrotendinous xanthomatosis
(CTX), 71, 204
biochemical studies, 204
clinical symptoms, 203–4
enzyme assay, 205
epidemiology, 203
genetic aspects, 205
neuroimaging, 204
neuropathology, 204
neurophysiology, 204
treatment, 205

CFD (cerebral folate deficiency), 71

Charlevoix-Saguenay. See autosomal
recessive spastic ataxia of
Charlevoix-Saguenay
(ARSACS)

check, disturbed, 44

chemical weapons, and cerebellar
ataxia, 165

chemotherapy
complications of, 143
for treatment of
ataxia-telangiectasia, 195
for treatment of cerebellar
metastases, 143
for treatment of ependymomas, 138
for treatment of Langerhans
histiocytosis, 146
for treatment of medulloblastomas,
135–6

cherry spot myoclonus syndrome
(sialidosis type I), 176–7, 217

Chiari malformations, 78–9, 83–4

childhood disorders, 70–1, 171

cholinergic inputs to cerebellum, 19

cisplatin, 162

CJD (Creutzfeldt-Jakob disease),
125–6, 127, 128

cladribine, 105

clinical scales
AS20
global disability score, 57
overview, 56
visual analog scale, 57
FARS
activities of daily living, 60–1

functional staging for ataxia, 60
instrumental testing, 64
lower limb coordination, 62
neurological examination, 61
overview, 59–60
peripheral nervous system,
62–3
upper limb coordination, 61–2
upright stability, 63–4
ICARS
kinetic functions, 54–5
oculomotor deficits, 55–6
overview, 53
posture and gait score, 53–4
speech assessment, 55
overview, 53
SARA
comparison between scales, 59
overview, 57–9
quantitative tests, 59
UMSARS, 64–7

clonazepam, 75, 114, 182

cMSA (cerebellar presentation), 71

cocaine, 96, 163

Cockayne syndrome, 194–5

coenzyme Q10 (CoQ10), 201–3
deficiency of, 232
synthesis of, 202
for treatment of Leigh syndrome,
232–3

cognitive abnormalities, 46–8

cognitive operations, 31

Composite Cerebellar Functional
Severity (CCFS) score, 59

computational models of cerebellar
function, 29–31

concussion, 149

congenital adrenal hyperplasia (CAH),
103

congenital disorders, 70–1

congenital disorders of glycosylation
(CDG; carbohydrate-deficient
glycoprotein syndromes), 84–5

Connexin 43 (Cx43), 10

contusions, 149, 150

copper metabolism disorders, 71

CoQ10. See coenzyme Q10

cortex, cerebellar. See cerebellar
cortex

cortical dorsal infarcts, 92

cortical-border zone infarcts, 92

corticobasal ganglionic degeneration (CBD)
  brain imaging, 133
  clinical features, 133
  differential diagnosis, 134
  neuropathology, 133–4
  neurophysiology, 133
  treatment, 134
corticosteroids, for treatment of MS, 105
Creutzfeldt-Jakob disease (CJD), 125–6, 127, 128
crossed atrophy of cerebellum, 155
CSF (cerebrospinal fluid) studies, 104
CTX. See cerebrotendinous xanthomatosis
cuneocerebellar tract (CCT), 13
Cx43 (Connexin 43), 10
cyanide, and cerebellar ataxia, 165
cyclosporin, 163
cysts, arachnoid, 84
cytosine arabinoside (Ara-C), 162

"dancing eyes" (opsoclonus), 38, 120
Dandy-Walker malformation, 82, 83
De Morsier syndrome (septo-optic dysplasia), 116
deafness, and cerebellar ataxia, 209
decomposition of movement, 43–4
deep brain stimulation (DBS) of thalamic nuclei (Vim), 185–6
deferiprone, 193
delayed-onset cerebellar syndrome, 151
delayed-onset intention tremor, 151
Delta, Serrate, and Lag-2 (DSL) ligands, 4
Delta-Notch-like EGF-related receptor (DNER), 4
dementia with Lewy bodies (DLB), 134
demyelination
  in Alexander, 218
  in infectious diseases, 120
  in MS, 102, 104
  in spinocerebellar ataxia
    type 2, 250
    type 7, 256
  in sulfatidoses, 215
dentate nucleus, 10–11, 14, 23, 25, 38

dentatorubral-pallidoluysian atrophy (DRPLA)
  clinical presentation, 256
  epidemiology, 256
  genetic and molecular aspects, 257
  neuroimaging, 256
  neuropathology, 257
  neurophysiology, 257
depression, 32
dermoid tumors, 141
DES (dysequilibrium syndrome), 211
desferioxamine, 193, 214
desmopressin, 182
developmental abnormalities, with fluid collections, 84
dexamethasone, 142
diabetes, and cerebellar ataxia, 116
diabetes insipidus, juvenile diabetes mellitus, optic atrophy, and deafness (DIDMOAD) syndrome, 209
diagnosis of cerebellar disorders, age as function of, 70–1
  ataxia in elderly, 71–3
  ataxias in young adults, 71
  blood studies, 70
  congenital and childhood disorders, 70–1
  cutoff for age, 70
  genetic testing, 73
  obtaining detailed genealogy, 69
  role of brain imaging, 69
DIDMOAD (diabetes insipidus, juvenile diabetes mellitus, optic atrophy, and deafness) syndrome, 209
diffuse axonal injury, 149
DISAS (dominantly inherited spastic ataxia syndromes), 274
disorders of pursuit, 38, 55
disorders of saccades, 39
dissection of vessel wall, 150
disturbed check, 44
DLB (dementia with Lewy bodies), 134
DNER (Delta-Notch-like EGF-related receptor), 4
dominant ataxias. See also spinocerebellar ataxia
  dentatorubral-pallidoluysian atrophy (DRPLA)
    clinical presentation, 256

  epidemiology, 256
  genetic and molecular aspects, 257
  neuroimaging, 256
  neuropathology, 257
  neurophysiology, 257
dominantly inherited spastic ataxia syndromes (DISAS), 274
episodic ataxias (EAs)
  clinical presentation, 270
  differential diagnosis, 271–3
  genetic aspects, 271
  neuroimaging, 270
  neurophysiology, 271
  treatment, 273–4
dominantly inherited spastic ataxia syndromes (DISAS), 274
dorsal spinocerebellar tract (DSCT; Flechsig tract), 11–13
Down-beat nystagmus, 39
D-penicillamine, 213
DRPLA. See dentatorubral-pallidoluysian atrophy
drugs, as toxic agents
  amiodarone, 162
  anticonvulsivants
    carbamazepine, 161
    other anticonvulsivants, 161–2
    phenytoin, 160–1
  antineoplastics
    5-FU (5-fluorouracil), 162
    Ara-C (cytosine arabinoside), 162
    cisplatin, oxaliplatin, taxol, 162
    methotrexate, 162
    oxaliplatin, 162
    taxol, 162
  brimonidine tartrate, 163
  cyclosporin and other calcineurin inhibitors, 163
  drug abuse
    cocaine, 163
    herbs, 164
    heroin, 163
    methadone, 163
    phencyclidine, 163–4
  lithium salts, 162
  metronidazole, 163
  procainamide, 162
DSCT (dorsal spinocerebellar tract; Flechsig tract), 11–13
DSL (Delta, Serrate and Lag-2) ligands, 4
Duret hemorrhage, 151

dysarthria, 40, 49, 56

dysdiadochokinesia, 37, 44

dysequilibrium syndrome (DES), 211

dysmetria, 37, 41

dysprosody, 40

dysrythmokinesia ("arrhythmokinesis"), 44

early-onset cerebellar ataxia with retained tendon reflexes (EOCARR; Harding ataxia)
    clinical description, 207
    epidemiology, 207
    genetic and molecular aspects, 207
    neuroimaging, 207
    neuropathology, 207
    neurophysiology, 207

EAs. See episodic ataxias

ECG (electrocardiographic) studies, 98

EGL (external granular layer), 2

elderly, ataxia in, 71–3

electrocardiographic (ECG) studies, 98

embryology
    generation of cerebellar neurons, 2
    genes, signaling, and development of cerebellum, 3–4
    imaging and fetal development, 5
    neurotrophins, 5
    origin of cerebellum, 2
    vertebrobasilar system embryogenesis, 3

emotional disorders, 46–8

endocannabinoids, 17

endocrine disorders
    cerebellar ataxia and diabetes, 116
    cerebellar ataxia and hypogonadism, 116
    parathyroid disorders, 115–16
    thyroid disorders
        drug-induced dysfunction of thyroid gland, 115
        Hashimoto ataxia, 113–14
        hyperthyroidism, 113
        hypothyroidism, 113
        overview, 113

environmental causes of cerebellar ataxia
    carbon monoxide, 165
    chemical weapons, 165
    consumption of edible morels, 166
    cyanide, 165
    eucalyptus oil, 166
    heavy metals
        lead, 164
        mercury, 164
    hyperthermia, 164–5
    insecticides, herbicides, 165
    polychlorinated biphenyls (PCBs), 165–6
    saxitoxin (shellfish poisoning), 166
    toluene benzene derivatives, 164

enzyme replacement therapy, 99

EOCARR. See early-onset cerebellar ataxia with retained tendon reflexes

ependymomas, 138

epidermoid tumors, 141

epidural hematoma, 150

episodic ataxias (EAs)
    clinical presentation, 270
    differential diagnosis, 271–3
    genetic aspects, 271
    neuroimaging, 270
    neurophysiology, 271
    treatment, 273–4

EPO (human recombinant erythropoietin), 193

Erdheim-Chester disease, 146–7

essential tremor (ET), 43
    clinical features, 184
    diagnostic criteria of, 185
    environmental factors, 185
    epidemiology, 184
    genetic studies, 185
    neuroimaging studies, 184
    neuropathology, 185
    neurophysiological studies, 184
    treatment of, 185–7

ethanol, 158–9

eucalyptus oil, 166

excessive rebound, 44

external granular layer (EGL), 2

extra-cerebellar disease, 40

extra-cerebellar lesions, causing hemiataxia, 94–5

eyeblink conditioning, 28, 29, 49

eyes, 25 See also index entries beginning with "ocular"

Fabry disease, 96

familial adult myoclonic epilepsy (FAME), 177

FARR (Friedreich ataxia with retained reflexes), 190

FARS (Friedreich Ataxia Rating Scale)
    activities of daily living, 60–1
    functional staging for ataxia, 60
    instrumental testing, 64
    lower limb coordination, 62
    neurological examination, 61
    overview, 59–60
    peripheral nervous system, 62–3
    upper limb coordination, 61–2
    upright stability, 63–4

fast nose-finger (dysmetria) test, 62

fastigial nucleus (FN), 13, 23

fatal familial insomnia, 126, 128

fetal development, imaging of, 5

finger taps test, 62, 65

finger-to-finger test, 40, 61–2

finger-to-nose test, 40

fixation deficits, 38

flocculus, development of, 2

fluid collections, developmental abnormalities with, 84

fluorocortisone, 182

Flynn and Aird syndrome, 209

FN (fastigial nucleus), 13, 23

FOXP2, 4

fragile X tremor ataxia syndrome (FXTAS), 71
    brain MRI and gait analysis in, 240
    clinical deficits in, 239
    clinical presentation, 238
    diagnostic criteria of, 239
    genetic and molecular aspects, 239
    neuroimaging, 238–9
    neuropathology, 239–40
    neurophysiology, 239
    treatment, 240

Friedreich ataxia (FRDA), 70
    biochemical aspects, 191
    clinical description, 189–90
    diagnostic criteria of, 190
    differential diagnosis of disorders associated with cerebral iron accumulation, 192–3
    molecular genetics, 191
    neuroimaging, 191
    neuropathology, 191–2
    neurophysiological investigations, 190
    pathology of heart, 192
    prognosis, 193
    treatment, 193

Friedreich Ataxia Rating Scale. *See* FARS

Friedreich ataxia with retained reflexes (FARR), 190

frontal ataxia, 45

fucosidosis, 216

Fukuhara disease. *See* myoclonic epilepsy with ragged-red fibers

FXTAS. *See* fragile X tremor ataxia syndrome

GABA, 17–18

gabapentin, 161, 185

GAD. *See* glutamic acid decarboxylase

GAD-Ab. *See* anti-GAD antibodies

gait, 26–7, 45
  in acute intoxication, 157
  in Ataxia Scale on 20 points, 56
  deficits in, 45–6
  in EOCARR, 207
  in fragile X tremor ataxia syndrome, 239
  in FXTAS syndrome, 240
  in gluten ataxia, 106
  ICARS score, 53–4
  psychogenic gait ataxia, 45–6
  in Scale for Assessment and Rating of Ataxia, 57
  in spinocerebellar ataxia
    type 6, 254
    type 10, 258
    type 20, 265
  in Unified Multiple System Atrophy Rating Scale, 65

ganglionic (monolayer) of cerebellar cortex, 8

gangliosidoses, 214–15

Gaucher disease (GD), 215

gaze
  in ataxia with oculomotor apraxia, 200
  checking stability of, 37
  in EOCARR, 207
  in multiple system atrophy, 179
  in spinocerebellar ataxia type 3, 251

gaze-evoked nystagmus (gaze-paretic), 39, 207

GD (Gaucher disease), 215

genealogy, and diagnosis of cerebellar disorders, 69

genes, and development of cerebellum, 3–4

genetic testing, 73

Gerstmann-Sträussler-Scheinker disease, 128

Gillespie syndrome, 210

Glatiramer acetate, 105

gliomas, brainstem, 136–8

Glut1 deficiency syndrome, 71

glutamic acid decarboxylase (GAD)
  ataxia with anti-GAD antibodies
    blood studies, 106
    clinical presentation, 106
    neuroimaging, 106
    neuropathology, 106
    overview, 106
    treatment, 106

gluten ataxia, and celiac disease
  blood studies, 107
  clinical presentation, 106–7
  neuroimaging, 107
  overview, 106
  pathogenesis, 107
  small bowel biopsy, 107
  treatment, 107

GM2 gangliosidosis type I (Tay-Sachs disease), 214

Golgi cells, 10

Gower tract. *See* ventral spinocerebellar tract

graft-versus-host disease (GVHD), 109

granule cells, 2, 8–10

granule neurons, 2

great toe-finger test, 41

Guillain-Barré syndrome, 121–2

GVHD (graft-versus-host disease), 109

Harding ataxia. *See* early-onset cerebellar ataxia with retained tendon reflexes

Hashimoto ataxia, 113–14

Hashimoto encephalopathy, 126

headaches, 36

heavy metals, and cerebellar ataxia
  lead, 164
  mercury, 164

heel along shin slide test, 62

heel-knee-shin test, 65

heel-to-knee test, 41

heel-to-shin tap test, 62

hemangioblastomas, 138

hemiataxia, extra-cerebellar lesions causing, 94–5

hemispheres, cerebellar, 2

hemorrhage, cerebellar, 96–7

herbicides, cerebellotoxic, 166

herbs, 164

heredopathia atactica polyneuritiformis. *See* Refsum disease

heroin, 163

hindbrain, malformations of, 78–82, 83–4

histiocytosis X. *See* Langherans histiocytosis

Holmes ataxia, 208

human prion diseases
  clinical presentation, 125–6
  CSF studies, 128
  differential diagnosis, 126
  genetic aspects, 128
  neuroimaging, 126
  neuropathology, 128
  neurophysiology, 126
  overview, 125
  treatment, 128

human recombinant erythropoietin (EPO), 193

Hurst disease, 121

hyperammonemia, 271–2

hypermetria, 41

hyperparathyroidism, 115–16

hyperthermia, and cerebellar ataxia, 164–5

hyperthyroidism, 113

hypoglossal artery, 3

hypogonadism, and cerebellar ataxia, 116
  blood studies, 208
  clinical description, 208
  differential diagnosis, 208–9
  genetic and molecular aspects, 208
  neuroimaging, 208
  neuropathology, 208
  neurophysiology, 208
  ophthalmologic investigations, 208
  treatment, 209

hypoparathyroidism, 115

hypoplasias, 78, 82–3, 84–5

hypothyroidism, 113, 114

hypotonia, 43

ICARS (International Cooperative
        Ataxia Rating Scale)
    kinetic functions, 54–5
    oculomotor deficits, 55–6
    overview, 53
    posture and gait score, 53–4
    speech assessment, 55
idebenone, 193, 232
idiopathic hypertrophic
        pachymeningitis (IHPM),
        140
idiopathic late-onset cerebellar ataxia
        (ILOCA), 73
IGL (internal granular layer), 2
IHPM (idiopathic hypertrophic
        pachymeningitis), 140
ILOCA. *See* idiopathic late-onset
        cerebellar ataxia
immune diseases
    ataxia with anti-GAD antibodies
        blood studies, 106
        clinical presentation, 106
        neuroimaging, 106
        neuropathology, 106
        overview, 106
        treatment, 106
    celiac disease and gluten ataxia
        blood studies, 107
        clinical presentation, 106–7
        neuroimaging, 107
        overview, 106
        pathogenesis, 107
        small bowel biopsy, 107
        treatment, 107
    multiple sclerosis (MS)
        cerebrospinal fluid (CSF) studies,
            104
        clinical manifestations, 102
        diagnostic criteria, 102–3
        differential diagnosis, 103
        neuroimaging, 104
        neuropathology, 104
        neurophysiology, 103–4
        overview, 102
        pathogenesis, 104
        treatment, 104–6
index-to-index test, 40
index-to-wrist test, 41
indomethacin, 182
infantile-onset spinocerebellar ataxia
        (IOSCA)
    clinical description, 206
    genetic and molecular aspects,
        207
    neuroimaging, 206

neuropathology, 206–7
neurophysiology, 206
infantile sialic acid storage disease
        (ISSD), 217
infarctions, cerebellar
    AICA infarctions, 89
    border zone infarctions (watershed),
        92
    extra-cerebellar lesions causing
        hemiataxia, 94–5
    lacunar infarctions, 92
    mechanisms of, 95
    outcome of, 95
    overview, 89
    PICA infarctions, 92
    SCA infarctions, 89
    territorial, symptoms in, 92
infectious diseases
    bacterial infections
        clinical presentation, 120
        differential diagnosis, 122–4
        infectious agents, 120
        investigations, 121–2
        neuroimaging, 118–19
        overview, 118
        pathogenesis, 120–1
        prognosis, 125
        treatment of cerebellar abscesses,
            119
        treatment of cerebellitis, 124–5
    in cancer patients, 143
    human prion diseases
        clinical presentation, 125–6
        CSF studies, 128
        differential diagnosis, 126
        genetic aspects, 128
        neuroimaging, 126
        neuropathology, 128
        neurophysiology, 126
        overview, 125
        treatment, 128
inferior cerebellar peduncle, 7
inferior olivary complex, 11, 25
inhibitory interneurons, 10
insecticides, 165, 166
internal granular layer (IGL), 2
International Cooperative Ataxia
        Rating Scale. *See* ICARS
isometrataxia, 44–5
ISSD (infantile sialic acid storage
        disease), 217

JC virus (papovavirus), 123, 124
Jeune-Tommasi disease, 209

Joubert syndrome and related
        disorders (JSRD), 79–81
juvenile pilocytic astrocytoma,
        136

kava, 164
Kayser-Fleischer ring, 211–12
Kearns-Sayre syndrome, 234
Kikuchi-Fujimoto disease (KFD;
        histiocytic necrotizing
        lymphadenitis), 109
kinetic functions, ICARS scale, 54–5
kinetic tremor, 41
Kinsbourne syndrome
        (opsoclonus-myoclonus), 38,
        122, 124
knee-tibia test, for deficits in limb
        movements, 41
Koletzko syndrome, 209

lacunar infarctions, 92
Lafora disease, 174–5
lamotrigine, 161
Langerhans histiocytosis, 145–6
late-onset Friedreich ataxia (LOFA),
        71
late-onset Tay-Sachs disease (LOTSD),
        214
lateral posterior inferior cerebellar
        artery (1PICA), 88
lateral reticular nucleus (LRN), 13
LCMV (lymphocytic choriomeningitis
        virus), 121
L-DOPS (L-threo-3,
        4-dihydroxyphenylserine), 182
lead, and cerebellar ataxia, 164
learning, 27–8
Leigh syndrome (subacute necrotizing
        encephalopathy), 231–2, 233
lesions
    and bilateral ataxia, 95
    in cancer, 136
    and contralateral hemiataxia, 95
    effect on posture and gait, 26
    in Erdheim-Chester disease, 147
    extra-cerebellar, causing hemiataxia,
        94–5
    of Guillain-Mollaret triangle, 151
    and hemangioblastomas, 138
    in multiple sclerosis, 103

lesions (*cont.*)
   resulting in oculomotor disorders, 37–8
   symptom mapping, 48
   in von Hippel-Lindau disease, 138

leukoencephalopathy, 163

levodopa-induced dyslinesias, 179

levothyroxine, 113

Lhermitte-Duclos disease, 85, 142

Lichenstein-Knorr syndrome, 209

limb movements, control of, 26, 40–5, 61–2

limbic cerebellum, 15

limbic system, 15

lipohyalinosis, 96

lithium salts, 143, 162

LLRs (long-latency reflexes), 27

lobules of cerebellum, 5, 7

LOFA (late-onset Friedreich ataxia), 71

long-latency reflexes (LLRs), 27

LOTSD (late-onset Tay-Sachs disease), 214

Louise-Bar syndrome, 194

LRN (lateral reticular nucleus), 13

L-threo-3, 4-dihydroxyphenylserine (L-DOPS), 182

Lugaro cells, 10

lymphocytic choriomeningitis virus (LCMV), 121

lymphomatosis cerebri, 126

lysosomal enzyme deficiency, 177

lysosomal storage diseases
   alpha-mannosidosis, 216
   cerebellar ataxia with elevated cerebrospinal free sialic acid (CAFSA), 217
   cystinosis, 217
   diagnosis of lysosomal storage disease, 217
   differential diagnosis, 217–18
   fucosidosis, 216
   gangliosidoses, 214–15
   Gaucher disease (GD), 215
   infantile sialic acid storage disease (ISSD) and salla disease, 217
   Niemann-Pick disease type C (NPC), 215–16
   overview, 214

sulfatidoses, 215
treatment, 218
Type I sialidosis, 217

macrocerebellum, 85

macrosaccadic oscillations, 38

malformations
   affecting predominantly cerebellum and derivatives, 82–3
   affecting predominantly lower hindbrain, 83–4
   of both midbrain and hindbrain, 78–82
   classification of, 78
   developmental abnormalities with fluid collections, 84
   pre-natal–onset degeneration, 84–5
management of cerebellar disorders
   medical treatment, 75–6
   overview, 75
   rehabilitation and assistive therapy, 76–7
   surgery, 76
   treatments under investigation, 77

maple syrup disease, 271

Marinesco-Sjögren syndrome (MSS)
   clinical symptoms, 203
   genetic aspects, 203
   neuroimaging, 203
   neuropathology, 203
   neurophysiology, 203
   treatment, 203

Marr-Albus-Ito theory, 24

Math1 gene, 4

medial posterior inferior cerebellar artery (mPICA), 88

medical treatment of cerebellar disorders, 75–6

medulloblastomas, 135–6

mega-cisterna magna, 84

memory, 27

meningiomas, 135, 138–40

meningoencephalitis, 121

mercury, and cerebellar ataxia, 164

MERRF. *See* myoclonic epilepsy with ragged-red fibers

metastases, 142–3

methadone, 163

methotrexate, 162

methylprednisolone
   for treatment of cerebellitis, 125

for treatment of Hashimoto ataxia, 114
for treatment of multiple sclerosis, 105

metronidazole, 163

microcephalin, 4

microneurosurgery, for treatment of cerebellar metastases, 143

microsurgery, for treatment of schwannomas (neurinomas), 140–1

midbrain, malformations of, 78–82

middle cerebellar peduncle (brachium pontis), 7

midodrine, 182

Miller Fisher syndrome, 121

mitochondrial disorders
   brain imaging, 232
   brain MRI and MR spectroscopy in, 235
   classification of, 230
   common symptoms in, 229
   defects of mtDNA, 229
   deficits of nucleo-mitochondrial signaling, 229–31
   differential diagnosis, 232
   introduction and classification, 229
   nuclear gene defects, 231–2
   treatment, 232–3

mitochondrial neurogastrointestinal encephalomyopathy (MNGIE), 231

mitoxantrone, 105

MNGIE (mitochondrial neurogastrointestinal encephalomyopathy), 231

Möbius syndrome, 84

molar tooth sign, 79

monoclonal antibodies, for treatment of MS, 105

monocular bobbing, 40

monolayer (ganglionic) of cerebellar cortex, 8

mood, 32, 155

morels, and cerebellar ataxia, 166

movement, decomposition of, 43–4

mPICA (medial posterior inferior cerebellar artery), 88

MS. *See* multiple sclerosis

MSA. *See* multiple system atrophy

MSS. *See* Marinesco-Sjögren syndrome

multiple sclerosis (MS)
    cerebrospinal fluid (CSF) studies, 104
    clinical manifestations, 102
    diagnostic criteria, 102–3
    differential diagnosis, 103
    neuroimaging, 104
    neuropathology, 104
    neurophysiology, 103–4
    overview, 102
    pathogenesis, 104
    treatment, 104–6

multiple-system atrophy (MSA)
    assessment of autonomic nervous system, 180
    autonomic symptoms in, 180
    diagnostic criteria, 179
    differential diagnosis, 180
    epidemiology, 179
    neuroimaging, 179–80
    neuropathology, 181–2
    overview, 179
    signs not suggestive of, 180
    symptomatic treatment in, 182
    treatment, 182

muscle tone, disorders of, 43

muscle weakness test, 62–3

mutism, 40, 47–8, 120

myelination, 5, 113 *See also* demyelination

myelinolysis, 157

myoclonic epilepsy with ragged-red fibers (MERRF; Fukuhara disease), 175–6

NBS (Nijmegen breakage syndrome), 194

NCLs (neuronal ceroid lipofuscinosis), 176

necrotizing lymphadenitis (Kikuchi-Fujimoto disease), 109

neocerebellum, 5

nerve growth factor (NGF), 5

net torque (NET), 26

neurinomas (schwannomas), 135, 140–1

neuroferritinopathy, 262

neuromodulators, 15, 17

neuromyelitis optica (NMO), 103

neuronal ceroid lipofuscinosis (NCL), 176

neurons, generation of, 2

neuropsychiatric symptoms, 46

neuropsychological deficits, 155

neurosteroids, 19

neurotransmitters, 15, 19

neurotrophin 3 (NT-3), 5

neurotrophins, 5

NGF (nerve growth factor), 5

Niemann-Pick disease type C (NPC), 215–16

Nijmegen breakage syndrome (NBS; ataxia-telangiectasia variant v1-AT-v1), 194

nitric oxide (NO), 19

NMO (neuromyelitis optica), 103

NO (nitric oxide), 19

nose-finger test, 58, 62

Notch proteins, 4

NPC (Niemann-Pick disease type C), 215–16

NRTP (nuclear reticularis tegmenti pontis), 13

NT-3 (neurotrophin 3), 5

nuclear neuroblasts, during cerebellar development, 2

nuclear reticularis tegmenti pontis (NRTP), 13

nuclei, cerebellar. *See* cerebellar nuclei

nucleus prepositus hypoglossi, 14

nutritional deficiencies, 158

nystagmus, 39–40, 77

occupational therapy, 76

ocular bobbing, 39–40

ocular tilt reaction (OTR), 38

oculomasticatory myorhythmia, 124

oculomotor deficits, 38, 55–6

oculomotor disturbances, 37–40

olivary hypertrophy, 151

olivary neurons, 25

olivopontocerebellar atrophy (OPCA), 180

opsoclonus ("dancing eyes"), 38, 120

opsoclonus-myoclonus (Kinsbourne syndrome), 122, 124

orthostatic symptoms, 65, 67

orthostatic tremor, 43

OTR (ocular tilt reaction), 38

oxaliplatin, 162

oxybutynin, 182

PACAP (pituitary adenylate cyclase-activating polypeptide), 16

palatal tremor, 43

paleocerebellum, 5

pancreas transcription factor 1A (PTF1A), 4

papovavirus (JC virus), 123, 124

paradichlorobenzene (PDB), 164

paramedian reticular nucleus (PRN), 13

paraneoplastic cerebellar degeneration (PCD), 143–5
    antibodies found in, 144
    recommended investigations in, 145

paraneoplastic disorders and tumors
    brainstem gliomas, 136–8
    cerebellar astrocytomas, 136
    cerebellar metastases, 142–3
    complications of chemotherapy, phenytoin, lithium salts, 143
    ependymomas, 138
    epidermoid and dermoid tumors, 141
    Erdheim-Chester disease, 146–7
    hemangioblastomas, 138
    infections, 143
    Langerhans histiocytosis, 145–6
    Lhermitte-Duclos disease, 142
    medulloblastomas, 135–6
    meningiomas, 138–40
    overview, 135
    paraneoplastic cerebellar degeneration (PCD), 143–5
    primary lymphomas of CNS (PCNSL), 141
    schwannomas (neurinomas), 140–1
    stroke, 143
    superficial siderosis, 143

parathyroid disorders, 115–16

Parkinson disease, 179, 180

PCBs (polychlorinated biphenyls), 165–6

PCD. *See* paraneoplastic cerebellar degeneration

PCNSL (primary lymphomas of CNS), 141

PDB (paradichlorobenzene), 164

penicillamine, 213

peripheral nervous system, FARS scale, 62–3

phencyclidine, 163–4

phenytoin, 160–1, 174
    complications of, 143
    for treatment of episodic ataxias, 273

PHP (pseudohypoparathyroidism), 115

physical therapy, 76–7

phytanic acid oxidase deficiency. *See* Refsum disease

PICA (posterior inferior cerebellar artery), 3, 88, 89, 93, 95

pinceau, 10

pituitary adenylate cyclase–activating polypeptide (PACAP), 16

plasma exchanges
    for treatment of aceruloplasminemia, 214
    for treatment of ataxia with anti-GAD antibodies, 106
    for treatment of MS, 105

plasmapheresis, 114

PME. *See* progressive myoclonic epilepsies

PML (progressive multifocal leukoencephalopathy), 123

PNET (primitive neuroectodermal tumors), 135–6

polyarteritis nodosa, 108

polychlorinated biphenyls (PCBs), 165–6

polycythemia, 138

pontine nuclei, 14

ponto-cerebellar hypoplasias, 84–5

position sense test, 63

posterior fossa trauma
    bilateral subdural hematoma of, 152
    clinical presentation, 149
    epidural hematoma of, 153

evaluation of, 151
investigations, 150–1
late complications, 151–5
management, 151
overview, 149
results of imaging studies in, 152
treatment of, 155
types of, 149, 150

posterior inferior cerebellar artery (PICA), 3, 88, 89, 93, 95

postural tremor, 42

posture, 26–7
    deficits in, 45–6
    ICARS score, 53–4
    in Unified Multiple System Atrophy Rating Scale, 65

pregabalin, 185

pre-natal–onset degeneration, 84–5

primary lymphomas of CNS (PCNSL), 141

primidone, 185

primitive neuroectodermal tumor (PNET), 135–6

prion disorders, 73

prism adaptation, 28

PRN (paramedian reticular nucleus), 13

proatlantal artery, 3

procainamide, 162

progressive multifocal leukoencephalopathy (PML), 123

progressive myoclonic epilepsies (PME), 174–7
    causes of, 175, 177
    differential diagnosis of, 175
    drugs commonly used in, 177
    genetics of, 175

progressive supranuclear palsy (PSP), 134

propranolol, 185

pseudohypoparathyroidism (PHP), 115

PSP (progressive supranuclear palsy), 134

psychogenic gait ataxia, 45–6

PTF1A (pancreas transcription factor 1A), 4

Purkinje cells
    during cerebellum development, 2

description of, 8
and GAD-Ab, 106
heat-induced injury of, 164–5

Purkinje neuroblasts, during cerebellum development, 2

Purkinje neurons, 8
    activities of, 24–5
    and cerebellar nuclei, 10–11
    during cerebellum development, 2
    description of, 8
    and neurosteroid formation, 19

pursuit, disorders of, 38, 55

pyruvate dehydrogenase (lipoamide) alpha 1 (PDHA1), 237

quinacrine, 128

radiation therapy
    for treatment of ataxia-telangiectasia, 195
    for treatment of cerebellar metastases, 143
    for treatment of ependymomas, 138
    for treatment of medulloblastomas, 135, 136
    for treatment of meningiomas, 140

radiosurgery
    for treatment of cerebellar metastases, 143
    for treatment of essential tremor, 187
    for treatment of schwannomas (neurinomas), 140–1

RCH (remote cerebellar hemorrhage), 97

rebound, excessive, 44

reelin, 4

Refsum disease (phytanic acid oxidase deficiency; heredopathia atactica polyneuritiformis)
    blood studies, 205
    clinical description, 205
    differential diagnosis, 206
    genetic and molecular aspects, 205–6
    neuroimaging, 206
    neuropathology, 206
    treatment, 206

rehabilitation, 76–7

remote cerebellar hemorrhage (RCH), 97

repetitive transcranial magnetic stimulation (rTMS), 106

reticular nuclei, 13–14

retrocerebellar arachnoid cyst (Blake pouch cyst), 84

Rett syndrome, 171, 172

rhombencephalosynapsis, 81–2

Richards-Rundle syndrome, 209

RNAi therapies, 270

rosettes, 8

rostral spinocerebellar tract (RSCT), 13

rTMS (repetitive transcranial magnetic stimulation), 106

saccades, disorders of, 39, 56

saccular aneurysms, 96

salla disease, 217

SARA (Scale for Assessment and Rating of Ataxia)
  comparison between scales, 59
  overview, 57–9
  quantitative tests, 59

saxitoxin (shellfish poisoning), 166

SCA (superior cerebellar artery), 88–9, 94, 95

SCA Functional Index (SCAFI), 59

SCAFI (SCA Functional Index), 59

Scale for Assessment and Rating of Ataxia. See SARA

SCAN1 (spinocerebellar ataxia with axonal neuropathy), 208

SCAs. See spinocerebellar ataxias

schizophrenia, 48

schwannomas (neurinomas), 135, 140–1

scorpions, and cerebellar toxicity, 166

seizures
  cerebellar fits, 43
  in dentatorubral-pallidoluysian atrophy,
  in Hashimoto ataxia, 114
  in Lafora disease, 174
  in progressive myoclonic epilepsies, 177
  in SCAs, 268
  in spinocerebellar ataxia type 10, 258

sensorimotor delays,

sensory ataxia, causes of, 46

sensory processing, 29

septo-optic dysplasia (De Morsier syndrome), 116

serial reaction time tasks (SRTT), 27

shellfish poisoning (saxitoxin), 166

SHH (Sonic hedgehog), 2, 3, 4

Shy-Drager syndrome, 180

sialidosis type I (cherry spot myoclonus syndrome), 176–7, 217

siderosis, superficial, 143

signaling, and development of cerebellum, 3–4

sildenafil, 105

skew deviation, 38

SLOS (Smith-Lemli-Opitz syndrome), 4, 85

small deep infarcts, 92

Smith-Lemli-Opitz syndrome (SLOS), 4, 85

Sonic hedgehog (SHH), 2, 3, 4

speech
  control of, 25–6
  examination of, 40
  ICARS scale, 55
  in Scale for Assessment and Rating of Ataxia, 58
  therapy for, 77
  in Unified Multiple System Atrophy Rating Scale, 65

spinocerebellar ataxia with axonal neuropathy (SCAN1), 208

spinocerebellar ataxias (SCAs), 46–7
  age of onset of, 71
  brain MRI of patient with, 247
  clinical presentations of, 243
  clues for diagnosis of, 242
  inclusions in, 244
  infarctions, 89
  overview, 242–5
  therapeutical strategies under investigation in, 269
  therapies of
    clinical trials and observations, 269
    general recommendations, 268–9
    polyglutamine repeat disorders under investigation, 269–70
  treatment of, overview, 75
  type 1 (SCA1)
    animal models of, 248
    clinical deficits in, 245
    clinical presentation, 245

    genetic and molecular aspects, 247–8
    neuroimaging, 245
    neuropathology, 248
    neurophysiology, 247
  type 2 (SCA2)
    clinical deficits in, 248
    clinical presentation, 248
    genetic aspects, 249
    neuroimaging, 248–9
    neuropathology, 249–50
    neurophysiology, 249
  type 3 (Machado-Joseph disease – MJD)
    animal models of, 252
    clinical deficits in, 251
    clinical presentation, 250–1
    genetic and molecular aspects, 252
    neuroimaging, 251
    neuropathology, 252
    neurophysiology, 251–2
  type 4 (SCA4)
    clinical presentation, 252–3
    electrophysiology, 253
    genetic and molecular aspects, 253
    neuropathology, 253
  type 5 (SCA5)
    clinical presentation, 253
    genetic and molecular aspects, 253–4
    neuroimaging, 253
    neuropathology, 254
  type 6 (SCA6)
    clinical presentation, 254
    electrophysiology, 254
    genetic and molecular aspects, 254
    neuroimaging, 254
    neuropathology, 255
  type 7 (SCA7)
    clinical presentation, 255
    genetic and molecular aspects, 255–6
    neuroimaging, 255
    neuropathology, 256
    neurophysiology, 255
  type 8 (SCA8)
    animal models, 258
    clinical presentation, 257
    genetic and molecular aspects, 257–8
    neuroimaging, 257
    neuropathology, 258
  type 10 (SCA10)
    clinical presentation, 258–9
    genetic and molecular aspects, 259

spinocerebellar ataxias (SCAs) (cont.)
   type 10 (SCA10) (cont.) 258
    geographical distribution,
    neuroimaging, 259
    neurophysiology, 259
   type 11 (SCA11)
    clinical presentation, 259
    genetic aspects, 259
    neuroimaging, 259
    neuropathology, 259–60
   type 12 (SCA12)
    clinical presentation, 260
    electrophysiology, 260
    genetic and molecular aspects,
     260
    neuroimaging, 260
   type 13 (SCA13)
    clinical presentation, 260
    genetic and functional aspects,
     260–1
    neuroimaging, 260
   type 14 (SCA14)
    clinical presentation, 261
    genetic and functional aspects,
     261
    neuroimaging, 261
   type 15–type 16 (SCA15-16)
    clinical presentation, 261
    genetic and functional aspects,
     261
    neuroimaging, 261
   type 17 (Huntington disease–like 4
    [HDL4]), 262
    clinical presentation, 262
    differential diagnosis, 262
    epidemiology, 261–2
    genetic and molecular aspects,
     263
    neuroimaging, 262
    neuropathology, 263
    neurophysiology, 262–3
   type 18 (SCA18)
    clinical presentation, 263–4
    genetic aspects, 264
    neuroimaging, 264
    neurophysiology, 264
   type 19 (SCA19) and type 22
    (SCA22)
    clinical presentation, 264
    genetic aspects, 264
    neuroimaging, 264
    neurophysiology, 264
    neuropsychological findings, 264
   type 20 (SCA20)
    clinical presentation, 264–5
    genetic aspects, 265
    neuroimaging, 265
    neurophysiology, 265
   type 21 (SCA21)

    clinical presentation, 265–6
    genetic aspects, 266
    neuroimaging, 266
    neuropathology, 266
    neurophysiology, 266
   type 23 (SCA23)
    clinical presentation, 266
    genetic aspects, 266
    neuropathology, 266
   type 25 (SCA25)
    clinical presentation, 266–7
    genetic aspects, 267
    neuroimaging, 267
    neuropathology, 267
    neurophysiology, 267
   type 26 (SCA26)
    clinical presentation, 267
    genetic aspects, 267
    neuroimaging, 267
   type 27 (SCA27)
    animal models, 267–8
    clinical presentation, 267
    genetic aspects, 267
    neuroimaging, 267
    neurophysiology, 267
   type 28 (SCA28)
    biochemical assays, 268
    clinical deficits in, 268
    clinical presentation, 268
    genetic aspects, 268
    neuroimaging, 268
    neurophysiology, 268
   type 30 (SCA30)
    clinical presentation, 268
    genetic aspects, 268
    neuroimaging, 268
spinocerebellar tracts, 11–13
SRTT (serial reaction time tasks), 27
stance
   ataxia of, 45
   in Scale for Assessment and Rating
    of Ataxia, 57–8
stellate cells, 10
steroids
   for treatment of cerebellar abscesses,
    119
   for treatment of cerebellar
    metastases, 142
   for treatment of Hashimoto ataxia,
    114
   for treatment of infectious diseases,
    125
   for treatment of MS, 105
Stewart-Holmes test, for deficits in
   limb movements, 41
striato-nigral degeneration, 180

stroke
   anatomy of cerebellar vessels,
    88–9
   in cancer patients, 143
   cerebellar hemorrhage, 96–7
   cerebellar infarctions
    AICA infarctions, 89
    border zone infarctions
     (watershed), 92
    extra-cerebellar lesions causing
     hemiataxia, 94–5
    lacunar infarctions, 92
    outcome of cerebellar infarctions,
     95
    overview, 89
    PICA infarctions, 89
    SCA infarctions, 89
   cerebellar vein thrombosis, 97
   diagnosis of cerebellar stroke,
    97–8
   management of, 98
   pathogenesis of cerebellar infarcts,
    95–6
   techniques and ancillary tests used
    for, 98
   treatment of cerebellar stroke,
    98–9
subacute necrotizing encephalopathy
   (Leigh syndrome), 231–2, 233
subarachnoid hemorrhage, 149
subdural hematoma of posterior fossa,
   150
sulfatidoses, 215
superficial siderosis, 143
superior cerebellar artery (SCA), 88–9,
   94, 95
superior cerebellar peduncle
   (brachium conjunctivum), 7
superior rhombic lip, development of,
   2
superior vermis, development of, 2
surgery, 76
   for treatment of aneurysms, 108
   for treatment of cerebellar abscesses,
    119
   for treatment of cerebellar
    metastases, 142–3
   for treatment of Chiari II
    malformation, 79
   for treatment of essential tremor,
    187
   for treatment of MS tremor, 105
   for treatment of schwannomas
    (neurinomas), 140–1
   for treatment of stroke, 99

symptoms of cerebellar disorders, 36
  ataxia, defined, 37
  classification of clinical signs
    autonomic signs, 46
    cognitive abnormalities and emotional disorders, 46–8
    deficits in gait posture, 45–6
    deficits in limb movements, 40–5
    dysarthria and mutism, 40
    oculomotor disturbances, 37–40
    overview, 37
  clinical signs and sagittal zone affected, 37
  lesion-symptom mapping, 48–9
  overview, 36–7
synaptogenesis, 5
systemic lupus erythematosus, 108

tachykinins, 17
tapping test, 40
taxol, 162
Tay-Sachs disease (GM2 gangliosidosis type I), 214
thalamocortical projections, 14
thiamin deficit, 158
thiamin supplementation, for treatment of PDAH1, 237
thrombosis, cerebellar vein, 97
thyroid disorders
  drug-induced dysfunction of thyroid gland, 115
  Hashimoto ataxia, 113–14
  hyperthyroidism, 113
  hypothyroidism, 113
  overview, 113
thyroidectomy, 114
tick-borne diseases, 121
timing, and cerebellum, 29
toluene benzene derivatives, 164
topiramate, 185
toxic agents
  animal-related cerebellar toxicity, 166
  drugs as
    5-FU (5-fluorouracil), 162
    amiodarone, 162
    Ara-C (cytosine arabinoside), 162
    brimonidine tartrate, 163
    carbamazepine, 161

cisplatin, 162
cocaine, 163
cyclosporin and other calcineurin inhibitors, 163
herbs, 164
heroin, 163
lithium salts, 162
methadone, 163
methotrexate, 162
metronidazole, 163
oxaliplatin, 162
phencyclidine, 163–4
phenytoin, 160–1
procainamide, 162
taxol, 162
environmental causes of cerebellar ataxia
  carbon monoxide, 165
  chemical weapons, 165
  consumption of edible morels, 166
  cyanide, 165
  eucalytpus oil, 166
  heavy metals, 164
  hyperthermia, 164–5
  insecticides, herbicides, 165
  polychlorinated biphenyls (PCBs), 165–6
  saxitoxin (shellfish poisoning), 166
  toluene benzene derivatives, 164
tremor
  action, 41–3, 65
  affecting limbs, 44
  delayed-onset intention tremor, 151
  drugs for, 77
  essential, 43
  kinetic, 41
  in MS, treatment for, 105
  orthostatic, 43
  palatal, 43
  postural, 42
  at rest, 65
  treatment of, 75
  in Unified Multiple System Atrophy Rating Scale, 65
trigeminal afferents, 19
trigeminal artery, 3
tumors and paraneoplastic disorders
  brainstem gliomas, 136–8
  cerebellar astrocytomas, 136
  cerebellar metastases, 142–3
  complications of chemotherapy, phenytoin, lithium salts, 143
  ependymomas, 138
  epidermoid and dermoid tumors, 141
  Erdheim-Chester disease, 146–7

hemangioblastomas, 138
infections, 143
Langerhans histiocytosis, 145–6
Lhermitte-Duclos disease, 142
medulloblastomas, 135–6
meningiomas, 138–40
overview, 135
paraneoplastic cerebellar degeneration (PCD), 143–5
primary lymphomas of CNS (PCNSL), 141
schwannomas (neurinomas), 140–1
stroke, 143
superficial siderosis, 143

UMSARS (Unified Multiple System Atrophy Rating Scale), 64–7
uncal or tonsillar herniation, 149
Unified Multiple System Atrophy Rating Scale (UMSARS), 64–7
unipolar brush cells, 10
Unverricht-Lundborg disease, 174
up-beat nystagmus, 39–40
upper limb, coordination of, 61–2
upright stability, 63–4

vagus nerve stimulation (VNS), 106
valproate, 75
vasospasm, 99
vein thrombosis, cerebellar, 97, 98
ventral spinocerebellar tract (VSCT; Gower tract), 13
ventricular neuroepithelium, 2
vertebrobasilar system embryogenesis, 3
vertigo, 120
very low density lipoprotein receptor (VLDLR), 4
vessel wall, dissection of, 150
vestibular afferents, 13
vestibular nucleus, 23
vestibulocerebellum, 5
vestibuloocular reflex (VOR), 25, 27–8, 37
vibratory sense test, 63
vigabatrin, 161
visual afferents, 19
vitamin supplementation, 196, 197

VLDLR (very low density lipoprotein receptor), 4

VNS (vagus nerve stimulation), 106

Vogt-Koyanagi-Harada disease, 109

von Hippel-Lindau disease, 138

VOR (vestibuloocular reflex), 25, 27–8, 37

VSCT (ventral spinocerebellar tract), 13

Wallenberg syndrome, 89

watershed (border zone infarctions), 92

Wernicke-Korsakoff syndrome, 157, 158

Whipple disease, 124

Wilson disease, 71
    blood studies, 212

clinical description, 211–12
clinical signs in, 212
epidemiology, 211
genetic and molecular aspects, 212
liver biopsy, 212
neuroimaging, 212
neurophysiology, 212
pathogenesis, 212–13
slit-lamp examination, 212
treatment, 213
urinary studies, 212

Wolfram syndrome, 209

xanthomas, 204

xeroderma pigmentosum (XP), 195

X-linked ataxias
    differential diagnosis and treatment of PDHA1, 237
    fragile X tremor ataxia syndrome (FXTAS)

clinical presentation, 238
genetic and molecular aspects, 239
neuroimaging, 238–9
neuropathology, 239–40
neurophysiology, 239
treatment, 240
    overview, 237

X-linked Pelizaeus-Merzbacher disease, 194

XP (xeroderma pigmentosum), 195

young adults, ataxias in, 71

zinc acetate, 213

zinc finger family of transcription factors (ZIC), 4

zinc sulfate, 214

zinc transporters (ZnT), 19